Essential Neurology

CONCISE TEXTBOOK SERIES

- *Essential Neurology, Third Edition,* William Pryse-Phillips, M.D., and T.J. Murray, M.D.

- *Psychiatry, Fifth Edition,* Merrill T. Eaton, Jr., M.D., Margaret H. Peterson, M.D. and James A. Davis, M.D.

- *Acute Internal Medicine,* Laurence B. Gardner, M.D.

- *Gynecology,* Ralph W. Hale, M.D., and John A. Krieger, M.D.

- *Endocrinology, Third Edition,* Ernest L. Mazzaferri, M.D., ed.

- *Pediatric Allergy, Third Edition,* Michael R. Sly, M.D.

- *Rheumatology,* Robert A. Turner, M.D., and Christopher M. Wise, M.D.

- *Infectious Diseases,* Robert H. Waldman, M.D., and Ronica M. Kluge, M.D.

- *Clinical Nuclear Medicine Imaging, Third Edition,* P. Matin, M.D., ed.

IN PREPARATION:

- *Obstetrics,* Ralph W. Hale, M.D., and John A. Krieger, M.D.

- *Pediatrics,* Raymond M. Russo, M.D.

- *Dermatology,* James W. Patterson, M.D., and W. Kenneth Blaylock, M.D.

- *Anesthesiology,* Thomas J. DeKornfeld, M.D., ed.

A CONCISE TEXTBOOK

Essential Neurology
Third Edition

William Pryse-Phillips, M.D. (Lond.), F.R.C.P., F.R.C.P.(C)
Professor of Medicine (Neurology)
Memorial University of Newfoundland
St. John's, Newfoundland

T.J. Murray, M.D., F.R.C.P.(C), F.A.C.P.
Dean of Medicine (Neurology)
Dalhousie University
Halifax, Nova Scotia

With a Foreword by

H.N.A. MacDonald, M.D., F.R.C.P.(C)
Professor of Medicine (Neurology)
Dalhousie University
Halifax, Nova Scotia

Medical Examination Publishing Company

Medical Examination Publishing Company
A Division of Elsevier Science Publishing Co., Inc.
52 Vanderbilt Avenue, New York, New York 10017

Library of Congress Cataloging in Publication Data

Pryse-Phillips, William.
    Textbook of essential neurology.

    Includes bibliographies and index.
    1. Nervous system – Diseases. 2. Neurology.
    I. Murray, T.J. II. Title. [DNLM: 1. Nervous System
    Diseases. 2. Neurologic Examination – methods.
WL 100 P973e]
RC346.P795   1986   616.8   86-1069
ISBN 0-444-01008-4

Current printing (last digit)
10 9 8 7 6 5 4 3 2 1

Manufactured in the United States of America

Contents

Foreword   vii
Preface   ix
Acknowledgments   xi

PART I   NEUROLOGICAL ASSESSMENT   1

Chapter   **1**   History and Examination of Mental Status   5
         2   Examination of the Nervous System   13
         3   Scanning Neurological Examination   52
         4   Neurological Examination in Children   54
         5   Neurological Examination in the Elderly   65
         6   Examination for Functional Disorders   68
         7   Examination of the Comatose Patient   75
         8   Neurological Investigations   85

PART II   LOCALIZATION IN THE NERVOUS SYSTEM   125

Chapter   **9**   Localization of Disease   129

PART III   AN APPROACH TO NEUROLOGICAL SYMPTOMS   165

Chapter   **10**   Reduction in Conscious Level   169
         11   Delirious States   185
         12   Dementia   193
         13   Disturbance of Memory   204
         14   Disorders of Speech   211
         15   Epileptic Seizures   221
         16   Raised Intracranial Pressure   241
         17   Headache   253

18 Sleep and Related Disorders   270

19 Disorders of Smell and Taste   278

20 Visual Disorders   280

21 Ocular Problems   290

22 Facial Pain and Numbness   308

23 Facial Palsy   318

24 Deafness, Vertigo, and Tinnitus   323

25 Bulbar and Pseudobulbar Palsy   335

26 Weakness   338

27 Muscle Cramps, Stiffness, and Pain   346

28 Clumsiness   351

29 Disorders of Movement   354

30 Pain in the Back   361

31 Scoliosis   372

32 Abnormalities of Gait   374

33 Abnormalities of Micturition   378

34 Impotence   383

35 Patterns of Sensory Deficit   386

36 Pain Syndromes   393

PART IV   **IMPORTANT NEUROLOGICAL DISORDERS   401**

Chapter   **37** Strokes   405

38 Head Injuries and Spinal Trauma   438

39 Cerebral Palsy and Mental Retardation   453

40 Infectious Diseases of the Nervous System   472

41 Neoplastic Disease   507

42 Neurological Complications of Systemic Disease   529

43 Toxic Damage to the Nervous System   560

44 Disorders of the Peripheral Nerves   586

45 Diseases of Muscle   610

46 Parkinson's Disease and Other Diseases of the Basal Ganglia   635

47 Motor Neuron Disease   651

48 Diseases of Myelin   659

49 Diseases of the Cerebellum   672

50 Spinal Diseases   682

51 Depression and Anxiety   696

INDEX   705

Foreword

In the past two decades there has been a huge increase in neurological knowledge. With this, the traditional role of the neurologist has changed considerably. The neurologist was always considered an intellectual who, as a result of an extensive knowledge of neuroanatomy and neurophysiology, was mainly interested in the intricacies of localization of lesions and the diagnosis of obscure diseases. Although neurologists were often criticized as physicians who could make peculiar diagnoses but offer no treatment, they did not play a large part in the mainstream of general medicine but maintained an ivory-tower image, and were called upon by their colleagues to sort out mysterious symptoms and findings. Tremendous advances in the neurosciences have redefined the role of neurologists, giving them a much wider dimension in the care of patients. Coupled with imaginative diagnostic techniques, these advances have furthered the art of neurology and have led to enviable breakthroughs in medical, surgical, and rehabilitation therapy of neurological patients.

With these advances in the art and science of neurology, there is an increasing responsibility for the neurologist in teaching. It is trite to state that rare diseases still exist, but that common disorders are seen more often. Many of the patients presenting to the family physician complain of symptoms referable to the nervous system. It therefore becomes a great challenge to the neurologist involved in teaching students to make them aware of common neurological symptoms. Medical students will have been exposed to neuroanatomy and neurophysiology, and to some degree to neurochemistry, and they are often bewildered by the vast amount of material. It becomes a challenging responsibility for the neurologist to show these students how to apply this knowledge to the analysis of symptoms and the examination of patients.

As very capable clinicians, the authors are extremely dedicated and aggressive teachers who present their book in a unique, personal fashion. By no means will the book supplant the many excellent standard textbooks of neurology, to which the inquisitive student will always refer.

Essential Neurology, however, is exceedingly well set out. The thoughtful student will find that neurology is not an abstruse specialty; he will gain considerable satisfaction in recognizing neurological manifestations of general medical disease, and will be capable of making a more intelligent referral for those patients that require a specialist neurologist.

It has been a pleasure for me to have been asked by the authors to review this book, and I would like to congratulate them for having produced a concise, readable, and understandable treatise, which sets out the essential facts of neurology.

Hugh N.A. MacDonald, M.D., F.R.C.P.(C)

Preface

Traditionally, the medical student is required to learn a great body of information before obtaining clinical experience.

All manner of experts (academics, researchers, subspecialists, and others) pour this information onto the student, with the implication that it must *all* be known; but as the student becomes more and more involved in clinical medicine, most of the irrelevant information begins to atrophy from disuse, and throws into sharp relief the store of knowledge needed to understand and solve problems.

After outlining an examination of the nervous system and a method of localizing problems, we discuss some of the most common symptoms presented to the physician. We dwell upon the approach to symptoms because patients present with symptoms, not with strangely named diseases. In selecting those to be discussed, we have chosen those that are common, that are treatable, that require urgent management, that aid in understanding the nervous system, or that illustrate important advances in recent years.

We recognize that this approach is a personal one and it does not take into account many other approaches to clinical neurology. We do not expect that our decisions concerning what to include and what to leave out will find favor with everyone, but we feel that this is inevitable. We wrote the first edition for the student and the family practitioner, but were surprised and delighted to find how well received it was by medical and neurological residents and by practicing neurologists.

We find it easier to write in the style of the second person, since this is how we teach; but we would be sorry if a reader thought of us as lecturing from a podium. We would prefer to be visualized as on the other side of the patient's bed, as this book is designed for the clinical situation.

By tradition, we use the masculine gender throughout, even when the feminine would be equally appropriate.

We do not presume in any way to supplant the major and comprehensive works on basic neuroscience and clinical neurology. As teachers however, it is our experience that students do not read these books, except for occasional reference. We would be glad if a graduating medical student confidently knew how to employ the principles set out in this book. Most students are unnecessarily anxious about neurology, but neurology is no more than the application of neuroanatomy and neurophysiology to an intelligent and meticulous history and a competent examination. We hope that, in this book, we have eliminated much of the pedantry of classic neurology and have presented a practical approach to the subject. With the information that is here, we think that a student should be able to solve most neurological problems at an acceptable level.

W.P.P.
T.J.M.

Acknowledgments

Our colleagues have assisted us greatly by their constructive criticism of the third edition; particularly Dr. Ian Bowmer, Dr. Martin Tweeddale and Dr. Andrew Kertesz.

Ackowledgments for illustrations are provided with each. We are particularly grateful to Dr. Brian Byrne and Dr. Virgilio Sangalang who contributed many new illustrations for this edition, and again acknowledge with gratitude the kindness of all our colleagues who have lent illustrations.

The immense task of typing and retyping was borne unflinchingly by Gertrude Dowden and Jean MacLean. It is impossible to thank them enough for their uncomplaining and very capable secretarial asssistance and advice.

We felt that students would probably better understand diagrams drawn by other students, and we were lucky to have Dr. Wiliam Maloney and Dr. Robert Bartlett, formerly of Memorial University Medical School, to provide illustrations. We also thank the Medical Audio-Visual Services of Memorial University, Dalhousie University, and Camp Hill Hospital for their skilled assistance. Rene Fogarty spent hours preparing hundreds of photographs for this edition and we are very grateful for her work and her skill.

This book arose from questions asked of us and answers given to us by patients and by medical students in our clinical and teaching practices. Those questions and answers are the raison d'être of the book, which is for students and about patients. We thank them all for the stimulus which they have given us to write it.

I
NEUROLOGICAL ASSESSMENT

INTRODUCTION TO PART I

In most medical schools, the skills of the neurological examination are taught at the same time as a neurosciences course, or immediately after. The neurological examination is an exercise in applied neuroanatomy and neurophysiology, and it depends upon knowledge of both. Neurological examination therefore is the basis of clinical neurology, for it enables you to localize the lesion often more accurately than the history does and may demonstrate signs of which the patient was unaware.

Chapter 1 surveys the headings under which the history is taken. Here, we briefly mention the *kinds* of complaints that patients bring to us: the analysis of these complaints is the subject of Part III. Because history taking is a skill that comes with practice and example, clinical examination takes much more space than the history in Part I.

But the importance of the history can hardly be exaggerated, and if you are not quite sure *what* is going on, and more or less *where,* by the time you stop asking questions and pick up the ophthalmoscope, then the examination usually will not help you very much. You must listen to the patient for, as Osler suggested, he is telling you the diagnosis; and you must go on listening when you examine, and observe physical signs during the interview. Patients often talk more freely when the doctor is not holding a pen, when they feel that the formal inquisition is over.

So stop while testing; give yourself and the patient a rest, and amplify or clarify anything that you did not understand completely. A full neurological examination can be tiring and it is never necessary to do *all* the maneuvers described in Chapter 2. For instance, once you have recognized a cerebellar syndrome, not every test for ataxia needs to be performed. Many similar tests are described, but only so that if the result of one is equivocal, you can turn to another. If the patient gets tired, you can always examine again later, and you should, since the results become unreliable if anyone's attention is less than complete.

Remember that the *whole* patient is there to be examined and do not restrict yourself to the presenting complaints. When you are examining, do the tests properly. Lackadaisical, imprecise, and uncontrolled tests are no more than diagnostic gestures and dangerously misleading wastes of time. *Think* as you examine or you will miss obvious signs. *Look* for specific signs or you may miss them completely.

Tell your patient what you are going to do, especially if it hurts. Do your examination in order, any order, but make sure that it is always the same one so that you will not leave anything out. We suggest an order of testing, but if you want to devise your own scheme, that is fine, as long as it is efficient and you stick to it.

Do not be put off by what from these pages seems to be a long and complicated ritual. The proper screening neurological and general physical examination should be completed in 10 min. To the novice this may seem impossible, but when the examination is done in a thoughtful manner after many patient encounters, it is entirely reasonable. Our screening examination is efficient enough to be included in every physical examination.

A sloppy examination is worse than none. We find it far more acceptable to read "CNS not examined" than "CNS — no abnormality," because the latter usually means that it was examined inadequately.

Brief sections on the examination of children and the elderly and a suggestion for a scanning examination are also supplied to reinforce our points that the range of normal variation is quite wide and that the central nervous system (CNS) can be assessed quickly.

Finally, the main investigations in neurology are described not only so that you know what tests to ask for and how to interpret the results reliably, but also so that you can tell your patients what is going to happen to them. Reassurance without explanation, though well tried in politics, has no place in medicine.

1
History and Examination of Mental Status

The neurological history and examination are used to decide

1. Whether there is a lesion in the CNS and if so, what level is involved (muscle, end-plate, nerve, cord, brainstem, hemisphere)
2. What type of process is involved (pathology)
3. What has caused the process to occur (etiology)
4. What management is required (emergency, urgent, or elective therapy)

In most instances these questions may be answered based on the history alone and only confirmed by the examination. In other situations the examination yields telling results that answer many questions arising from the interview. An experienced neurologist however gets most information from a careful history and relies on the examination to confirm his clinical suspicions; he is seldom surprised by the physical signs.

In what follows, the most practical and efficient methods used in the examination of patients will be mentioned. The significance of the abnormalities found are best learned in the clinical situation. It is most important that when you perform any clinical maneuver, you know exactly what you are testing. You perform the test to examine a part of the nervous system and to see if it is functioning normally, not as a rote part of the "neurologic examination." The order in which the tests are performed is not so important, but it is sensible to learn one sequence of tests and to stick to it to avoid leaving anything out. Errors result more from lack of observation than from lack of knowledge.

HISTORY

Throughout history taking, assess the patient's ability and desire to communicate and try to form an estimate of his intelligence, reliability, character, and mood. While taking the history, observe the patient carefully.

Pay particular attention to *speech;* is there dysphasia or dysarthria? Bearing in mind that brain disease may distort or falsify memories, ask yourself whether what the patient is saying is inherently likely, or could some of his statements be errors or confabulations? Note if he repeats words or phrases unnecessarily or out of context. The actual use of words, construction of sentences, ability to use vocabulary, and other facets of verbalization are described in the section on dysphasias (see Chap. 14).

Look at the patient's clothes, expression, posture, and mobility. Decide whether or not there are abnormal movements or actions, whether the overall amount of activity is increased or reduced.

Chief Complaint

Ask for the symptoms that are most troublesome and note their exact time and speed of onset. Has anything similar ever happened before? Then trace the progression of all symptoms through time, up to the present. Questions such as "How did that affect you at work?" and "What did you do when it came on?" often allow a better estimate of severity than the patient's own emotional description of his symptoms.

Most symptoms can be analyzed in the same way as pain is analyzed, with commonsense alterations. With any pain, including headaches, ask about

1. Character, severity
2. Situation, localization, paths of reference
3. Frequency, duration, special times of occurrence
4. Aggravating and relieving factors
5. Associated symptoms
6. Effect on the patient and his life patterns

After examining all the presenting symptoms in turn, you have to ask leading questions, remembering that questions such as "Do you get a pain in the back of your neck when you pass water?" suggest to the patient what answer you might like to receive, but by adding the words ". . . or not," you will present a second choice with less chance of suggesting symptoms.

Nervous System Review

In a complete history you might ask about the following, but be selective and try to decide whether questions are appropriate and which can be left out. Ask about

Mood. Are there any special worries or problems of a personal, circumstantial, economic, or other nature? Is he at all depressed; does he sleep well, and are appetite and energy normal? Is his weight stable? Are there any symptoms of anxiety or agitation? If you have any doubts about the patient's mood level, use the outline given under Examination of Mental State to search for further evidence of a psychological illness.

Memory, both recent and remote; *concentration* and *attention; energy* (see the following and Chaps. 12 and 13).

Epileptic fits, faints, or any forms of attack in which similar symptoms occur repeatedly (such as migraine, muscle spasm, tic douloureux). If there is any suggestion of epilepsy, find out if the patient had any warning of the impending attack and go into the symptoms in order and in detail: what happened before, during, and after the fit. If he does not know the details of an episode of unconsciousness, find out by talking to someone who does (see Chap. 15).

Headache (see Chap. 17).

Smell and *taste* (see Chap. 19).

Vision, including inquiry about recent change in glasses and if there has been any double vision or unusual visual perception (such as flashes of light, color, complex hallucinations) (see Chaps. 20 and 21).

Deafness, tinnitus, vertigo. If the last occurs, ask what brings it on, and whether there is any headache, nausea, or vomiting (see Chap. 24). Giddiness and *dizziness* are terms often used by patients to mean faintness, anxiety, vertigo (which is an illusion of movement of the self or the environment), nausea, headache, and indeed almost anything else. Get the patient to describe *exactly* what he does mean if he uses these terms.

Difficulties in *speaking* or *swallowing* (see Chap. 25).

Pain (see Chap. 36).

Muscle spasm, tremors, twitching, or other involuntary movements; alteration in writing and in the *motor skills* of the hands (which are usually mainly noticed at work); the patient's ability to move about, walk, and work; and about the timing of such symptoms (see Chaps. 9 and 29).

Loss of strength, muscle wasting, clumsiness. The last may be a symptom of upper motor neuron, cerebellar, proprioceptive, or muscular lesions. Ask about handedness. Do not ask about bodily deformity; it is unkind and unnecessary, as you will see what there is when you examine the patient (see Chaps. 26 and 28).

Sensory symptoms. The patient may have noticed defects of touch, pain, or temperature sensation, or he may complain of numbness, tingling, paresthesia (pins and needles), heaviness, deadness, clumsiness, or uselessness of a limb (see Chap. 35).

Family History

Enquire if anyone in the family has ever had symptoms that were anything like those of the patient. A history of epilepsy, diabetes mellitus, muscle disease, thyroid disorder, or psychiatric disorder in the family is obviously relevant. In addition, a previous history in the family of cerebrovascular disease and hypertension is important. If looking for a family history of neuromuscular disease and none is obviously forthcoming, ask the patient if anyone in his family has had "arthritis," trouble with walking, or "weakness," because gait disturbance, peripheral neuropathy, or familial myopathy may be interpreted as joint or other disease by the family. If positive results are obtained with this line of questioning, draw a family tree.

Personal History

Ask about the jobs the patient has had and his present occupation. Then inquire about consumption of alcohol and about any drugs taken, and why. Do not use only the word "drug" but also ask about "medicines," "pills," and "medications." In the case of a suspected "hard" drug taker, or possible alcohol dependence, ask when he *last* had any; this tends to stop him troubling to deny his addiction.

Smoking habits also must be noted accurately; "I don't smoke" often means "I gave up again last week." Ask about the largest number of cigarettes smoked daily and the period over which this occurred. Remember that use of drugs and cigarettes is often higher in youth; of alcohol, in middle life.

Past Medical History

Obviously the questioner must elicit a full medical history, including operations, accidents, and allergies. In the case of a child, get the details of early life and development from a parent. Note all hospitalizations and serious illness, injuries, and pregnancies. The patient who has a chronic disease can usually give a good account of the diagnoses and the years of occurrence of illnesses and operations. These should be noted and charted, preferably in the form of a graph or chronological table.

Bodily Functions

Ask about sleep patterns, weight and appetite changes, and menstruation. Be sure to find out about any alteration in bladder or bowel function and describe these in detail. Also ask about sweating, warmth of hands and feet, and (if the subject is in context) about sexual activity.

Information from Others

By now you should know your patient quite well, but it may be important to see a relative to clarify, illuminate, or confirm the history. Sometimes useful information is divulged such that you wish that you had seen the relative to begin with. Important data may also be obtained from the patient's friends, workmates, the police, or anybody else who may have observed his illness. Ambulance drivers are often fruitful sources of important information during emergencies.

Information from others is important in situations suggestive of epilepsy, syncope, personality change, dementia, depression, and hysteria.

EXAMINATION OF MENTAL STATE

The examination of the mental state can be as long or as short as one pleases, but it seldom needs to be prolonged unless history taking or the interview suggests that a cerebral lesion may exist or that there is an abnormality of mental status. There are six major aspects of functioning that need to be assessed in a patient whose mental state is to be clinically examined in detail.

1. Intelligence
2. Behavior
3. Emotional status
4. Perceptions and thought processes
5. Physiological abnormalities
6. Premorbid personality

Obviously, if there is a speech disturbance or any reduction in the level of consciousness, the testing will be not only difficult but unreliable. As always, it is better to select a few general high-yield tests assessing certain functions and to use these regularly, having a backup store of additional tests that can be used if the occasion seems to be appropriate. There follows a selection of the clinical observations that may be made; most of these can be supplemented and quantified by the use of more sophisticated psychological testing.

Intelligence

Intelligence is an indefinable concatenation of capabilities that may be assessed by means of tests of various functions.

Memory and Concentration (see Chap. 13).

> *Digit span forward:* Normal patients can repeat seven digits forward, right after they have heard them.[*]
> *Digit span reversed:* Normal patients can reproduce four digits in reverse order to that in which they were given. This is not only a test of memory and concentration but also tests the ability to handle abstract concepts, in this case numbers. A variation, which is a useful test of diffuse cerebral dysfunction, is to ask the patient to spell "world" backwards.
> *.100 - 7 test:* The normal subject will be able to subtract 7s serially from 100 down to 2 correctly in less than 60 sec with three or fewer mistakes. The test is excellent when repeated examinations have to be performed because 101 minus 7, 102 minus 7, and so on can be substituted with equal value. It is important to continue to the end because mistakes often become evident only as the test continues.
> *Three objects:* A normal subject will repeat three objects (e.g., 23 Broadway, pen, rose) correctly 5 min after an appropriate warning about being retested later on. The interval between giving the three objects and asking for their recall may be filled by other tests.
> *Remote events:* If a patient has a normal level of consciousness he will certainly know his birthday (the day, month, and year), and if married, the date of his marriage. Birthdays of children will probably be remembered, particularly of the eldest.

The patient with a disorder of the limbic system may *confabulate,* which means that he gives incorrect answers to questions and often is extremely suggestible. Rather than lying, he responds with memories in a disturbed temporal sequence. If asked if he was out for a walk this morning, he may say that he was and will describe elaborate experiences if encouraged, the "memories" coming from various times in the past.

Orientation

The normal subject will know the approximate time of day, and the day, date, month, and year, as well as where he is, his home address, his name, job, and the occupation of his examiner, i.e., the doctor.

---

[*]North American telephone systems realize that; hence seven-digit codes — but use your office number.

Comprehension, Reasoning, and Planning

These tests should not be introduced out of context but in a conversational way in which subjects of current interest are introduced and the patient's opinion sought, e.g., a recent political or sporting event, how the patient feels about recent news items, and so on. Questions about hospital food usually provoke a spirited response. If conversational gambits fail, introduce other questions with an explanation that you are going to be testing some aspects of the way in which the patient thinks, and use questions such as "Why do we have to pay taxes?" and "Why are traffic rules needed?"; or you can ask for explanations of *proverbs* such as "Shallow brooks are noisy," "Strike while the iron is hot," or "A bird in the hand is worth two in the bush."

The patient may also be asked about *similarities,* e.g., between an egg and a seed, wood and alcohol, air and water, an axe and a saw, a coat and a dress; or *differences,* e.g., between ice and glass, a wall and a fence, a child and a dwarf. Record the reply *exactly* as given. Similarities are more difficult than differences to the patient with cerebral dysfunction.

Arithmetic

Simple arithmetical tasks $(5 + 9 + 7 + ?, 8 + 5 - 7 = ?)$ will be performed particularly badly when patients have a dominant parietal lobe lesion but usually do not have localizing value and are a function of intelligence. Also, use the $100 - 7$ test or the $21 - 3$ test to assess the patient's subtraction ability.

General Knowledge

The normal subject will know the names of two or three people in high public office in his country, state, or province; and should be able to recall the names of at least four monarchs, prime ministers, or presidents without difficulty; the dates of recent wars, and six cities in his country or six towns in his state or province should be known too.

Intellect

During the history taking, you will have learned about the patient's educational and work records and will have noticed the extent of his *vocabulary;* all are sensitive indicators of his poor intellectual abilities.

Behavior

It is unlikely that you will apply formal tests to assess behavior, but many aspects of distorted behavior may be apparent if you are unaware that they exist or don't look for them. The general level of *motor activity* is graded from immobility through retardation, poverty of movement, normality, and overactivity, up to mania with or without abnormal movements, and continuous motor restlessness (akathisia). The patient's distractibility, his lack of persistence with any task in hand, and easy fatigability or boredom should be obvious.

Not only the content but also the form of his *speech* is important; the latter may vary from aphonia, through retardation, up to pressure of speech. (The content of speech is considered in Chap. 14.) A patient's reaction to tasks that he cannot do should normally be resigned but with a slight concern; a *catastrophic* reaction with weeping and refusal to continue is a nonspecific sign and of no localizing value, but it suggests diffuse brain disease. Some demented patients are not untidy but rather the opposite and show *organic orderliness* in which they have fallen back upon obsessional routines to protect themselves against the difficulties of change with which they cannot cope. *Perseveration* is a nonspecific, nonlocalizing sign, again indicating diffuse brain disease (except in children and very old people in whom some perseveration is normal).

Finally, the patient's drive, ambition, and work performance may be assessed from histories taken from his friends, workmates, or relatives.

Emotion

The most common emotional disorders seen in neurological practice are *anxiety* and *depression*. In the history you will already have reviewed those by asking direct questions about the patient's affect (see Chap. 51). Somatic symptoms and signs include:

1. Difficulty in falling asleep, restlessness, and disturbed sleep with waking during the night; waking in the early hours of the morning without sleeping again.
2. Slowness of thought, speech, or activity.
3. Restlessness associated with anxiety.
4. Muscle tension with tremor; sweating; indigestion; palpitations; heartburn; frequency of urination; constipation or diarrhea; anorexia; nausea; backache; loss of energy and fatigability; heaviness in the limbs, back or head; loss of libido; menstrual disturbances; weight loss; and diurnal variation of mood.
5. A depressed mood level with a gloomy attitude, pessimism about the future, feelings of sadness, and a tendency to weep, coupled with self-reproach or ideas of guilt or inadequacy.
6. Suicidal ideas, ranging from feelings that life is not worth living, through a wish for death up to suicidal ideas and suicidal attempts. These must always be inquired for in a patient suspected of having depressive illness.
7. Hypochondriasis, loss of insight, depersonalization, and paranoid symptoms may also occur, usually in marked depressive illnesses.

Mood may be unusually labile, or blunted and flat, frequently a result of frontal lobe disease, but these mood alterations do not have definite localizing value. The patient's emotional experience and his emotional expression are not always the same and many patients with bilateral upper motor neuron lesions producing *pseudobulbar palsy* give every impression of overpowering sadness with sudden weeping and facial grimacing, but on questioning they deny feelings of unhappiness. This condition is known as *pathological emotionally*.

Perceptions and Thought Processes

Hallucinations are perceptions without any adequate objective stimuli. *Illusions* are false perceptions of objective stimuli, and *delusions* are false beliefs alien to the patient's social background, tenaciously held against logical argument. *Over-valued ideas* are mild form of delusions.

Primary delusions are those that cannot be explained in terms of the patient's mood level, e.g., delusional perceptions and delusional ideas; *secondary* delusions can be explained in terms of mood. These may include, for example, a delusion that his guts have turned to concrete, which is not an uncommon complaint of patients with severe constipation in association with a depressive illness.

Physiological Changes

Organic mental illness and depressive diseases are frequently associated with changes in bowel habits, loss of weight, sweating, tremor, wide palpebral fissures, tachycardia, palpitations, anorexia, nausea, vomiting, diarrhea, frequency of micturition, loss of energy, and diminution of interests. Sleep changes include initial insomnia, interrupted sleep, early-morning waking, and nightmares. Other physiological changes include general retardation in speech, movement, and thought.

Premorbid Personality

This is difficult to assess, particularly as we do not know precisely what personality really means. Without using any of the current psychiatric vocabulary one may achieve some idea of the patient's premorbid personality by asking about education; about what jobs he has had, how frequently he has changed them, and why; about the amount of alcohol and drugs he uses; about sexual orientation and activity; and about hobbies and interests.

In the case of younger patients, whose parents can be interviewed, a history of early occurrence of nightmares, temper tantrums, food fads, thumbsucking, naitbiting, prolonged enuresis or initial difficulty in toilet training, and delay in motor milestones may suggest a liability to later "neurotic" symptomatology. It is probably unwise to label people with single epithets marking out personality types such as explosive, aggressive, unstable, paranoid, obsessive, compulsive, sensitive, hysterical, and so forth. Information should be obtained from the family and friends of the patient because it is unlikely that people will give reliable information about their own appearance to others.

Perhaps most important is the history of a *change* in the patient's personality toward more or less self-care, alterations in his temper and frustration tolerance, alterations in his aggressiveness, ease in relationships with other people, interest in former hobbies, and the like. Any problems presented in this line will alert you to the background characteristics of the patient and may suggest the presence of organic disease.

BIBLIOGRAPHY

Hamilton, M. A rating scale for depression. *J. Neurol. Psychiat.* 23:56, 1960.

Strub, R.L., Black, F.W. *The Mental Status Examination in Neurology.* Philadelphia, F.A. Davis Co., 1977.

2
Examination of the Nervous System

GENERAL EXAMINATION

The examination of the other major systems may be performed before or after the examination of the nervous system. However, most clinicians have a set pattern of doing a general physical and neurological examination that enables them to scan all areas and systems quickly but efficiently (Fig. 2-1).

Observation of experienced clinicians shows that the history varies in each case according to the circumstances, but the examination is similar in all cases. Good problem-solving physicians develop a highly efficient approach that scans all systems but only assesses specific areas in depth. This method allows the physician quickly to pick up abnormalities that may be present, to assess areas with abnormalities expected from the history or observation, and to prevent forgetting or omitting aspects of the examination.

General Observations

As you took the history you should have noted any obvious signs such as abnormal posture, wasting of hands, tremors, ptosis, squint, facial or limb weakness, or involuntary movements. If you get the chance, and if it seems appropriate, watch the patient preparing himself for examination and climbing onto the examining couch; the actions of the person who does not know he is being watched are sometimes surprisingly effortless. Begin the formal neurological examination with the skull, neck, and spine.

The Head and Neck

Look at the shape and size of the skull. Feel for deformity and fractures, and note whether or not the temporal arteries pulsate and whether or not they are tender.

13

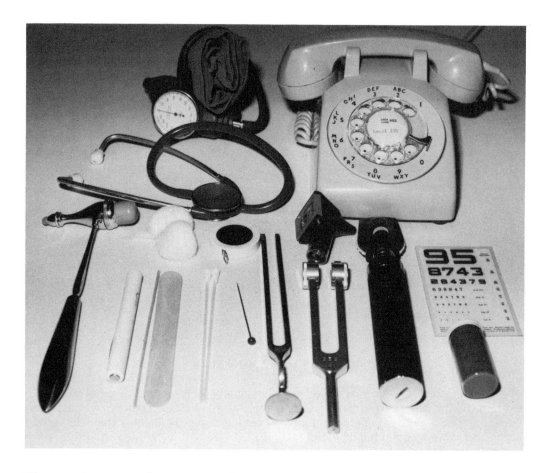

Figure 2-1   Tools of the neurological examination. The telephone is included as a reminder of its importance in history-taking.

Look for dilated veins over the surface of the skull. Note the level of the hairline. Listen for bruits over both carotids and also over the eyes. To eliminate background noise from eyelid movement when listening over the eye, have the patient gently close the eye, keeping the other one open and looking down. (Figs. 2-2A to C.)

Meningeal Irritation

Three tests can be done to assess meningeal irritation.

1. *Neck stiffness:* Place both hands below the occiput and gently, then more firm-ly, flex the neck; local pain and spasm of the neck muscles occur with menin-geal irritation, increased intracranial pressure, and cervical spondylosis (Fig. 2-3A, B). Knee flexion may also occur (Brudzinski's sign, Fig. 2-3C).
2. *Kernig's sign:* Flex the knee as far as it will go and then flex the hip to 90° (Fig. 2-3B, C). Try to extend the knee fully. Spasm of the hamstrings suggests root lesions or meningeal irritation.

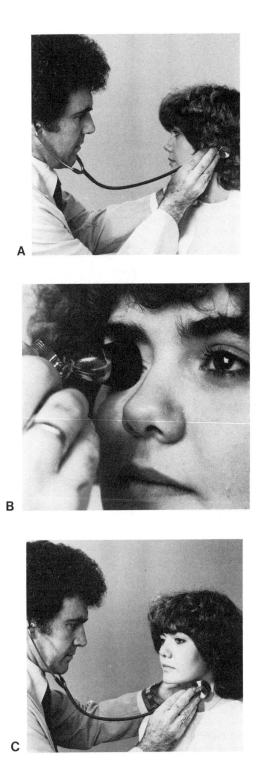

Figure 2-2A, B, C   Auscultation of the head and neck.

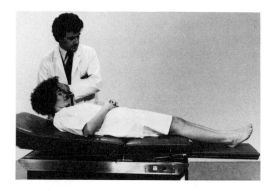

Figure 2-3A   Meningism: neck stiffness.

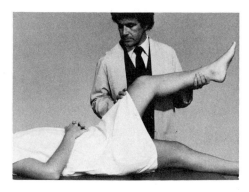

Figure 2-3B   Meningism: Kernig's sign.

3. *Straight-leg raising* (Fig. 2-4): Compare the angles obtained on each side when the hips are flexed with the knee extended. Unilateral restriction suggests root irritation.

The Spine

With the patient sitting (and later standing) observe the curves of the spine and look for deformity. A patch of hair or horizontal "silver striae" in the low lumbar area may be associated with an underlying bony defect. Finally, note the range of movement (flexion, extension, lateral flexion to the right and left, and rotation) in the cervical and lumbar spine and feel for *crepitus* (a grating sensation), which suggests arthritis of the spine.

An electric shocklike sensation felt running down the back on neck flexion indicates irritation of, or pressure upon, the posterior columns and is known as *Lhermitte's sign* (see Fig. 9-14).

Peripheral Nerves

Certain of the superficial nerves of the body can be both seen and felt. These include the greater auricular, supraclavicular, superficial radial, ulnar, common peroneal, and anterior tibial. Using an oblique light source to view the skin shadows, look for and then feel for these if a neuropathy is suspected, because enlargement

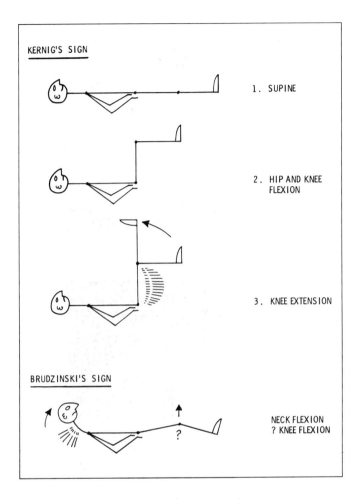

Figure 2-3C   Diagram of clinical tests for meningism.

indicates that the patient has a *hypertrophic* neuropathy. Paresthesias felt in the distribution of a nerve when it is tapped with the finger indicates regeneration after damage to that nerve *(Tinel's sign)*.

Cranial Nerves

1 Olfactory Nerve

Ask whether or not the patient tastes and smells his food normally. Then test each nostril separately, closing the opposite nostril (Fig. 2-5); coffee, cinnamon, and lemon are probably the best to use because they are available and do not irritate the fifth nerve, which supplies the nasal mucous membranes. The fifth nerve may be stimulated if odors such as ammonia or strong aromatics are employed, and this might mistakenly be interpreted as indicating normal olfaction. Determine if the patient can smell with each nostril; actual identification of the odors is not necessary.

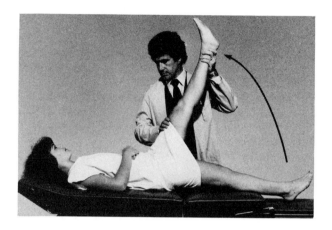

Figure 2-4   Straight-leg raising.

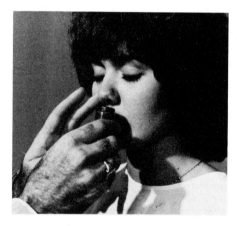

Figure 2-5   Olfactory testing.

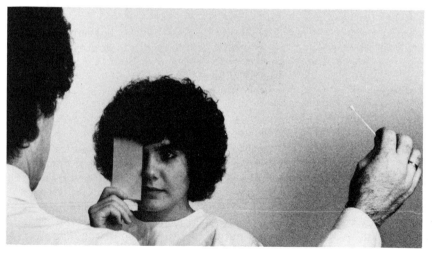

Figure 2-6A   Visual fields.

II Optic Nerve

There are four parts to the examination of the optic nerve.

Visual Acuity: Visual acuity should be examined with a test card (e.g., the Snellen chart for distant vision). For near vision, a Jaeger or similar card should be used. Newspaper print can be read at 3 ft by the normal-sighted individual. Record acuity in each eye separately, with the patient's glasses on.

Visual fields: Test the peripheral fields and blind spot, comparing the patient's visual field in all four quadrants with your own. Confrontation is tested with a white object or moving fingers in all quadrants of the visual fields (Fig. 2-6A). An efficient way is to hold up one or two fingers of your hand, to the right and left of the patients gaze, asking him to count the total number raised. The two upper and lower quadrants are tested one after another, the other eye being occluded. The blind spot is outlined using a small white test object. If there appears to be any defect on visual field testing, arrange for further testing on a tangent screen or with a perimeter. In cases where you suspect a cortical lesion, test for visual inattention *(extinction)* by presenting the subject with simultaneous stimuli on the two sides. If there is extinction, then a finger movement that is perceived when given alone will not be noticed when a similar movement occurs simultaneously on the opposite side.

Fundi: Examine these in a dim light with the patient focusing on a distant point so that the pupils are dilated (Fig. 2-6B). It is sometimes necessary to dilate the pupils with 0.5% tropicamide, but this might be dangerous in patients who have glaucoma and in any situation where the pupillary signs could be important in the next few hours, as in a changing neurological picture or suspected intracranial mass le-

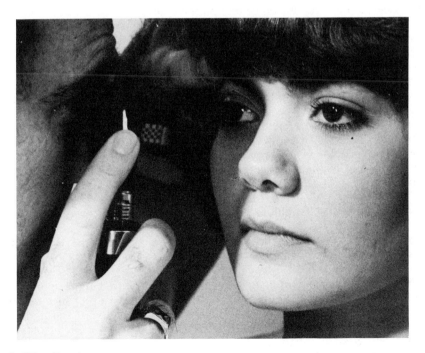

Figure 2-6B   Fundoscopy.

sion. Get someone more experienced to have a look before you use mydriatic drops; thus you may get the information you need without altering a very important neurological sign. In the situation where drops *are* needed, mark clearly on the chart (and on the patients forehead) what drops were instilled, and when. Otherwise somebody is bound to interpret the unilaterally dilated pupil as a sign of third nerve compression, an emergency situation.

First, with the ophthalmoscope in your eye, stand back from the patient and look at both eyes through the aperture of the machine. You should be able to see a *red reflex* coming out of both pupils, indicating that the cornea, lens, and vitreous are clear. Then go close to the patient (always using your *right* hand to hold the ophthalmoscope to your *right* eye when examing the patient's *right* eye and your *left* and and *left* eye when examining the patient's *left* eye) and search for the optic disks, finding them by tracing the vessels back to their origin at the disk head.

Note the color and shape of the disks, the distinctness of their edges and the depth of the physiological cup; this you can do by altering the focus of the ophthalmoscope, noting how many diopters of difference there are between the focus at the disk edge and that in its center. Usually, the nasal side of the disk is slightly blurred, whereas because of the presence of the maculopapillar bundle, the temporal side looks paler than the rest of the disk.

The major abnormalities to be seen in the optic nerve head are papilledema and optic atrophy. *Papilledema* is swelling of the optic nerve head caused by increased pressure of CSF in the subarachnoid space surrounding it. The disk is swollen, sometimes engorged, and the physiological cup is filled in. If you look carefully at the veins running back to the disk in the normal retina, you will see that they pulsate gently against the pale background of the disk, but in papilledema this pulsation is lost. Hemorrhages and exudates may occur in the fundus in association with optic nerve head swelling. *Optic atrophy* signifies abnormal disk pallor, which can only be assessed on the basis of experience.

Next, look at the distribution of any pigment on the retina and then pay attention to the vessels running NE, NW, SW, and SE from the disk, noting relative size, caliber, regularity, and tortuosity. Look for hemorrhages and exudates.

Then ask the patient to look at your light, which brings his macula into view so that you can assess the presence of degenerative changes, pigmentation, vascularity, and the presence of any hemorrhage there.

At this time it is convenient to examine the rest of the eye as well and in particular the lens, the media, the iris, and the cornea.

Color Vision: It is rarely necessary to test color vision. It is worth mentioning that if the visual field is tested with a red pinhead, it will be smaller than with a white one and that color vision is particularly decreased in patients with retrobulbar neuritis. Use of Ishihara's charts or common colored objects is seldom necessary clinically.

III Oculomotor Nerve, IV Trochlear Nerve, and VI Abducens Nerve

It is simplest to consider these three nerves together because they have similar functions involving eye movement.

External Ocular Movements: Ask the patient to follow a light up and down on both sides while you look at the eyes to see if there is any defect of eye movement (Fig. 2-7A, B). This will be shown on the asymmetric position of the light reflection from the cornea which shows as a little bright spot against the background of the black pupil. The position of the spot upon the pupil should be the same in the two eyes. If you use a light for the patient to follow rather than a finger, it will be

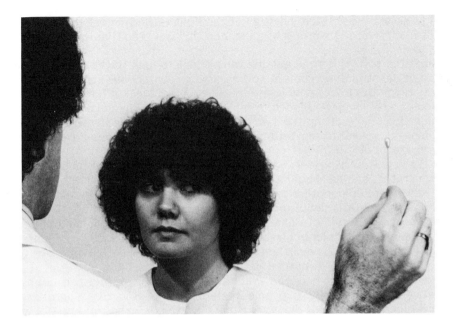

Figure 2-7A   External ocular movements.

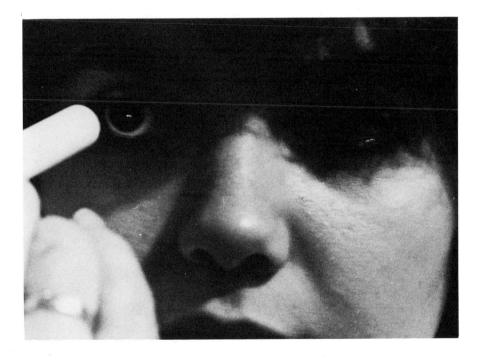

Figure 2-7B   Pupillary light reaction.

possible to assess the relative position of the light reflecting off the cornea on the two sides in different directions of gaze, and this is a sensitive way of detecting a squint.

Repeat the test, this time getting the patient to look to the sides, up and down, without a visual stimulus; you are now assessing *spontaneous* and not *reflex* gaze. Enquire if the patient sees double at any time. If he does, determine if the diplopia is monocular or binocular. *Binocular* diplopia is relieved by covering either eye. *Monocular* diplopia resulting from an abnormality of the eye itself, such as a dislocated lens or corneal lesion, will remain when the other eye is covered, but if it is of psychogenic origin, the effects of covering the eye vary.

Next, the patient is asked to indicate in which direction the images are most widely separated, and he should also say whether they are horizontal, vertical, or oblique relative to one another and which image is less clear. The extramacular image (the one from the deviating or abnormal eye) is less distinct. To document diplopia and the direction of image separation more clearly, you can use a red disk in front of one eye or diplopia glasses, which cover one eye with a red glass and the other with a green one. The patient then indicates the direction of separation of the red and green lights. A normal patient sees only one light source.

A *concomitant squint* is one in which the ocular axes are not parallel but the angle between them remains the same in all directions of gaze. A *paralytic squint* is one in which movement of one eye in one direction is impaired, usually by a lesion of the third, fourth, or sixth cranial nerves (although theoretically, the muscles could be primarily involved) (Fig. 2-8). The ocular axes are thus parallel in some directions of gaze and not in others.

If the axes are *not* parallel, either the patient "suppresses" one of the two images he sees, or he sees double. The separation of images is always greatest in the direction of action of the affected muscle. The peripheral image, displaced vertically, horizontally, or diagonally from the other, comes from the eye with the weak muscle.

To detect a squint that is "latent" or very slight, cover the eyes alternately back and forth with a piece of card (cover test). If there is a squint, the covered eye will drift away from the direction of fixation, so that when it is uncovered and the other eye is covered up, it moves to the correct gaze position. This test will not be of any value if the sight in one eye is so defective that the patient cannot fixate.

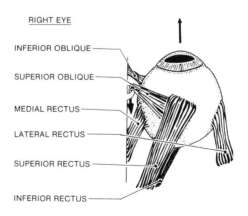

RIGHT EYE

INFERIOR OBLIQUE

SUPERIOR OBLIQUE

MEDIAL RECTUS

LATERAL RECTUS

SUPERIOR RECTUS

INFERIOR RECTUS

Figure 2-8   Oculomotor muscles.

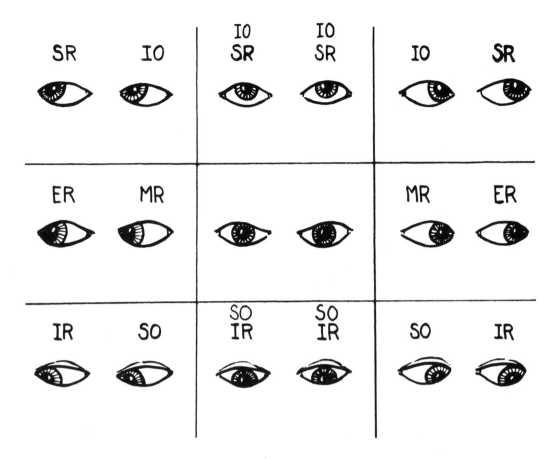

Figure 2-9   Muscles responsible for eye movement to different positions of gaze.

In the event of any oculomotor nerve paralysis, the patient will hold his head in such a position as to diminish the severity of the diplopia. Thus with a right sixth nerve palsy, he may hold it turned to the right and with a right fourth nerve palsy, the head tilts to the left and down, the face turns to the right, and the chin moves downwards.

The six muscles controlling the movements of the globe are arranged in three pairs, the two muscles in each pair acting antagonistically (Fig. 2-9). Thus the lateral and medial recti abduct and adduct the eye, respectively. The superior and inferior obliques act as pure depressors and elevators when the eye is adducted, the recti when it is abducted.

So far you have examined for evidence of a lower motor neuron lesion by attending to the function of muscles. You should also examine *gaze,* for this is a function of the upper motor neuron. (In general, the lower motor neuron controls *muscles,* the upper motor neuron controls *movements*). By gaze is meant the process of turning the eyes in any direction in parallel. If, for instance, neither eye can turn to the right but both can look to the left, then this is a disturbance of conjugate gaze. It is not likely to be due to a lesion of nerve or muscle since for the two eyes to look to the right requires the combined action of the right lateral rectus and the left medial rectus, and it is unusual for these two muscles to be affected by themselves. Similarly, partial lesions of the right sixth and the right third nerves would also be very unlikely. (For a further analysis of diplopia, see Chap. 21.)

Nystagmus: Nystagmus is a disorder of ocular posture in which the eyes repeatedly and rhythmically move from the position of fixation and then return quickly to it to correct this drift. Usually there is a fast and a slow phase, this form being called *jerk nystagmus.* In another type, *pendular nystagmus,* the speed of movement of the eyes is the same in each direction. Do not hold the test object further than about 45° from the midline, because after that point, binocular vision is lost and physiological searching movements that look like nystagmus may result (end-point nystagmus; see also Chap. 21).

The eyelids: While you are examining vertical gaze, look for *lid lag* as the patient follows your finger downwards after having gazed upwards. Look also for *proptosis* by standing above and behind the patient, looking down over his forehead to see if the eye is pushed forward relative to the other.

Ptosis: Finally, look for *ptosis,* which means drooping of the upper eyelid. It will usually be apparent when the eyes are examined with the patient sitting upright but will probably be missed when he is lying down. It may occur in association with sympathetic, or third nerve lesions. In the former instance, other manifestations of *Horner's syndrome* are likely to be present — a small pupil, and possibly vasodilation and decreased sweating on the same side of the face. With a *third nerve palsy,* there will probably be deviation of the eye and the pupil will be dilated, because the parasympathetic fibers that constrict the pupil run with the third nerve. Watch the eyelids during blinking because you may see a difference in the completeness of the blink or a difference in the timing on the two sides. If the lower lid on the side of the ptosis is lower than the other one, a primary muscle disease or myasthenia gravis is likely. As a test for myasthenia, ask the subject to look upward for 60 sec and determine if there is any drooping of the lid after that time. (For further discussion of ptosis and its analysis, see Chaps. 9 and 21.)

Pupils: Record the size of the pupils in millimeters and look carefully for even slight degrees of inequality and irregularity (see Chap. 21). Then shine a flashlight obliquely into the eyes, one at a time (see Fig. 2-7B), and note whether or not the pupil constricts on the side tested, and on the other side (consensual response). Finally, ask the patient to gaze into the distance and then to focus on your finger held about a foot in front of his nose. When he does so, the eyes should converge and the pupils constrict — the accommodation response.

V Trigeminal Nerve

Motor Functions: Test the power of jaw opening and sideways deviation against the resistance of your hand. Weakness of one side will cause the open mouth to deviate *toward* that side. Feel the contraction of the temporalis and masseter muscles while the patient bites on a tongue depressor (Fig. 2-10A, B). Test the *jaw jerk;* if it is increased (i.e., visible or palpable) this suggests a bilateral upper motor neuron lesion above the level of the fifth nerve motor nucleus which is situated in the posterior part of the mid-pons.

Sensory Functions: Test the corneal reflex by lightly touching the cornea *(not the conjunctiva)* with a wisp of cotton wool (Fig. 2-10C). Test pinprick, light touch and temperature over the three divisions of the nerve on either side and on the bridge of the nose. This nerve also gives sensation to the nostril and the mucosa of the mouth anteriorly, including the gums. The skin over the angle of the jaw is supplied by the greater auricular nerve (C2).

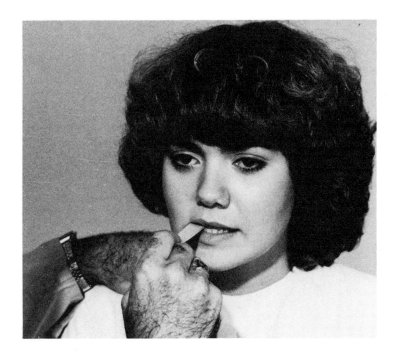

Figure 2-10A   Fifth nerve: bite.

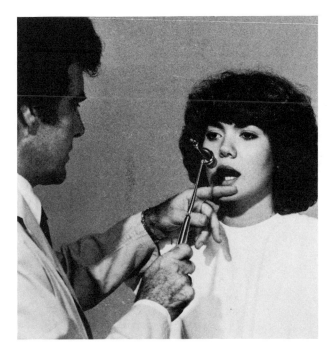

Figure 2-10B   Fifth nerve: jaw jerk.

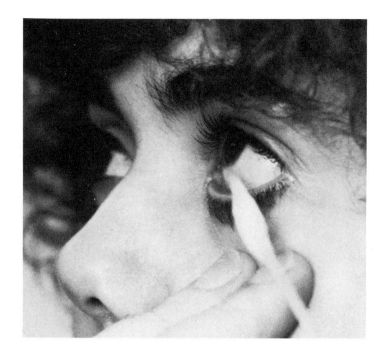

Figure 2-10C   Fifth nerve: corneal reflex.

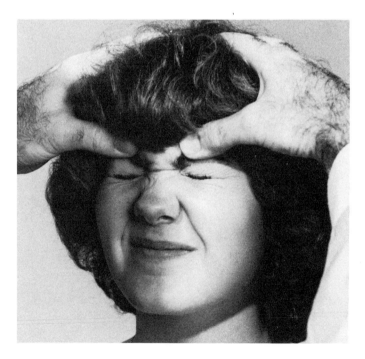

Figure 2-11   Seventh nerve: tight eye closure. Other movements such as baring the teeth should also be examined.

VII Facial Nerve

The motor functions of the facial nerve are tested by observing any asymmetry of the face at rest and when the patient speaks, bares the teeth, raises the eyebrows to wrinkle the forehead, screws up the eyes, or tenses the muscles of the neck. Another way to assess spontaneous facial movement and mimetic function is to ask the patient to whistle. Almost everyone will smile when asked, and this is more valuable to watch carefully than the whistling. Test power yourself by trying to overcome his resistance to your attempt to open his closed eyes or compressed lips. Watch his facial grimace as he resists you; this often reveals asymmetry that did not show on the other tests (Fig. 2-11).

Fibers running in the chorda tympani, which runs with the facial nerve, carry impulses from taste receptors on the anterior two-thirds of the tongue. One may test their function by moistening a cotton swab with dilute solutions of sugar, salt, quinine, or vinegar, and applying them to the tongue, which is kept outside the mouth. Test the two sides separately, and allow the patient a glass of water between each stimulus to erase traces of the last.

The nervus intermedius carries secretomotor fibers to the submaxillary and lacrimal glands. Functional testing simply requires observation of the production of tears and of mucous saliva. Absence of these may indicate nerve or gland dysfunction.

Other physical signs involving the facial nerve include

> *Chvostek's sign:* In cases of hypocalcemia or hypomagnesemia, and sometimes in normal people, tapping over the facial nerve in the parotid gland will cause the facial muscles on that side to twitch.
>
> *Myokymia:* This is a fine writhing contraction of the facial muscles on one side or the other. Common in states of anxiety and fatigue, it may occasionally be seen in brainstem disease, e.g., multiple sclerosis. The common eyelid twitch everyone experiences is due to tiredness.
>
> *Reflex eye closure:* A sudden, threatening movement of your hand before the patient's face will produce immediate blinking (the menace reflex). This is usually used as a test of visual fields rather than of facial nerve function.
>
> *Bell's phenomenon:* When you close your eyes, they normally turn upward under the lids. In cases of facial palsy, the eye may not be able to close so the upward turning of the eyeball can be clearly seen.
>
> *Glabellar tap:* Repetitive tapping over the bridge of the nose produces blinking at each tap for the first few taps, after which blinking ceases. In patients with diffuse cortical disease, such fatigue of reflex blinking does not occur.

VIII Auditory Nerve

Vestibular Division: The presence of nystagmus of the peripheral type (see Chap. 21) will indicate that there is an abnormality of function, as also may complaints of vertigo, imbalance, nausea, vomiting, or gait disturbance, but any of these symptoms may also be produced by disease of other parts of the brain. The most useful tests are *cold caloric tests* (see Chap. 7 on the examination of the comatose patient) and *positional testing* (Fig. 2-12A, B). To do the latter, get the patient to look to the left and then bend him backwards quickly while supporting the head in your hands, so that his head lies over the side of the couch and 45° below the horizontal. Maintain him in that position with his eyes turned to the left for 30 sec and look for nystagmus, at the same time asking for any complaint of vertigo.

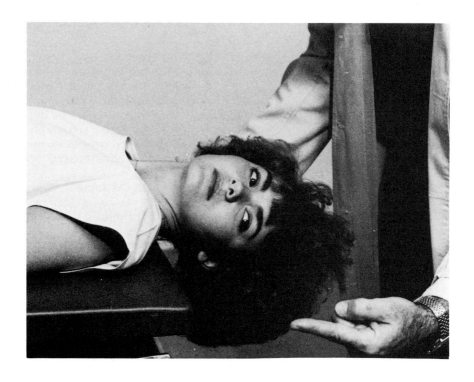

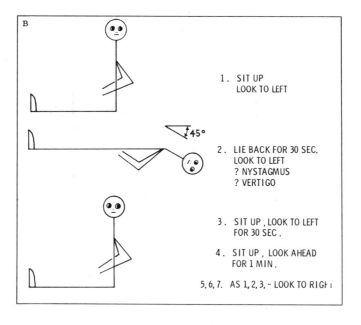

Figure 2–12A, B   Positional testing.

Then allow him to sit up, still with the head turned to the left for half a minute and continue observation. After any vertigo or nystagmus has ceased (about a minute) repeat the procedure with the head and eyes turned to the opposite side. Nystagmus and vertigo occurring with a 10 to 20 sec *latent period* and with *fatigue* of the response when the test is repeated two or three times suggest a lesion situated in the peripheral vestibular apparatus. With central lesions, no latent period and no fatigue of the response occurs (see Chap. 24). With peripheral lesions, the nystagmus and accompanying vertigo will probably be more severe than with central disease, and other signs of brainstem involvement will be absent. In such cases, vertigo and nystagmus are usually present together, and when vertigo is absent, nystagmus is usually also absent. Spontaneous nystagmus without vertigo suggests a central lesion.

Auditory Division

Acuity: Acuity is easily tested by rubbing the fingers together beside the ear or by using a watch, the whispered voice, or a tuning fork (256 Hz). Compare the patient's two ears using yourself as a control (Fig. 2-13).

Weber's test: Place a tuning fork on the center of the forehead and ask the patient if it is heard equally in both ears. In the presence of nerve deafness on one side, it will probably be heard most easily in the other, but with unilateral middle-ear deafness, it may be heard more loudly on that side. (Fig. 2-14A.)

Rinne's test: This test compares air and bone conduction. The vibrating tuning fork is placed on one mastoid process and then held with its tip beside the auricle. The patient with normal hearing or mild nerve deafness will say that it is louder in the latter position, while with middle-ear (conductive) deafness, it will be heard louder than when on the mastoid bone (Fig. 2-14B, C).

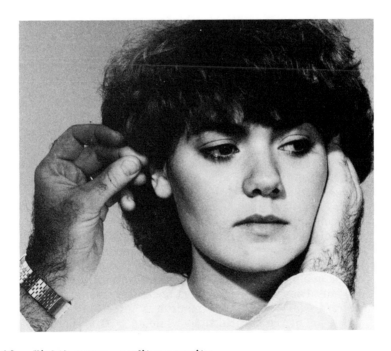

Figure 2-13 Eighth nerve: auditory acuity.

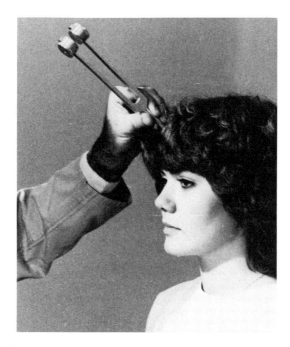

Figure 2-14A   Eighth nerve: Weber's test.

IX Glossopharyngeal Nerve and X Vagus Nerve

These are complex nerves with multiple components. Not all can be tested in the clinical situation.

1. Autonomic motor functions include the supply of secretomotor fibers to the parotid gland (which is best assessed by asking about salivation) and the whole of the parasympathetic supply to smooth muscle, heart, and glands, except for that emerging in the sacral outflow at S2, 3, 4.
2. Voluntary motor fibers innervate the pharynx and larynx. Test *phonation, coughing,* and *swallowing,* and note any drooling of *saliva* from, or pooling in, the mouth. The palate should rise symmetrically on phonation of, for example, *ee* or *r,* and should close off the nasopharynx when one sounds *k-k-k.* Any drawing-up of the palate to one side indicates weakness on the *opposite* side (see also tongue weakness, discussed later).
3. Afferent fibers supply common sensation to the posterior part of the tongue and pharynx, easily tested by touching the back of the throat with a tongue depressor and noting the gag reflex. Unilateral loss of the gag reflex is always abnormal, but in some normal subjects, stimulation on either side fails to produce gagging. Also, scarring from tonsillectomy often results in asymmetric elevation of the uvula, which has to be differentiated from paresis.
    Although not always safe and seldom necessary, one can also test the *carotid sinus reflex* (afferent fibers in nerve IX, efferent in nerve X) by unilateral compression of the carotid sinus while an ECG is running; a positive reflex is shown by bradycardia and/or marked hypotension.
4. Special sensory fibers bring taste sensation from the same areas of the tongue and pharynx and are not usually tested.

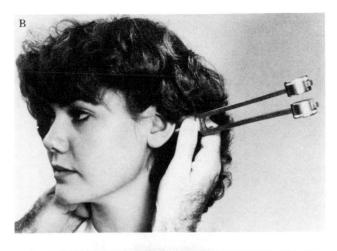

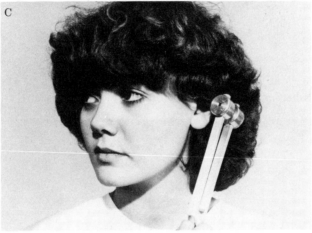

Figure 2-14B, C   Eighth nerve: Rinne's test.

XI Spinal Accessory Nerve

The cranial part of this nerve may be considered to be included within the ninth-tenth nerve complex. The spinal part, containing fibers from C2, 3, 4, supplies the trapezius and sternomastoid muscles. Test the power of shrugging the shoulders and of turning the head to one side against resistance; recall that the right sterno-mastoid turns the head to the left (Fig. 2-15A, B).

XII Hypoglossal Nerve

The hypoglossal nerve supplies motor fibers to the intrinsic muscles of the tongue. Damage to the lower motor neuron at any site may produce wasting of the tongue on that side, fasciculations, and weakness. If the patient is asked to push the tongue into the cheek or against a tongue depressor, power may be tested by press-ing against it and comparing the two sides (Fig. 2-16A, B).

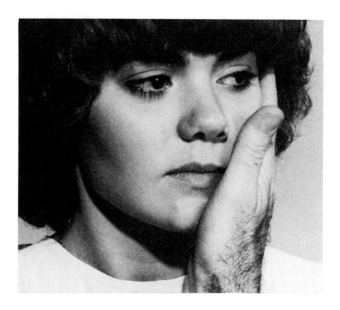

Figure 2-15A   Ninth nerve: sternomastoid power.

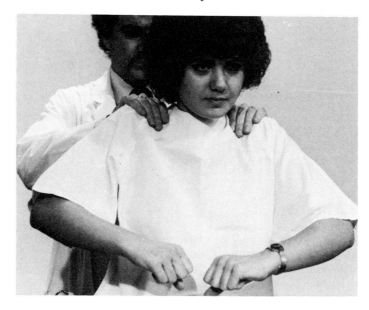

Figure 2-15B   Ninth nerve: trapezius power.

In facial paralysis, the mouth will not open symmetrically and deviation of the tongue will result even though it may not be weak. Another word of warning concerns abnormal tongue movements; it is hardly possible to keep the tongue still when it is outside the mouth, so only judge whether fasciculations are present or absent on inspection of the tongue *inside* the mouth.

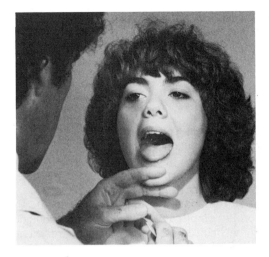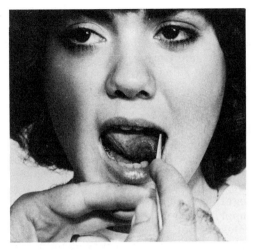

Figure 2–16A, B Twelfth nerve. (A) Inspection of the tongue; (B) Tongue power. (N.B. Examination of pharyngeal and palatal functions may also be performed at this time.)

A bitten tongue is a suggestive sign of trigeminal sensory loss or of a recent epileptic seizure.

The Motor System

The leading questions to be answered by examination of the motor system are

1. Is there any reduction in power?
2. If there is weakness, is it due to disease affecting upper or lower motor neutons, endplate or muscle?
3. Is there any evidence of abnormal movements or incoordination?

Inspection

Look carefully at the temples, limbs, and the pelvic and shoulder girdles to detect any wasting, fasciculations, or muscle hypertrophy. If atrophy is seen, decide whether this is localized or part of a generalized wasting process. Assess also the patient's state of nutrition, and look for scars, deformities, and contractures. Also assess vasomotor tone and look for evidence of Raynaud's phenomenon.

Tone

Tone is muscular resistance to passive stretch and must be evaluated using quick movements of the limb when the patient has achieved a state of good voluntary relaxation. Tone in the arm can be assessed by shaking the forearm and seeing how floppy the hand and wrist are, or by rapid supination-pronation of the relaxed forearm. Leg tone can be assessed by suddenly lifting the leg from under the knees. The relaxed limb flexes at the knee and the heel drags along the bedclothes. The spastic leg may stay stiff, so that the heel rises off the bed.

Spasticity is an increasing resistance to the stretching force, building up to a point and then giving way. The resistance felt in rigidity is increased more than normal but is consistent.

Decide whether the tone is normal, increased, or diminished, comparing the two sides; then if it is increased, determine whether there is spasticity (the "clasp-knife" phenomenon) or rigidity (which may be of the "plastic" or "cogwheel" type). At the same time it is a good idea to note whether or not the muscles are at all *tender* on palpation.

Power

Decrease in power may be manifest as weakness of a *movement* (indicating that the upper neuron system is damaged) or of one or more *muscles,* in which case the lesion is likely to be of the lower motor neuron. Depending upon the early findings, you will want to concentrate on weakness of one or the other. In the latter instance you will need to refer to a chart, such as Table 2-1, that details the muscles that together produce certain joint movements, with their innervation and segmental supply. Obviously such a detailed examination is complicated; it is seldom required unless a root or nerve lesion is thought likely. A briefer evaluation of power is most often sufficient on a survey examination (Figs. 2-17A to L, 2-18 A to F).

If weakness of any kind is detected however, it should be graded using a scale such as the following:

0 = Total paralysis.
1 = Only a flicker of contraction is seen.
2 = Movement is possible only if gravity is eliminated.
3 = Movement is possible against gravity only, not against any added resistance.
4 = Movement can be overcome by resistance.
5 = Full power.

This scale is bottom-heavy; one may want to subdivide category 4 into 4-, 4, and 4+. Crude as this type of grading may be, it is a far cry from the meaningless terms often used to describe weakness.

If cooperation is not perfect and you feel that the patient is not trying as hard as you would wish, try putting his limb in the position he is trying to achieve and getting him to resist your attempts to move it, rather than getting him to bring the limb to the desired position against resistance.

Most individuals feel that their dominant hand and arm are significantly stronger than the other. In fact, there is little difference in strength, but there is greater agility in the dominant hand. Do not accept as normal a measurable difference in strength just because the stronger limb is the dominant one.

Shorter Form of Testing Power: It is seldom necessary to examine the whole of the muscular system (see Table 2-1) to determine the degree of weakness present. If there seems to be an upper motor lesion, then the examination may well just include examination of those movements most likely to be affected — those performed by the extensors in the upper limb and the flexors in the lower limb. With a pyramidal lesion, then, expect to find most weakness in shoulder abduction, elbow extension, and wrist and finger dorsiflexion. In the leg, hip and knee flexion and ankle and toe dorsiflexion (really *extensor* movements) will be weaker than their opposing movements.

Scanning tests to identify any weakness include having the patient hold his arms extended with palms up and eyes closed for 30 sec. Slight rotation of the hand and falling of the limb indicates a minor loss of power. Then have the patient lower his arms to his lap and then snap them back to the horizontal. The mildly weak arm will be slightly slower in rising. To pick up mild leg weakness, have the patient lift both legs together off the bed. The weak leg will rise more slowly and be held lower than the normal one.

Table 2-1   Muscle Innervation

Joint	Movement	Main Muscles	Nerve	Main Roots
Shoulder	Adduction	Latissimus dorsi	Thoracodorsal	C(6),7,8
		Pectoralis major	Pectoral	C6-T1
	Abduction	Supraspinatus	Suprascapular	C5(6)
		Deltoid	Axillary	C5(6)
	Flexion	Deltoid		
	Extension	Deltoid		
		Latissimus dorsi		
	Internal	Latissimus dorsi		
	Rotation	Subscapularis	Subscapular	C5,6
	External	Teres minor	Axillary	C4,5
	Rotation	Supraspinatus		
		Infraspinatus	Suprascapular	C5(6)
Elbow	Flexion	Brachialis	Musculocutaneous	C5,6
		Biceps	Musculocutaneous	C5,6
		Brachioradialis	Radial	C5,6
	Extension	Triceps	Radial	C6,7,8
	Supination	Biceps		
		Supinator	Radial	C(5)6(7)
	Pronation	Pronator teres	Median	C6,7
Wrist	Flexion	Fl. carpi radialis	Median	C6,7
		Fl. carpi ulnaris	Ulnar	C7,8
	Extension	Ext. carpi radialis		
		longus and brevis	Radial	C6,7(8)
		Ext. carpi ulnaris	P. interosseous	C7,8
Metacarpo- phalan- geal	Flexion	Lumbricals	Median and ulnar	C8-T1
		Interossei	Ulnar	C8-T1
	Extension	Ext. digitorum	Radial	C7,8
Interpha- langeal	Flexion	Fl. digitorum sublimis	Median	C(7),8-T1
		Fl. digitorum profundus	Median and ulnar	C7,8-T1
	Extensor	Ext. digitorum		
		Lumbricals		
	Adduction	Interossei		
	Abduction	Interossei		
Thumb	Flexion	Fl. pollicis longus	Median	C7,8-T1
		Fl. pollicis brevis	Median	C8-T1
	Extension	Ext. pollicis longus	P. interosseous	C7,8-T1
		Lumbricals		

Table 2-1 (continued)

Joint	Movement	Main Muscles	Nerve	Main Roots
Thumb (cont'd)	Adduction	Interossei		
	Abduction	Interossei		
	Flexion	Fl. pollicis longus	Median	C7,8-T1
		Fl. pollicis brevis	Median	C8-T1
	Extension	Ext. pollicis longus	P. interosseous	C7,8-T1
		Ext. pollicis brevis	P. interosseous	C8-T1
	Adduction	Add. pollicis	Ulnar	C8-T1
	Abduction	Abd. pollicis longus	P. interosseous	C7,8
		Abd. pollicis brevis	Median	C8-T1
	Opposition	Opp. pollicis	Median	C6-7-8
Trunk		Diaphragm	Phrenic	C3,4,5
		Rhomboids	Dorsal scapular	C5
		Serratus ant.	Long thoracic	C5,6,7
		Sacrospinalis gp.	Segmental at all levels	
		Intercostals	Segmental	T1-12
		Rectus abdominis	Segmental	T5-12
		Levator ani	Pudendal	S3,4,5
Hip	Flexion	Iliopsoas	Femoral	L2,3
		Tensor fascia lata	Sup. gluteal	L4,5
	Extension	Gluteus max.	Inf. gluteal	L5-S1,2
		Hamstrings	Sciatic	L5,S1,2
	Adduction	Adductor gp.	Obturator	L2,3,4
	Abduction	Gluteus med. Gluteus min.	Sup. gluteal	L4,5-S1
Knee	Flexion	Hamstrings		
	Extension	Quadriceps	Femoral	L2,3,4
Ankle	Plantar flexion	Gastrocnemius	Tibial	S1,2
		Soleus	Tibial	L(5)-S1,2
		Tibialis post.	Tibial	L5-S1
	Dorsiflexion	Tibialis ant.	Tibial	L4,5
	Inversion	Tibialis post.		
	Eversion	Peronei		
Toe	Plantar flexion	Fl. digitorum long.	Tibial	L5-S1(2)
		Fl. digitorum brev.	Tibial	L5-S1(2)
	Dorsiflexion	Ext. digitorum long.	Peroneal	L4,5-S1
		Ext. hallucis long.	Peroneal	L5-S1,2

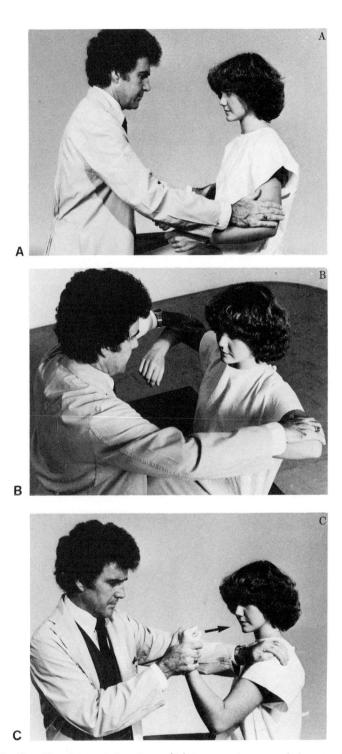

Figure 2-17A-C Shoulder abduction. (A) Supraspinatus; (B) Deltoid; (C) Elbow flexors (biceps, brachialis).

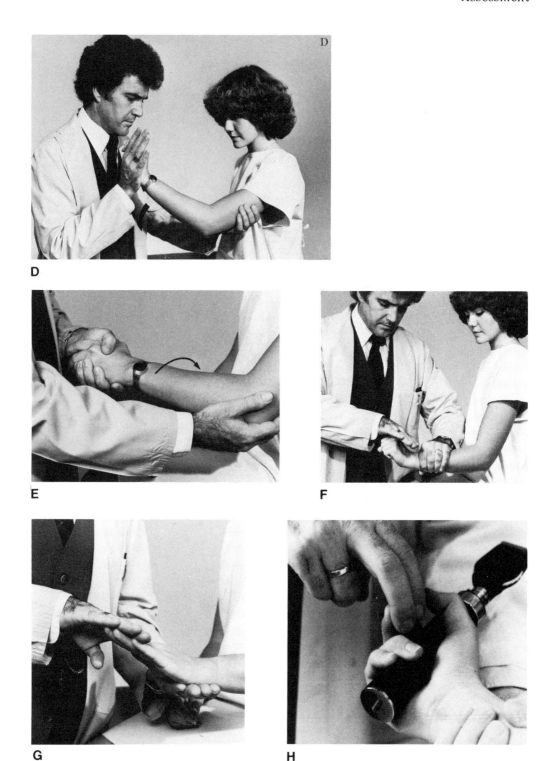

Figure 2-17D-H   (D) Elbow extensors (triceps); (E) Elbow rotators (supinator, biceps, pronators); (F) Wrist extensors; (G) Finger extensors; (H) Finger flexors.

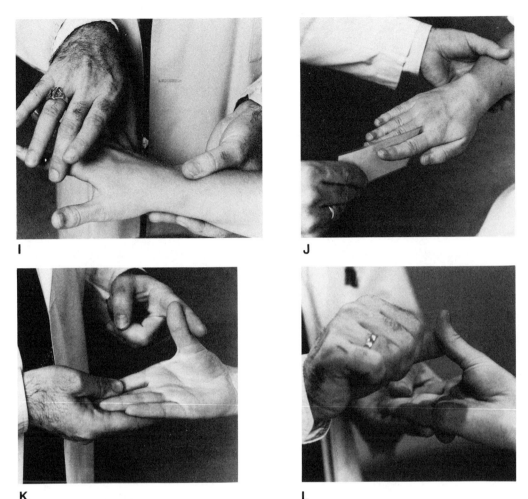

I

J

K   L

Figure 2-171-L   (I, J) Dorsal and palmar interossei;   (K) Thumb adductors;   (L) Thumb adductor.

If there is a suggestion of a root lesion, examination of certain muscles will help you to determine which root(s) are affected. These are

Arm: C5 deltoid
      C6 biceps
      C7 triceps
      C8 long finger flexors
      T1 interossei
Leg: L1 iliopsoas
      L2 hip adductors
      L3 quadriceps
      L4 ankle dorsiflexors
      L5 dorsiflexors of hallux
      S1 gastrocnemius/soleus

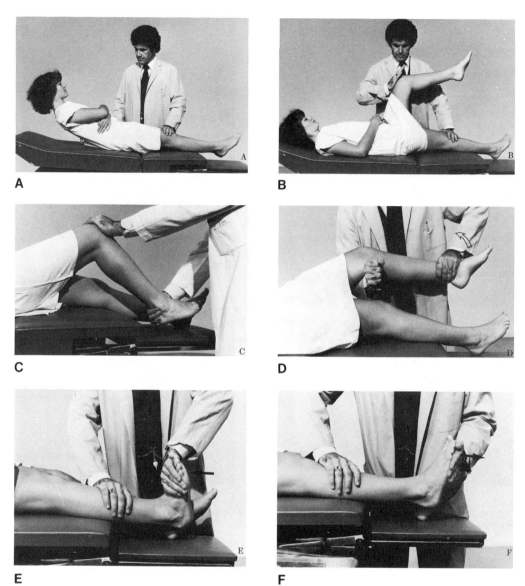

Figure 2-18A-F (A) Trunk flexors; (B) Hip flexors (iliopsoas); (C) Knee flexors (hamstrings); (D) Knee extensors (quadriceps); (E) Ankle dorsiflexors (tibialis anterior/peronei); (F) Ankle plantar-flexors (gastrocnemius).

This scheme represents a convenient approximation rather than absolute truth, since there are other roots contributing to each of the muscles or muscle groups mentioned.

Coordination

Many factors influence the smoothness and accuracy of movements. There will seem to be incoordination if there is any weakness, pain, involuntary movement, or joint disorder, and also if there is any abnormality of position sense or perhaps of vision. These should all be excluded before you decide that there is a cerebellar lesion. The more important tests are as follows:

Outstretched Arms: Ask the patient to stand or sit with his arms out horizontally in front of him and with his eyes closed; look for falling away or deviation of one arm to the side. This is not diagnostic of a cerebellar disorder if it occurs; it may also be seen with proprioceptive deficits and with weakness from any cause. (However the arm in cerebellar disease tends to *drift,* in proprioceptive disorders tends to *elevate,* and with pyramidal or myopathic weakness tends to *fall*). When the patient has his eyes open and his arms outstretched horizontally, press upon one hand, asking him to maintain the arm in the same position. If you take your hand away suddenly and the arm shoots up in the air an abnormal distance, this is known as *rebound.* This is a form of failure to make a rapid correction of movement, usually caused by cerebellar disease.

Finger-Nose and Heel-Shin Tests (Fig. 2-19A, B): In the finger-nose test, the patient is asked to touch in rapid succession the examiner's finger (held at arm's length in front of him) and his own nose, using his right and then his left index finger. Cerebellar disease results in overshooting *(past-pointing),* and the movement will be irregular and lack smoothness. *Decomposition of movement* may also be seen. This is the breaking up of the orderly coordinated sequence of minor movements required to produce a smooth, flowing voluntary action into its component parts as if each joint was moved in sequence rather than together. *Intention* or *action tremor* is also common in cerebellar disease. This is a coarse, side-to-side movement of the hand and arm that increases as the hand is moved out farther. It can be regarded as yet another form of failure to make rapid and exact course corrections when the various proprioceptive monitors and the visual system provide information that the arm is drifting off course from the target. The corrections that are made are faulty in *range, force,* and *direction.* In performing the heel-shin test, the subject is asked to raise his extended leg as high as he can while lying

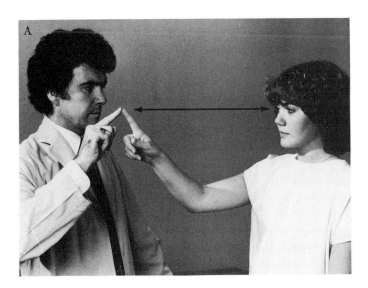
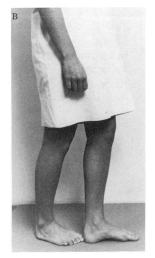

Figure 2-19   Cerebellar testing. (A) Finger-nose test; (B) Heel-toe gait. The many other tests are not shown.

on his back. He then flexes the knee and places the heel on the opposite knee, holding it on top of the patella: next he taps the heel on the patella, and runs it down the shin to the ankle. The same faults may be observed here. The heel reaches the patella in a jerky, irregular movement, cannot be held on the patella, is very irregularly tapped, and then shakily moves down the shin.

Rapid Alternating Movement: Get the patient to pat the palm of one hand with the palm and dorsum of the other hand alternately; to pronate and supinate the hands rapidly; or to oppose the thumb to each finger backward and forward in turn. Rapid tapping on the table with the index finger or with the four fingers of one hand (making a sound like a horse cantering) allows auditory as well as visual monitoring of the patient's ability to make rapid movements in a regular, rhythmic, and coordinated manner. The dominant hand usually performs slightly better than the nondominant. In cerebellar disease these tests all show irregularity and lack of smoothness.

Functional Abilities: Ask the patient to pick up pins or coins from a flat surface using one hand, to do up buttons or zip fasteners, strike a match, or write.

Tandem Stance and Gait: The previous tests are mainly indicators of the functions of the lateral lobes of the cerebellum. The vermis and the flocculonodular lobe are mainly concerned with vestibular function, i.e., the patient's position in space. Therefore see if he can sit up in bed unsupported, can stand with his feet together or placed one in front of the other, and can walk a line heel-to-toe. Have him walk, looking for a lurching, drunken, or staggering gait with a tendency to fall to one side or other, usually to the side of maximal cerebellar involvement. If this does appear to be present but very slight, ask him to walk around a chair placed in the center of an open space. With a right-sided cerebellar lesion, the patient will fall inward towards the chair when he walks around it clockwise, but outwards and away from it when he walks in the opposite direction.

Reflex Activity

Tendon Reflexes: Tap firmly one or two times with the reflex hammer over the tendon (see Figs. 2-20A to F) and assess the degree of reflex muscle contraction.

Jaw jerk	V3
Biceps	C5, 6
Brachioradialis	C6 mainly
Triceps	C7 mainly
Knee	L3, 4
Ankle	S1

The results should be recorded.

0	=	Absent.
±	=	Just present
+	=	Slightly diminished.
++	=	Normal.
+++	=	Overactive or brisk.
++++	=	Markedly overactive. If the reflex merits this rating there will probably be clonus.

If deep reflexes are sluggish or absent, get the patient to clench his teeth or squeeze his fingers together while you repeat the test. This is *Jendrassik's maneuver* (see Fig. 2-20F) and may "reinforce" the reflex so that it appears when it was formerly absent.

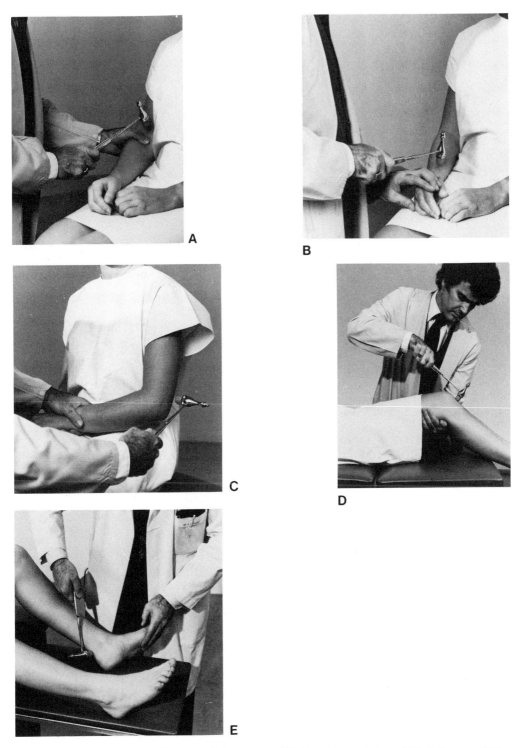

Figure 2-20 Tendon reflexes. (A) Biceps, (B) Brachioradialis; (C) Triceps; (D) Knee; (E) Ankle.

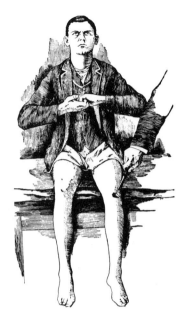

Figure 2-20F   Tendon reflexes. Jendrassik's maneuver (From: Dana C.L. *Textbook of Nervous Diseases,* 6th Ed., New York, Wood, 1894).

With pyramidal lesions, deep reflexes are increased, superficial reflexes often abolished, and the hallux turns upward rather than the normal downward movement with plantar stimulation.   Reflexes are diminished or absent with any damage to the reflex arc.

Superficial Reflexes: Look for contraction of the abdominal wall when you scratch it lightly with a pin or applicator stick in the four quadrants;   or of the dartos muscle of the scrotum on scratching the inner upper thigh.

Abdominal	T7-10
	T10-12
Cremasteric	L1
Plantar	S1-2

The plantar response (Fig. 2-21) is best tested with an applicator stick or a broken tongue depressor,[*] stroking slowly up the lateral side of the foot and then across the sole to the ball of the foot (Babinski's[†] test).   If the patient is ticklish, try Chaddock's test, stroking behind and below the lateral malleolus and along the dorsolateral side of the foot.   If the response is equivocal, try the Chaddock's and

---

[*]English consultant neurologists may insist that the best instrument is a Rolls-Royce or Bentley key, but we feel this relates more to their seniority and experience than to the instrument itself.   We prefer the applicator stick, because if one uses too much pressure, it breaks, and the patient's skin is not scored nor actually cut.   Besides, neither of us has a Rolls-Royce or a Bentley.

[†]Josef Babinski (1857-1932), a Parisian of Polish origin, described the famous abnormality of plantar response seen in disorders involving the corticospinal tracts in a series of short articles beginning in 1896.

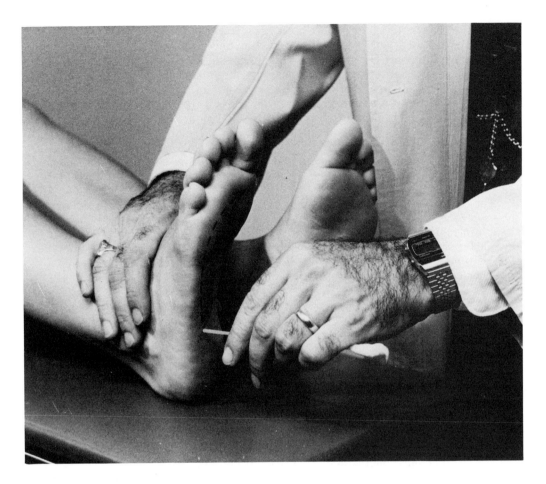

Figure 2-21   The plantar response.

Babinski's together. Babinski's test should be done with a *potentially* painful stimulus, but it does not have to *be* painful. Never use pins or needles to do the test. Be especially gentle and careful in patients with diabetes or peripheral vascular disease.

The normal response is for the big toe to go down. In disorders of the spinal cord, brainstem, or hemispheres involving the corticospinal (pyramidal) pathways, the toe will go up and the other toes may spread in a fanlike movement. Remember that this reflex is a mass reflex, and with a marked response, results in dorsiflexion of the great toe, fanning of the other toes, dorsiflexion of the ankle, and flexion of the knee and hip. Indeed, the first muscles to contract in the Babinski's response are the hamstring and adductor muscles of the thigh.

For a discussion of the primitive reflexes present in diffuse cerebral dysfunction see Chapter 12.

The Sensory System

If this examination is to have diagnostic or localizing value, it must be done properly. Casual or muddled testing is a waste of time and effort of the patient and for yourself. If any deficit is found, it must be demarcated exactly. Look for a level; for the point, if any, where *abnormal* sensation becomes *normal* again. However, screening for a sensory deficit may be performed quite quickly.

If any sensory deficit is found, the responsible lesion could be in the cerebral cortex; in the ascending fiber tracts in the brainstem, thalamus, or corona radiata; in the spinal cord; in the emerging posterior roots or the dorsal root ganglia; or in the peripheral nerves. In other words, it could be cortical, thalamic, long tract, segmental, or neural. The importance of defining the modalities involved and the exact boundaries of the area affected is thus paramount. The patient can usually do this better than you can and should be asked to outline with his fingers the area of sensory abnormality, but be careful not to suggest to him any type or area of sensory involvement.

The sensations to be examined may be divided between the *exteroceptive* and the *proprioceptive*. *Exteroceptive* refers to those sensations that give the body some information about external events, including pain, temperature, and light touch. *Proprioception* refers to innate bodily sensations including deep pain, and the position of joints in space. Vibration sense is conventionally accepted as a posterior column function but may actually ascend in the dorsal spinocerebellar tract.

Pinprick, heat and cold, crude light touch, tickle, and itch sensations are all transmitted by the same pathways, and if one is affected, the others probably are. *Cortical sensory loss* combines features of exteroceptive and proprioceptive function, and it is best to consider it separately (Figs. 2-22(A-D), 2-23, 2-24).

Exteroceptive Sensations

Pinprick Pain: Test for pain sensation with a pin, comparing side with side, proximal with distal, segment with segment. Never use a very sharp (e.g., hypodermic) needle, because this might draw blood, and if used again could transmit hepatitis. Because of its sharpness and small area of stimulation it might miss pain spots, giving rise to misinterpretation of sensory deficiency.

Temperature: Test for temperature sensation with cold steel or with tubes filled with water about 30°C and 45°C. The latter are more accurate, but less convenient.

Light Touch: Test for light touch sensation with cotton wool, applying it in dabs rather than stroking movements.

These sensations are mediated predominantly by thin, slowly conducting fibers in the peripheral nerves, and the second-order neurons travel upward in the anterior and lateral spinothalamic tracts. Tickle and itch sensations are mediated by the same fibers.

Proprioceptive Sensations

Position of Joints in Space: Test this function by getting the patient to oppose the fingers of the two hands with his eyes closed or by putting one limb in a certain position and getting him to make the same position with the other limb, with his eyes closed.

Passive Movements: Ask the patient to close his eyes and identify the direction in which you are moving the terminal phalanx of a finger or great toe (up or down). Before you do this however, demonstrate which movements you are going to test. Hold only the sides of the digit being moved because the differential pressure provided by your grip on top of and underneath the digit will give more clues.

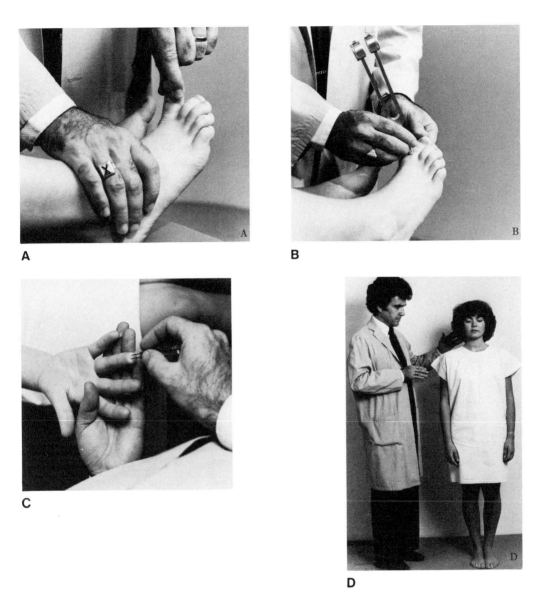

Figure 2-22   Sensation. (A) Joint position sense; (B) Vibration; (C) Two-point discrimination; (D) Romberg's test.

Deep Pressure and Deep Pain: Observe the patient's reaction when you squeeze the Achilles tendon, and assess the interval between the application of the painful stimulus and the patient's response, whether verbal or facial. If the fast-conducting (thick) fibers are severely damaged, the pain response may be delayed up to 2 or 3 sec.

Vibration: Introduce the patient to this test by placing the vibrating tuning fork (128 Hz) on the chest wall and letting him feel the vibration. Then test by placing it on toes and fingers, but be sure that it is *vibration* and not *pressure* that he is feeling in each situation. To compare the two sides, place the vibrating tuning fork on the extremity, damp it gently with your fingers, and ask the patient to

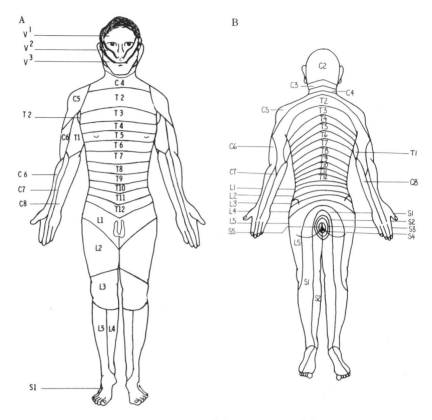

Figure 2-23   The sensory dermatomes. (A) Anterior; (B) Posterior.

tell you as soon as he no longer feels the vibration. Then quickly transfer the fork to the other side and see if it is felt there.

With the possible exception of vibration, these sensations are mediated by thick, rapidly conducting contralateral fibers passing upward in the posterior columns with one relay, to the opposite ventroposterior thalamic nucleus and thence to the parietal cortex. In older patients, symmetric diminution of the sense of vibration peripherally may not be pathological.

Romberg's Test: Get the patient to stand with his feet together for half a minute, then ask him to close his eyes. A positive Romberg's test occurs when the patient can stand with the eyes open but *falls* when they are closed.* It indicates a proprioceptive lesion and is not a test of cerebellar function, a common misconception. With midline cerebellar disease, the patient has difficulty standing with the eyes open as well as them closed.

Cortical Sensory Loss

Even though peripheral sensory mechanisms and pathways may be normal, correct interpretation of sensory stimuli requires that the parietal cortex be functioning normally. If there is a possibility of cortical impairment, test stereognosis, tactile

---

*Make sure that you are there to catch him.

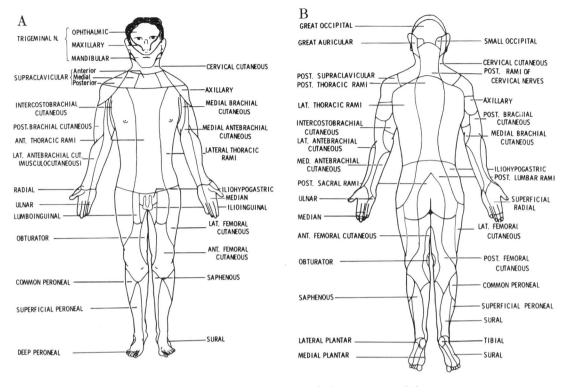

Figure 2-24   Distribution of superficial nerves. (A) Anterior; (B) Posterior aspect.

localization, and sensory competition, but be aware that in the presence of any major degree of sensory loss (light touch, pinprick, deep pressure, etc.), tests of cortical sensory loss may be invalid.

Stereognosis is the ability to discriminate shape, size, weight, texture, and form. Test by tracing figures or numbers (graphesthesia) on the palm of the hand, by getting the patient to identify coins or similar objects in his hand without seeing or hearing them (stereognosis), and by testing two-point discrimination, using the blunted ends of a compass placed on the sides of the fingers or toes. A separation of 5 mm on the fingertips is usually taken as normal, while double or treble will be acceptable in the feet. Other tests include the ability to discriminate cotton from silk, a sheet from a blanket, or paper from cardboard. Obviously these tests should be given to the patient with his eyes closed.

To test *tactile localization,* ask the patient to point out the place on the hands, arms, and legs that you touched, again with his eyes closed.

Sensory competition can be assessed if simultaneous bilateral touches are given, e.g., to both hands, both sides of the face, and so on. Even though the subject may be able to perceive such stimuli given separately, if they are given both at the same time one may be ignored, suggesting a contralateral cortical lesion. This test can only be acceptable if peripheral sensation is normal.

Autonomic Function

Pupillary function, salivation, and tear formation will have been noted already. Ask about faintness, and test for postural hypotension by recording the blood pressure in the standing and lying positions. Questions about bladder, bowel, and sexual functions will have been put during history taking. Note the strength of the patient's glasses, and ask about accommodation for near vision. Ask about, and look for, sweating, pallor, and flushing of the skin. Reflex sweating may be tested by heating the patient with a body cradle, using starch powder and iodine on the skin.

The *ciliospinal reflex* is tested by pinching the skin of one side of the neck; a normal response is for the homolateral pupil to dilate a little and suggests normal brainstem and sympathetic function on that side.

The pulse rate may be followed during a *Valsalva maneuver;* this is best done with an ECG running. It is difficult to monitor the blood pressure clinically without major instrumentation, but a change can be recorded in most patients with a blood pressure cuff.

The *cold pressor response* is done by immersing an arm in cold or ice water and recording an increase in pulse rate and blood pressure. The best way to record a change is again to use an ECG machine to document the pulse rate before, during, and after the test. Because of the discomfort, most patients will not tolerate the ice water more than 1 or 2 min.

Finally, *axon reflexes* may be assessed using intradermal histamine or by scratching the skin with an orange stick and noting whether or not the three components of the triple response all appear. Some other tests are mentioned in Chapter 44.

Gait

Get the patient to stand on one leg, then to mark time on one spot, and to rock on his toes and heels. Then observe him walking, noting particularly how steady he is on turning. If there is any chance that he might fall, accompany him. Finally, ask him to walk heel-to-toe along a straight line. Look at his shoes for evidence of scuffing of the toes or excess wear. Abnormal gaits are described in Chapter 32.

Finally, watch the patient unobtrusively while he is moving about in the interview and examining room. Often you will see that the gross signs, present when the patient first came into the office, have lessened at the end of the examination when the need to impress you with their genuineness and the anxiety of coming to the office both have passed. On the other hand, some abnormalities of function will become more evident because of fatigue.

Most of the tests previously mentioned are simple and all are potentially informative, but this is not to say that they will all be needed when a patient is seen for the first time. The selection of tests can only be made on the basis of experience, and students will be well advised to practice as many of them as possible to get to know their limitations and meanings, as well as the routine of the full neurological examination, while time still permits.

BIBLIOGRAPHY

Aminoff, M.J., Wilcox, G.S. Assessment of autonomic function in patients with a parkinsonian syndrome. *Br. Med. J.* 4:80-83, 1971.

Bickerstaff, E.R. *The Neurological Examination in Clinical Practice,* 4th Ed. London, Blackwell Scientific, 1980.

DeJong, R.N. *The Neurological Examination,* 4th Ed. Hagerstown, Md., Harper & Row, 1979.

Mayo Clinic, Department of Neurology. *Clinical Examinations in Neurology,* 5th Ed. Philadelphia, W.B. Saunders Co., 1981.

Medical Research Council. *Aids to the Diagnosis of Peripheral Nerve Injuries.* London, H.M.S.O., 1976.

3
Scanning Neurological Examination

A "formal" neurological examination is an indispensable part of the assessment of every patient suspected of having a neurological problem. What about the patient who has a nonneurological problem? What kind of rapid examination can we use to test the nervous system to make sure that nothing is being missed? It must be practical, efficient, and brief, and must give a high yield of information. The method taught to medical students in the past regarded the neurological examination as a necessarily *complete* survey; it often took the novice an hour to do. When out of the neurologists' sight, in the emergency room, on the wards, or in practice, not knowing an efficient way to do it, it was thus omitted altogether.

In developing your examination skills you must be *competent* to do the tests and assessments correctly. Then develop *confidence* as you get more and more experience and recognize that you are getting good at examing the nervous system. Next you must be *efficient* in doing an examination whenever it is required and *reliable* so that your conclusions are correct; when you say that the plantar reflexes are abnormal, they *are* abnormal; when you say the strength is normal, it *is* normal. Finally, you must use in your examination the tests and techniques that are most likely to demonstrate the abnormalities present to yield the most information.

We offer the following as a rapid scan of the nervous system; we think that in 5 min the nervous system can be tested with little likelihood that significant lesions will be missed. It is brief but should identify almost all abnormalities. Do it on every patient you see and you will become competent, confident, efficient, and reliable.

SCANNING EXAMINATION

History Taking

During history taking you will be able to assess

1. Level of consciousness
2. Mental status
3. Speech and sight

Cranial Nerves

1. Examine fundi and visual fields by confrontation.
2. Check pupils and eye movement; look for nystagmus.
3. Touch over the three divisions of the face with cotton wool, rating both touch and tickle sensations.
4. Test the jaw jerk.
5. Test facial muscles by observing tight eye closure and the smile.
6. Rub fingers together next to the ear to test hearing.
7. Ask the patient to open the mouth widely, say "Ah," and then protrude the tongue.

Motor Functions

1. Test deltoids, biceps, triceps, wrist extensors, and grip. Observe arms extended for 20-30 sec with the palms toward the ceiling and eyes closed.
2. Test hip, knee, and ankle flexors and extensors.
3. With patient standing, test plantar flexors and extensors; ask the patient to hop on toes of each foot; and to hold up the toes while standing on the heels.
4. Test coordination by the finger-nose and the heel-shin tests.

Reflexes

1. Test deep tendon reflexes (biceps, triceps, brachioradialis, knee, and ankle) and plantar responses.

Sensation

1. Touch over face, tip of the shoulder, forearm and hand, thigh, lateral side of the foot, and great toe, all on each side.
2. Move (touch or pin) from the toe toward the thigh asking about any change in sensation.

Stance and Gait

1. Observe normal and heel-toe walking.
2. Perform Romberg's test.

4
Neurological Examination in Children

Many students shy away from examining the nervous system in infants or small children because of a feeling that, if the examination is difficult in the adult, it must be impossible in a baby.

It is true that the infant cannot help you with the history nor add subjective responses to your examination, and is often crying and in continuous motion, but by careful observation and simple examination techniques, you should be able to obtain most of the data that you require. After the age of 5 or 6 years children can cooperate with a standard CNS examination, but before that age, it must be kept brief and simple. To an even greater extent than in the adult, the examination of the child depends upon observation of spontaneous movement and activity.

EXAMINATION IN INFANTS

Examination of infants can be carried out under six major headings.

1. Observation
2. Head, spine
3. Eyes
4. Hearing and lower cranial nerves
5. Developmental reflexes
6. Motor system

Observation

As much of the examination as possible is done without actually touching the child, who may be observed while lying in a cot, on the examination table, or on his mother's or nurse's lap. The most satisfactory observation is carried out while the infant is quietly feeding.

Such matters as *level of consciousness* can be assessed in the same way as in adults, but the child's *responsiveness* to touch, noise, or light stimuli and the degree of *irritability* should be noted too. The tremulous baby who startles easily and has exaggerated tendon jerks is described as showing cerebral irritation. This stage precedes cerebral depression, in which the infant sleeps excessively, is hard to arouse, shows little spontaneous movement, and has depressed tendon jerks. A newborn child should lie symmetrically with the head rotated to one side and with the arms flexed, the legs often extended. Movements should be seen on both sides of the body; they will be jerky and of wide amplitude. *Lack of movement* on one side, *abnormal postures,* and *abnormal movements* can all be seen without disturbing the child. The ability to swallow will be obvious if he is sucking at a bottle.

The pattern of *respiration* may be useful: apart from abnormalities seen in the respiratory distress syndrome or caused by pneumonia, "diaphragmatic breathing" with little or no contribution from the intercostal muscles may occur in infantile spinal muscular atrophy and with cervical injury following obstetric trauma.

Head, Spine

The largest occipitofrontal circumference must be *measured* and compared with a graph of normal head size (Fig. 4-1A, B). If the head circumference is smaller than 2.5 standard deviations below the mean for the gestational age, then there is a high probability of subsequent developmental retardation. If the head is abnormally large for the gestational age, then this is to be due to excess fluid distending the ventricles *(hydrocephalus),* replacing the cerebral hemispheres *(hydranencephaly),* or forming a *cyst.* Enlargement can also be due to intracranial hemorrhage or to the presence of excessive brain tissue. In all cases of likely intracranial disease, particularly if there is any asymmetry of the skull or if hydrocephalus or a subdural effusion are suspected, *transillumination* should be carried out using a flashlight shone down a cardboard tube* placed on the side of the head while the child is in a dark room. The amount of light glowing around the tube can be assessed and compared on the two sides. Large amounts of clear fluid will transilluminate.

The *shape* of the head must be observed. A long, boat-shaped head may be due to premature fusion of the sagittal suture, a tall or tower-shaped head may mean fusion of the coronal suture, and an asymmetric head can result from unilateral coronal synostosis (fusion of sutures). Although these features are usually more obvious at a few months of age, they should be recognized as early as possible, because the younger the infant is when neurosurgical intervention is carried out, the better the outcome. The anterior fontanel should be palpated, as should the space (if any) between the cranial sutures. At this age a tense fontanel, suture separation, and a "cracked-pot" note heard when the skull is tapped are the best signs of acutely raised intracranial pressure (papilledema is an unusual finding in infants).

---

*There's one in the bathroom.

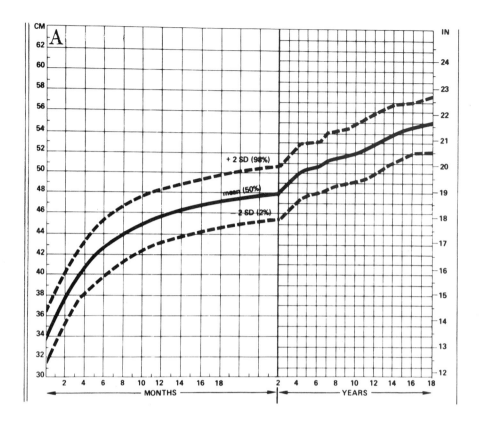

Figure 4-1A   Normal values of head circumference in girls.

Meningism is best detected using Brudzinski's test because neck stiffness may not be demonstrable in infants. *Congenital defects* anywhere in the musculoskeletal system (e.g., syndactyly, high-arched palate, prognathism, pes cavus, hip dislocation), but particularly over the spine (skin clefts, hair tufts, cysts), may also be noted at this time.

Eyes

Fundoscopy can usually be carried out when the baby is feeding because the eyes are often kept open, but do not use too bright a light or the infant will reflexly close his eyes. Attempts to open them forcibly will be futile. At the end of the examination, having assessed the pupillary responses, it is occasionally necessary to dilate the pupils with phenylephrine to see the fundi. One is looking for choroiditis in "congenital" viral infections; retinal hemorrhages in cases of intracranial bleeding (retinal hemorrhages can be found in at least 10 percent of normal neonates, if sought for carefully); or colobomata and other congenital anomalies of the retina when blindness is suspected. Visual *fields* can be assessed by menace (flicking the hand in front of the eyes) or by dangling a toy in the periphery of vision; even when being fed, the child will follow a light or turn the head and eyes toward one, provided it is held only 1 to 2 ft away. *Strabismus* is not necessarily abnormal up to the age of 6 months. In children with hydrocephalus, the eyes may appear to be looking down, with an expanse of sclera showing above the pupil (the "sunset" sign). The function of the extraocular muscles may be assessed by noting spontaneous movements of the eyes or by performing the doll's head maneuver (see Chap. 7).

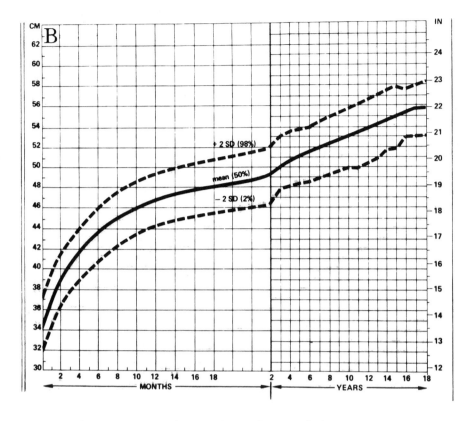

Figure 4-1B Normal values of head circumference in boys.

Hearing and Lower Cranial Nerves

The *corneal reflex* and *facial sensation* can be tested, and the child's ability to *suck* and *swallow* will have been noticed already. Hearing can be tested by assessing responses to quiet, then louder sounds (see later discussion) and by eliciting a startle response (extension of the arms and legs, stiffening, or blinking) to a sudden loud noise. In the same way as a visual stimulus must be given silently, so must an auditory stimulus be given outside the child's field of vision. At a later age, the baby turns his eyes toward the sound and the pupils may dilate; he will also turn toward his mother's voice and may vocalize or cease crying when she speaks. *Facial movements* are best assessed when the child cries. Facial asymmetry and inequality of the palpebral fissures suggest facial weakness when the baby is at rest. Involvement of the ninth and tenth nerves should be suspected if the alert infant's cry and sucking are weak, and if the gag reflex is absent. The most common cause is cerebral depression from anoxia, but neonatal myasthenia and myopathies may present in this manner. Weakness, wasting, or fasciculations of the tongue indicate a twelfth nerve lesion, but these are rare.

Developmental Reflexes

Although scores of reflexes have been described in small children, only a few need be known. The *Moro reflex* consists of a sudden extension and abduction of the arms with opening of the hand, followed by slow flexion of the arms across the midline

(Fig. 4-2). It can be elicited by a sudden loud noise or by allowing the baby's head to drop suddenly 3 or 4 in. as hand support is temporarily removed. It is most often absent in cerebral depression or asymmetric because of brachial plexus palsy, a fractured clavicle, or cerebral palsy.

The *flexor withdrawal* reflex is seen in the leg with sudden and brief stimulation of the sole of the foot. It normally should be present.

A *tonic neck* reflex (turning of the head to one side causes extension of that arm and flexion of the opposite one) is normal up to the age of about 4 months, but retention thereafter suggests generalized cerebral dysfunction.

To elicit the *parachute reflex,* hold the child horizontal in the prone position with your hands on the chest/abdomen and low back. Raise him 2 or 3 ft and then

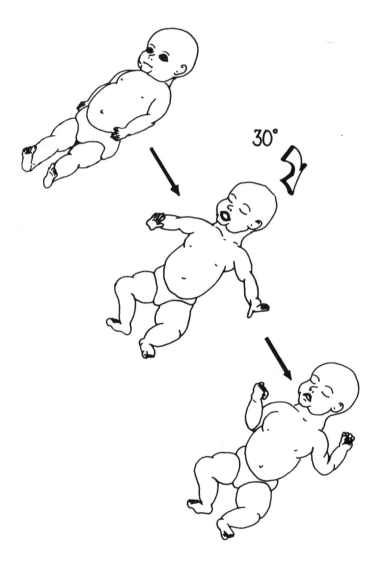

Figure 4-2   Diagram of the Moro reflex. The examiner suddenly causes the head to fall back, at which the infant's legs flex and the arms extend.

suddenly let him drop in your hands about 1 ft. All four limbs should extend symmetrically.

Constant gentle pressure in the palm or on the sole of the foot should normally elicit flexion of the fingers or toes, the plantar and palmar *grasp reflexes,* normally present up to 6 months. In each case, asymmetric responses or the persistence of such responses after the usual age indicate an abnormality.

Motor System

Inspection has already been mentioned; we might repeat that it is seldom possible to see fasciculations or wasting in young children because of the subcutaneous fat. *Tone* can be assessed as in the adult, whereas an assessment of *power* is usually impossible except by noting which limbs the child uses, or by eliciting the Moro or parachute reflexes. If a child persistently makes a fist on one side and not on the other, a pyramidal lesion is likely on that side. The deep tendon *reflexes* are usually present in the legs, and normally there may be a few beats of ankle *clonus* in the newborn child; reflexes in the arms are not usually so easily detectable. The *plantar responses* are frequently said to be upgoing but this is probably a withdrawal response which may be seen up to the age of 12 to 18 months.

EXAMINATION OF YOUNG CHILDREN

Examination of the young child is simple and valuable if the child is cooperative and both difficult and unreliable if he is not. Flattery, persuasion, bribery, and pleading sometimes work; intimidation never does. If it is possible to turn the tests into a kind of game or competition, children respond much better, and the same is true if they are given interesting objects to play with under your close scrutiny. Depending upon the age of the child, examination may more resemble that of infants or of adults. Do not undress the child until it is absolutely necessary, and if possible, give frequent small rewards and certainly praise for cooperation and good behavior.

Smaller children are best examined on their mother's lap opposite the seated examiner. As with infants, examination can proceed under six headings.

1. Observation.
2. Head and spine, meningism, and congenital defects.
3. Cranial nerves.
4. Motor and sensory examination.
5. Persistence of infantile responses.
6. Developmental assessment. (In the child who is not acutely ill, but who may have a developmental problem, this can be done first.)

Observation

Again, the child's motility and the presence of a limp may be noted as he comes into the room. Lack of *limb growth* on one side or the other (Fig. 4-3), *deformities,* and *handedness* can be assessed, as can the use he makes of his limbs while climbing onto a chair, the examination table, or his mother's lap. His *cooperation* and *activity level,* his *mood,* and the development of his *speech function* can similarly be evaluated before the examination proper begins.

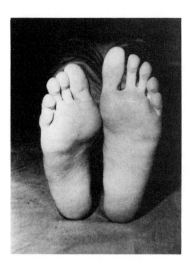

Figure 4-3   Asymmetry of the feet in a teenager with right spastic hemiparesis caused by cerebral palsy.

Examination of the Head and Spine

Examination of the *head* and *spine,* inspection for *congenital defects* mainly in the musculoskeletal system, and the examination for *meningism* are the same as in adults.

Cranial Nerves

Vision and *hearing* tests must be included with examination of the ears, nose, and throat. One can test for hemianopia by noting whether or not the patient turns to objects such as a reflex hammer brought in from the periphery of either visual field, but more precise assessment is difficult at this age. When testing hearing, quiet sounds — rustling paper, rubbed fingers — may be presented first, and then progressively louder stimuli introduced, looking for evidence that the sounds have been heard, such as turning of the eyes or head or extension of an arm toward the sound. Visual acuity may be tested as in young children by getting the child to follow a moving object, but other tests — naming or picking up small objects, use of matching cards, and so forth — may also be valuable in detecting impairment of sight. Fundoscopy can only be performed in a cooperative child and is often best left until the end of the examination when the child's confidence has been given. When testing pupillary function, bring the light up from below because this causes less blinking and eye closure. *External ocular movements, facial power* and *sensation,* and *bulbar functions* can be assessed in most children in the same way as in adults.

Motor and Sensory Testing

Inspection for repetitive abnormal movements and examination of tone and of reflexes can proceed in most cases just as in adults. It is not always easy to test power and great heed should be taken of the way in which the child uses his limbs, noting any particular limb preference. *Coordination* may be assessed by having the child pick up a number of objects, such as coins, blocks, or candles, and by watching him walk or run. *Sensory testing* relies, in younger children, upon their involuntary responses to light tickling, for example games in which they have to say where they have been touched, and upon vibration, in which the sensation of vibration may be introduced as resembling the purring of a cat.

Gait and *stance* usually are best tested by getting the child to follow his mother walking around the room. All forms of gait disturbance and difficulty in turning will be obvious. The hemiparetic gait with the plantar reflexes, inverted foot, and adducted, flexed posture of the arm becomes most evident when the child runs. The lordotic waddling gait resulting from weak hip and spine extensors, such as seen in muscular dystrophy, is readily apparent and can be made more so by having the child rise from the lying or sitting position so that he performs Gower's maneuver of "climbing up his legs" to spare the weakened hip extensors.

Persistence of Infantile Responses

In children with definite motor deficits, certain of the reflexes may persist longer than normal, whereas others may not appear when they should. The flexor withdrawal, tonic neck, and Moro reflexes should have disappeared by 5 to 6 months, whereas plantar grasp may be present for somewhat longer.

Developmental Assessment

There are a number of charts outlining the gross and fine motor, language, or personal/social capacities of children at various ages. Most of these require training in their administration and interpretation. We reproduce here one such chart (Table 4-1) that can be used for reference as a simple guide to the usual abilities of children because it demands little but careful observation of their uncomplicated activities. Such developmental assessments are sometimes of importance in general practice, but children who require extended evaluation should be under a specialist's care. Since developmental screening may show up abnormalities even before they become obvious on formal neurological examination, every family physician should have at least working knowledge of this chart or of the Denver Developmental Screening Test.

Table 4-1   Developmental Assessment

Age (Months)	0-3	3-6
Motor	Prone, lifts head (1)* Eyes follow to midline (1) Eyes follow past midline (3)	Sit, head steady (4) Rolls over (5) Reaches for object (5)
Language	Responds to sound (1) Vocalizes, not crying (2)	Laughs (3) Squeals (5)
Adaptive-social	Regards face (1) Smiles responsively (2)	Smiles spontaneously (5)

Age (Months)	12-18	18-24
Motor	Walks holding on to furniture (13) Walks alone well (14) Neat pincer grasp of object (15)	Tower of two cubes (20) Walks up steps (22) Kicks ball forward (24) Dumps object from bottle, demonstrated (24)
Language	*Dada* or *mama,* specific (13)	Three words other than *mama, dada* (21) Points to one named body part (21)
Adaptive-social	Plays pat-a-cake (13) Plays ball with examiner (16)	Imitates housework (20) Removes clothes (22) Uses spoon (24)

*Numbers in parentheses indicate age in months at which most normal children will achieve task.
From: Swaiman, K.F., Wright, F.S. In *Clinical Neurology.* Baker, A.B., Baker, L.H. (eds.). New York, Harper & Row, 1975. Modified and reporduced with permission.

6-9	9-12
Pull to sit, no head lag (6)	Pulls self to stand (10)
Transfers cube (1") hand to hand (7)	Thumb-finger grasp (11)
Sits without support (8)	Gets to sitting (11)
Turns to voice (8)	*Dada* or *mama,* nonspecific (10) Imitates speech sounds (11)
Feeds self cracker (8)	Plays peek-a-boo (10)
Works for toy out of reach (9)	Resists toy pull (10)

24-36

Scribbles spontaneously (25)
Builds tower of four to six cubes (26)
Jumps in place (36)
Pedals trike (36)
Imitates vertical line within 30° (36)

Combines two different words (28)
Names one picture (30)
Follows two of three simple
 directions (32)

Puts on shoes, not tied (36)

BIBLIOGRAPHY

Arriel-Tyson, C., Grema, A. *Neurologic Evaluation of the Newborn and the Infant.* Paris, Masson, 1982.

Baird, H.W., Gordon, E.C. *Neurological Evaluation of Infants and Children. Clin. Dev. Med.* No. 84/85, Oxford, Blackwell Scientific, 1983.

Swaiman, K.F., Wright, F.S. *The Practice of Pediatric Neurology,* Vol. I and II. St. Louis, C.V. Mosby Co., 1975.

5
Neurological Examination in the Elderly

Unless the student is aware of the progressive changes that occur with age, confusing problems can result when he applies to the aged the standards of the normal neurological examination in the younger person. Whether or not one can regard many of the changes of aging as being "normal" is a moot point, but for the purposes of this discussion we will comment on alterations that are commonly seen during the process of aging but which do not necessarily imply classic "disease." Although the terms *elderly* and *geriatric* are applied to those over aged 65, most of the problems to be discussed are only major problems to those over 75.

The psychological changes of the impaired elderly are well known. We have all seen the elderly gentleman sitting on the front steps talking about going over the trenches in World War I or detailing the happy adventures of his misspent youth, even though he does not know what day it is, cannot remember if he has had breakfast, and has no idea of where his pipe is. The normal elderly often seem to live in the past because it is the time they remember best. Emotional changes are also frequent, the elderly sometimes become more withdrawn, depressed, irritable, and less patient.

Anatomical changes accompany these psychological and emotional alterations. The brain decreases in weight after the sixth decade and the neurons progressively decrease in number. Pigmentation occurs in the neurons, and senile plaques and neurofibrillary tangles begin to appear. Vascular changes include endothelial proliferation, medial fibrosis, and hyalinization. In the peripheral nerves there is an increase in both the endo- and perineurium and a reduction in the number of nerve fibers.

Cerebral blood flow progressively decreases after the age of 20, cerebrovascular resistance progressively increases, and the rate of cerebral oxygen consumption falls.

Nerve conduction velocity decreases with age in most nerves, probably because of a progressive reduction in the number of large, myelinated, rapidly conducting nerve fibers.

NORMAL VARIATIONS ON EXAMINATION

Most people over the age of 65 will have at least some of the following changes on neurological examination.

Mental Status

Patients are often forgetful, with involvement of recent more than of past memory.[*] Rigidity, resistance to change, and withdrawal are common. They learn less well and more slowly. They sleep less and waken earlier than younger people. Abnormal responses on the diffuse dysfunction battery (see Chap. 9) increase markedly after the age of 70.

Cranial Nerves

The senses of smell and taste are often blunted and vision tends to be less acute. The elderly often have difficulty with visual tracking and holding fixation on lateral gaze (impersistence). Pupils are often irregular, sluggish in their reaction to light, and smaller than in youth. Arcus senilis is common and the patient may appear to have slight ptosis. Limitation of upward and downward gaze is common in the elderly and convergence is poor. There may be decreased tone in the face and neck muscles.

Motor Examination

There is a decrease in muscle bulk generally, particularly of the small muscles of the hands and feet. This is most obvious over the back of the hand where guttering can be noticed. Despite this, strength is often preserved. This small muscle atrophy probably results from dropout of peripheral nerve fibers, but it may be contributed to by the cervical spondylosis that is seen in virtually all patients over the age of 70 years. Minor basal ganglia signs are very common and a mild parkinsonian picture characterizes the "typical" aged person. Most actors asked to play the part of an octogenarian will assume a flexed posture and move in a slow, stiff, parkinsonian manner. The elderly may show some resistance to passive movements (paratonia) in arms and legs.

Sensory Examination

Most elderly patients have decreased peripheral sensation, particularly of vibration, touch, and position senses. This usually begins in the feet and slowly ascends. The

---

[*] "Loss of recent memory" really refers to a failure of an early step in memorization, the creation of a short-term memory trace, and thus of more permanent traces later. Because this problem is a late development, it is the memory for *recent* events that is defective, while older-established memories remain intact until changes are marked throughout the cerebral cortex.

sensory changes develop slowly during adulthood and old age in men, but they begin to develop in women after the menopause. Such changes are consistent with degeneration of peripheral neurons. Meissner's corpuscles and other peripheral nerve structures also atrophy with age. Although vibratory sense is the most prominent modality lost, pain, touch, and temperature are also diminished in some patients. These sensory changes, often associated with paresthesia, are often asymptomatic.

Reflexes

Reflexes become less brisk with age, and many elderly patients lose their ankle jerks. Primitive reflexes may be noted, with an increase in the jaw jerk, the appearance of palmomental reflexes, and occasionally a Babinski sign. Evidence of diffuse cerebral dysfunction may become evident by testing nuchocephalic, glabellar, blink, and sucking reflexes.

Stance and Gait

With increasing age, the gait tends to be less brisk, and the stride shorter and more cautious. Patients move *en bloc* and take many small steps when turning. Their postural reflexes are poor and they tend to get off balance easily. Some develop a parkinsonian gait, without the full-blown syndrome, and they may have the greatest difficulty in taking the first step.

An interesting occurrence in some elderly people is a peculiar fear of walking even though no specific abnormalities can be found to explain their apprehension (astasia trepidante). Occasionally, they may be so fearful of walking that they refuse to take a step and "freeze"; when encouraged to step out, they may clutch onto things or even drop to their knees.

A disturbing problem in older people is the *multisensory syndrome,* in which the patient has mild difficulty orienting himself in space. We know where we are in space because of our peripheral proprioceptors, our labyrinthine system, and our vision. Elderly patients often have poor proprioception, degeneration in the labyrinth and eighth nerve, and poor vision. They thus have difficulty orienting themselves in space and may complain of "dizziness" although they really mean a feeling of unsteadiness or swaying.

BIBLIOGRAPHY

Adams, G. *Essentials of Geriatric Medicine.* Oxford, Oxford Medical Publications, 1977.

Albert, M.L. *Clinical Neurology of Aging.* New York, Oxford, 1984.

Katzman, R. and Terry, R.D. *The Neurology of Aging.* Philadelphia, F.A. Davis Co., 1983.

6
Examination for Functional Disorders

Hysteria has something in common with the elephant: it is almost impossible to define, but we can recognize it when faced with it. What we tend to identify more easily is the *hysterical personality* rather than any particular hysterical manifestation. The definition of the term hysteria is a current controversy, but in general it refers to the symptoms resulting from a dissociative or conversion reaction.

Hysterical symptoms were recorded on Egyptian papyri 4000 years ago, but the word itself first appeared in writings attributed to Hippocrates and reflected the belief that the womb floated about in the body, causing symptoms wherever it came to rest.

The essence of hysteria is the patient's failure to cope with some aspects of life and his attempts to solve the conflict resulting from this failure by using the mental mechanism of dissociation. *Dissociation* involves a splitting of consciousness so that certain painful mental contents are removed from the patient's awareness, leaving the patient brittle but calm. Should such mental conflicts manifest as physical symptoms, these are regarded as *conversion symptoms.*

The patient derives some secondary gain from hysterical symptoms because they remove an unbearable conflict from consciousness, get him more sympathy or attention, or allow the manipulation of family, friends, medical personnel, or environment. Often it will be apparent to others that the gain is slight and offers no permanent solution to the stresses that provoked the conversion symptoms. One may be able to see more efficient ways of resolving these stresses, but it is important to remember that the hysterical illness, however bizarre, is the best solution that the patient can manage at the time. One aim of treatment is to help the person to find a more effective solution.

The capacity to use dissociation and conversion mechanisms is latent; for everyone there is some level of stress beyond which he can no longer make adaptive adjustments. Use of the mechanisms to handle stress and conflicts has strong social, cultural, and ethnic influences, and was an accepted and common way of handling even minor stresses in the Victorian Age. It is seen much less now and appears to be decreasing.

The attributes of the "hysterical personality" are controversial. It has been said that patients possessing it tend to be immature and dependent; they try to appear more than they are to impress those on whom they depend; and they are exhibitionistic and suggestible, showing rapid but short-lived mood changes. Their interest and enthusiasm for both things and people tend to be superficial and fleeting. They often show emotional insecurity by marked possessive traits and emotionally demanding behavior. Females with the hysterical personality are often sexually frigid, but by their behavior and dress they appear sexually provocative. Such people are said to enjoy being the center of attention, whether in dress, in speech, or in behavior, and their conversation tends to be loaded with superlatives. They often seem immune to the repercussions of the stormy scenes they have created.

Despite this description, many patients with hysterical symptoms do not have these personality traits. There is also an important differentiation to be made between the person who has hysterical conversion symptoms, for whom we shall use the term *hysteric,* and another who has *histrionic* behavior, the latter term being applied to the person who really shows only excessive emotional display.

It is also important to differentiate the *malingerer* from the hysteric. The malingerer is practicing deception and knows it. The hysteric, on the other hand, has little insight into his problem and feels that he is ill, because the phenomena are produced unconsciously. He is practicing self-deception and does not know it. If asked, both will say that they would prefer that the symptoms were not there. But hysterical patients, unlike malingerers, do not resent repeated examination, may transiently appreciate reassurance, will comply with the physician's suggestions, usually take their medications, and may even undergo surgery. While they tend to be honest with the physician, they are very suggestible and their history often changes from hour to hour. Malingerers, on the other hand, have made up their story, have rehearsed it carefully, and have it word perfect each time. They know that they are not ill and therefore refuse or object to repeated examinations, investigations, and procedures, seeking without delay the benefit they expect to gain from their symptoms.

NEUROLOGICAL CONVERSION SYMPTOMS

Unlike the bad actress who was once described as "running the gamut of emotions from A to B," there is hardly any symptom of organic disease that cannot be simulated by the hysterical patient. The symptoms that may be manifestations of a conversation reaction are legion. In addition, it has been said that virtually any sign may have a hysterical basis, except for papilledema. Before discussing some of the more common ones, we would point out that it is important to differentiate the physiological hysterical responses. Such physiological responses occur normally in anyone undergoing severe stress or anxiety and include such symptoms as vomiting, sweating, tremor, palpitations, dizziness, weakness, and paresthesias.

There are a number of points that one may notice during the initial history and examination of patients with conversion symptoms. There is often a history of previous hysterical reactions, sometimes among their family members as well. It is common to find that the mother has had "nervous trouble." The patient has often had repeated hospitalizations, operations, or visits to doctors. The abdomens of some hysterical patients look like battlefields, with most dispensable organs gone. It is always enlightening to ask such a patient when they were last healthy; they may then describe a life-long history of one problem after another. The functional inquiry is particularly colorful in these patients and you often get a positive response to every leading question asked.

Whatever the presenting problem, there are certain features that are common on examination. The patients often appear humorless, and overanxious to do the right thing. They jump onto your examining table or lie down before instructed to do so, are eager to tell their story, and may talk endlessly about their symptoms and many other problems. They continually seem to observe the physician for his reaction and often have a sheepish smile as they tell of their "horrible" or "excruciating" problems with overuse of superlatives.

Common features on examination are blepharospasm in the orbicularis oculi muscles and a tendency not to look directly at the examiner. They do not seem to be as distressed by their symptoms as one would normally expect *(la belle indifference),* but still tend to jump with most stimuli, including touch or smell. Because they appear to aim at excessive accuracy, some testing is difficult to interpret and becomes more confusing the more it is tried. This is particularly so with the sensory examination.

Disorders of Consciousness

A patient who appears to have a lowered level of consciousness as a manifestation of a conversion reaction will have a normal waking EEG with an obvious alpha rhythm. The corneal and gag reflexes will probably be present.[*] The patient will usually appear to be asleep but stimuli that would normally cause awakening will not awaken him. The single best test of "hysterical coma" is the cold caloric test, which results in nystagmus when the patient's eyes are held open. The presence of nystagmus indicates that the patient is conscious. He may also be noted to have flaccid limbs, but if the arm is held above the face and dropped, it will fall but miss the face each time; a comatose patient's arm will fall and hit the face. There are many bizarre forms of drowsiness, stupor, and coma simulated by the hysterical patient; sometimes their nature is obvious, but at other times they are difficult to recognize.

Attacks of Loss of Consciousness

Hysterical "fits" may follow an emotional crisis and usually occur only in the presence of other people. The attacks may be prolonged to impress the spectators; complete recovery may be delayed for days. The patient's color is normal in the attacks and incontinence is rare. Usually a fall does not result in injury and the tongue is seldom bitten in the "seizure." Limb movements tend to be spectacular and thrashing without the typical tonic-clonic-flaccid sequence. The corneal reflexes will be present and the plantar responses will be flexor. Again, the EEG will be normal, with alpha activity present and no slow activity after the attack.

Minor attacks tend to be of the motor type, and often movements are more tremulous than jerky. The sensory or psychomotor features commonly seen in focal seizures are seldom seen. Patients who have bilateral motor activity of the clonic type as part of a true seizure discharge will lose consciousness, but often a hysterical patient will have bilateral jerky movements but can be shown

---

[*]But some normal people do not have a gag reflex.

to be still conscious and aware. Some of these patients can describe their entire seizure.

Remember that subjects with marked anxiety symptoms may well exhibit hyperventilation which in turn can result in respiratory alkalosis, cerebral ischemia, and seizures. The most difficult clinical situation occurs when an epileptic has hysterical seizures, which is not uncommon. In fact, seizures as conversion symptoms are uncommon *except* in patients with epilepsy. Videotape monitoring of the patient and the EEG is the best diagnostic strategy.

Loss of Smell

Patients who have anosmia on hysterical basis will probably say that they cannot *smell* but that they can *taste* things, not recognizing that most of the discriminating aspects of taste are contributed to by smell. True anosmia enables patients to taste only sweet, sour, bitter, and salt. These patients will also deny that they can smell ammonia when it is presented to them, but most of the reaction to ammonia fumes is mediated through trigeminal afferents inside the nostril. If the patient says he cannot smell ammonia and does not react to it, then he either has both the first and fifth nerves involved (a highly unlikely combination) or is suffering from hysterical anosmia.

Blindness

Hysterical blindness is often hard to evaluate. However, the pupils will react to light directly and consensually, and external ocular movements will be full. A normal visual pathway can be demonstrated by evoking optokinetic nystagmus with a tape measure (a striped band is not necessary). You can also do a cold caloric test which shows nystagmus, demonstrating that the patient is able to correct for the tendency of his eyes to deviate toward the cold stimulus. A simple procedure might be to just flip the hand in front of the eyes, which results in sudden involuntary blinking (but be careful not to allow wind from the waving hand to stimulate the corneal reflex).

Diplopia

Double vision is a common conversion symptom. Some patients even complain of seeing three, four, or more objects. A patient with hysterical diplopia will often indicate that the objects seem just as far apart when they are held close as when they are distant; they *should* move further apart when the object is held further away. If the separation of images is plotted in different directions, particularly using red–green glasses, the pattern of separation will be inconstant and unphysiological. Psychogenic ptosis is accompanied by depression of the eyebrow.

Facial Numbness

The most common observation of value in hysterical facial numbness is that the sensation is decreased over the whole face and also the angle of the jaw, which is supplied not by the fifth nerve but by the C2 and C3 roots. The corneal reflex will be present and normal when the face is supposedly completely numb. The patient can often be shown to have an exact sensory split down the center of his face, which is unphysiological; if there is true hemianesthesia, the line of demarcation should be toward the affected side because of overlap by nerves from the opposite side. With hysterical numbness one may demonstrate grimacing when a vibrating tuning fork is touched to the nostril or a tickle reaction when a wisp of cotton wool is placed inside the nostril. This does *not* suggest that the patient is malingering, simply that his conception of body image does not follow exact anatomical guide-lines.

Deafness

A vibrating tuning fork placed on top of the head when a finger occludes one ear will cause the vibration to be heard more loudly in the occluded ear by a normal person. The malingerer will often say that it sounds louder in the unoccluded ear because it seems more logical that way; but the patient with hysterical unilateral deafness will not. This test is not diagnostic of malingering because the patient with nerve deafness may give the same answer. Sudden noise will tend to produce an eyeblink and pupillary dilation in normal subjects and also in the patient who has hysterical deafness. An audiogram should be done in all patients with hearing loss; the findings in hysterical deafness are characteristic.

Aphonia

Aphonia is not likely to be of organic origin if the patient can cough. The gag re-flex is too frequently absent in normal people to be of much value in testing for hysterical anesthesia of the ninth nerve. The patient may be caught off guard if you peer down the throat using a tongue depressor and casually ask him to say "ah." Some hysterical patients have a complete inability to communicate verbally and just open and close their mouths. In organic aphonia (a very rare entity) the patient can still whisper and usually can make some sounds.

Weakness

Resistance may suddenly "give" on muscle testing, and variable grip and strength responses are often found. Even though the patients may demonstrate weakness when you test them, afterward they can be seen using their limbs normally, per-haps unknowingly, in some functions.

If a normal patient is asked to raise his good leg off the bed, there will be some downward pressure of the opposite leg, and a hand placed below that heel should feel it. The patient with hysterical weakness will not lift the leg, but a lack of pressure downward on the other heel indicates that he is not trying.

A patient with hysterical weakness should have normal deep tendon and super-ficial reflexes. Usually there is no differentiation between weakness in proximal and distal muscles or between flexor and extensor groups.

Some patients may change the side of their weakness if they are turned onto their stomachs and quickly retested. Often it is possible to show that isometric contraction is relatively strong when isotonic contraction is weak. If, for example, the patient has not been able to raise his arms to the abducted position, he may be able to maintain the abducted posture if his arms are placed there by the examiner, and they then may even retain their position against resistance.

Sir William Gowers described a test for hysterical paralysis of both legs, which we do not recommend that you use unless you have discussed it first with your hos-pital administrator and your lawyer. It involves spreading the patient's knees apart and then suddenly grabbing a handful of pubic hair. The legs will immediately snap together.

Abnormal Gait

It is not possible to characterize the hysterical gait because it may take many colorful and dramatic forms. However it usually does not conform to any well-recognized pattern but is bizarre, inconsistent, and variable. The gait may become even more markedly abnormal when the patient knows he is being watched. Even though the gait may be wild and poorly controlled, the patient usually does not fall but heads for walls or for the examiner. If falling to the wall on the right when going one way, he may fall toward the same wall, now on his left, when he returns.

Sensation

The sensory examination is the most variable and frustrating area of testing, and it is common to note an unphysiological pattern of sensory impairment that may have been suggested by the method of examination, even if the problem was not there originally. Doing Romberg's test the patient may tend to fall consistently toward the examiner or toward the bed, even if turned in the opposite direction, as with gait. The ankles may show a "dance of the tendons," a dramatic swaying of the body with maintenance of stance, which demonstrates excellent balance.

In hysterical hemianesthesia,* the patient often will not feel the tuning fork when it is placed on the affected side of the sternum, but *will* feel vibration when the fork is placed on the opposite side, a few centimeters away. This should not occur, because the vibrations will be transmitted across the sternum and therefore are felt through the normal sensory pathways on the opposite side. Always test sensation in the supine and in the prone positions: often the sensory "loss" changes sides.

The sensory loss in nonorganic cases will not follow the distribution expected with root or peripheral nerve involvement, and the cutoff point with "glove-and-stocking" anesthesia tends to be at the thigh and shoulder and is sharply demarcated, quite unlike the findings in peripheral neuropathies in which the transition between normal and abnormal is gradual over a few centimeters. If the sensory level is in the thorax, the normal slope (following the ribs) will not be found. Occasionally, patients will complain of a "stovepipe" loss of sensation in a limb in which the sensation is normal proximally and distally but with a central loss of sensation involving the whole limb in its midportion.

DIAGNOSIS

The diagnosis of a conversion reaction is extremely important because treatment is much easier in the initial stages, before the symptoms become deeply ingrained. However one must not make this diagnosis only because a particular clinical picture is puzzling, bizarre, or difficult to explain; but in the presence of such symptoms, and with knowledge that the patient has used conversion mechanisms before, is young, has current major stresses and a potential for secondary gain, and has shown typical personality characteristics, this diagnosis may be reasonable.

There are a number of clinical situations in which the diagnosis of hysteria is always dangerous and often incorrect. Any patient over the age of 35 developing what appear to be conversion symptoms for the first time should be suspected of having an organic illness. *Never* diagnose hysteria on the basis of one single complaint because hysterical patients usually have many complaints. In our experience, a patient with what appears to be monosymptomatic hysteria usually turns out to

---

*Strangely, almost always on the left side.

have neurological disease. Beware of the patient who has no previous history of hysteria or psychiatric abnormalities. With no wish to be chauvinists, we would also suggest that one should be especially wary of making the diagnosis of hysteria in a male.

It is sobering to remember that in one-third of these patients diagnosed as hysterical by competent neurologists, an underlying neurological disorder is ultimately found. It is worth remembering that there is often a reason why the hysteric has selected the area affected; sometimes it is because of some underlying pathology in that area.

MANAGEMENT

Hysterical symptoms require immediate management, because the longer they remain, the more deeply ingrained they become and the harder they are to treat.
If such symptoms are based on an acute anxiety state or depression, then they may be treated and resolution of the nonorganic features awaited. As stated earlier, careful investigation for organic disease is frequently required even if the symptoms *are* caused by conversion mechanisms. In all cases one should attempt to discover the underlying conflicts and other stresses that have induced the symptoms.

Reassurance based on explanation and a strong positive supportive approach are important in therapy, and one may make use of the fact that these patients are extremely suggestible. Hypnosis is sometimes effective in reducing and eventually relieving these symptoms, but psychotherapy is the mainstay of treatment. Intravenous amobarbital sodium (Sodium Amytal) can be a valuable method of treatment, but this should not be given unless the person giving it is willing to provide both the immediate and long-term psychotherapy that the patient will require.

In closing, remember the axiom that one's failure to understand a condition is no proof that it has a psychogenic basis.

BIBLIOGRAPHY

Gulick, T.A. et al. Pseudo-seizures: Ictal phenomena. *Neurology 32*:24-30, 1982.

Keane, J.R. Neuro-ophthalmic signs and symptoms of hysteria. *Neurology 32:* 757-762, 1982.

Merskey, H. *The Analysis of Hysteria.* London, Bailliere Tindall, 1979.

Weintraub, M.I. *Hysterical Conversion Reactions. A Clinical Guide to Diagnosis and Treatment.* Lancaster, MTP Press Ltd., 1983.

7

Examination of the Comatose Patient

The patient in coma presents a diagnostic challenge, which can in large part be met by careful consideration of the events leading up to the coma and of the patient's physical signs. Although it is predominantly the nervous system that will be investigated, the usual nervous system examination is not appropriate in a comatose patient whose cooperation is impossible and in whom certain physical signs depend upon the patient's depth of coma and upon whether this is deepening, lightening, or remaining the same; upon whether a structural lesion or a metabolic cause is responsible; and (if the former is true) whether it is situated supra- or infratentorially and on which side it is.

Examination of the patient is unlikely to help much in determining the pathogenesis of the coma unless abnormal physical signs are noted in other major systems. However it is vital to take a history from a relative, friend, or workmate of a comatose subject, and if none appears then the police should be asked to contact and summon anyone who can give any background information. One would of course be most interested in a recent history of trauma, the circumstances in which the patient was found, the speed of onset of the reduction in conscious level, its progress, and the duration to date. It will be important to know if the patient has a history of psychiatric disease, epilepsy, diabetes, or any endocrine or metabolic disease and if he has had previous cardiac or cerebrovascular disease. Important information may be found in hospital records, in the patient's family doctor's office, or at his place of work. Try to find out if he has access to any drugs and ask the patient's relatives to search his residence for drugs or empty containers and to bring them for inspection and identification.

Because management may have to precede neurological examination, we include it here. A discussion of the procedure to determine cerebral death is found in Chapter 10.

EMERGENCY MANAGEMENT

1. First, guard the airway. If the patient is vomiting he must be turned on his side and the examination carried out in that position.* Clear the airway by suction. Sometimes a pharyngeal airway is all that is necessary to keep the airway clear, but if breathing is shallow, irregular, or obstructed, an endo-tracheal tube must be passed *at once* before further examination. Decide if a respirator is required, if necessary by measuring tidal volume and blood gases.
2. Repeatedly document vital signs, including the patient's *temperature, pulse,* and *respiratory rate,* using a low-reading thermometer for the rectal temp-erature, if necessary. The *blood pressure* should be taken in both arms and circulatory failure should be excluded. Shock never results from a head injury alone.
3. *Signs of injury* must be sought for, particularly those that involve the spinal column, the skull, and abdominal viscera. Look carefully for signs of bleeding, remembering that large amounts of blood can be lost into a body cavity or tissues with little external evidence.
4. The *odor* of acetone, alcohol, or other poisons or products of metabolic dys-function may be smelled on the breath.
5. After these initial assessments, it is wise to take blood for hemoglobin, hema-tocrit, white cell count, blood sugar level, electrolytes, calcium, pH, $PaCO_2$, and standard bicarbonate tests. If there is any suggestion of poisoning, blood and urine samples for salicylates, alcohol, bromides, barbiturates, and other tests may be taken; these are invaluable for medicolegal purposes. Other poisons such as carbon monoxide may be detected by blood spectroscopy. Un-less it seems likely that the patient is in diabetic coma, will have a prolonged reduction in conscious level, or is in shock, a catheter need not be inserted at this stage. Having taken blood, give 20 ml of 50% glucose IV (unless you are quite certain that the patient could not have hypoglycemia) and set up an IV line.

EXAMINATION OF THE
NERVOUS SYSTEM IN COMA

Six major areas are examined to determine the level at which the brain is involved, the nature of the pathology, and the direction the process is taking. These are

1. State of consciousness
2. Respiration
3. Pupils and fundi
4. Brainstem reflexes
5. Motor responses
6. Meningism

---

*"If the patient is positioned facing towards heaven, he will soon be in it."

The State of Consciousness

There are many loose and meaningless terms used to describe changes in consciousness, the most vague being the commonly used *semiconscious* which has no specific meaning at all. The terms used by Plum and Posner in their excellent monograph on coma are

> Alert wakefulness: The patient responds immediately, fully, and appropriately to all stimuli.
> Lethargy: A state of drowsiness, inaction, or indifference with delayed or incomplete responses; increased stimulation may be needed to get a response.
> Obtundation: An even duller state in which the patient maintains his wakefulness, but little more.
> Stupor: A state in which the patient can be aroused only by vigorous stimuli.
> Coma[*]: A state in which psychological and motor responses are lost.

As a working rule it may be stated that, except in the case of deep coma, each of the other categories can be "shifted up" one level with adequate stimulation. In deep coma there will be no response by the patient to any form of stimulation, whereas in light coma, restlessness or semipurposive movements such as grunting or arm or leg avoidance movements may occur if unpleasant stimuli are given.

With stimulation, the comatose patient makes only reflex responses, but the stuporous patient makes some kind of defensive response. The obtunded patient vocalizes, the drowsy one verbalizes. Repeated charting is necessary so that one is able to comprehend the progress of the disease.

Respiration

Different levels of CNS involvement in coma induce different respiratory patterns. That of the comatose patient should therefore be carefully assessed. Although the respiratory centers are in the pons and medulla, there are important influences from higher areas; thus the forebrain activates normal breathing in situations where CO_2 is reduced. A deep lesion in the hemispheres, in the region of the diencephalon, will cut off this forebrain influence and the patient will no longer breathe when CO_2 levels are low, resulting in *Cheyne-Stokes* respirations. This is a regular waxing-and-waning respiration, governed by the CO_2 level.

A lesion in the midbrain may be accompanied by *neurogenic hyperventilation* which is characterized by a very regular, rapid respiration rate.

A lesion in the pons may result in *apneustic* breathing, with long pauses at full inspiration.

A lower pontine lesion may result in *ataxic* breathing, which is irregular and variable. *Cluster* breathing may also occur with regular groups of respirations, but without the waxing and waning, characteristic of *Cheyne-Stokes* respiration.

With a medullary lesion, respiration becomes more erratic and *gasping* and may eventually decrease and then stop.

---

[*]The Glasgow Coma Scale, now generally accepted as one reliable and simple measure of the course of coma, is shown in Table 7-1.

Table 7-1   Glasgow Coma Scale[a]

Eye opening	Spontaneous To speech or shouting To painful stimulation None
Verbal response	Oriented to place, person, and time Confused conversation but attention held Inappropriate speech, random or shouting, etc. Incomprehensible sounds, moaning, etc. None

Best motor response
 	
(Take the best response
in any limb)
	Obeys commands
	Localizes; limb moves to prevent noxious
	  stimulus
	Flexor response, hemiplegic or decorticate
	  posturing
	Extensor response
	None

[a] Repeated observations are necessary, charted on a graph. This scale has been widely adopted and is simple and reliable for both nursing and medical use. *Adapted from:* Teasdale, G., Jennet, B. Assessment of coma and impaired consciousness: A practical scale. *Lancet* 2:81-84, 1974.

Therefore observe the respiratory pattern because it may be a clue to the level of CNS involvement in coma, and it will reflect any progression downward or upward. Various respiratory patterns are shown in Figure 7-1.

Pupils and Fundi

Examination of the cranial nerves is limited in coma, but certain of the usual tests should be performed and the pupils and brainstem reflexes are of major importance.

Optic Nerve

Assess the fundi first, looking particularly for diabetic or hypertensive retinopathy, for venous pulsations at the margins of the optic disks, and for papilledema. If the eyes can be kept open, assess the *menace reflex*, bringing your hands suddenly up to the patient's eyes from the left and from the right field, in each case looking for blinking.

Pupils

Next observe the reactions of the pupils to light. A brief review of neuroanatomy is necessary here to understand the changes that occur at different levels of brain damage. The sympathetic fibers originate in the hypothalamus and travel down to the lateral part of the brainstem to exit in the thoracic area. These fibers synapse in the cervical sympathetic ganglia, and the postganglionic fibers travel to the eye

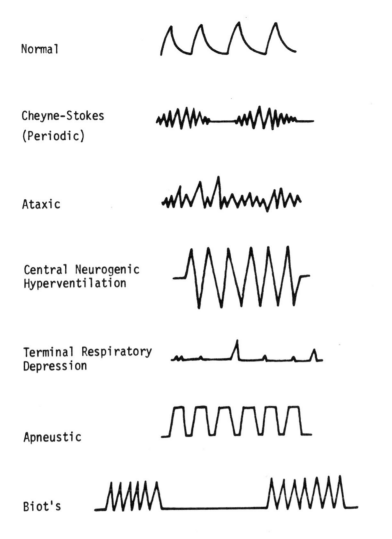

Normal

Cheyne-Stokes
(Periodic)

Ataxic

Central Neurogenic
Hyperventilation

Terminal Respiratory
Depression

Apneustic

Biot's

Figure 7-1   Patterns of respiratory abnormality in comatose patients. The pattern seen varies with the level of brain stem involvement.

along the wall of the carotid and ophthalmic arteries. The parasympathetic fibers travel down from the hypothalamus to the midbrain and then exit with the third nerve fibers.

The afferent pathway for the light reflex is retina, to optic nerve, to lateral geniculate body, to the midbrain pretectal area. The efferent side of the reflex runs from the Edinger-Westphal nucleus through the parasympathetic fibers in the third nerve to the pupillary constrictors (see Chap. 21).

Pupillary abnormalities in comatose patients can be of great localizing value. A lesion in the hypothalamus may cause a Horner's syndrome (small pupil, ptosis, decreased sweating on the same side of the face) resulting from sympathetic fiber involvement. Midbrain damage may cause loss of the light reflex, with midpositioned, regular pupils that do not respond to light. A lesion of the third nerve removes parasympathetic influences and the resulting sympathetic dominance causes fixed dilation of the pupil. Pontine lesions interrupt the sympathetic but leave the parasympathetic fibers undamaged; thus the pupil is pinpoint. A lesion in the lateral medullary or cervical regions may also cause Horner's syndrome.

Brainstem Reflexes

Brainstem reflexes include the

1. Oculocephalic or doll's head reflex (Fig. 7-2A, B)
2. Oculovestibular reflex (caloric stimulation) (Fig. 7-3)
3. Corneal, gag, cough, and blink reflexes

The first two reflexes have essentially the same pathway. In each case, we stimulate the vestibular receptors, and the reflex arc includes the vestibular part of the eighth nerve, the vestibular nuclei at the pontomedullary junction, and fibers running through the pons in the median longitudinal fasciculus. The efferent pathways are through the oculomotor nerves. As the reflex arc runs through a large part of the brainstem, a significant local destructive lesion will usually disrupt it. Thus, these are useful tests of brainstem function in comatose patients.

The *oculocephalic,* or doll's head, reflex is elicited by holding the patient's head from underneath in your right hand, keeping the upper eyelids raised with your left thumb and index finger, and turning the head quickly to the left and then to the right. In coma resulting from metabolic causes or supratentorial disease without brainstem involvement, the response will be a "lagging behind" of the eyes so that if the head is suddenly turned to the left, the eyes will deviate temporarily toward the right before returning to the central position. The eyes thus seem to keep looking in the original direction for a second or so after the head is suddenly turned. If the vestibular structures or brain stem have been damaged, the reflex may be lost and the eyes will turn with the head.

Caloric stimulation is simply performed with a 10-ml syringe fitted with a rubber catheter tip and containing ice-cold water. Check the ear canals and drums first to make sure that the canals are not blocked by wax or the drums perforated. Irrigate one external auditory meatus with ice water (10 ml) with the patient's head raised 30°. Normally, this vestibular stimulation causes the eyes to drift toward the cold stimulus. An alert patient corrects for this by fast eye jerks (nystagmus) in the opposite direction. In coma however, the eyes come over to the side of the cold stimulus and stay there without any such correction. The eyes return to the midline position in a few minutes. When they have done so, irrigate the opposite side. Deviation of the eyes demonstrates that the reflex arc through the brainstem is intact. If it is disrupted by a brainstem lesion, the eyes will not move on caloric stimulation. Because comatose patients show only deviation of the eyes without nystagmus, caloric testing is a simple way to differentiate true from hysterical coma because the hysterical patient will develop nystagmus when caloric testing is performed. Asymmetric responses of the eyes may be due to a third or sixth nerve lesion. So watch *both* eyes carefully.

The doll's head maneuver and caloric stimulation are rapid and simple tests of brainstem function and should always be performed in comatose patients.

The *corneal reflexes* and the *jaw jerk* can always be tested too, and sometimes patients may make voluntary movements in response to pinprick pain over the cheeks showing that fifth nerve function is intact.

The *ciliospinal reflex* is evoked by a painful stimulus such as pinching the skin of the neck which results in dilation of the pupil, a normal phenomenon. If the reflex is absent there is a disruption in the brainstem fiber pathway (Fig. 7-4).

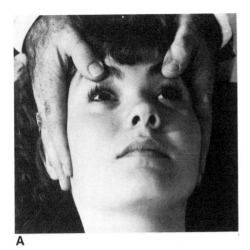 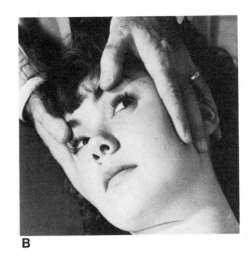

A   B

Figure 7-2 Doll's head movements. (A) Head central, eyes central; (B) Head rotated to the right, eyes "lag-behind" momentarily, indicating normal brainstem function.

Facial movements may be assessed, if the patient is breathing spontaneously, by holding his nose and noting any puffing out of the cheeks on either side or by giving noxious stimuli elsewhere and watching for a facial grimace.

A sudden loud noise normally causes widening of the palpebral fissure and dilatation of the pupils, and is an easy test to perform, again assessing brainstem function.

The *gag* and cough *reflexes* can be tested if no airway has been inserted. One of the best ways is to suction the laryngopharynx using a soft catheter.

Examination of Motor Functions

Examination of motor functions follows the same lines as in the conscious patient. *Inspection* may show an abnormal posture. Thus the head or eyes may be turned *to* the side of the lesion in the brain (i.e., away from the hemiparesis), or as with an acute brainstem lesion, the head and eyes may turn *away* from the side of the lesion in the brain. If one leg is everted compared with the other, this suggests a hemiparesis affecting that side (or a fractured neck or femur).

The *decorticate posture* is one in which the arms are flexed and the legs extended, indicating isolation of the brainstem and spinal cord from cortical influences. The *decerebrate posture* is that in which both the arms and legs extend, especially when painful stimuli are given. It indicates that the lesion is in the midbrain, isolating only the lower brainstem and spinal cord from influences above the midbrain center. If the head is grasped gently between the hands and rotated slowly to one side and then to the other, the arm and leg on the side to which the head is turned may extend, a tonic neck reflex, again indicating at least partial *decortication* (Fig. 7-5A, B).

At this time also, an examination for *meningism* should be made looking for positive Kernig's and Brudzinski's signs and also for neck stiffness. Tapping over the lower lip may produce a *snouting response* and stroking of the lips a *suck response,* both signs of diffuse frontal lobe impairment.

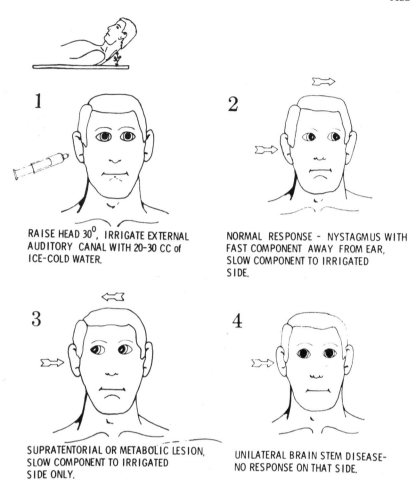

Figure 7-3   Ice-water caloric tests in normal subjects (1 and 2) and in comatose patients with normal (3) and abnormal (4) brainstem function.

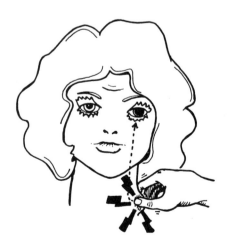

Figure 7-4   The ciliospinal reflex.

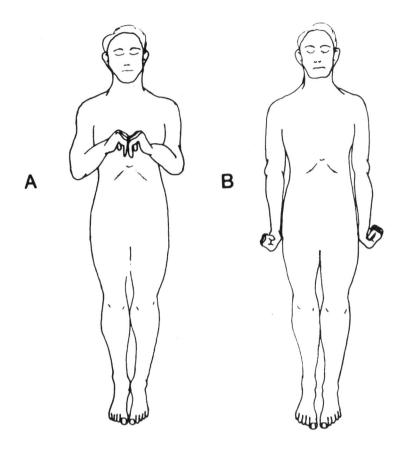

Figure 7-5   (A) Decorticate; and (B) Decerebrate postures.

Any seizures seen should be described in full, particularly as to the part of the body in which they started.

Tone (muscular resistance to passive stretch) must be examined with great care in all four limbs; flaccidity, spasticity, or a semivoluntary obstruction of your movements by the patient (paratonia or *gegenhalten*) may be found.

All the deep tendon *reflexes* and obviously the plantar reflexes should be examined.

It is not usually possible to assess *power* in a patient with any marked degree of impairment of consciousness, but often a hint of the palsied side may be gained by the patient a deep pain stimulus (e.g., pressing on the sternum or over the supra-orbital regions with your knuckles) and noting any response on one or other side.

Sensory testing involves an examination of response to pinprick pain and deep pain, the latter tested as above. Other forms of sensory assessment are not really of great value in the patient with reduced consciousness.

Meningism

Neck stiffness may indicate a local problem, fracture or dislocation, in a trauma patient and may occur because of raised intracranial pressure. Examination for neck stiffness and for Kernig's sign are both necessary in all cases.

BIBLIOGRAPHY

Miller Fisher, C. The neurological examination of the comatose patient. *Acta Neurol. Scand.* Suppl. 36, 1969.

Plum, F., Posner, J.B. *The Diagnosis of Stupor and Coma.* 3rd Ed. Philadelphia, F.A. Davis Co., 1980.

Teasedale, G., Jennett, B. Assessment of coma and impaired consciousness. A practical scale. *Lancet,* 1974, 2:81–84.

8
Neurological Investigations

SKULL X-RAYS

The oldest noninvasive neurological investigation, an x-ray of the skull, may contribute a good deal to diagnosis, but the indications for ordering it are limited and specific.

Four views are most often requested: posteroanterior (PA), lateral, basal, and Towne's. The main bony landmarks are identified in Figures 8-1 to 8-4.

Abnormalities seen include

Changes in bony structure: e.g., Paget's, osteolytic lesions, fibrous dysplasia, and hyperostosis (Tables 8-1, 8-2).

Fractures of the vault or base.

Intracranial calcification: See Table 8-3 for a list of causes. The patterns of calcification however are seldom diagnostic of the underlying pathology, although "tramline" calcification in the Sturge-Weber syndrome and stippled flecks of calcium in oligodendrogliomas are fairly typical. The basal ganglia may calcify in hypoparathyroidism, and this may also occur as an autosomal-dominant characteristic in certain family members in whom there are not necessarily any physical signs. See Table 8-3 for a list of causes. Calcification may be normal in the pineal gland, where this is a reasonably good indicator of any shift of the midline structures. Calcium may also be seen normally in the falx and choroid flexus.

Raised intracranial pressure: With raised intracranial pressure, a number of changes occur of which by far the most important is decalcification of the posterior clinoid process. A "doubling" of the floor of the pituitary fossa and so-called copper-beating of the whole of the vault are other signs of less specificity. In children, suture separation is important evidence of raised intracranial pressure.

85

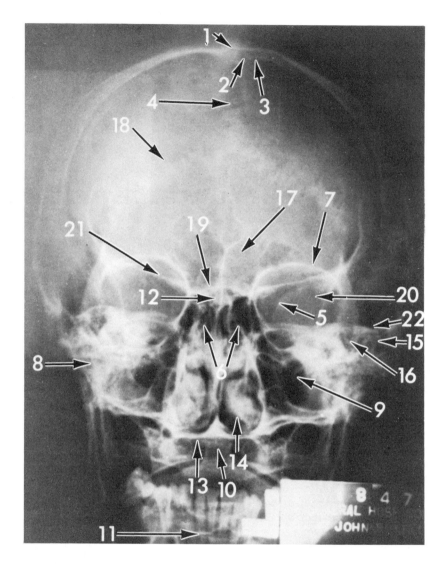

Figure 8-1   Frontal view of skull. (1)Outer table; (2) Inner table; (3) Diploe; (4) Sagittal suture; (5) Superior orbital fissure; (6) Ethmoidal sinuses; (7) Margin or orbit; (8) Head of mandible; (9) Maxillary sinus; (10) Odontoid; (11) Mandible with teeth; (12) Nasal septum; (13) Palate; (14) Inferior concha; (15) Petrous part of temporal bone; (16) Zygomatic bone; (17) Frontal sinus; (18) Lamboid suture; (19) Granger's line (plaum sphenoidale); (20) Greater wing of sphenoid; (21) Lesser wing of sphenoid; (22) Petrous ridge.

Craniostenosis: This is a condition of abnormally early fusion of sutures leading to failure of growth of the skull. The coronal, lambdoid, and sagittal sutures, or any combination of these, are usually involved. If the skull cannot expand, intracranial pressure rises and other signs appear as listed previously.

Venous lakes: These are small translucencies usually seen at or close beside the midline sagittal suture. They have no pathological significance.

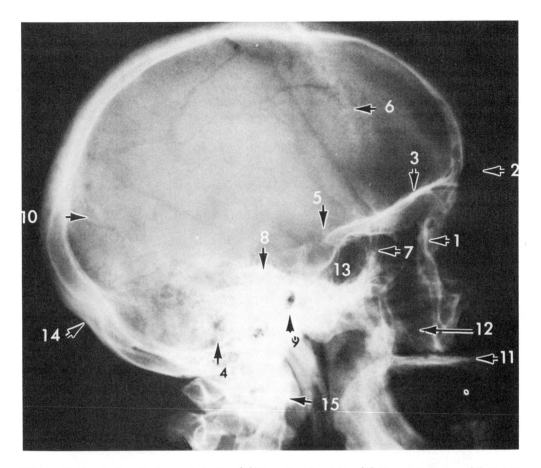

Figure 8-2   Lateral view of skull. (1) Margin of orbit; (2) Frontal sinus; (3) Orbital plates of frontal bone; (4) Mastoid air cells; (5) Tuberculum sellae with anterior clinoid process, sella turcica, and posterior clinoid process behind; (6) Coronal suture; (7) Anterior wall of middle cranial fossa; (8) Petrous part of temporal bone; (9) External auditory meatus; (10) Lamboid suture; (11) Hard palate; (12) Maxillary sinus; (13) Sphenoidal sinus; (14) Occipital bone (inion); (15) Odontoid process of axis.

Petrous temporal bone changes: Towne's view and other views particularly directed to showing the mastoids, the petrous temporal ridges, or the internal auditory meati, may be helpful in the diagnosis of mastoiditis, petrous osteitis, or a cerebellopontine angle tumor.

Pituitary expansion: This is common with intrasellar neoplasms, usually chromophobe adenomas. Craniopharyngiomas also may distort the sella and often contain calcium flecks.

Sinus changes: Sinus x-rays and special views including tomograms to show the nasopharyngeal spaces may be indicated in certain circumstances to confirm the presence of infective or neoplastic pathologies.

Congenital or acquired disorders of the skull base: Basilar invagination is encroachment upward into the posterior fossa by the atlas bone of the cervical spine, with resulting protrusion of the odontoid peg of the axis. This may be

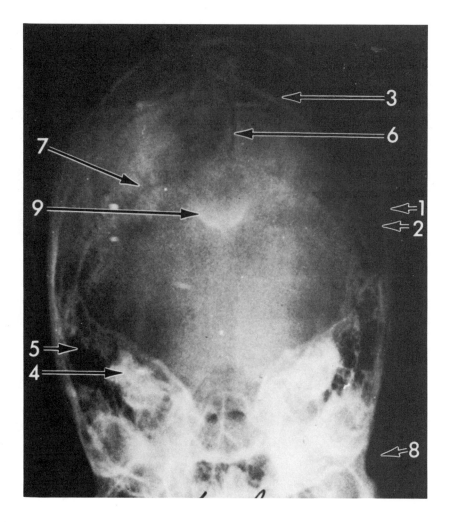

Figure 8-3 Inclined AP (Towne's) view of skull. (1) Outer table; (2) Inner table; (3) Lamboid suture; (4) Petrous pyramids; (5) Mastoid air cells; (6) Sagittal suture; (7) Coronal suture; (8) Head of mandible; (9) Internal occipital protuberance (inion).

seen now to project above the line drawn straight back along the level of the hard palate. Such an abnormality may be *congenital,* often associated with the Arnold-Chiari malformation, or *acquired,* a result of primary bone disease that causes softening (Paget's, osteomalacia, etc.).

Because x-rays are cheap, safe, repeatable, noninvasive, and painless, they are often requested on uncertain grounds, the main indication being, it seems, the presence of any symptoms suggesting intracranial disease. This attitude is reminiscent of that of Mr. Micawber, who lived in everlasting hope that "something would turn up," and (as in his case) appears to be entrenched, a triumph of hope over experience. With the modern investigations now available, the skull x-ray will be done only as an accessory test or where it shows abnormalities more reliably, e.g., skull fractures.

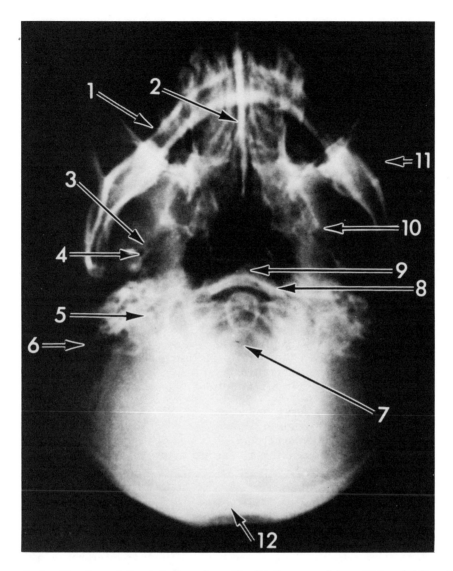

Figure 8-4 Verticosubmental view (basal). (1) Ramus of mandible; (2) Nasal septum; (3) Foramen ovale; (4) Foramen spinosum; (5) Petrous part of temporal bone; (6) Mastoid air cells; (7) Odontoid process of axis; (8) Anterior arch of atlas; (9) Clivus; (10) Lesser wing of sphenoid; (11) Zygoma; (12) Inion.

Table 8-1   Causes of Bony Defects on Skull Films

Burr holes
Venous lakes
Secondary carcinoma
Myelomatosis
Osteomyelitis
Fibrous displasia
Eosinophilic granuloma

Table 8-2   Causes of Hyperostosis on Skull Films

Benign "hyperostosis frontalis interna"
Paget's disease
Fibrous dysplasia
Meningioma
Cephalohematoma
Syphilis
Acromegaly
Chronic osteomyelitis

Table 8-3   Causes of Abnormal Intracranial Calcification

Neoplasms	Meningioma
	Craniopharyngioma
	Slowly-growing glioma
Infection	Cerebral abscess
	Toxoplasmosis
	Cytomegalic inclusion body disease
	Tuberculoma
	Fungal infections

Chronic subdural hematoma
Hypoparathyroidism
Sturge-Weber syndrome
Atheromatous internal carotid artery

SPINAL X-RAYS

X-rays of the spine are, like those of the skull, difficult to interpret unless the changes are striking. Not only structures such as the bodies, pedicles, spine, and laminae of the vertebrae, but also their spatial relationships have to be examined (Figs. 8-5 to 8-7). The intervertebral disk spaces, the foramina, the canal width, and the bodies' alignment must all be scrutinized carefully. Changes that might be seen include:

Congenital lesions: Fusion of the vertebrae, usually in the cervical region, as in the Klippel-Feil syndrome, or lumbosacral, will show as bony bridging.
Syringomyelia is often associated with a widened cervical canal.
Tuberculosis: Tuberculosis is still the most common primary infective disease of the spine. Loss of disk spaces or paravertebral abscesses may be identified in midthoracic or cervical regions.
Trauma: Trauma may cause crush fractures of the vertebrae, with wedging or angulations; or fractures of the transverse processes, usually in the lumbar region. Fracture-dislocation may be seen as a crush fracture with displacement of one vertebral body forward upon another, but with the more serious extension injuries, only the vertebral misalignment may be present.

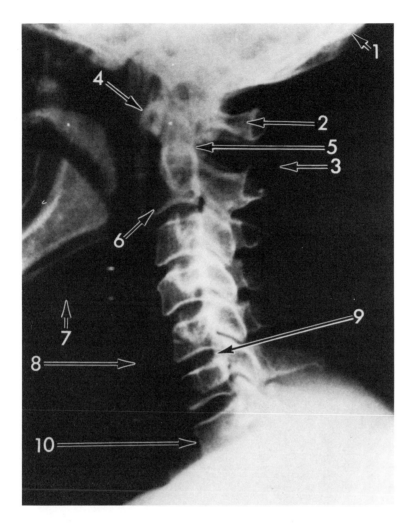

Figure 8-5 Lateral view of cervical spine. (1) Occipital bone; (2) Posterior arch of the atlas; (3) Spine of axis; (4) Anterior arch of atlas; (5) Odontoid process; (6) Body of axis; (7) Hyoid bone; (8) Thyroid cartilage; (9) C5-6 disk space; (10) Body of C-7.

Spondylolisthesis, a forward slipping of one vertebral body over another, is another effect of (remote) trauma and occurs mainly in the lumbosacral region; but it may also be congenital.

Tumors: Intraspinal tumors may cause pressure erosion of bone and thus widen the canal. Secondary tumors are usually seen in the bodies and pedicles of the vertebrae; on an AP view the pedicle may not be seen. Primary bone tumors are uncommon in the spine.

Metabolic bone disease: Paget's disease, osteoporosis, and osteomalacia produce characteristic changes in both the density of bone and in vertebral position because of bony softening. Basilar invagination is one example.

Degenerative disk disease: The most characteristic change caused here is a reduction in the intervertebral disk space. Bony outgrowths (osteophytes) extend from the anterior and posterior surfaces of the vertebrae beside the disks

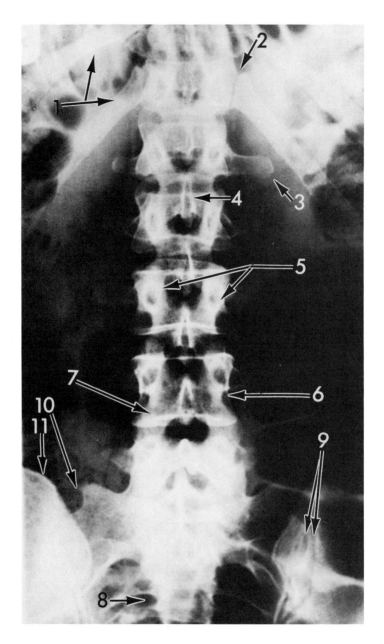

Figure 8-6 AP view of lower thoracic, lumbar, and sacral vertebrae. (1) Eleventh and twelfth ribs; (2) Costovertebral joint; (3) Transverse process of L-1; (4) L-2 spine; (5) Pedicles of L-3; (6) Vertebral body of L-4; (7) Lamina of L-4; (8) Sacral foramina; (9) Sacroiliac joint; (10) Lateral mass of the sacrum; (11) Iliac crest.

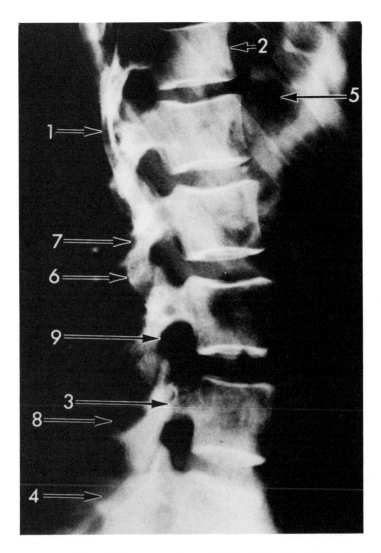

Figure 8-7 Lateral view of lumbar spine. (1) Twelfth rib; (2) Body of T-12; (3) Pedicle of L-4; (4) Iliac crest; (5) Gas in colon; (6) Superior articular process L-3; (7) Inferior articular process L-2; (8) Spine of L-4; (9) Intervertebral foramen for exit of fourth lumbar root.

and may encroach upon the foramina. Periarticular osteosclerosis of the vertebral bodies may also be seen. Both at cervical and lumbar levels, osteo- phytes, disks, and enlarged laminae may narrow the sagittal diameter of the canal (spinal stenosis).

LUMBAR PUNCTURE

A lumbar puncture (LP) is only indicated in situations in which it can give appro- priate information. To use the test indiscriminately in any "neurological" situation diminishes its yield, causes the patient increased risk and discomfort, and often adds only confusing data. For instance, it is common for an LP to be suggested to see "if the protein might be a little raised," even though it is of little help in diag- nosis to know whether the protein is normal or slightly elevated.

Contraindications

Although contraindications to LP are seldom absolute, there are some very strong *relative* contraindications. *Raised intracranial pressure* is one — because an LP still has to be performed in a patient with papilledema who is suspected of having meningitis. It is usually safe in patients with benign intracranial hypertension, al- though LP in a patient with raised intracranial pressure should be performed only when a neurosurgeon has been notified and would be immediately available.

In the presence of an *intracranial mass* lesion, particularly in the posterior fos- sa, an LP could produce herniation and would be dangerous. *Skin infection* around the lumbar puncture site is a strong contraindication because it might introduce infection into the CSF. Patients with an *hysterical personality* or those complaining of a long history of back pain for which no structural cause has yet been found may complain stridently of the unwanted effects of the LP and ascribe to it all manner of later symptoms. In patients on *anticoagulants,* an LP should be performed only after anticoagulation has been reversed.

Technique

Before performing a lumbar puncture, you really must explain the procedure step by step to patients so that they are aware of what is about to happen behind their back, and why. Most patients will cooperate when the understand clearly what is to be done and why it is important. They must be reassured that it *is* important and not necessarily uncomfortable, as most have heard terrible tales about spinal taps and can tell stories about the friend of a friend who has continuous back pain or never walked again after one. It is advisable not to overemphasize the possibility of a post-LP headache, although if it does occur, they may be reassured that it is not uncommon and will decrease with time and bed rest.

The patient lies on his side on a hard bed or table, his back exposed and verti- cal to the floor (Fig. 8-8). The low lumbar area is cleaned with an antiseptic solu- tion and the area draped. The patient is asked to bend his knees up toward his chest and the head should be flexed down toward the knees. When he is thus curled up in a ball, it is important that the flat lumbar area should remain vertical, the pelvis tilted neither toward nor away from you. Feel the posterosuperior iliac spine. A line dropped from this point to the vertebral column crosses the spine at L-4. The needle should be inserted just above this landmark in the L3-4 space.

Inject local anesthetic into the spot, making a small wheal under the skin. You could use a lumbar needle to infiltrate the track which the LP needle will take, but

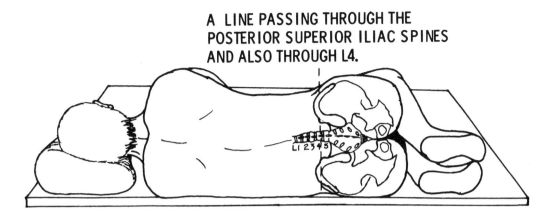

A LINE PASSING THROUGH THE POSTERIOR SUPERIOR ILIAC SPINES AND ALSO THROUGH L4.

Figure 8-8   Position for lumbar puncture.

this is often more painful than the LP itself. (When you become expert, the least painful puncture is done by anesthetizing only the skin and subcutaneous tissues.) Wait for a minute for the anesthetic to work, reassure the patient, and continue to explain each step as you proceed. Then insert the LP needle with the bevel flat so that it *separates* rather than *cuts* the longitudinal dural fibers. Aim the needle towards the umbilicus. As it enters the subdural space and you feel the membrane "give," withdraw the stylette. If no fluid runs back, rotate the needle slowly. If you are up against bone, withdraw the needle slowly, enough to be able to realign it, and insert it again. If you are not sure of your technique, try only three or four times and then get somebody more experienced to help; if you continue to jab at the patient you will become increasingly frustrated, and the patient will become more and more upset and may refuse to have the test done by anybody. Do not be too discouraged if you miss because even the most experienced LP swordsmen miss now and then, and they had to acquire their ability through experience.

When the needle is in, allow only one drop of CSF to escape, verifying that the needle is truly in the subarachnoid space. Reinsert the stylette quickly so that the pressure does not change significantly, and tell the patient that the discomfort is now over and that he can straighten out his legs gently and bring his head up. Have him relax and breathe slowly. After a minute or so, you can take the pressure using a manometer. The most common mistake when doing an LP is to take the pressure with the patient still rolled up tightly because this posture increases the intraabdominal, and thus the CSF, pressure. Therefore make sure that the patient is straightened before the pressure is read.

The Queckenstedt test is done by compressing the jugular veins in the neck, causing the CSF pressure to increase in the manometer if there is no spinal cord block. This test is horribly dangerous if there is any increased intracranial pressure, and there are always better ways of making a diagnosis of spinal block (e.g., a myelogram). Forget that you ever heard of this test. If he had been called Smith, you never would have.

If the pressure is above normal (180 mm of CSF), collect the fluid which is in the manometer and remove the needle if the fluid is clear. If it is cloudy (i.e., if you think the patient has meningitis), take 5 ml and then withdraw the needle. If the pressure is normal, collect a large enough sample to give the laboratory enough CSF to perform the tests that you have ordered. You can then remove the needle *without* measuring the closing pressure which is of absolutely no clinical value.

If the CSF is bloody, note if it tends to clear as you take the samples into three tubes. If it is bloody initially and clears quickly, then the blood came from trauma to a vein during the procedure. If it is bloody throughout, this then suggests a subarachnoid hemorrhage. It is always important to spin a bloody CSF sample in a centrifuge to see if the supernatant fluid is yellow (xanthochromic). If it is, then the blood has been present for at least 4 hr before the LP was done, which indicates previous subarachnoid bleeding rather than a traumatic tap. Do not delay in doing this; a small centrifuge is usually available.

Finally, remove the LP needle quickly, press on the area to prevent local bleeding, and put a small dressing over the puncture site. The patient should then be asked to remain lying down for the next few hours, preferably in the prone position. After this he may get up, but if any headache persists, may remain on his stomach for a day.

Cells

Up to 10 mononuclear cells are allowable in adults without assuming pathology; in children the figure may be somewhat higher. A stained smear of a spun deposit is examined for the differential count. If you suspect that malignant cells may be present, the fluid may be put through a Millipore filter and the cell concentrate examined by a cytologist.

Sugar

Never estimate a CSF sugar without taking a blood sugar level *simultaneously*. The normal CSF value is about 20 mg/dl below the blood sugar level but many patients having LPs have an IV glucose drip running. The normal figure is 45-80 mg/dl. It is reduced in association with an CNS infection, whether purulent, bacterial, tuberculous, fungal, syphilitic, or granulomatous; and also in carcinomatous meningitis, mumps, and herpetic meningoencephalitis (Table 8-4). In association with systemic hypoglycemia and following subarachnoid hemorrhage, CSF values also may fall.

Protein

The normal figure is 380 ± 100 mmol/L; thus the normal range (mean and 2 SD) is 180-580 mmol/L. The normal content of immunogammaglobulin (IgG) is less than 13% of total protein and this figure rises in demyelination from any cause and with neurosyphilis. A rise in protein otherwise is of no specific diagnostic importance, occurring in association with any type of infection, spinal block, cerebral tumor (either benign or malignant), cerebrovascular accident, and diabetes mellitus. However a normal CSF protein does not completely rule out any of these diagnoses. Very high protein levels produce a yellowish color in the fluid (xanthochromia) (Table 8-5).

Chlorides

The normal CSF chloride is 120-130 mmol/L. This is about 20 mmol/L above the serum value, which it always reflects. It falls in any type of infection of the meninges, but usually reflects serum changes.

Table 8-4   Causes of CSF Lymphocytosis

Meningitis	Viral	Brucellar
	Partly treated bacterial	Tuberculous
	Leptospiral	Rickettsial
	Syphilis	Protozoal
	Fungal	
	Chemical	Carcinomatous
Parameningeal infections	Mastoiditis, epidural abscess, etc. Sinus thrombophlebitis	
Other CNS infections	Poliomyelitis	Encephalitis
	Herpes zoster	Cerebral abscess
Postinfective encephalitis		
Miscellaneous	Cerebral tumor Multiple sclerosis Following: ischemic infarction subarachnoid bleeding cerebral trauma Lead poisoning Collagen-vascular diseases Sarcoidosis	

Table 8-5   Causes of CSF Xanthochromia

Recent subarachnoid bleeding
Spinal block*
Guillain-Barré syndrome*
Acoustic neuroma*
Subdural hematoma
Purulent meningitis

*In these conditions the cell count will be normal.

Bacteriology

The Gram, Ziehl-Neelsen, and Wright stains all may give important information. Certainly, the first two should be performed if the patient is suspected of having any form of meningitis. If fungal infection is suspected, an India ink preparation should be requested. Dark-ground illumination will be required to identify spirochetes. Otherwise the usual culture media are employed as indicated.

Serology

The VDRL and FTA-ABS tests for syphilis are easily performed on the CSF.

ELECTROENCEPHALOGRAPHY

The electroencephalogram (EEG) records alterations in the electrical activity of the brain. Because the scalp and skull are between the electrodes and the surface of the brain, the potentials recorded are very small and the only significant electrical changes are a summation of potentials from cortical dendrites. The discharge of a single neuron will never be recorded by the scalp EEG electrodes. The largest voltage alterations arise from masses of neurons with their fiber tracts oriented toward the surface of the scalp. A mass discharge in the tract will be recorded as a high-voltage discharge on the EEG. Artifacts from muscles, from movement of the patient, and even from the heart are easily picked up by the EEG because of the sensitivity of the apparatus and the tremendous amplification used to record the brain's electrical activity. The procedure takes 45 to 60 min, with a usual recording time of about 20 min.

A pattern of electrodes is placed on the scalp. These may be glued on with collodion or very fine needles can be inserted just under the skin. Up to 20 electrodes are usually placed on defined regions of the scalp and the electrical potential fluctuation between any pair of these electrodes is amplied and recorded permanently. Eight, twelve, or sixteen channels are displayed on moving paper as the EEG is performed. During the procedure the patient lies quietly on a bed or reclining chair, being carefully watched by a technician who notes any movement, swallowing, eye blinks, or talking that may cause artifacts on the recording. Stimulation techniques are commonly used to bring out abnormalities not present in the resting record. These include *hyperventilation* to blow off CO_2, causing mild cerebral vasoconstriction and ischemia, and *photic stimulation* using a bright flickering strobe light at varying frequencies. Other techniques occasionally employed include the insertion of electrodes through the nose into the pharynx to record from the anterior and inferior aspect of the temporal lobe *(nasopharyngeal electrodes)* or the insertion of a long needle through the side of the face to lie by the sphenoid bone *(sphenoidal electrodes)*. The end of the needle contains an electrode that can better pick up abnormalities from the medial temporal lobe region. If the brain is exposed during an operation, electrodes can be placed within its substance or on the surface for more accurate recording.

A patient requires little preparation for an EEG. However he should not be fasting unless one is looking for evidence of electrical abnormality from hypoglycemia. Medications should *not* be stopped before the recording, particularly not anticonvulsants, because the advantages far outweigh the complications of discontinuing therapy. The electroencephalographer should be informed of the clinical state of the patient and the questions that you are asking by doing the test. He should know what drugs have been prescribed.

When reading the 100 to 200 ft of EEG recording, the electroencephalographer pays particular attention to the basic wave forms present, the symmetry of the cerebral activity seen, transient discharges, and the response to stimulation techniques.

Basic Wave Forms

Alpha rhythm (Figs. 8-9A-D) is a regular, almost sinusoidal rhythm, between 8 and 13 Hz (cycles per second) seen in the posterior aspect of the head when the eyes are closed and the patient mentally alert but relaxed. Alpha activity tends to be suppressed when the eyes are open or if the individual engages in mental tasks such as arithmetic.

Beta activity is a wave form between 14 and 30 Hz. It is most likely to be associated with anxiety, depression, or sedative medications.

Theta activity is regular activity between 4 and 7 Hz, seldom of much diagnostic significance unless it is definitely asymmetric.

Delta activity is a slow-wave form between 0.5 and 3.5 Hz and is usually abnormal except in small children and during sleep. If present over only one portion of the brain, delta activity often indicates an underlying destructive process such as a tumor or cerebral infarction.

Transient Discharges

Some transient discharges are of little significance, whereas other types indicate abnormal cerebral electrical activity. *Spikes* are brief, high-amplitude discharges which may indicate an underlying epileptic focus. *Spike-and-wave* discharges are bursts of stereotyped cerebral activity in which a slow wave is followed by a spike. These may occur at very regular intervals, often three per second. *Artifacts* caused by eye blinking, movement, etc., inducing a transient burst of activity on the EEG are usually easily recognized as being such.

The four stages of slow-wave sleep and the state of rapid eye movement (REM) sleep cause characteristic EEG changes. Sometimes a sleep recording is done particularly to show epileptic discharges which may only appear at this time.

Indications

The EEG is one of the most abused tests in neurology. It is frequently called upon to answer questions that it is not capable of answering, and it is commonly used in the evaluation of conditions in which it does not show characteristic patterns of abnormality. It is also not commonly understood that the electrical diagnosis does not necessarily correspond to the clinical diagnosis.

The EEG can be extremely valuable in certain circumstances, but it is a poor test in many others. For example, it is almost useless in the elucidation of "spells" or "attacks" which are not thought clinically to be epileptic. It cannot by itself differentiate fits from faints, and it is highly unlikely that it will give any useful information in the evaluation of patients with headaches, if they have no abnormal physical findings. It is of spurious value as medicolegal evidence in most instances, and it shows few, if any, diagnostic features in psychiatric disease. Finally, the EEG interpretation is only of value if the clinician who is giving his opinion has had some information on the clinical status of the patient and the reason for doing the test.

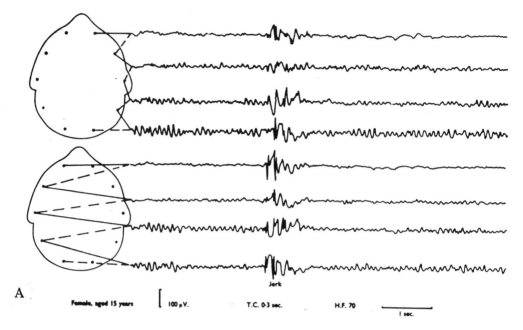

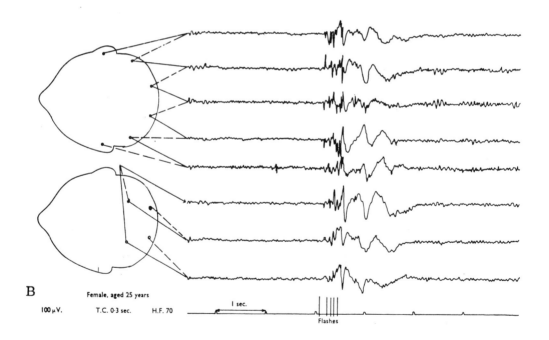

Figure 8-9 Eight-channel EEGs. (A) Myoclonus. Irregular, bilateral spikes and slow waves accompanying a brief muscular jerk. Note preceding and following normal alpha rhythms posteriorly. (B) Photosensitivity. Irregular spikes and slow waves occurring only with flashes of light (bottom markings).

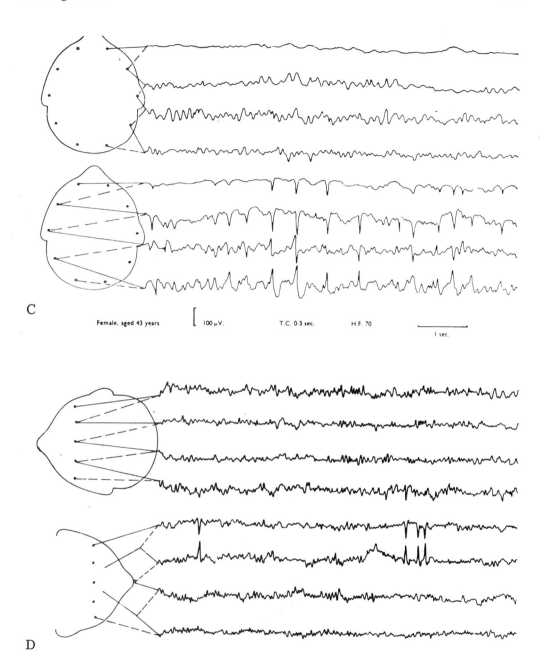

C   Female, aged 43 years   [100 μV.   T.C. 0·3 sec.   H.F. 70   _____
                                                                                      I sec.

D   Female, aged 37 years   [50 μV.   T.C. 0·3 sec.   H.F. 100   _____
                                                                                      I sec.

Figure 8-9   Eight-channel EEGs. (C) Focal spike discharges, arising from the left temporal regions and phase-revising to the point of origin. (D) Sphenoidal lead recording. Wires have been inserted through the cheek to lie below the lesser wing of the sphenoid and thus close to the anterior and inferior temporal lobe. Spikes are seen arising from the left sphenoidal region. Prominent fast activity is due to barbiturate sedation. (Reproduced from Bayliss, S.G. In *Epilepsy*, W.E.M. Pryse-Phillips.) Bristol, John Wright & Sons, 1969. By courtesy of the author and publishers.)

The EEG can be useful in some circumstances. The following are some indications.

1. To localize and assess changes that result from cerebral damage caused by trauma, neoplasm, infection, or vascular disease. Change in these situations are usually asymmetries of normal background rhythms or increased cerebral activity in the theta or delta range. In a subdural hematoma, slow activity or diminished amplitude of the background cerebral rhythms may be seen on the side of the lesion, but there is no diagnostic EEG pattern in this disorder. The EEG is always markedly abnormal in cases of cerebral abscess and is frequently so with encephalitis and meningitis. With vascular and neoplastic disease, the EEG only localizes pathology.

2. To localize the origin and identify the type of epilepsy present: Generalized epilepsy will often show symmetric single or multiple bursts of spikes or sharp waves. With petit mal epilepsy, the classical three per second spike-and-wave pattern may be recorded in almost all subjects even when the patient appears to be normally alert. Careful observations may show that there are attention lapses during these brief periods or that there is brief myoclonus associated with the discharge. In "partial" or focal epilepsy spikes or sharp waves may be recorded from a discrete region of the brain with or without similar wave forms on the opposite side. Although not diagnostic of epilepsy, all such changes may be useful in differentiating a seizure from hysterical activity, because in the latter the EEG will probably be normal. Needless to say, the more definite the clinical diagnosis of epilepsy, the greater the chance of the EEG showing typical abnormalities. The value of the EEG in epilepsy lies not in making the diagnosis (which is entirely a clinical matter) but in helping to establish the nature of the seizure and its site of origin.

3. To assist in the diagnosis of coma: Although loss of the basic cerebral rhythms, such as the alpha rhythm, will occur in nearly all cases of coma, asymmetric abnormalities or the presence of certain discharge patterns may localize an underlying lesion or give support to a clinical diagnosis of the cause of the coma, e.g., in hepatic or uremic cases, diffuse slow-wave changes with "triphasic" waves are commonly seen.

4. In patients with subacute sclerosing panencephalitis and sometimes in herpes simplex encephalitis (Chap. 40): Periodic complexes with diffuse irregular slow activity suggest the diagnosis.

5. In patients with dementia or organic brain syndromes: Many elderly patients who are becoming demented may appear to be only depressed. The EEG may be of value because demented patients are likely to have a low-amplitude record with a great deal of slow activity; depressed patients will not produce any delta activity while awake.

6. In the evaluation of the treatment of hepatic coma: In this situation there is a lot of slow-wave activity bilaterally with brief triphasic discharges mainly over the frontal region. These are correlated closely with the severity of the encephalopathy. Serial recordings can be of great value in following the patient's response to therapy and later indicate any tendency to develop a recurrence of the encephalopathy.

7. Alpha activity is usually suppressed when a patient's eyes are open or when he pays visual attention to his surroundings. In patients who are blind, the alpha activity will probably be recorded at all times unless they are performing some mental task such as arithmetic. However patients with hysterical blindness should suppress their alpha rhythm when their eyes are open.

8. To assess the value of steroid therapy in infantile spasms: Children with this
    abnormality have a chaotic EEG appearance known as *hypsarrhythmia*.
9. To assist in the diagnosis of cerebral death (see Chap. 10).

In conclusion, 10 percent of thoroughly normal and healthy individuals have an
EEG that is electrically "abnormal." Even though a higher proportion of patients
with migraine or psychopathic personality disorders have abnormal records, compared with patients without these conditions, the EEG is of no diagnostic value in
such disorders. The test may be properly used to answer a certain limited number
of questions. It will probably answer these quite well. In all other conditions it
will probably contribute nothing but confusion.

EVOKED POTENTIAL (EP) STUDIES

Research on evoked potentials (EP) has rapidly advanced in the past 10 years and
has produced much new information about how the nervous system receives and
transmits sensory inputs. Three forms of EPs are recorded in the clinical diagnostic
laboratory: visual, auditory (brainstem), and somatosensory (see Fig. 8-10A, B).

In each case, repetitive stimuli are presented to the nervous system (visual pattern, auditory click, or electrical skin stimulation), and electrodes on the skin over
the spine or skull record the resulting cerebral electrical activity. Because these
tiny evoked responses would be lost in the random background activity of the normal functioning brain, the apparatus includes a computer which records cerebral
activity immediately following hundreds of stimuli. Thus random activity is "averaged out," only responses to the stimuli remaining as a constant wave pattern.
These are superimposed to give a composite graph of the cortical potentials evoked
by the stimulus.

Visual evoked potentials are best recorded with an alternating black and white
checkerboard stimulus. Various other patterns have been used as well. The test is
of particular value in multiple sclerosis because slowed conduction in demyelinated
optic nerve fibers alters both the wave forms and their timing.

Brainstem auditory evoked potentials (BAERs) are recorded when clicks are
presented to each ear separately. This test is of value in assessing coma and
cerebral death, in multiple sclerosis, and in posterior fossa tumors and other brainstem disorders, because the wave forms are altered in different ways by lesions
at different sites from the eighth nerve, through the brainstem, to the cortex.

Somatosensory evoked potentials (SEPs) are evoked by a mechanical or electrical stimulus given peripherally. The responses over a more proximal part of the
nerve, over the cord, or over the scalp are then recorded and averaged. The stimulus and recording sites depend upon the type and localization of the suspected lesion. The test is of value in the identification of rough quantitation of nerve, cord,
and brainstem lesions. It is most commonly used in determining cord lesions in tumors and demyelination and in determining the extent of damage in traumatic cord
damage.

EMG AND NERVE CONDUCTION STUDIES

Electromyography (EMG) refers to the recording of the electrical potentials associated with the contraction of muscle fibers. Nerve conduction studies examine the
ability of nerves to conduct electrical potentials along their length in both motor
and sensory nerve fibers. These tests are performed by stimulation of a peripheral

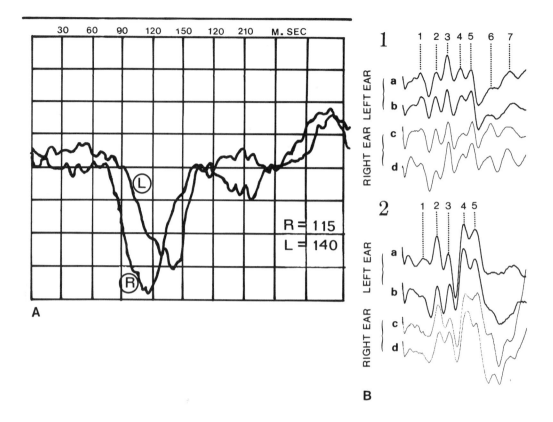

Figure 8-10 (A) Visual evoked potentials in right and left eyes following alternating checkerboard stimuli. Note delay and lower amplitude of waves from left eye. (B) Brain stem auditory evoked potentials. 1000 clicks were used as the stimulus at 10 clicks/sec. The wave form results from a superimposition of the consistent response occurring after each click. The background EEG and random electrical activity is averaged out. The waves illustrated occur at different levels throughout the auditory system, from ear to auditory cortex. Two tracings from each ear were taken from two patients (1 and 2). (Courtesy of Dr. D.M. Regan.)

nerve, usually in more than one site, recording the muscle action potential or the sensory action potential resulting. The decision about what type of study is required, which nerves or muscles should be examined, and what special studies should be performed must depend upon the results of a careful history and clinical examination by the electromyographer himself. To ask for an EMG study, therefore, is also to ask for a consultation.

Electromyogram

Although spontaneous and evoked muscle action potentials can be recorded through the skin using surface electrodes, the most widely used way of measuring these is with a concentric needle electrode, consisting of an insulated platinum wire inserted into a hollow needle.* The potential difference between the center of the needle

---

*This is thus a bipolar electrode. Monopolar electrodes are favored in some EMG laboratories.

and the outside is amplified to be displayed on an oscilloscope (Fig. 8-11A-D) and is also fed to a loudspeaker for auditory interpretation of sound produced by such potentials. Since most nerve disorders have their greatest effect in the periphery, a distal muscle will usually be chosen for a needle examination if denervation is suspected. Specific nerve injuries, as in a root lesion or mononeuropathy, would require selection of the area to be examined depending upon the findings on examination. Most of the muscles of the body, including paraspinal, girdle, and facial muscles, can be examined by EMG. In cases where a primary disorder of muscle is suspected, proximal muscles will probably be examined.

Normally, no motor activity is recorded when the needle is inserted into the resting muscle. If denervation is present, abnormal spontaneous potentials may be seen and heard. *Fibrillations* are regularly recurring, brief, small-amplitude potentials that occur 10 to 14 days after a muscle has lost its motor nerve supply, and they continue until it is completely atrophic or else reinnervated. Except perhaps in the tongue, fibrillations cannot be seen clinically. They arise from single muscle fibers that now contract in response to circulating cholinergic substances, to which they have become unusually sensitive. Since similar potentials may be recorded from myopathic muscles, fibrillations cannot be regarded as diagnostic of denervation.

Fasciculations are single, irregularly occurring electrical discharges within all the muscle fibers of a motor unit and are usually caused by disease of the anterior horn cell. They are thus much greater in amplitude and have a longer duration than fibrillations and correspond to the physical twitching of a muscle, which can be seen clinically.

Needle movement should produce little electrical discharge from the fibers traumatized by the needle, but occasionally in primary muscle disease repetitive *irregular discharges* may occur, referred to as muscle *irritability*. When the patient contracts the muscle gently, single *action potentials* can be seen that are separated from each other well enough for the examiner to note the number of phases, normally four or less. An excess of polyphasic units indicates either denervation with some reinnervation occurring or a primary muscle disease. Brief, abundant, small-amplitude potentials are commonly seen in primary muscle disease while *giant units* 2 to 10 times normal size may occur during the repair process following denervation.

The patient is then asked to contract his muscle as strongly as he can, and the size of the recruitment pattern is estimated. The baseline is normally obliterated by this maximal contraction and a full-throated roar is heard from the machine, indicating a full pattern with activation of all motor units. It is a matter of experience and judgment to decide if the pattern produced and the sound of the motor units are normal.

Although the most important diagnostic use of EMG is the demonstration of changes of denervation or myopathy, there are a few other diagnostic situations that are of interest. *Myositis* is associated with the usual changes of a primary myopathy primarily in proximal muscles, often with fibrillations. In *myotonic* diseases, a characteristic, high-frequency but decelerating discharge of potentials occurs, sounding like a motorcycle.

Fatigability of muscles can be shown by continuous recording of the recruitment pattern, which will be seen to diminish in amplitude as the rate of firing and number of units activated both decrease, as in myasthenia gravis.

The EMG can seldom differentiate one type of myopathy from another, although it may be diagnostic in myositis, myotonia, and myasthenia. It is of no value in demonstrating changes with disuse atrophy or with a corticospinal lesion.

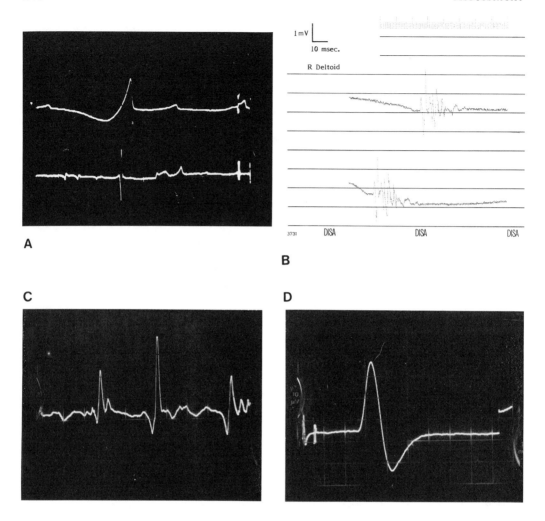

Figure 8-11   (A) Fibrillation potentials and positive sharp waves in a denervated muscle; (B) Large polyphasic unit recording twice from the right deltoid muscle, following reinvervation; (C) Normal motor unit potentials during minimal contraction; (D) Normal sensory action potentials from the index finger after stimulation of the median nerve at the wrist; 20 traces averaged.

Electromyography is dangerous in patients with bleeding disorders, such as hemophilia, and will cause a rise of serum creatine kinase (CK) for the next 1 or 2 days. If a muscle biopsy is taken from a site formerly needled during EMG, microscopic changes suggesting myositis may be reported by the pathologist.

Nerve Conduction Studies

Many peripheral nerves can be stimulated through the site. This produces a sensation somewhere between discomfort and pain, which can usually be borne without difficulty for a short period. The nerve studies will depend upon the clinical findings, but commonly examined areas are the supraorbital branch of the fifth nerve, the seventh nerve, fibers of the brachial plexus, the median, ulnar, radial, and the

sciatic, common peroneal and medial popliteal, saphenous, posterior tibial, and sural nerves (Fig. 8-11D).

The motor conduction velocity is calculated from two sites of stimulation because there is a very definite delay at the neuromuscular junction and the influence
of this has to be obviated by making it common to both measurements. The different latencies of these responses represent the time taken for the impulse to go
from the proximal to the distal site. When the distance between them is measured,
the velocity of the impulse can be calculated. In sensory fibers however, no such
delay occurs and one can therefore stimulate the nerve at one point and record
from it at another.

Three types of abnormality may be found. First, there may be slowing of motor
or sensory conduction velocity along a nerve, and this may be more pronounced distally. If this slowing reduces the conduction velocity to a figure still over 75 percent of normal, then it is likely that the neuropathy is of the axonal or "neuronal"
type, in which there is a generalized lesion affecting larger and smaller fibers together. Second, slowing may be detected which is of a much greater degree so that
the speeds are often much less than 75 percent of the normal speeds. This suggests
a more selective lesion, affecting particularly the large fibers which conduct more
quickly, as seen in a demyelinating neuropathy. Remember that the thickest nerve
fibers are the ones with the most myelin and are the ones that conduct the fastest.
Thus a demyelinating lesion will affect these fibers the most and the slowing of conduction speed will be greatest. Third, there may be localized slowing of conduction
within a nerve at a certain area, the conduction velocity above and below that lesion being within normal limits or nearly so. Such is the case with nerve compression occurring at numerous sites.

The value of nerve conduction studies is primarily to determine the presence
of a neuropathy and to demonstrate whether it involves one, more than one, or perhaps all peripheral nerves. It is also useful to show whether mainly motor or sensory fibers are involved and whether the degree of slowing suggests an axonal or
demyelinating neuropathy. The studies are also able to show the exact site of a
conduction block and can be used to demonstrate the site of severe root trauma.
Repetitive stimulation studies are useful for confirming the diagnosis of myasthenia
gravis and the myasthenic syndrome associated with oat-cell carcinoma of the
lung. Occasionally the EMG is used to demonstrate a brainstem lesion by measuring the blink response to stimulation of the supraorbital nerve.

Use of the EMG machine is an extension of the clinical examination and more
than any other investigation in neurology is entirely dependent upon the clinical decisions of the investigator, in whose hands it is an extremely useful tool with which
to refine his clinical observations.

NERVE AND MUSCLE BIOPSY

Biopsy procedures are simple and safe when done properly and yield a surprising
amount of important information when done for selected indications. Who does the
biopsy varies. The neurologist often does it because he best knows which site to
select. The pathologist sometimes does it because he knows exactly how to minimize the artifacts that often are seen under the microscope. A surgeon sometimes
asks to do all biopsies so that he becomes expert in the technique. Whoever does
the biopsy, he must be aware of the immense fragility of the specimens and the
special care that must be taken with the tissue.

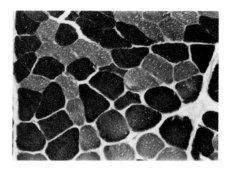

Figure 8-12   Normal muscle biopsy, stained with ATPase to show the differential staining of type 1 and type 2 fibers.

Muscle Biopsy

Local anesthetic is employed for a muscle biopsy (Fig. 8-12) in adults and infants and only rarely is a general anesthetic necessary. If a biopsy is to be performed under general anesthesia, the anesthetist should be on guard to detect the sudden development of *malignant hyperthermia* (Chap. 45).

The biopsy should be taken from a muscle affected by the disease but not totally atrophic. The area selected should not have been tested by EMG needles because these cause significant artifactual changes in the tissue. In general, a patient suspected of having a myopathy will have the biopsy taken from a proximal muscle, such as the deloid or quadriceps. The specimen obtained is prepared for histochemical study and light and electron microscopy.

Muscle biopsy may be of value in

1.   The evaluation of proximal or distal muscle weakness or muscle wasting without sensory loss. It may also be used in the evaluation of congenital weakness when it is not known whether the disorder is primarily myopathic or neurogenic.
2.   The diagnosis of lipid and glycogen diseases, sarcoidosis, primary vascular disease (vasculitis), and polymyositis.
3.   The search for particular microscopic changes, as may be found in myasthenia gravis, myotonia, hyperthyroidism, and congenital myopathies.

Nerve Biopsy

The sural and superficial radial nerves are most likely to be selected. The sural nerve is larger and almost entirely sensory, supplying only the outside edge of the foot. A fascicular biopsy from this nerve leaves a very small area of sensory impairment which is not a significant problem to the patient.

A standard technique requires local anesthesia, identification of the nerve, and the isolation of one or more fascicles, which are removed and prepared for light and electron microscopy or histochemical study, if appropriate, and for staining with osmic acid (which colors the myelin black). This allows visualization of the nerve in transverse and longitudinal sections under the light microscope and also, after maceration in glycerine, allows single nerve fibers to be teased out and examined.

Nerve biopsy may be of value in

1.   Differentiating between axonal and demyelinating neuropathies

2. Showing infiltration of peripheral nerves as in myeloma, carcinoma, sarcoidosis, amyloidosis, vasculitis, and leprosy
3. Characterizing congenital hypertrophic neuropathies
4. Identifying lipid storage diseases and leukodystrophies

It is not a commonly used diagnostic technique in clinical neurology because clinical and electrodiagnostic examination usually give enough data for diagnosis, but it is a valuable research method and may be warranted in difficult diagnostic problems.

BRAIN SCAN

With the intravenous injection of a radionuclide such as technetium ($_{99m}$Tc), rapid circulation to the whole body occurs, but the isotope will not cross an intact blood-brain barrier. If a scintiscan is taken of the head at any time after the injection, marked uptake will be seen from the scalp, from the mucosa of the sinuses, from all the bones of the head, and from the superior sagittal and transverse sinuses. Uptake may also be recognized within the choroid plexuses, but if the patient is premedicated with potassium chlorate, the ability of the choroid plexus to secrete the isotope is diminished and this particular artifact is removed. The brain itself however will not take up and retain the isotope unless in some area the blood-brain barrier is demolished; brain scans therefore are essentially maps of the areas where that has occurred (Fig. 8-13).

The isotopes generally used are well accepted by certain lesions — meningiomas, malignant gliomas, metastases, and abscesses, for example — but may not be accepted by benign or low-grade malignant tumors. Indications for the test are

To demonstrate the site and size of suspected intracranial neoplasms any area of focal brain disease such as abscess, herpes simplex encephalitis, or the area of brain around an AV malformation.

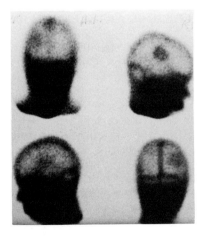

Figure 8-13   Isotope brain scan, showing a right posterior frontal glioma

To differentiate between tumor and stroke. Immediately after an apparent stroke the scan should be negative, becoming positive in 4 to 7 days and remaining so for some 6 to 8 weeks, after which it again reverts to negative. This is probably because of damage to the blood-brain barrier in the area surrounding the infarct, this ischemic zone taking up the isotope and retaining it only some days after the accident has occurred. If *immediately following* apparent stroke the brain scan is positive, an AV malformation or tumor may be suspected as the actual cause of the patient's symptoms and signs, and further investigations will probably be required.

With the technique of bolus intravenous injection and rapidly repeated initial scans, some ideas of intracerebral blood flow may be achieved, the side on which flow is slowest showing less radioactivity in the early stages and continuing to show uptake for some seconds after the other, normal side has cleared. In the case of very vascular lesions (AVM), these may show up early and clear more quickly than the other, normal brain areas.

The isotope brain scan is almost redundant where NMR scans are available.

ISOTOPE CISTERNOGRAPHY (RISA SCAN)

This investigation consists of the injection of radioiodinated serum albumin (RISA) into the lumbar subarachnoid space. The RISA will follow the flow of CSF up to the basal cisterns and will then pass out over the cerebral convexity to be absorbed by the arachnoid granulations into the superior sagittal sinus. Because the flow of CSF is out of the ventricular system through the foramen of Magendie, the RISA will not normally enter the ventricles. If there is an abnormality of flow over the cerebral convexities and the RISA enters the ventricles and stays there instead of passing up toward the superior sagittal sinus, the picture is almost diagnostic of normal pressure hydrocephalus.

The RISA scan may be able to pinpoint the leak causing CSF rhinorrhea after head injury.

The patency of shunts inserted to relieve hydrocephalus or subarachnoid block may be assessed by injecting the RISA into the shunt or the subarachnoid space and scanning over the venous or peritoneal end of the tube.

CEREBRAL ARTERIOGRAPHY

Cerebral arteriography is a method of visualizing the intracranial vascular system by injecting radiopaque material into the bloodstream (Fig. 8-14A-C). The injection may be made directly into a carotid or vertebral artery by needle puncture, but more often a catheter is passed up from the femoral artery into the arch of the aorta. From here, the catheter can be selectively directed into the right innominate, subclavian, or common carotid arteries or into the subclavian or carotid arteries on the left side. Injection of a radiopaque substance can then be made selectively into any, or all, of these vessels, as indicated. An arteriogram will not only show the arterial vascular tree but also, as the dye passes on, will allow some appreciation of the capillary and venous phases on the rapid series of x-rays taken following the injection. Usually, films are exposed in two planes (anteroposterior and lateral) at the same time. The arterial phase best outlines the major arteries and the gross structure of the brain. The capillary phase enables one to take note of any area of generally increased vascularity, while the venous phase best demonstrates the deep cerebral structures and the ventricles. The technique of arteriography of the spinal cord has now developed to the point that it is being used to

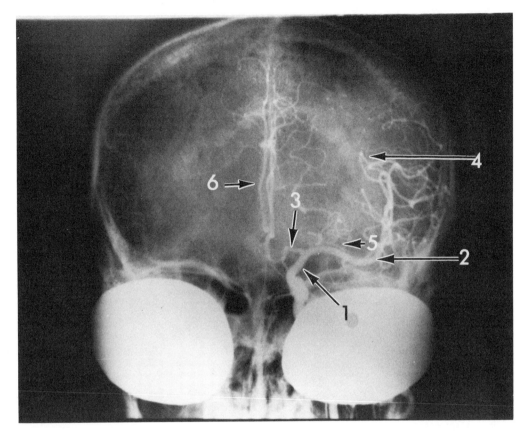

Figure 8-14A   Left carotid angiogram (AP view). (1) Internal carotid (ICA); (2) Middle cerebral (MCA); (3) Anterior cerebral (ACA); (4) Sylvian point; (5) Lenticulostriate arteries; (6) Right and left pericallosal arteries.

demonstrate some spinal cord lesions, chiefly those of a vascular nature. Again, a selective catheter technique is most frequently used.

Indications

Arteriography is a good method of demonstrating the following abnormalities, most of which are vascular.

1.   Aneurysms
2.   Arteriovenous malformations
3.   Tumors[*]
4.   Occlusive vascular diseases, including arteriosclerosis and other diseases of the major extracranial vessels and their origins
5.   Subdural and intracerebral hematomas[*]
6.   The "subclavian steal" phenomenon

---

[*]These intracranial lesions are better visualized however by CT scanning.

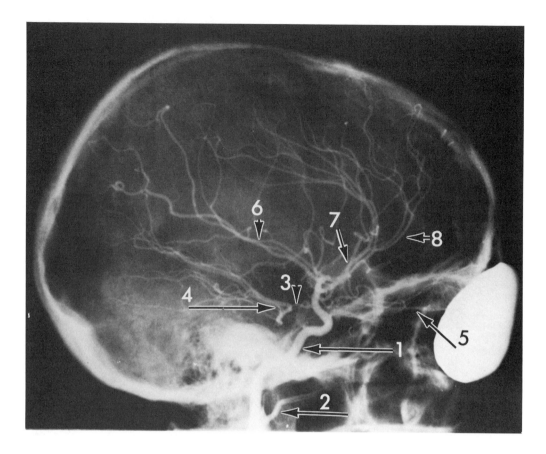

Figure 8-14B   Left carotid angiogram (lateral view). (1) Internal carotid; (2) Maxillary branch (ECA); (3) Posterior communicating artery (ICA); (4) Posterior cerebral; (5) Ophthalmic (ICA); (6) Middle cerebral (MCA); (7) Right and left cerebral (ACA); (8) Frontopolar branch of ACA.

Arteriography is most useful in demonstrating the site and location of both intra- and extracerebral occlusive vascular disease. This is important because the role of the extracranial vessels in providing a source of emboli to the intracranial vasculature is now recognized, and both medical and surgical treatments are available. One looks for disease of the arterial wall, particularly in the extracranial vessels; for evidence of midline shift; for compression of the brain by an extracerebral mass such as a subdural hematoma; for occlusion of a vessel; and for aneurysms.

Although cerebral angiography is usually performed under local anesthesia, the experience of the loud clatter of the x-ray machinery and the rapid change cassettes, the unpleasant, hot flushing sensation when the dye enters the cerebral vasculature, and the fact that everybody in the room except the patient vanishes behind lead screens during the worst part of the whole procedure may make general anesthesia preferable in some patients. As with any investigation, it is important to describe clearly the test procedure to the patient beforehand because informed consent must be obtained.

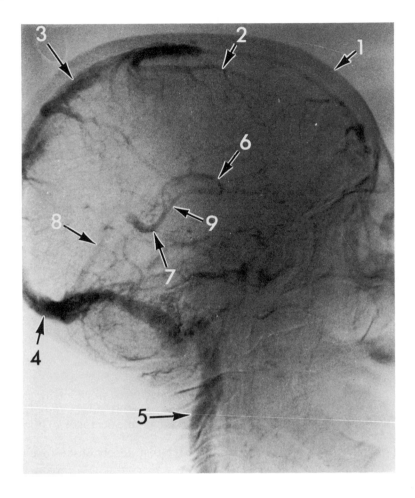

Figure 8-14C   Common carotid angiogram, venous phase (subtraction). (1) Frontal bone; (2) A superficial ascending cortical vein; (3) Superior sagittal sinus; (4) Transverse sinus; (5) Internal jugular vein; (6) Thalamostriate vein; (7) Great vein of Galen; (8) Straight sinus; (9) Internal cerebral vein.

Complications

Cerebral arteriography is not embarked upon lightly; complications are more frequent in patients who are seriously ill, elderly, hypertensive, diabetic, or suffering from other serious disease. The usual radiation hazards apply, naturally. Any contrast medium may induce allergic or even anaphylactic reactions; some physicians test the patient for sensitivity to a medium by injecting a small amount intravenously for a few minutes before carrying out the procedure. Direct arterial puncture in the neck may actually produce emboli if the vessel is very atheromatous. Bleeding is a further hazard. Transient blindness may occur during vertebral arteriography when dye replaces blood in both occipital lobes. The intramural injection of dye is uncommon since selective procedures have become widely used, but it is feared because it may obstruct the vessel.

There is some pain at the injection site, and the area is often tender following the procedure. With selective catheter techniques there is a particular danger of bleeding in the area of the injection, and pressure must be maintained there for some minutes after the catheter is withdrawn to prevent a hematoma. Local spasm of the arterial injection site may be a problem, particularly if there is already circulatory impairment in that limb, and monitoring of the pulses is wise for a period after the injection.

Digital Subtraction Angiography

Digital subtraction angiography (DSA) is another use of computers to produce images. An injection of 40 ml of iodinated contrast material into the antecubital vein is observed to flow into the major vessels of the neck by pulsed fluoroscopic exposures every 1.5 sec. These images are converted instantaneously into numbers (digitalized) by a computer and stored. The computer then separates numbers in the images without contrast from those with contrast. The resultant subtraction pictures show contrast in the vessels with the bones and other structures subtracted.

The technique is potentially powerful but the image is not yet clear enough to give us confidence to make decisions regarding surgery, and one cannot see small intracerebral vessels. It is used primarily to see if major vessel obstruction is present and to verify that vessels remain open postoperatively.

PNEUMOENCEPHALOGRAPHY

Pneumoencephalography (PEG) is a radiological procedure in which air is injected into the lumbar subarachnoid space to outline the cavities within the brain, the cisterns at the base of the brain, and the spaces over the surfaces of the hemispheres (Fig. 8-15).

The CT scan has fortunately made this nasty test nearly obsolete.

VENTRICULOGRAPHY

Ventriculography is a method of injecting air directly into the lateral ventricles. It is usually done when clinical signs and arteriography have suggested raised intracranial pressure or imminent herniation through the tentorium of foramen magnum, as with tumors of the posterior fossa. Again, CT scanning has largely replaced it. The lateral ventricles, foramina of Munro, and the third ventricle are usually seen well, but it is more difficult to outline the aqueduct and fourth ventricle. It visualizes only the ventricular outline and not the basal cisterns nor the surface of the brain (Fig. 8-16A).

MYELOGRAPHY

If positive contrast material is injected into the lumbar subarachnoid space, the fluid can be made to flow upward or downward by tilting the patient. The outline of the inside of the spinal cord and the negative shadow of the spinal cord can be seen by this method (Figs. 8-16B; 8-17A, B). Screening under television control precedes the exposure of film which gives a permanent record of the appearance.

Myelography is contraindicated if lumbar puncture is contraindicated, or if the subject is allergic to iodine. Water soluble media (such as metrizamide) are

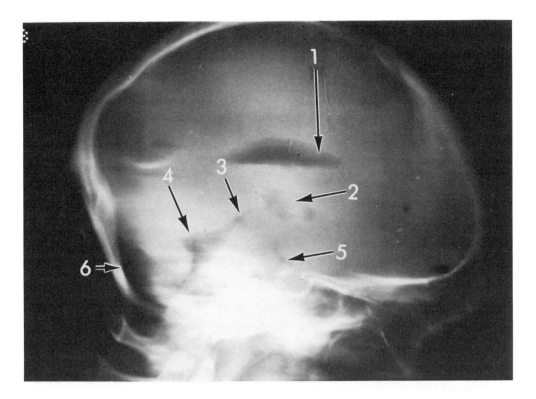

Figure 8-15 Normal pneumoencephalogram (autotomogram focusing on midline structures). (1) Partly-filled lateral ventricle; (2) Partly-filled third ventricle; (3) Aqueduct; (4) Fourth ventricle; (5) Interpeduncular fossa; (6) Cisterna magna.

preferable but are used cautiously in patients with hepatic or renal dysfunction, chronic alcoholism, asthma, multiple sclerosis (MS), or epilepsy — the last because of the epileptogenic potential of the substance. To minimize the change of a seizure, a patient who has had a metrizamide myelogram lies supine with the head raised for 24 hr, and as a result, postlumbar puncture headaches are frequent. If there is a suggestion of spinal block, a neurosurgeon should be at hand so that if the contrast medium converts the *partial* into a *total* block, this can be relieved by immediate operation. The indications for myelography are to

1. Localize known intraspinal pathology before surgery, e.g., prolapsed inteverte-bral disk, spinal tumors
2. Demonstrate significant canal narrowing in cases of lumbar or cervical spondylosis
3. Differentiate between an intramedullary and an extramedullary lesion, and in the latter case, to show whether it is inside or outside the dura
4. Delineate lesions of the craniovertebral junction and in the posterior fossa
5. Demonstrate cord widening in syringomyelia

The decision to perform myelography should usually be made by a neurologist, a neurosurgeon, or an orthopedic surgeon. Myelography using air rather than positive contrast materials may be useful in the diagnosis of syringomyelia.

Because CSF is removed during myelography, it is available for any appropriate tests. It must be taken *at the start* of the procedure however, or the cell count will show a false elevation.

COMPUTERIZED AXIAL TOMOGRAPHY
(CT SCAN)

This technique represents the most sophisticated employment of x-rays in diagnosis since their discovery. The patient lies on a table, his head inside a circular chamber around which an x-ray source and a detector crystal are placed diametrically opposite one another. A thin beam of x-rays (in newer models, a spreading fan of x-rays) crosses the patient's head and the energy not absorbed by the intracranial structures in its pathway is sensed by the detector. After the x-ray emission, the tube rotates 1° and another exposure is made until 180° have been covered, when every point in the head has been examined. Usually 8 to 10 "slices" of the head are examined. Horizontal, sagittal, and coronal views may be taken (Figs. 8-18A-F).

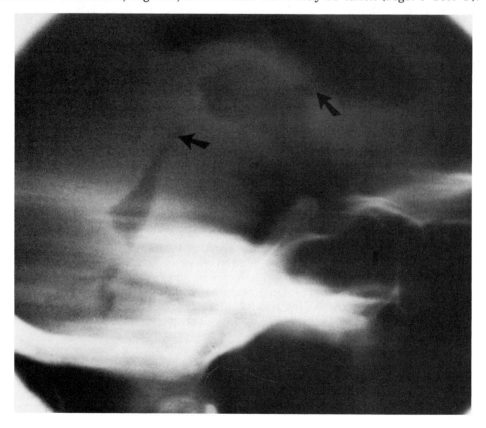

Figure 8-16A   Air ventriculogram. Arrows point to foramen of Munro and aqueduct.

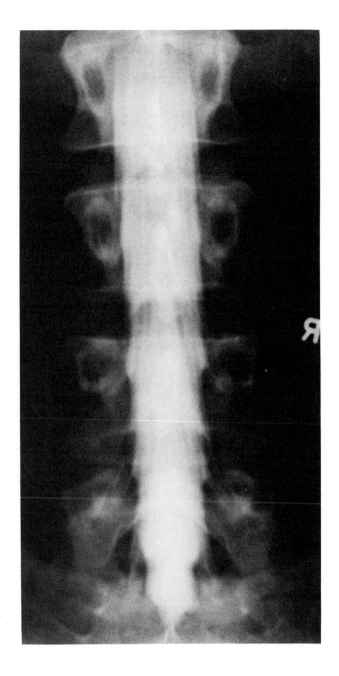

Figure 8-16B Lumbar myelogram with metrizamide; AP view. The "fir-tree" pattern of the cauda equina roots is well shown.

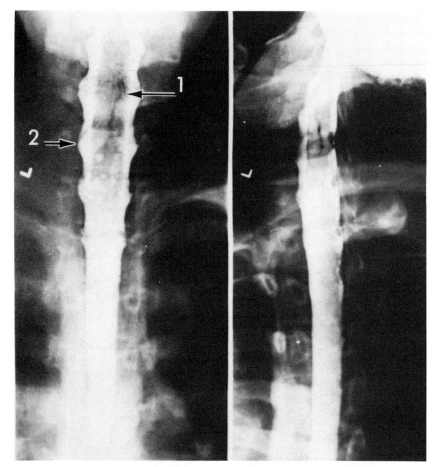

Figure 8-17A Cervical myelogram. AP and oblique views. (1) Negative shadow of cervical cord, demarcated by contrast medium; (2) Downward-angled cervical root.

The radiodensity of each point is calculated by a linked computer according to the distribution of densities plotted on a point matrix. Thus a "map" of a slice of the intracranial contents, 3-12 mm thick, is generated and displayed on a cathode ray oscilloscope (CRO) or on photographic film.

Bone has a high absorption coefficient, CSF and water are in the midrange, and air is low. Most cranial lesions have densities varying somewhat from the surrounding brain parenchyma; thus blood, calcium, and tumors have high densities and fluid or gas-filled cysts have low densities. Not only can these be localized; often one can make the pathological diagnosis from the appearances on the film.

On the image created, the eyes, orbits, second nerve, pituitary fossa, falx, and gray and white matter, ventricles and CSF spaces, and the blood vessels all can be examined. Such abnormalities as gliomas, acoustic neuromas, and other tumors; abscesses; infarcts and intracerebral or subarachnoid hemorrhages (all of which it can differentiate); cerebral atrophy; acute sub- or extradural hematomas and brain edema are all well shown. The test is both sensitive and reasonably specific.

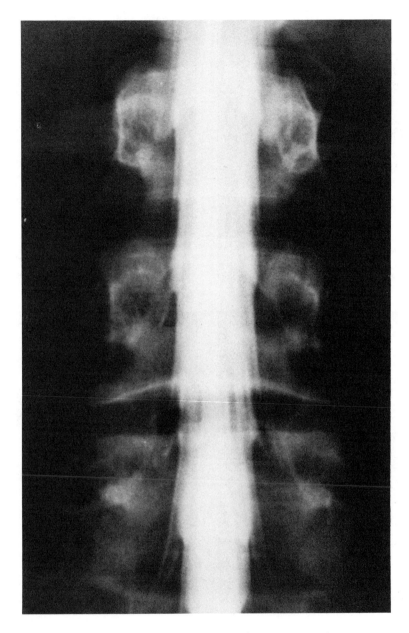

Figure 8-17B Normal lumbar myelogram showing nerve roots.

Intravenous iodinated contrast medium is frequently given after the initial scans have been made; this enhances the image of the blood vessels, both normal and abnormal, and of the falx. It also shows up any area in which the blood-brain barrier has been damaged such as around a tumor, or in an area of cerebral edema.

Naturally, some cautions are necessary. The CT scan is not as good at showing small lesions close to dense, (e.g., bony) structures; some subacute or chronic

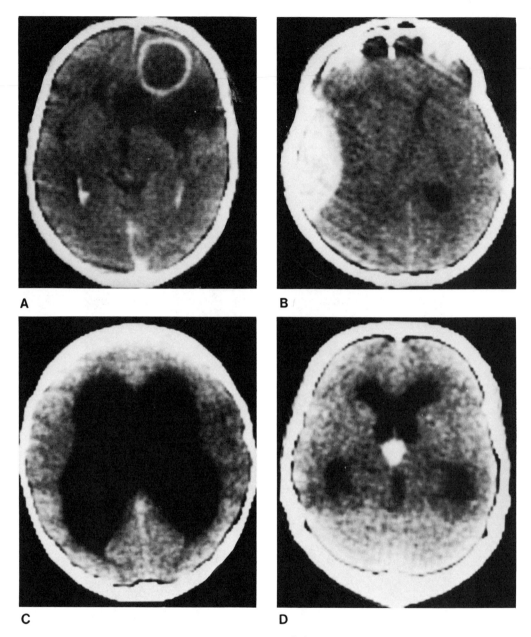

Figure 8–18A–D   Representative CT scans. (A) Cerebral abscess with edema; (B) Epidural hematoma; (C) Hydrocephalus; (D) Colloid cyst.

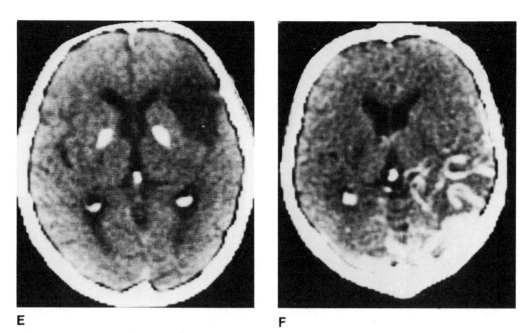

Figure 8-18E-F   (E) Cerebral infarction. Note calcification of basal ganglia, pineal and choroid plexus; (F) Arterial venous malformation.

hematomas are isodense with respect to the brain. Liaison between the responsible clinician and the radiologist is essential, both in planning the test and in interpreting the results.

POSITRON EMISSION TOMOGRAPHY

Positron emission transverse tomography is an experimental investigation combining the use of radioisotopes and a scanning device. The patient inhales, e.g., oxygen tagged with a positron-emitting isotope with a short half-life, and the detector follows the activity of the compound and displays a dynamic map of the chemical activity within the brain. Even the brain's metabolic changes accompanying reading can be assessed by this method, but the price tag makes the CT scanner look cheap. It is likely that this procedure will remain an important research tool but not become a routine investigation.

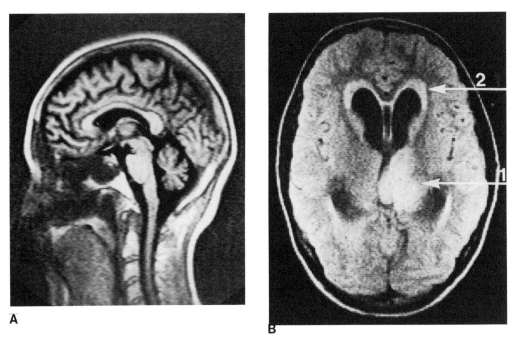

Figure 8–19 (A) Cerebellar atrophy shown by NMR scanning. (B) Thalamic glioma in an 8-year-old boy (arrow 1); the rise of interventricular pressure has led to transudation of CSF into the brain (arrow 2) shown by NMR scanning.

NUCLEAR MAGNETIC RESONANCE IMAGING
(NMR)

Nuclear magnetic resonance imaging is an advanced method of displaying the magnetic properties of the hydrogen atom nucleus, the proton. (The NMR spectral displays have been used in chemistry for 25 years). The patient is placed in a magnetic field and radiofrequency energy is applied from a coil surrounding the head, exciting the protons. By applying a second magnetic field or time-varying the fields, a NMR response may be induced from precise areas of the head. The images are computer processed like the CT scans. (Figures 8-19 A and B.)

Nuclear magnetic resonance has advanced rapidly, and the images are giving us information we did not have with other techniques. The NMR and CT scanning are different techniques imaging different physical properties, hence each has its uses; however the CT scan is likely to remain the investigative procedure for most routine investigations. Where NMR seems particularly useful is in displaying MS demyelination plaques, tumors, and vascular infarction changes, partly because it can differentiate gray and white matter (Fig. 8-20). The place of NMR in specific clinical situations will become clear over the next few years as experience grows and the technology advances.

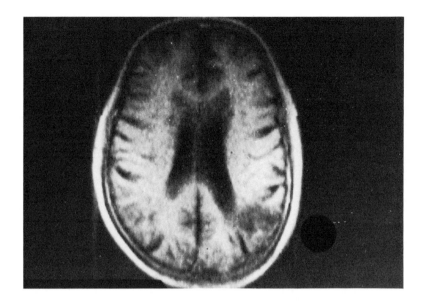

Figure 8-20   Nuclear magnetic resonance image showing posterior right cerebral infarction.

BIBLIOGRAPHY

Buonanno, F. (Ed.). Symposium on Neuroimaging; Neurologic Clinics. 2. Philadelphia, Saunders, 1984.

Dubowitz, V., Brooke, B.H. Muscle biopsy: A modern approach. In *Major Problems in Neurology,* Vol. 2. J.N. Walton (ed.). Philadelphia, W.B. Saunders Co., 1973.

Halliday, A.M. (Ed.). *Evoked Potentials in Clinical Testing.* Edinburgh, Churchill Livingstone, 1982.

Kiloh, L.G., McComas, A.J., Osselton, J.W. *Clinical Electroencephalography.* 3rd Ed. London, Butterworths.

Kimura, J. Principles and pitfalls of nerve conduction studies. *Ann. Neurology 16:* 415-429, 1984.

Locoge, M., Cumings, J.N. The cerebrospinal fluid in various diseases. *Br. Med. J. 1:*618, 1958.

Starr, A. Sensory evoked potentials in clinical disorders of the nervous system. *Ann. Rev. Neurosci. 1:*103-127, 1978.

Toole, J.F. (Ed.). *Special Techniques for Neurologic Diagnosis.* Contemporary Neurology Series. No. 4, Philadelphia, F.A. Davis Co., 1970.

II

LOCALIZATION IN THE NERVOUS SYSTEM

INTRODUCTION TO PART II

In this part of the book, we describe the meaning of the data acquired from the patient, partly by history but mainly by examination. Thus we include little about pathology and less about disease, but rather we are concerned with the sites in the nervous system that, when damaged, produce physical signs.

Localization is often difficult and some physical signs cannot be said to point to disease of any single brain part: memory is bilaterally represented; dementia is a diffuse disorder; coma implies reticular activating system (RAS) or generalized cortical disorders. However, many physical signs do allow one to say confidently that a particular nucleus, tract, or nerve is affected. Even then, as with loss of joint position sense in the left foot, the pathway along which the lesion lies may be 6 ft long and added signs are needed to enable one to say *where* along this path the problem lies. Long-tract signs are helpful, but a lower motor or first sensory neuron lesion affecting cranial or spinal nerves is the best guide to the precise level of the pathology.

Having elicited two signs, for example, a right third nerve palsy and a left pyramidal syndrome, localization is easy; the lesion is presumably where the right third nerve and corticospinal tract fibers destined for the left side are adjacent; in other words, in the midbrain on the right. Such is the basis of all localization. In this part, these principles will be described.

9

Localization of Disease

CEREBRAL HEMISPHERES

The cerebral hemispheres are two anatomical mirror images, consisting of a central core, mainly composed of white matter, and the basal ganglia overlaid by a convoluted covering of gray matter, the cortex. The basal ganglia and cortex are made up of neuronal cell bodies and the fibers that connect them. The white matter is made from medullated nerve fiber tracts that connect parts of the same hemisphere (association fibers), that connect the two hemispheres (commissural fibers), or that descend to or ascend from the brain stem and spinal cord (projection fibers).

In the last century, a concept developed of *centers* in the brain that are responsible for certain functions. We now recognize that there are indeed areas that subserve certain functions primarily but only because of their interconnection with other areas of function. Thus

A lesion in a hemisphere will cause loss of function because of destruction or alteration of the neurons or their long axons. This might show as paralysis, when the function of movement is no longer possible, or as excessive activity (a release phenomenon) such as clonus or spasticity, because the cells destroyed had formerly inhibited other neurons. Sometimes, clinical manifestations represent a compensatory mechanism whereby one part hyperfunctions to compensate for the failure of another.

Less commonly, a lesion in a hemisphere causes excitation or stimulation of neurons, which would cause activation of whatever function the area in question normally performs. A motor seizure would be an example of this.

An important principle in delineating a cerebral lesion is the concept of *contralaterality*; one hemisphere controls the opposite side of the body. Thus the right

129

hemisphere controls the motor and sensory function of the left side of the face and the left arm and leg. A second principle, that of *cerebral dominance,* states that certain functions are preferentially handled by one or the other hemisphere. Speech is a left hemisphere function in all right-handed people, and most left-handed, too. However the right hemisphere is dominant for the appreciation of nonlanguage sounds and visuospatial functions. Yet other activities are handled by both hemispheres — memory for example.

THE FRONTAL LOBES

The frontal lobes extend back from the frontal poles to the central sulcus. Their anterior portions are sometimes regarded as "silent areas" because the clinical effects of lesions there are subtle, but the posterior portions contain the motor strip where lesions cause paresis or paralysis[*] on the contralateral side of the body (Fig. 9-1A-C).

The motor strip is subdivided into areas that are more or less specifically involved with initiating movement of individual parts of the body on the other side. The body is topographically represented upside-down (see the diagrammatic homunculus, Fig. 9-2). The area activating the pharynx and larynx is lowest, just above the Sylvian fissure; above it, in ascending order, are the areas responsible for movement in the palate, mandible, tongue, lips, mouth, face, eyelids, forehead, neck, thumb, fingers, hand, wrist, forearm, arm, shoulder, upper thorax, diaphragm, lower thorax, abdomen, bladder, rectum and genitalia, thigh, leg, foot, and toes. The areas for the tongue, face, and digits are especially large and each finger is represented individually. This is undoubtedly the basis for the complex and isolated movements of these parts. The motor area gives rise to the corticobulbar and corticospinal (pyramidal) tracts, which descend through the internal capsule to the brainstem and spinal cord. A lesion damaging these pathways will result in weakness that mainly involves the distal parts; fine, skilled volitional movements are most affected. Because of the simultaneous involvement of the so-called extrapyramidal pathways (which arise from areas mainly anterior to the motor strip as well as from the basal ganglia), spasticity is added to the paralysis. The larynx, pharynx, palate, upper face, trunk, diaphragm, rectum, and bladder receive innervation from both hemispheres so are little affected by unilateral cortical lesions. If the lesion irritates neurons rather than destroys their function, then focal motor seizures may result.

Important fiber tracts from the middle frontal convolution, anterior to areas 7 and 8, run to the cerebellum. If they are damaged, gait disturbance is prominent (Brun's gait apraxia) and cerebellar signs appear, on the opposite side.

Area 8 in the frontal lobe is called the *frontal eye field.* It is the center for voluntary control of conjugate eye movement. Stimulation of this region induces deviation of the eyes to the opposite side, accompanied by turning of the head and trunk in the same direction. If the upper portion of this area is stimulated, the eyes deviate upward and to the other side; if the lower portion, the eyes move down and across. With this, the eyes may open wide and the pupils dilate. If these areas of cortex are destroyed — by a stroke, for example — the eyes will deviate *toward* the side of the lesion, being turned that way by the unopposed tonic action of the other, normal hemisphere.

The lowermost part of the motor and premotor regions on the dominant side is the motor speech or *Broca's* area. Lesions here cause dysphasia (see Chap. 14) which is predominantly expressive in type, although there is always at least some difficulty in speech comprehension.

---

[*]These terms are almost interchangeable but in common usage, paresis means weakness and paralysis a total loss of power.

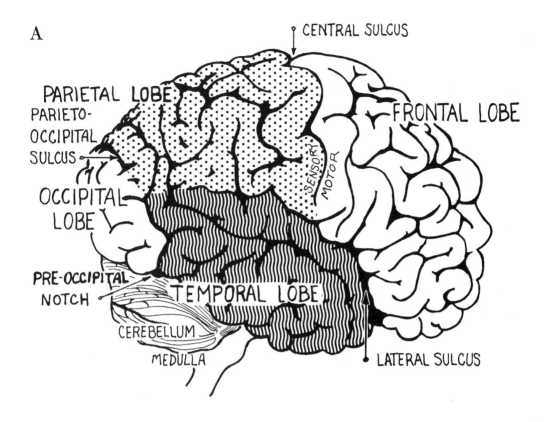

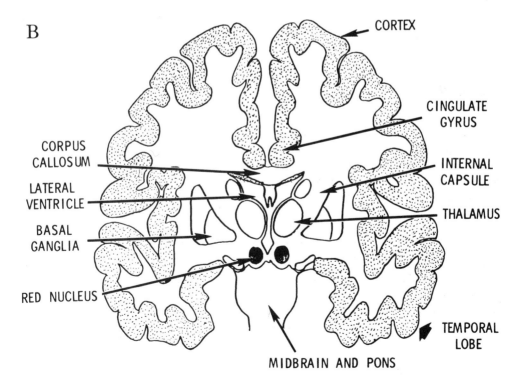

Figure 9-1 (A) Lateral aspect of the brain; (B) Coronal section of the brain.

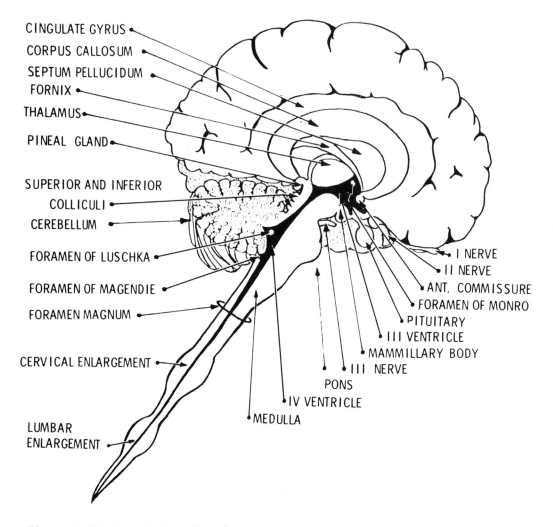

Figure 9-1C   Saggital section of the brain.

The large area of the frontal lobes lying anterior to the frontal eye field and speech area has wide connections with the visual, auditory, and other sensory areas by way of association fibers, and with the thalamus and hypothalamus by means of projection fibers. This frontal association area is often referred to as the prefrontal region — a poor term. It is conspicuously developed in man and has long been considered the seat of higher intellectual functions such as memory, judgment, foresight, and reasoning power, and of various perceptual, associative, and executive mental functions. This part of the brain is hard to study because experimental stimulation produces variable results, and destruction causes either subtle disturbances, or none at all.

The first indications of the functions of the frontal lobes was given in 1848, when a powder explosion blew a tamping iron through the left frontal lobe of a 25-year-old man, Mr. Phineas Gage, hitherto described as pious, quiet, responsible, and hard working. The missile made its exit just to the right of the coronal suture. The man lived another 13 years, and once traveled in Barnum's circus but was said

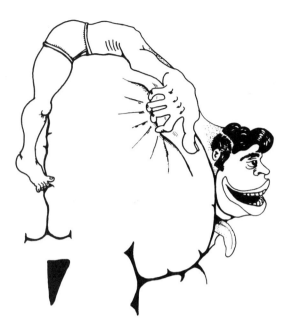

Figure 9-2   The motor homunculus.

to be now irreverent, profane, impatient of restraint, and unable to hold a job or make plans for his future. He was ". . . a child in his intellectual capacities, but with the general passions of a strong man."

Patients with frontal lesions, particularly bilateral ones, show diminished inhibition of affective responses, jocularity or euphoria, restlessness, loss of initiative, disturbed intellectual processes, loss of memory for details, and difficulty with mental associations. About a fifth of them will also show personality changes and a marked increase in appetite and weight. The personality changes may not interfere with normal social existence, but intellectual work is impaired. With unilateral frontal lobe lesions, no changes at all may be found, or there may be slight loss of initiative, and impaired imagination and abstract thought. The symptoms seem more marked if the left frontal lobe is removed from a right-handed individual.

Striking frontal lobe syndromes are seen in patients with degenerative conditions affecting the cortex diffusely, such as Alzheimer's disease. With the frontal cortical atrophy there occur loss of new-learning capacity, impaired judgment, e.g., in social and ethical situations, and loss of those patterns of behavioral restraint instilled over years of childhood training. Thus there may be demonstrated an increase in both natural and unnatural appetites, carelessness of dress and personal hygiene, sexual promiscuity, and loss of shame. The ability to perceive abstract relationships is impaired early, and these patients have great difficulty coping with new problems and situations. With shortened attention span, distractibility may be marked. Initiative, decision making, and ambition are impaired. Emotional lability is common, with quickly changing moods and outbursts of rage, weeping, or laughter. A striking frontal lobe sign (when it is present) is an euphoric affect with an increased sense of well-being, facetiousness, levity, and silly joking and punning, a state known by the German word *witzelsucht*. Primitive reflexes (see later discussion) are often released.

Thus the frontal association areas govern the higher intellectual and social development of man, being concerned in memory, judgment, association, reasoning, mental syntheses, abstract thinking, and restraint over emotional expression. The more automatic aspects of intelligence — such as remote memory and the ability to perform previously learned tasks — may be unaffected.

All lesions of the frontal lobe reduce seizure thresholds. Depending upon the site of focal damage, typical upper motor neuron lesions may be found. Lesions on the underside of the lobe may compress the olfactory nerve, causing anosmia.

One other localizing sign with frontal lesions is *urinary incontinence*. The para-central lobule on the medial aspect of the frontal lobes is involved in the control of bladder function, primarily by inhibiting the spinal reflexes controlling micturition. As a result, a lesion of the medial aspect of the frontal lobes, such as a parasagittal meningioma, may produce both the changes mentioned earlier and incontinence of urine. This is involuntary, and the patient may be surprised and embarrassed by it — unlike the patient with diffuse cortical atrophy, who, because of a lack of re-straint or control, does not seem to care.

Thus a patient suspected of having frontal lobe disease must be examined for his

1. *Mood:* Euphoric or depressed, irritable, often labile.
2. *Forward planning:* He may now be unable to do crosswords, to play chess, bridge, or any game of skill effectively; to plan his life for the next day, month, or year; or to foretell the consequences of actions put to him.
3. *Concentration:* Impersistence is common. The 100 − 7 test is useful here.
4. *Consistency:* His abilities in all aspects of activity may vary markedly from day to day.
5. *Memory:* This is frequently poor, mainly because of failure to attend to the material to be learned in the first place.
6. *Behavior:* Because lack of attention to the higher socializing rules of inter-personal behavior and of self-conduct is common, some of the patient's con-duct may be offensive, inappropriate, or ill regulated; and his level of personal care may decline. Focal motor, adversive, or grand mal seizures may also occur.

Formal testing may show

1. Reduction in all spheres of general awareness and knowledge of current events
2. Expressive speech disorder
3. Pyramidal tract dysfunction
4. Urinary incontinence

In addition, a number of signs of diffuse cerebral dysfunction may be detected. Those most useful in diagnosis have been identified by Jenkyn and his colleagues.*

1. Nuchocephalic reflex: The shoulders of the standing subject, whose eyes are closed, are turned briskly to the left/right and the position of the head is noted. The reflex is inhibited (normal) if the head actively turns in the direction of shoulder movement after a lag period of half a second or so. The reflex is dis-inhibited (abnormal) if the head remains in the original position. Movement of

---

*The descriptions of the tests given here are reproduced with slight adaptation from the work of Jenkyn et al. (see Bibliography) and are reproduced with his permission and that of the Editor of the *Journal of Neurology, Neurosurgery* and *Psychiatry.*

the head and shoulder en bloc, as may be seen with cervical spondylosis, obscure the reflex and prevent its assessment.

2. Glabellar tap: Persistent blinking is abnormal.
3. Suck reflex: The knuckle of the examiner's flexed finger is firmly placed between the patient's lips; there should be no response. Pursing of the lips or sucking is abnormal.
4,5. Conjugate gaze: The subject tries to follow the examiner's finger in all directions of gaze. Normally, at least 5 mm upward and 7 mm downward deviation of the globe from the midposition will be seen.
6. Visual tracking: The subject is asked to hold his head still, and to follow the examiner's finger as it moves between the extremes of horizontal gaze. The eyes should be seen to move smoothly; irregular, hesitant, or jerking saccades are abnormal.
7. Lateral gaze impersistence: The subject fixes his gaze on a finger held to the side for 30 sec. One deviation of gaze from the finger, or more than one deviation in each field, right and left, is abnormal.
8,9. Gegenhalten (paratonia): This has been described previously. It must be assessed in both arms and both legs.
10. Limb placement: The examiner holds the subjects arm up and tells him to relax, leaving the examiner to bear all the weight. He then releases his support, at which the patient's arm should fall. Any delay in dropping the arm suggests diffuse cortical damage, as long as the patient does not have parkinsonism or spasticity.
11. Three-item recall: The examiner enunciates three items (e.g., red, table, 23 Broadway) and asks the subject to repeat them. If this is found difficult, the words may be presented three times. The subject is told to remember them. They should be reproduced correctly both at the end of the learning period and 3 min later. Do not help by saying how many items there were.
12. Memory: Ask the subject to name past presidents, monarchs, or prime ministers of his country in reverse order from the present. Although this test is a function of age, most people should be able to recall the names of heads of state in their country since they were about 10 years old.
13. Spelling reversal: Ask the subject to spell the word *world* forward and backward.

Many other signs such as the grasp, palmomental and snout reflexes, and the plantar response, are also abnormal in diffuse cerebral dysfunction but they are less discriminatory than those just listed, and we have faith in this test battery. A patient with two or more positive responses needs formal psychological evaluation; more than seven indicates marked disturbance of cognitive function.

THE TEMPORAL LOBES

Destructive lesions may cause difficulty with equilibrium and a predominantly receptive dysphasia caused by involvement of Wernicke's area. The superior temporal gyri are the cortical areas concerned with the reception and analysis of auditory stimuli. A unilateral lesion does not cause deafness, but bilateral lesions may do so, rather uncommonly. Much of the temporal lobes are "silent" but this is largely because their functions are often shared bilaterally. Thus with memory, a unilateral lesion may have little effect, while bilateral damage leads to complete inability to retain new information for longer than a few seconds, which is a crippling mental deficit.

It was first shown by the late Dr. Wilder Penfield that stimulation of parts of the temporal lobes produces perceptual illusions; auditory, olfactory, and tactile hallucinations; automatisms; emotional responses; and vivid "memories" in conscious subjects at operation.

The uncus is a gyrus on the inferior and medial aspect of the temporal lobe. It is the cortical projection area for the sense of smell; thus seizures that emanate from this region may begin with an olfactory hallucination. In the analysis of focal seizures (type 2 in our classification) many of the symptoms elicited will be due to activation of temporal lobe structures, whether or not the seizure actually started there. Most of the symptoms listed under the heading *Psychological* in Chapter 15 have their origin in the temporal lobes. The same is true of automatisms, which are complex, formed patterns of movements that occur, outside the patient's control, as a result of the abnormal electrical discharge. The epigastric aura, and both visceral and some general sensory symptoms are similarly based on abnormal activation of this region.

The temporal lobes have lower thresholds for seizure activity than other areas of the brain. The events resulting from endogenous (i.e., epileptic) stimulation and variously known as *psychomotor, uncal,* or *complex partial* seizures include all those mentioned as occurring with electrical stimulation at operation; they are described in detail in Chapter 15.

THE PARIETAL LOBES

The parietal lobes are primarily sensory areas. The postcentral gyrus, just posterior to the central sulcus, is the primary sensory receptive area — the sensory strip, corresponding to the motor strip on the anterior lip of the sulcus and with a similar topographic representation. It receives a large projection from the thalamus in which impulses are relayed from the posterior columns, spinothalamic and trigeminal tracts, and from the reticular activating system (Fig. 9–3). These ascending fibers run upward in the posterior limb of the internal capsule and then radiate out to the sensory cortex. Behind the primary receptive area is the sensory association area that receives association fibers from the sensory strip and projection fibers from various thalamic nuclei.

The parietal lobes are largely involved with the reception, correlation, analysis, and elaboration of sensory impulses derived from the thalamus. Irritative lesions often result in dysesthesias, felt as tingling sensations in the contralateral half of the body. If irritation leads on to a focal sensory epileptic discharge, a pins-and-needles sensation or even lightninglike pains may be felt, as may an hallucination of movement of the limbs. Sometimes a Jacksonian march occurs, in which the abnormal sensations travel from their original site to other areas on that side of the body. *Destructive* lesions may cause loss of sensation or complex disturbances of sensory perception or interpretation. Some of these are unusually intriguing.

The Effects of Parietal Lobe Lesions

1. Appreciation of the *position* of the limbs in space is affected, particularly if the lesion is posterior. The outstretched arm and hand will droop or adopt an unusual posture, and the limb may show *sensory ataxia.* Appreciation of *passive movement* is also impaired, but *vibration* sense usually remains intact unless the lesion extends deeply.
2. *Tactile discrimination* is impaired. The patient will fail to identify objects placed in the hand *(astereognosis),* to identify figures drawn on his palm (loss of *graphesthesia),* to discriminate two closely-spaced points applied to a finger, and to discriminate the weight or texture of objects held in the hand.

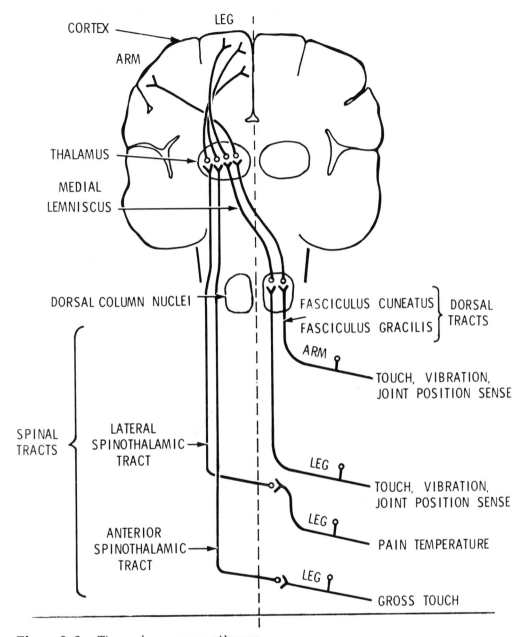

Figure 9-3   The main sensory pathways.

3. Tactile illusions and hallucinations may occur.
4. When localization of stimuli is impaired, the patient will fail to state where he was touched, e.g., by the examiner's finger.
5. Some complex problems occur with parietal lobe lesions. One tests for *tactile inattention* by stimulating two symmetric parts of the body at the same time. It is more often found with a right parietal lesion; the patient fails to perceive the stimulus given to the left side but is aware of that on the right, although he

would be aware of the left-sided stimulus were it given alone. These inattention or extinction phenomena also may be manifested in the visual and auditory
modalities. *Tactile perseveration* exists when a stimulus is applied repeatedly
and then stops, but the patient experiences a hallucination of the touch continuing; or the sensation of an object persists after it has been removed from the
hand. If a stimulus to one hand is projected to a corresponding point on the
other hand, it is known as *tactile projection*. The stimulus may be projected to
other parts of the body as well — thus the patient may say that he was touched
on the cheek. The most striking *disturbance of body image* is anosognosia, a
denial of the other side of the body and of its neurological deficit. Some patients merely use the side less, or ignore it, for instance shaving or applying
cosmetics only to the right side of the face (this is a sign seen with right-sided
parietal lesions). Others are unconcerned about their left hemiparesis, ration-
alize its existence, or they act as though unaware of it. Outside the body, the
ability to interpret correctly the relative positions of objects in space leads to
disorientation, to failure to localize familiar places on a map, and to maintain
normal "figure-ground" discriminations.
6. Gerstmann described a syndrome of
    a) Inability to recognize and name fingers
    b) Difficulty in distinguishing right from left
    c) Difficulty with writing
    d) Difficulty with calculations
    This syndrome results from lesions of the dominant (left) angular and supra-
    marginal gyri and the contiguous parts of the occipital lobe. Although there
    has been controversy about whether Gerstmann's syndrome is a real phenome-
    non or an artifact of our testing methods, these signs are often found together
    with left parietal lobe disease.
7. Distortion of the shape, size, or form of objects (*metamorphopsia*), and distor-
    tion of the speed of the passage of *time,* are other problems encountered.

Finally, many parietal lobe lesions give rise to specific disturbances called
agnosias and apraxias, which will be discussed in the following sections.

Agnosias

Failure to comprehend the nature, use, or qualities of objects perceived, in the absence of dementia and of significant sensory deficits, are *agnosias*. Such failure
may affect any channel — visual, tactile, auditory — and may affect the patients
awareness of his own body image. Agnosias are to nonlanguage functions what receptive dysphasias are to those that do involve language. Some involve one parietal
lobe, some both, but most are due to disease affecting the dominant supramarginal
gyrus. They will be considered in four major groups.

Visuospatial Agnosia

The patient cannot recognize by sight objects or people known to him. Shown a
key, he may describe its color, shape, and size but does not know its function or
name until he touches it. When he does so, he will name it unless he is dysphasic.
If he *is* dysphasic, ask him whether what he feels is a watch, pen, coat, key, door,
or so on. If he agrees that it is a key, then he does not have agnosia. If he still
fails to recognize it as a key when the word, with others, is given to him, he probably has.

Test: Using common objects — key, book, pen, watch, tissues, etc. Subtypes of visual agnosia include

1. *Prosopagnosia:* An inability to recognize the faces of known people.
2. *Artistic agnosia:* A failure to recognize the content of pictures, photographs or simple drawings.
3. *Simultagnosia:* Also operative in the fields of sound, space, and touch, this problem lies somewhere between agnosia and hemianopia. If stimuli such as lights, moving hands, etc., are presented singly to each side, then they are perceived; but if they are presented on each side simultaneously, then that on the side opposite to the damaged cortex (usually the right) is ignored. This is also known as sensory competition, extinction, or visual inattention (see earlier discussion).
4. *Spatial agnosia:* If there is simultagnosia, then understandably (since the whole of the visual field is being presented to one all of the time) one-half of the field will extinguish the other — a state hardly distinguishable from hemianopsia. If, for example, the left field is thus extinguished, then objects on that side, e.g., the left side of a picture, will tend to be ignored in favor of those on the right side. Neglect of half of space results. (Fig. 9-4A.)

Test: By noting whether or not the patient can place a cross accurately on the center of a line; draw a clock face or a star (copying the latter); and identify objects in a field, such as random spots or stars on a piece of paper (see Table 9-1 and Fig. 9-4B).

The ability to identify a map of his country, province, or state, or to localize towns on such a map may also fail. Such geographical disorientation is another form of spatial agnosia, because we rely mainly on vision for spatial orientation.

Auditory Agnosia

Failure to identify objects or people by their sound is uncommon. In testing, non-language stimuli must be used.

Test: See if the patient can identify the sounds of paper crumpled or torn, money or keys rattled, or fingers snapped outside his field of vision or with the eyes closed. Recognition of musical themes or of people by their voices may also be impaired.

Body Image Agnosia

This occurs when the patient fails to recognize, accept, or identify his own or another's body part by sight or touch. Of the many signs, only a few will be mentioned.

1. Inability to point out specific fingers when given their names; this may apply also to the sides of the body, so that left and right sides are mistaken.
2. Failure to identify a finger or other part of the body named by the examiner.
3. Denial of the existence of half his body; if it is diseased — e.g., hemianopia or hemiplegia — he may deny that there is anything wrong with it. This agnosia is usually caused by a right-sided lesion (see previous discussion).
4. Inability to localize a single stimulus, or even more likely, stimuli presented to both sides simultaneously (again the phenomenon of extinction). This failure of localization is known as *autotopagnosia.*

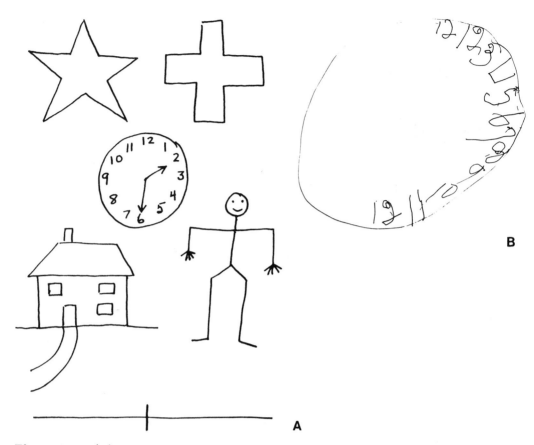

Figure 9-4 (A) Drawing tests useful in assessing parietal lobe function. (B) The clock here is drawn all on the right in a man with a right parietal syndrome causing neglect of the left side. Ask the patient to draw a star, open cross, clock face, house, and a stick man; and to divide a line which you have drawn, making a mark at it's center.

5. Rarely, a tactile stimulus is displaced so that if a patient's hands are placed on a table and one of them is touched by the examiner, the patient may claim that the examiner touched the table, not his hand.
6. Gerstmann's syndrome (discussed earlier) includes finger agnosia and right/left indiscrimination.

Tactile Agnosia

Tactile agnosia consists of failure to recognize and identify objects by touch. When they are seen or heard however, identification may be quite normal. This failure of recognition occurs in the absence of any impairment of common sensory or proprioceptive function. Such abnormalities can only be identified by determining that the patient is aware of the stimulus but fails to integrate the various qualities of the sensation to enable its interpretation. Thus he may describe the size, shape, weight, edge, surface, and temperature of a coin held in the hand but fail to identify it as a coin.

Table 9-1   Summary of the Main Tests for Agnosias

Visuospatial

> Visual recognition of objects and faces
> Bilateral visual stimulation
> Localization of places on maps
> Drawing a clock face, a star, a house

Auditory

> Recognition of simple sounds — money, paper, keys

Body image

> Naming fingers
> Pointing out named fingers
> Right-left discrimination
> Localization of tactile stimuli

Tactile

> Identification on numbers traced, or coins placed in the hand
> Two-point discrimination
> Simultaneous bilateral touch

Test: By asking for identification of such common objects as coins, pencils, a ring, and so on, placed in his hand (unseen and unheard); by asking for identification of numbers drawn on the palm of his hand with an orange-stick; or by testing two-point discrimination.

Again, presentation of double stimuli, e.g., touching both hands, cheeks, or legs simultaneously, may lead to extinction of one stimulus; thus the patient may feel only the touch given on the same side as the damaged cortex.

Apraxias

Apraxias are defects in the performance of motor actions in patients who have no weakness, incoordination, or sensory loss. Four types are usually described, but the differences between the first two are fine and of slight clinical importance.

Ideomotor Apraxia

While the subject may succeed in performing simple acts quite normally (such as scratching his nose, opening doors, or crossing his arms) this is so only when the motivation is internal. In other words, the movements are automatic. When he tries to imitate them on seeing them performed by the examiner, or to perform them on request, he will fail to conceptualize and thus to carry them out. The lesion is usually on the left, in the region of the angular gyrus.

Test: Ask the patient to do any of the things just mentioned; to imitate a meaningful gesture such as a salute, beckoning, or waving goodbye; or to mime such an activity as lighting a match or using a key to open a door.

Ideational Apraxia

In ideational apraxia, the patient is aware of what is to be done but cannot synthesize the movements required to do it, even though he is able to perform the various parts of the whole movement in isolation. Thus he may be able to grasp, or loop, or pull on a piece of string, but he cannot tie a knot on command.

This has been described as the disruption of the normal sequence of manipulation required for the use of common objects; even though the patient can understand the nature of the desired end result, he cannot conceive of how to do it in its entirety — to put together all those small movements that build up into meaningful action. Most patients with this problem also have some form of dysphasia, usually of the receptive type, and again, the lesion is usually in left parieto-occipital areas.

Test: Ask the patient to comb his hair, to use scissors, or use a toothbrush.

Constructional Apraxia

Here, subjects fail in tasks demanding the arrangement of two- or three-dimensional shapes to conform with patterns. As a result, they will be unable to draw a star, a man, or a house, etc., and to copy designs using matches or blocks. The whole problem may be based on a visuospatial agnosia, so it is not surprising that the lesion is in the right parietal lobe.

Dressing Apraxia

Possibly again no more than the expression of a body-image agnosia; usually caused by a lesion in the nondominant (right) parietal lobe, dressing apraxia constitutes a failure to fit clothes, a mold of the body, to the body itself.

Test: Ask the patient to put on his coat. To make it harder, if you feel sneaky, pull one sleeve inside-out before giving it to him. The sequence of activities required to produce a desired movement includes an understanding of the effect to be achieved, an ability to synthesize the pattern of movements that have to be performed, and a capacity actually to do them. The first fails in ideomotor apraxia, the second in ideational apraxia. The third fails with palsies or motor incoordination. All depend initially upon the patient's ability to comprehend the commands in the first place, so receptive dysphasia will negate any meaningful results of testing for apraxias.

OCCIPITAL LOBES

The occipital lobes are concerned with vision. The poles are the primary reception area for visual stimuli, and the interpretative cortex lies anteriorly, between the occipital, temporal, and parietal lobes. Homonymous hemianopia is the usual result of unilateral damage, with the saving grace of sparing the central 10° of (macular) vision in cases of stroke because of anastomoses between the posterior and middle cerebral arteries in the overlying pia mater. Such sparing is not found with other destructive lesions in the region.

Bilateral occipital ischemia, as with severe anoxia or bilateral posterior cerebral artery occlusions, leads to *cortical blindness,* in which state the patient cannot see, although he may deny it (Anton's syndrome). Normal pupillary reactions remain, since their pathway runs from the lateral geniculate body to the superior colliculi without involving the cortex. In mild ischemia, as with fainting, the visual loss may consist only of a "closing-out" of vision followed by brief subtotal loss.

Irritative lesions produce visual hallucinations — unformed flashes of light, spots, stars, etc., from the pole and more formed images such as shapes, or even faces or places when the damage is further forward. In one peculiar but memorable phenomenon the patient goes on seeing something after it has moved away or he has transferred his gaze from it. This persisting visual hallucinatory state has been called *palinopsia;* it is rare indeed.

NONSPECIFIC CEREBRAL SIGNS

Patients with localized, or with diffuse brain disease, may present with symptoms or signs which, although not localizing, do indicate cerebral damage. Many have been described previously. Others include *impaired concentration; disorientation in time, place, or person; poverty of speech and movement; slowness;* and *organic orderliness.* Perseveration is another such sign.

Perseveration

The continuation or repetition of an activity without the appropriate stimulus, so that the activity persists after the subject has consciously attempted to change it, is known as perseveration. This persistence of the primary activity is shown by a transient interference with the next activity. Among children, the aged, the people who are fatigued, dysphasic, clouded, or brain damaged from any cause, but especially those with frontal lobe disease, this is a common sign. It is usually first noticed by the examiner when the patient repeats words, phrases, or whole replies during the history, or when perseveration interrupts the physical examination if the patient persistently makes the same response to different directions.

One may document perseveration by getting the subject to write *S*s, followed by reversed *S*s, changing between ordinary and reversed letters at command. Another useful test is to ask him to find four or five coins which you have "hidden" (while he was watching) under books, bedclothes, etc. He may keep looking in the same place. Object naming, writing to dictation, and copying may also be useful because in each case the patient continues to make the same stereotyped response when it is no longer appropriate.

THE BRAINSTEM

The brainstem (medulla, pons, and mesencephalon) is located entirely in the posterior fossa. Crowded into this small area are the nuclei for cranial nerves III through XII, the sensory and motor pathways running between the cerebral hemispheres, cerebellum, and spinal cord, and the reticular activating system. Because the anatomy of this region is complex, with many structures crowded together, small and discrete lesions often produce devastating and widespread symptoms and signs. However for the same reasons, it often is quite easy to localize a lesion in this area.

A lesion in the brainstem will give rise to signs based on the structures involved (Fig. 9-5). The major structures can be classified as those that originate

1. In the brainstem and terminate elsewhere
2. Elsewhere and terminate in the brainstem
3. And terminate outside the brainstem
4. And terminate within the brainstem

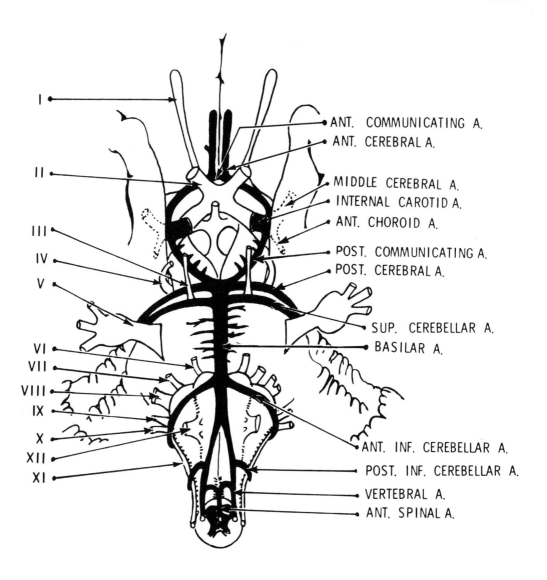

Figure 9-5   Cranial nerves and major blood vessels at the base of the brain.

Fibers that Originate in the Brainstem and Terminate Elsewhere

All of the cranial nerves except the first and second have their exit or entry in the brainstem. The presence of a cranial nerve lesion thus is an excellent guide to the precise level of the lesion.

Fibers that Originate Elsewhere and Terminate in the Brainstem

Supranuclear fibers arise in the cerebral hemispheres and descend through the internal capsule to the motor nuclei of the brainstem. These corticomesencephalic and corticobulbar pathways provide supranuclear control over cranial nerve motor functions. Most run to motor nuclei on *both* sides. Thus it requires bilateral cerebral lesions to cause the disturbance of motor function called *pseudobulbar palsy*. This results in an impassive face resulting from bilateral facial weakness (upper motor neuron type); difficulty in swallowing; dysarthria; weakness of tongue protrusion; and pathological emotionality — laughing or crying. This last is an explosive emotional outburst unaccompanied by the appropriate feelings in the patient who may weep but, when asked, denies any sad feelings.

The spinocerebellar pathways also terminate at this level but in the cerebellum.

Fiber Systems that Originate and Terminate Outside the Brainstem

Most important here are the *corticospinal tracts*. A lesion involving one of them will produce an upper motor neuron syndrome on the opposite side of the body. At the level of the medulla, the corticospinal tracts decussate, hence a lesion below this level will produce signs on the same side. Another important fiber system running through the brainstem is the *sympathetic* pathway. It originates in the hypothalamus and passes through the brainstem to the thoracolumbar cord. Damage to this system causes a Horner's syndrome (Chap. 21) on the same side.

The ascending fiber systems passing through the brainstem are the sensory pathways. The *medial lemniscus* carries impulses mediating position sense, tactile discrimination, and probably vibration; and the spinothalamic tracts carry impulses giving information about pain, temperature, and crude light touch. Both terminate in the thalamus. Fibers originating in the cerebellum and destined for the basal ganglia, motor cortex, spinal cord (and brainstem) also belong in this group. Lesions affecting them produce cerebellar signs, almost always on the same side (see the following).

Fibers that Originate and Terminate Within the Brainstem

Two intrinsic fiber systems descend to the cervical cord but return within the brainstem; these are the median longitudinal fasciculi and the spinal nucleus and tract of the fifth nerve. The *median longitudinal fasciculus* (MLF) is important as the coordinator of eye movements through the third, fourth, and sixth nerve nuclei of each side. A lesion of the MLF will result in a failure of coordinated eye movements, which may be shown as the characteristic internuclear ophthalmoplegia (see Chap. 21). Because the trigeminal *spinal nucleus and tract* extends down from the brainstem as far as C-3, brainstem or high cervical lesions may cause loss of pain and temperature sensation over that side of the face (other sensory modes are handled in the principal sensory nucleus of the fifth nerve, in the pons). Input from the ninth and tenth nerves also reaches this tract. The *reticular activating system* (RAS) is a diffuse, anatomically indistinct system of neurons and fiber tracts extending from the low brainstem up to the thalamus and above. It is a complex network with multisynaptic connections and is primarily involved in the maintenance of consciousness by activation of the cortex and in controlling sleep rhythm and muscle tone through the gamma system. It projects to the whole of the cortex and limbic lobes through the central tegmental tract as well as downward through the reticulospinal tract. Through the vestibular system it has both inhibitory and facilitatory effects on muscle tone. The RAS receives afferent input from all ascending sensory pathways as well as from the cerebellum, basal ganglia, and cortex.

FUNCTIONAL ANATOMY OF THE BRAINSTEM

At the *cervicomedullary junction* (Fig. 9-6) intrinsic lesions such as syringomyelia or ischemic infarcts may damage the pyramidal fibers, which are crossing at this point, producing upper motor neuron signs in either limb. This is below the level of the twelfth nerve nucleus, thus the tongue will be spared. Extrinsic lesions such as meningiomas or the Arnold-Chiari malformation may compress the eleventh (spinal accessory) nerve fibers ascending here and also cause pyramidal tract damage. At this level, the spinal nucleus and tract of nerve V contain only fibers from the first division of the nerve, so any pain and temperature loss will be confined to that area unless contralateral loss is caused by involvement of the adjacent ascending spinothalamic tract. The dorsal columns are often spared by lesions at this level. In the Arnold-Chiari syndrome (see Chap. 50) hydrocephalus and cerebellar signs may be expected, in addition, the latter resulting from tonsillar distortion rather than to spinocerebellar tract compression.

In the *low medulla* (Fig. 9-7) local lesions, such as infarcts, may involve the twelfth nerve and parts of the ninth-tenth nuclear complex, resulting in atrophy of the tongue and combinations of dysphonia, dysarthria, dysphagia, and sensory loss in the oropharyngeal and palatal regions. Myoclonus and alterations in blood pressure, consciousness, and respiratory rate and depth may also occur. If one pyramid is involved, upper motor neuron signs will be found on the other side, and as with lesions at the decussation, the arm or leg may be more affected. Sympathetic fiber involvement leads to Horner's syndrome of the same side. Sensory losses are due to lesions of the spinal nucleus and tract of the fifth nerve now affecting the first and second divisions of the nerve, and with spinothalamic tract damage, this all leads to *alternating thermoanalgesia* in which the face on the side of the lesion, and the trunk and limbs on the opposite side lose pain and temperature sensation. The medial lemniscus is formed here by the decussation of fibers arising from the gracile and cuneate nuclei, so proprioception may be involved on one or the other side.

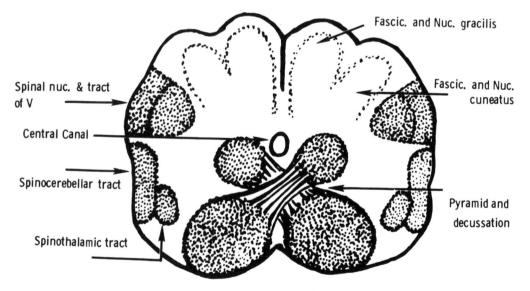

Figure 9-6   T/S Cervicomedullary junction.

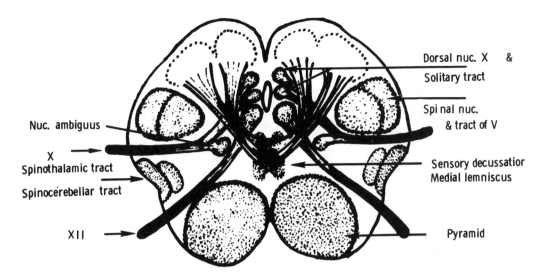

Dorsal nuc. X   &
Solitary tract

Spinal nuc.
& tract of V

Nuc. ambiguus

X
Spinothalamic tract

Spinocerebellar tract

Sensory decussation
Medial lemniscus

XII

Pyramid

Figure 9-7   T/S Low medulla.

At the *midmedullary* level (Fig. 9-8), pathologies include tumors, infarcts, encephalitis, and demyelination. Some vagal motor fibers are present at this level
(the superior salivary nucleus). The pyramids, medial lemnisci, and medial longitudinal fasciculi lie centrally and may be affected by some of these diseases. In
the *lateral medullary syndrome* they are spared. In this condition, infarction in the
territory of the posteroinferior cerebellar artery damages the inferior cerebellar
peduncle producing homolateral cerebellar signs; the descending sympathetic pathway (Horner's syndrome); the spinal nucleus and tract of nerve V and the spinothalamic tracts (alternating thermoanalgesia); and the vestibular nuclei (vertigo and
vomiting). Unilateral damage to the cochlear nuclei has little clinical effect, as
hearing functions are represented bilaterally, even at this low level. Damage to the
nucleus ambiguus is shown by dysarthria, dysphagia, and dysphonia. The olive usually escapes damage; if affected, more severe cerebellar signs are seen. Hiccups and
myoclonic jerks (see Chap. 15) are common although nonspecific signs of medullary
lesions.

At *midpontine* levels (Fig. 9-9), involvement of the sixth and seventh nerves
help to localize a lesion. Depending upon how central or peripheral it is, any combination of cerebellar and pyramidal signs occur. Involvement of the descending
sympathetic paths may occur, producing pinpoint pupils, and one or both MLFs may
be involved (internuclear ophthalmoplegia). Damage to the superior and lateral
vestibular nuclei again causes vertigo. Although also occurring with cerebellar lesions, ocular bobbing (oscillations of the eyes up and down at the same speed in
each direction) usually indicates the presence of a serious pontine lesion. Central
lesions damaging the RAS may cause coma or akinetic mutism (Chap. 10). Because
lesions here may damage the thermoregulatory center, high fever may occur.

Masses at the *cerebellopontine angle* compress and distort the fibers of the
fifth, seventh, and eighth nerves and of the middle cerebellar peduncle, but the
medial lemnisci and pyramidal fibers are spared, at least until the tumor attains
a huge size.

At a higher level still (Fig. 9-10) the ascending sensory tracts have begun to
form a crescent, migrating laterally so that the lateral and medial lemnisci are

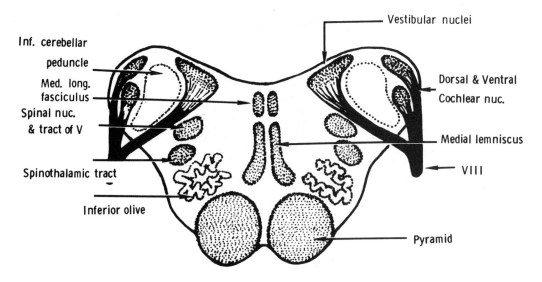

Figure 9-8   T/S Midmedulla.

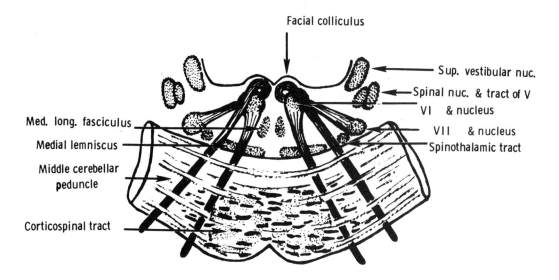

Figure 9-9   T/S Midpons.

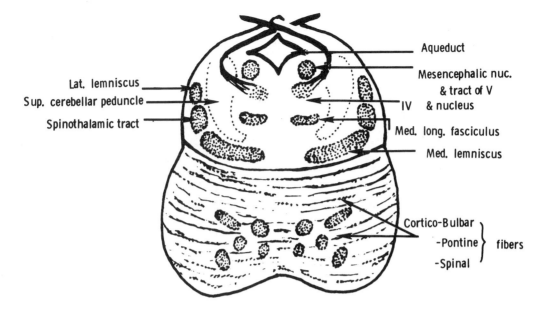

Figure 9-10   T/S Brainstem at pontomesencephalic junction.

now likely to be involved together, leading to sensory loss in all modalities on the opposite side of the face and body. Lesions of the anterior part (the tegmentum) of the *low mesencephalon* produce upper motor lesions in the cranial nerves caudal to this level and in the limbs on the other side because the corticobular and cortico-spinal pathways cross at lower levels. The superior cerebellar peduncle is another structure that may be damaged by lesions here; homolateral cerebellar signs result. Involvement of the MLF, sympathetic pathways, and the fourth nerve nucleus cause, respectively, internuclear ophthalmoplegia, Horner's syndrome, and isolated fourth nerve palsy on the opposite side.[*]

Extrinsic lesions here, as at the next higher level, may compress and obstruct the aqueduct with a resulting increase in intracranial pressure.

Many vessels supply the *midbrain* structures shown in Figure 9-11 and ischemic lesions are the most common problems here. A third nerve palsy is the prime local-izing sign. With damage to the cerebral peduncle, a contralateral hemiplegia re-sults. Because the third nerve palsy is on one side and the face and limb weakness on the other, this is known as an "alternating" hemiplegia. As with intrinsic lesions at any level of the brainstem, coma or at least some alteration of consciousness is likely because of involvement of the RAS. Damage to the red nucleus produces a rather gross static and kinetic tremor, like that of bad cerebellar disease. If the

---

[*] The fourth nerve decussates; no other cranial nerve does.

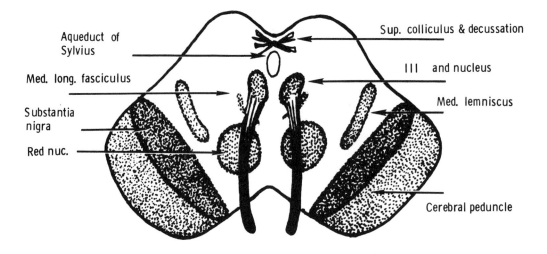

Figure 9-11   T/S Midbrain at the level of the superior colliculus.

parasympathetic nuclei associated with the third nerve (e.g., Edinger-Westphal) are
also affected, there will be impairment of the pupillary reactions to light and accomodation. Compression of the superior colliculi leads to paresis of upward gaze,
a useful localizing sign; another is the (rare) form of nystagmus in which the eyes
retract jerkily in their sockets — retraction nystagmus. The sensory fibers are all
gathered closely together as they approach the ventoposterior thalamic nuclei, and
sensory loss in all modes will be found on the other side of the face and body if the
lemniscus is involved. Damage to the substantia nigra is overshadowed by the involvement of the peduncles, hence parkinsonism will be seen with a compressive
lesion. This is one of the sites where a single small lesion, between the peduncles,
may cause bilateral corticospinal signs. Parasagittal masses and central cord lesions may do this as well.

THE CEREBELLUM

The cerebellum or "little brain" consists of paired hemispheres of convoluted folia
separated by an unpaired median vermis and some primitive — but vital — nuclei.
The cerebellum is primarily concerned with the control of postural tone and with
the coordination of movements.

The brain is often compared to a computer, but this is a poor analogy except
in the case of the cerebellum, which really does appear to function similarly. Coordination of movement is carried out by the cerebellum acting upon information
that it obtains from muscle spindles (degree of stretch and change in tension of
muscles), the vestibular apparatus (position and acceleration in space), and the cortex, i.e., conscious and unconscious proprioceptive information. Acting on this, the
cerebellum controls the *rate, range, direction, and force* of voluntary movements,
and through its close vestibular connections, it monitors and maintains the body's
upright position in space. If this cerebellar control is lost, then rapid and coordinated muscle movements are impossible, and the upright position may be unattain-
able.

Cerebellar lesions produce the following signs.

1. Hypotonia
2. Truncal ataxia
3. Nystagmus
4. Limb ataxia: dysmetria, dysdiadokokinesis, decomposition of movement
5. Scanning speech
6. Kinetic ("intention" or "action") tremor

Disease affecting the vestibular connections of the cerebellum, which are mainly with the flocculonodular lobe and the vermis, leads to the mild hypotonia commonly present with cerebellar disease. This is hard to assess by the usual method of suddenly moving joints and is best detected either by (1) having the patient put his elbows on a table, keeping the forearms vertical; the affected wrist will then droop more than the normal one; or (2) by eliciting the knee jerk with the leg hanging free; there will be prolonged swinging of the leg — the "pendular" reflex. Postural changes such as drooping of the affected shoulder and lateral tilt of the head are described but are easy to miss.

Truncal ataxia cannot be demonstrated when the patient is lying supine. However if he is asked to sit up in bed or to stand up, severe dysequilibrium prevents him from doing so, even with the support of his arms. In less severe cases, the gait suggests marked drunkedness such that the subject reels or staggers, predominantly to the side of the lesion, if this is unilateral. (In fact, because alcohol is a potent short-term as well as long-term cerebellar poison, the police are in the habit of testing cerebellar function as clinical, or at least roadside, evidence of alcohol intoxication.) Nystagmus of the central type (see Chap. 21) is traceable to damage of the flocculonodular lobe, but cannot be distinguished from that produced by damage to the brainstem vestibular nuclei, even by the police.

Ataxia of voluntary limb movements is a blanket term covering dysmetria (overshooting or past-pointing and falling short of targets), dysdiadokokinesis, and decomposition of movements. All of these result from the failure of cerebellar control over the rate, range, or force of voluntary movements. Any deviation from the course that the limb was programmed to take will be corrected late and either too much or too little. The resulting new course command will again be delayed and the resulting movement maladroit. In the finger-nose test, this causes the extended finger to over- or undershoot the target, or to veer to one side. This is *dysmetria.* Beware of calling a movement dysmetric however, if the patient does not have binocular vision.

Dysdiadokokinesis is a precious word in neurology.* The word signifies difficulty in performing alternating movements rapidly and accurately, because of lateral lobe disease. The finger-nose and heel-shin tests, rapid tapping or drumming of the fingers on a flat surface, and rapid supination and pronation of the forearm are the usual clinical maneuvers used to detect this evidence of failure of the central coordinating mechanisms that regulate precise voluntary movements. Decomposition of movement (which you can hear in *scanning speech*) is yet another result of the same failures in which movements are not flowing and smooth but rather disjointed and jerky, being split up into their components so that a simple action looks as though it were being performed by a badly-handled puppet.

---

* You may interpret "precious" as you wish. We regard the word *dysdiadokokinesis* as a neurological shibboleth (Judges XII, 4-6). It is derived from classic Greek words signifying difficulty, a follower, and movement.

Intention tremor reflects a failure of the lateral lobes to smooth out voluntary limb movements. Deviations from the required course are corrected excessively or inadequately. As a limb is extended, it oscillates over a wider arc until, when the target is finally reached and voluntary movement (as opposed to maintenance of a posture) ceases, the tremor ceases too. Failure of control of antagonistic muscle contraction and of deviations from the course set for a limb accounts for *rebound* that is seen, for example, when the patient stretches the arms out in front of him, one is pressed down by the examiner against the patient's resistance, and the pressure is suddenly removed. Now the arm flies up in the air, well above the other, because the compensatory halting of this upward movement is delayed; the movement is unchecked. Since all of these abnormalities are due to the loss of efferent control, no amount of afferent information (proprioceptive or visual) will be able to correct them. In this context, it is worth repeating that Romberg's test examines afferent proprioceptive and not efferent, cerebellar functions.

SPINAL CORD

In localizing a lesion of the spinal cord, one must ask three questions. First, where is the lesion in the longitudinal axis of the cord — what is the level of the lesion? Second, how much of the cord is affected — what is the horizontal extent of the disease? Third, is the problem intrinsic (within the cord) or extrinsic (outside it, either inside or outside the dura)? *Intramedullary* and *extramedullary* are terms with the same meaning.

Signs Determining the Level of the Lesion

Lower Motor Neuron Lesion

Examination may show muscle atrophy, possibly deformity, and trophic changes; diminution of tone and power involving *muscles* rather than gross *movements*; incoordination secondary to that lack of power; and reduction or loss of tendon reflexes (Fig. 9-12) at the level of cord involvement. Major muscle innervation and reflex root values are shown in Chapter 2.

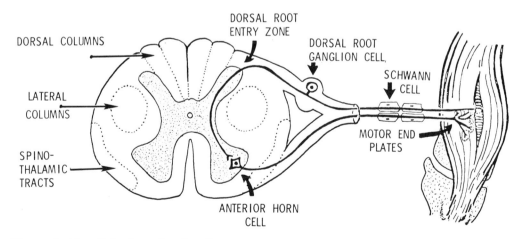

Figure 9-12   Spinal cord and reflex arc.

Upper Motor Neuron Lesion

Signs will be found on the same side below the level of the cord lesion because the corticospinal fibers crossed higher up at the decussation of the pyramids. If the cord lesion is, for example, at C6, then the biceps jerk will be normal, the brachioradialis diminished or absent, and the triceps, knee, and ankle jerks increased. The plantar response will be upgoing on that side.

Radicular Sensory Involvement

Sensory changes from cord or root involvement often cause *pain,* especially if the lesion is extrinsic rather than intrinsic. Girdle pain is sharp, stabbing, or burning and is referred in the area of the whole dermatome. The pain occurs spontaneously but is also precipitated by movement or by spinal percussion at the affected level. Sometimes coughing, sneezing, or straining will aggravate the pain by elevating CSF pressure; this in turn deforms the dura and stretches nerve roots. *Altered sensation* will be detected on the trunk only if the lesion affects a number of segments, because of the marked overlap of spinal nerves. In the limbs a single root lesion may well produce sensory change in the one dermatome. With some extrinsic spinal lesions such as neoplasms, herpes zoster (shingles) develops in the distribution of the affected root.

Sensory Level

A definite segmental level below which posterior column or spinothalamic sensations are diminished or lost is the single most helpful sign in localizing a cord lesion. The transition from abnormal to normal may be quite distinct and is especially easy to determine on the trunk. The sensory level with posterior column disease is at the level of the lesion; with spinothalamic tract lesions it may be one or two segments lower, because the entering fibers ascend for one or two segments on the same side of the cord before crossing to the other (damaged) side.

Vertebral Column Abnormalities

These include *deformity* such as angulation or scoliosis and *tenderness* on local percussion, which is a useful localizing sign with both intrinsic and extrinsic disease. Local *muscle spasm* is common but seldom of localizing value.

Signs Determining the Extent of Spinal Involvement

Motor

Corticospinal tract dysfunction leads to signs of an upper motor neuron lesion. On inspection, there may be abnormal posture such as shoulder adduction, elbow flexion, pronation at the wrist and finger flexion, and external rotation of the leg with hip and knee extension and plantar flexion at the ankle — the typical posture seen with pyramidal tract lesions. In the event of a long-standing cortical upper motor neuron lesion, failure of growth may occur in the affected limb. Tone will be increased *(spasticity)* and power will be dimished in pyramidal distribution. Thus as may be expected from the postural changes already described, there will be particular weakness of shoulder abduction, elbow extension, wrist dorsiflexion, and finger extension in the upper limb, and of hip and knee flexion and ankle dorsiflexion and eversion in the lower. The muscle groups antagonistic to these movements will also be weaker than normal but less markedly so. *Deep tendon reflexes* will be hyper-active, superficial reflexes lost, and *abnormal reflexes* may appear, such as the upgoing Babinski's plantar response. Lesions involving both sides of the cord may lead to urgency and frequency of *micturition* because of spastic bladder and to *impotence*. Such problems should not occur with unilateral lesions.

Sensory

Posterior column dysfunction is shown by diminished joint position, passive move-ment, tactile discrimination, and deep pain sensations in all regions of the body be-low the lesion on the same side. Vibration sense, probably carried diffusely and in the dorsal spinocerebellar tracts, is also reduced.

   With dysfunction of the *spinothalamic tracts,* crude light touch, sharp pain, scratch, tickle, and itch sensations are almost always involved together. Here, in-stead of the lesion producing signs on the same side, reduction or loss of these modalities will be found contralaterally, usually starting a couple of segments be-low the site of cord damage.

   With corticospinal tract damage, it is impossible to tell whether or not there is involvement of the spinocerebellar tracts. When they are affected, one may still be unable to detect cerebellar signs because of the multiple inputs into the cerebellum. Nevertheless, by putting together all of the long tract, radicular sen-sory, and lower motor enuron signs, one can usually assess the extent of the damage within the cord at the involved level.

Signs Differentiating Between
Intrinsic and Extrinsic Cord Lesions

It is often hard to tell the difference between an intrinsic and extrinsic cord lesion (Fig. 9-13). The following simple signs may help you to do so, but sometimes both kinds of problem occur together; for example, a tumor that compresses the cord may induce secondary hemorrhage within it. Because of this overlap, a myelogram and CT scan are usually needed to supplement clinical observation.

   Intrinsic lesions are more likely in the presence of

1. Lhermitte's sign
2. *Early* long-tract signs
3. *Early* bladder involvement
4. *Bilateral* signs
5. Involvement of anterior horn cells (fasciculations)
6. Dissociated anesthesia (see following)
7. Normal CSF indices

   Extrinsic lesions tend to produce

1. Root pain
2. Signs explicable on the basis of a unilateral lesion
3. *Later* appearance of long tract signs
4. *Later* appearance of bladder involvement
5. Abnormal CSF, and myelographic evidence of partial or complete spinal block

Dissociated Anesthesia

This is exemplified by the classic *Brown-Sequard syndrome,* caused by hemisection or lateral compression of the cord, in which dorsal column loss is present on one

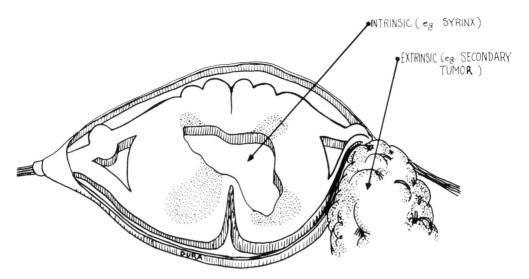

INTRINSIC (e.g. SYRINX)

EXTRINSIC (e.g. SECONDARY TUMOR)

Figure 9-13   Intrinsic and extrinsic cord lesions.

side of the body below a spinal lesion and spinothalamic loss is found on the other side. The term includes conditions in which loss of one set of sensory modalities is not accompanied by loss of the other set, from whatever cause.

Syringomyelia is another example. Here, the crossing spinothalamic fibers are damaged by the cavity in the cord, but the posterior columns are relatively spared. Anterior spinal artery occlusion produces a sudden, similar picture. In all three of these conditions, pyramidal and other cord signs may be expected.

At a higher level, the syndrome of the posteroinferior cerebellar artery (the lateral medullary syndrome) also causes dissociated sensory loss. Peripherally, some neuropathies (e.g., in diabetes) involve myelin damage; hence sensory impulses carried in heavily myelinated fibers are most affected (position, tactile discrimination, vibration) and those carried in thinner fibers are more or less spared. The opposite also occurs, such as when the small dorsal root ganglion cells are selectively damaged in some hereditary sensory neuropathies.

Syndromes of Cord Involvement at Different Levels

The presence of marked deformity of angulation of the spine, or of a tuft of hair, a lipoma, a midline cleft, or of a meningocele, meningomyelocele, or hemangioma in the skin make localization easy, but they are uncommon. A very short neck often suggests the presence of a high cervical lesion.

Foramen Magnum

If you suspect a lesion at this level, look for involvement if the spinal nucleus and tract of the fifth nerve, producing homolateral pain and temperature loss over the forehead; for involvement of the spinal accessory nerve (sternomastoid and trapezius weakness); and for signs of cerebellar dysfunction. Below the level of the lesion, any combination of long-tract signs may be found, but an upper level may be hard to define. Normal facial power, the absence of bulbar signs, and a normal jaw jerk are useful indicators that the problem is sited below the midmedulla.

Cervical

Patients may complain of pain or spasm in the neck muscles, the pain radiating to the head or shoulders. The sensation of tingling or electric shock radiating down the back on forward flexion of the neck is Lhermitte's sign (really a symptom), indicating the presence of intrinsic (e.g., multiple sclerosis) or extrinsic disease (e.g., compression by a tumor or cervical disk). Look for lower motor neuron signs in the hands, arms, and shoulder girdle, and for complaints of radicular pain with percussion of the spine (see Fig. 9-14).

There also may be segmental sensory hyper- or hypoesthesia, and below the level of the lesion, long-tract motor and sensory signs may be expected. With a cord lesion above C-3, diaphragmatic palsy will occur because the phrenic nerve arises from C-3, C-4, and C-5. The sympathetic pathway also can be damaged in cervical cord disease, although Horner's syndrome is most often caused by a lesion at C8-T1 or in the neck.

Thoracic

Signs at and below the level of the lesion are as expected from the descriptions already given, but they are hard to localize unless a sensory level is found because no reflexes can be elicited here and lower motor neuron lesions are hard to detect in the intercostal muscles.

Low Cord Lesions

The spinal cord extends down as far as the lower border of L-1 vertebra, while the subarachnoid space extends to S-1 or S-2. The terminal part of the cord (S-3, S-4, S-4, and coccygeal-1) is known as the conus medullaris. It is hardly ever involved alone; indeed, because of its central position, it may be unaffected despite marked cauda equina compression by a disk or tumor — *sacral sparing.*

Damage to the descending lumbar roots, which leave the cord at vertebral levels T-12 and L-1 and then descend to their exit foramina as the *cauda equina,* produce different findings. Radicular pain is common, usually referred to the back of the thigh and leg below the knee and maximal at night. Examination may show lower motor neuron signs, often asymmetric, with diminution of the knee, and loss of the ankle reflex, and weakness with wasting at levels below L-1. Involvement of rectal and urinary sphincters will occur only if the lower sacral roots are affected. Sensory changes, involving all modalities, are asymmetric and again can usually be localized within the affected dermatomes. Progressive lesions of the cauda equina tend in time to involve the lower sacral segments so that the initial sacral sparing is lost.

Damage to the conus medullaris produces urinary and rectal incontinence and impotence resulting from involvement of the emerging parasympathetic fibers at this level. *Saddle anesthesia* refers to the loss of sensation over the upper and inner thigh and perianal region, these areas being supplied by the lowest sacral segments. No muscles are innervated by these segments, so no somatic motor signs will be found. The conus is so small that any lesion tends to affect it on both sides; symmetric findings are to be expected.

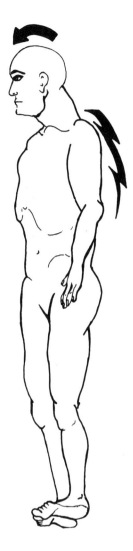

Figure 9-14   Lhermitte's sign.

PERIPHERAL NERVES

In Chapter 44 the clinical features of neuropathies are shown to be related to their pathology. Thus some neuropathies have predominant involvement of the larger, heavily myelinated fibers, some involve the thinner fibers, and some involve both to about the same degree. The clinical findings are to some extent dependent upon the type of pathology present because of this. The geographical patterns of deficit that may occur depend upon whether there is a discrete lesion of one or more nerves (*mononeuropathy* or *multiple mononeuropathy*) or else a generalized abnormality producing symptoms and signs initially in those nerves with the longest course (distal symmetric *polyneuropathy*). The nerve cell body supplies a nutritive and trophic function to its axons by axoplasmic flow distally down the fiber; thus the first effects of metabolic damage to the cell body will be manifested at the very end of the axon, perhaps a meter away.[*]

Because most of these lesions are metabolic, the signs are usually symmetric.

Clinical examination will reveal patterns of sensory loss or motor weakness that can either be anatomically localized to one or more particular nerves or that appear to be generalized and symmetric, extending to some point up the limb or on the trunk. Weakness caused by neural and myopathic diseases can be differentiated by clinical examination (see Table 9-2).

Findings in a disease of the *anterior horn cell* include *fasciculations,* which also occur with more distal damage to the axon. At least in the early stages, anterior horn cell and axonal diseases tend to be patchy and incomplete so that the usual signs of a lower motor neuron lesion may also be incomplete. Thus the reflexes may be preserved until late. They are depressed at an early stage with demyelinating neuropathies, and other motor signs tend to be symmetric and distal.

Nerves already damaged by an intrinsic pathology are especially vulnerable to added compression or other trauma, resulting in weakness and sensory change affecting all modalities in the distribution of that nerve. Therefore a total conduction block in a single nerve indicates a search for a mild generalized underlying neuropathy.

Common *sensory complaints* are paresthesias, numbness, heaviness, deadness, or tightness in a limb, and dysesthesia. This last term refers to both spontaneous pains and hyperesthesia — as may occur when gentle touch or mild temperature stimuli produce discomfort, e.g., in thin-fiber neuropathies (see Chap. 36).

Trophic changes are common when sensory loss is marked. They include perforating ulcers of the feet, painless burns, edema, coldness of the hands and feet, lack of sweating, hair loss, thickening of the skin, and Raynaud's phenomenon. Some of these changes are due to lack of perception of tissue damage by the patient, who will neither protect nor attend to the area when damage occurs. Others are due to involvement of sympathetic fibers running with the peripheral nerves. Joint deformity and destruction may result if deep pain sensation is lost, giving rise to the classic (if uncommon) Charcot's joints of syringomyelia, tabes, and hereditary sensory neuropathy. The nerves themselves can be seen or felt at many sites, where thickening may suggest nerve infiltration, as in some metabolic, infective, or hereditary neuropathies. Discrete swelling of nerves occurs in neurofibromatosis (see Chap. 40).

If a nerve is damaged at any site and begins to regenerate, tapping the nerve at the point of regeneration induces a tingling sensation felt distally in the distribution of that nerve. This is Tinel's sign, valuable evidence of the site of nerve damage and regeneration.

Proximal neuropathies are rare, and when they occur are usually motor, as in the Guillain-Barré syndrome. Symmetry is also usual, although in neuralgic amyotrophy and polio (Chap. 45) that is not true. Most generalized neuropathies, sensory, motor, or mixed, progress centrally from distal sites of onset. Of course the sites of mononeuropathies determine the area where symptoms appear.

It is seldom possible to decide clinically whether the pathology is axonal damage or demyelination; early reflex loss, major involvement of thick-fiber functions (vibration, proprioception), and nerve enlargement favor demyelination, while

---

[*]Much as empires, plagued by dissolution or decay in the capital, first withdraw from their most distant colonies: the longest lines of communication can no longer be maintained.

Table 9-2   Neurogenic and Myopathic Weakness

	Neurogenic	Myopathic
Distribution	Distal	Proximal
Symmetry	Variable	Usual
Facial involvement	Rare	Common
Fasciculations	Common	Rare
Wasting	Focal	Diffuse
Reflex loss	Early	Late
Sensory signs	Common	Not present

fasciculations and major involvement of pinprick pain and temperature are more suggestive of axonal neuropathies; but one is still seldom certain.

The clinical aspects of diseases of nerves are discussed in Chapter 44.

MYONEURAL JUNCTION

At the myoneural junction, quanta or "packets" of acetylcholine (ACh) are liberated from the nerve terminal and diffuse across the synaptic cleft to depolarize the end-plate. In the resting state, quanta are continuously liberated and produce miniature end-plate potentials (but no myofibrillary contraction); the arrival of a nerve impulse leads to much increased ACh release, enough to depolarize the postjunctional membrane. Contraction of the myofibril results.

In myasthenia gravis, a proportion of the end-plate receptors are engaged, blocked, and destroyed by anti-ACh receptor antibodies. As a result, ACh quanta released from the nerve terminal cross the synaptic cleft but find few receptors available for depolarization. Variable weakness and fatigability result. Fatigability however is not a specific sign of myasthenia because it also occurs (although less dramatically) in both motor neuropathies and primary diseases of muscle.

The leading symptom of end-plate disease is progressive weakness during the performance of a voluntary act, such as looking upward, holding the arms level with the shoulders, talking, chewing, and walking. Reversal of this fatigability may occur with the intravenous injection of edrophonium, a short-acting anticholinesterase, but even this test may be negative in myasthenia (particularly regarding the ocular muscles) and positive in patients with muscle or nerve problems. It is most dramatically positive when a patient is asked to count, to hold the arms up against gravity, or when ventilatory function tests are performed before, and again immediately after, the administration of edrophonium. The EMG appearance is of rapid reduction in the size of the muscle action potential evoked by rapid stimulation of the nerve supplying it.

Another end-plate disorder is the *myasthenic syndrome,* in which there is a decrease in the number of quanta liberated — a prejunctional abnormality. It is a pity that the term sounds so much like myasthenia because the two conditions produce different signs. In the myasthenic syndrome the patient gains strength for the first few seconds of a movement, fatiguing only then; while this may be hard to appreciate clinically, the EMG picture is of an increase in the size of the muscle potential with rapid stimulation of its nerve.

Diseases of the end-plate are discussed in Chapter 45.

MUSCLE

There are few symptoms or signs that are pathognomonic of muscle disease; almost all of the clinical features can also occur as a result of upper motor neuron lesions or systemic disorders. The following six items are particularly helpful in the diagnosis of myopathy.

Weakness

In most cases of primary muscle disease, weakness and wasting are proportionate, but that is not so in myasthenia, polymyositis, and the myopathy of osteomalacia, in all of which there may be no atrophy. In all but facioscapulohumeral (FSH) dystrophy, the signs are symmetric. Also in almost all cases, the proximal rather than the distal muscles are mainly involved. Myotonic dystrophy is the only common exception to this rule.

Sometimes, the pattern of involvement is helpful. In myotonic dystrophy, the face and eyelids, the neck muscles such as sternomastoids, and the distal muscles are affected. In scapuloperoneal and FSH dystrophies, appearances are as suggested by the names. The *eyes* are affected in myasthenia, ocular myopathies, and hyperthyroidism (in which the usual initial problem is in upward gaze). *Facial* weakness is seen in FSH, ocular, and myotonic dystrophies, and in myasthenia gravis. *Bulbar* involvement is common in polymyositis, ocular and myotonic dystrophies, and myasthenia. Bulbar and proximal limb weakness may also be found however in anterior horn cell diseases and with upper motor neuron lesions of all types.

Initial involvement of the *pelvic girdle* is common to most primary muscle diseases, including Duchenne and limb-girdle dystrophies, most congenital myopathies, and polymyositis, but the latter two conditions, with FSH and myotonic dystrophy, sometimes involve the shoulder girdle first.

The speed of onset of the weakness may be helpful diagnostically. Gradually increasing disability is usual with endocrine, metabolic, and collagen-vascular myopathies, as well as in genetically determined dystrophies and myopathies. Causes of weakness of rapid onset are discussed in Chapter 26. *Periodic and intermittent weakness* is seen in periodic paralyses and in myasthenia gravis, but it may be the presenting complaint of any early motor neuropathy or myopathy. Fatigability was discussed earlier.

Muscle Size

While severe, early, proximal, and symmetric muscle *atrophy* is the rule in genetic dystrophies, it is still a nonspecific sign of muscle disease because it also occurs in lower motor (and some long-standing upper motor) neuron lesions. Atrophy is often less marked in acquired muscle diseases. Muscle *hypertrophy,* again, is not specific. It may be due to long-standing excessive activity in the muscle, such as occurs in congenital myotonia, but it is also a feature of syndromes marked by involuntary movements such as dystonias and athetosis. In all such cases, true hypertrophy will be present. But muscles may be enlarged because of inflammation (polymyositis) or because of their infiltration with fat (e.g., Duchenne dystrophy), amyloid, or glycogen. In such cases the calves and tongue are most obviously affected.

Muscle Pain and Tenderness at Rest

The analysis of these complaints, and of *cramp,* will be found in Chapter 27. Pain usually signifies swelling of the muscle fibers and the distortion of pain-sensitive nerve endings in the endo- and perimysium. If the extent of muscle damage is great, myofibrils will be destroyed and their contents released into the circulation. A huge rise is serum CK and systemic liberation of myoglobin will result that is dangerous because it may precipitate in the renal tubules. Myoglobinuria is discussed in Chapter 45.

Abnormal Movements

Fibrillations,[*] even in the tongue, are invisible to the naked eye. *Fasciculations* are very visible, best with an oblique light. They may be benign (Chap. 45) or indicative of motor nerve lesions. These and other movement abnormalities are described in Chapter 29. *Delayed relaxation* of muscles is the classic complaint of patients with myotonic syndromes. They complain that they cannot let go of an object gripped in their hand, such as a doorknob, a toothbrush, or a corkscrew;[†] they may have trouble letting go when shaking hands if myotonia is severe, or if their hands are cold. Tapping muscles — especially those of the thenar eminence or the tongue — causes a dimple to appear and the thumb will rise up for a few seconds before settling down again. Patients with congenital myotonia will have no muscle weakness but will complain of trouble "getting going," although the symptom goes away when they are warmed up. They fail hopelessly in the hundred meters, but may well catch up in the mile! Most of the syndromes in which myotonia occurs are dominantly inherited, hence the family history is usually positive.

In hypothyroidism, the ankle jerk is characteristically "hung-up," again an example of delayed relaxation. In this context it is not due to electrical after-discharges, caused by a disorder of the muscle membrane, but to mechanical difficulties that prevent the myofibrils from sliding past each other normally during relaxation. In this form of *pseudomyotonia* no abnormal electrical activity can be recorded on the EMG.

Cardiac Signs

Cardiomyopathies producing cardiac failure, rhythm disturbances, and conduction defects, are part of the presentation of Duchenne and myotonic dystrophies and glycogen storage diseases. Because of autonomic dysfunction, serious cardiac problems may complicate certain neuropathies, e.g., the Guillain-Barré syndrome.

---

[*]Oscar Wilde said that artists, like Greek Gods, are only revealed to one another. Fibrillations are only revealed to the electromyographer.

[†]Or a hand grenade. Such patients should choose their occupations with care.

Family History

Faced with a patient who may have a muscle disease, a careful family history is essential. Where there is any doubt, family members should be examined as well and may need EMG and even muscle biopsy. Myotonias and FSH dystrophy are autosomal-dominant conditions, as are the ocular and some of the congenital myopathies. Duchenne dystrophy and its milder and rarer variant, Becker dystrophy, are sex-linked recessive traits. Most other genetic muscles diseases are inherited recessively.

Finally, any patient with a primary muscle disease also may have some other system involved. Cardiac disorders have already been mentioned, but in both genetic and acquired conditions, endocrine function and the condition of the skin need to be assessed, and often a search will have to be made for underlying metabolic or neoplastic diseases. The reasons that a full drug history must be taken are obvious on looking at Chapter 43.

TRANSIENT EPISODES OF
NEUROLOGICAL DYSFUNCTION

Although we have concentrated, so far, almost exclusively on the localization of lesions in space, the temporal characteristics of symptoms and signs also have the greatest diagnostic value, mainly regarding pathogenesis. As an example, let us consider visual disturbances.

A lesion irritating the visual cortex may produce flashes of light or formed hallucinations that have instantaneous onset and also usually disappearance, although these positive phenomena may leave a negative one — blindness in a sector of the visual field, a *scotoma* — afterward. The very sudden onset indicates an electrical cause.

If visual loss comes on over 5 to 30 sec, as if a blind were being drawn down over the eye, a vascular cause is likely; it takes a few seconds for the retinal cells to "run out" of substrate in the presence of ischemia, so although the vascular occlusion may be abrupt, visual loss is not instantaneous. Patients who awake with a paralyzed arm may think their stroke came on suddenly, but of course they were actually asleep at the time.

If vision takes a few minutes or hours to fail, suspect a metabolic problem such as hypoglycemia or nerve compression during a transient rise in intracranial pressure. Onset over a day or two is more characteristic of demyelinating disease; if it takes weeks or more, local (not primary neurological) causes or compression of the optic nerve by a tumor must be considered.

Thus it is not enough to identify a symptom and to localize its origin; precise delineation of its speed of onset and duration are also essential.

All such episodes in which neurological symptoms have a defined onset and termination, or recur with periods of normality in between, may be gathered under the heading *transient episodes of neurological dysfunction* (TENDS). All the examples following are discussed more fully elsewhere in this book. Almost anything can happen, from disturbance of higher cortical functioning to minor sensory loss, but most symptoms involve the level of consciousness, the cranial nerves, and the motor systems.

Electrical Causes

All forms of *seizure* have an instantaneous onset and termination, although deficits may remain to obscure the latter. The *narcolepsy* complex (brief episodes of irresistible sleep with cataplexy, sleep paralysis, and hallucinations) also "switches" on and off. Drop attacks may be a variation of either, or they may be caused by brainstem electrical disturbances secondary to ischemia. Neuralgic pains, e.g., of the fifth or ninth nerves or at spinal level ("lightning pains") are again electrically based, even though the reason for the abnormal discharge may be nerve fiber compression or irritation. Rather similar to these, but on the motor side, hemifacial spasm (and also flexor and extensor spasms and fasciculations) witness the tendency for electrical responses to be made to a variety of CNS pathologies. Benign positional vertigo and vestibular neuronitis are characterized by intermittent episodes of severe vertigo, probably because of irritation of the end-organ, which responds with a burst of electrical energy. In Ménières disease, excessive endolymphatic pressure sets off a similar excessive discharge.

Vascular Diseases

The pathogenesis of some forms of diminished cerebral blood flow is described in Chapter 10. The TENDs often are due to recurrent emboli, vasospasm, or temporary thromboembolic vascular occlusions. When they clear completely in a day, they are known as *transient ischemic attacks* (TIAs); slower resolution gives them the name of reversible ischemic neurological deficits (RINDs), a Humpty-Dumpty phrase still in vogue. In all cases, symptoms take an appreciable time to develop — seconds or minutes.

Metabolic and Toxic Disorders

Symptoms thus induced develop over minutes or hours, sometimes even longer. Hypoglycemia is symptomatic in minutes, whereas hyperglycemic coma may take hours, and that caused by liver failure progresses over days. Symptoms of other metabolic lesions — weakness in periodic paralysis or porphyria, muscle cramps in glycogen storage disease, alkalotic sensory symptoms, or tetany — take less than an hour to develop in most instances.

Demyelinating Disease

Multiple sclerosis is an important cause of transient symptoms, producing a whole range of clinical features that may be temporary and that progress over hours or days. Sometimes different pathologies interact; a patient with MS who can easily step into a hot bath may be unable to climb out 5 min later, heat somehow exacerbating the electrical block initially caused by the plaques of demyelination.

Mechanical Causes

Traumatic shock waves disrupt synapses to produce instantaneous brief coma in concussion, while a lucid interval and subsequent slow decline into delayed coma are classically described with extradural hematomas. Mechanical lesions compressing the nervous system cause slowly progressive functional loss over weeks unless: (1) they suddenly expand, as with hemorrhage into their substance, (2) they cause a seizure, or (3) they cut off the blood supply to part of the nervous system, as with a pressure palsy of a nerve, which is thus properly regarded as a vascular rather than a mechanical cause. Rarely, the ball-valve effect of a third or fourth ventricle tumor causes a rapid rise in intracranial pressure with headache and loss of consciousness. The genesis of these is probably a failure of cerebral blood flow consequent on the pressure rise intracranially that now exceeds perfusion pressure.

To conclude, do not be satisfied with an analysis of the nature of a symptom and of its spatial localization; examine its temporal characteristics also, for in doing so you will acquire data that may well enable you to give an opinion upon pathogenesis, and thus upon etiology.

BIBLIOGRAPHY

Gassell, M. False localizing signs. *Arch. Neurol. 4*:70, 1961.

Haymaker, W. (ed.). *Bing's Local Diagnosis in Neurological Diseases,* 15th Ed. St. Louis, C.V. Mosby Co., 1969.

Jenkyn, L.R. et al. Clinical signs in diffuse cerebral dysfunction. *J. Neurol. Neurosurg. Psychiatry 40*:956-966, 1977.

Spillane, J.D. *An Atlas of Clinical Neurology,* 3rd Ed. Toronto, Oxford University Press, 1983.

Walton, J.N. *Introduction to Clinical Neuroscience,* London, Bailliere, Tindall, 1983.

III
AN APPROACH TO NEUROLOGICAL SYMPTOMS

INTRODUCTION TO PART III

In the following chapters (10 to 36) we will discuss the neurological problems that the patient brings to your office. Patients do not present with uncal compression, McArdle's syndrome, or Korsakoff's syndrome. They present with headache, muscle pain, or memory disturbance. There are many textbooks covering the specific syndromes in neurology in fine detail, but as patients come to you with complaints and not with specific syndromes, we devote Part III to an approach to symptoms and signs. We hope that you will develop a practical approach to assessing and solving these general problems to arrive at a diagnosis, at which point you should probably go to a reference text (i.e., something heavier than this) for more detailed information: after reading this book, at least you should know where to look.

We also feel that an understanding of the common symptoms and signs of neurological disease that patients present to you enables you to handle the first contact quite adequately. After all, this is the approach that clinical neurologists take when assessing a problem; they do not just cast about for an appropriate eponym but have developed, through experience, an ability to assess a problem in terms of the most likely pathology in the sites affected. If they do not know what the trouble is after the history has been taken, the physical examination usually will not help much to clarify the problem.

In part IV we describe in summary form those neurological problems that the family practitioner should be able to recognize, because he will see them from time to time and will at least share in their management. But this section contains the basis of neurological practice; the assessment of the problems that patients bring to the doctor.

10

Reduction in Conscious Level

COMA

Consciousness has been defined as a primary element in experience that cannot be described in terms of anything else. This evasion of the problem however tells one nothing. Consciousness is not a thing but a process, an activity, an interaction, whereby the individual is aware of his internal and external environment.

As consciousness is reduced, fewer and fewer characteristics of the environment are attended to, summed up, comprehended, and remembered, and the contents of mind, awareness, and thought are diminished. In the earlier stages of reduction of consciousness, complex and abstract thought may be lost, whereas later on the content of thought is simpler still, until eventually only feeling remains; when even that is lost, the patient becomes unaware of the outside world, his internal bodily world, and the interactions of the two. Finally, even the reflex reactions of his body to external stimuli fade, becoming more and more primitive, and terminally they cease.*

Pathogenesis

Alertness depends upon the activity of the reticular activating system (RAS) in the upper brainstem (Fig. 10-1). The RAS receives collateral input from all incoming

---

*Thus to divide consciousness between the three traditional categories (awake, asleep, and dead) is an oversimplification, ignoring the vital necessity of grading the conscious level.

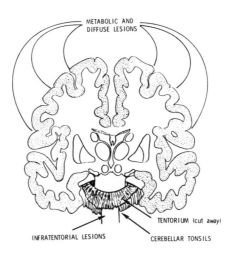

Figure 10-1   Pathogenesis of coma. Infratentorial lesions directly damage the brainstem, but to cause coma supratentorial lesions must be diffuse and bilateral unless, (a) they compress the brainstem themselves, or (b) they are associated with raised intracranial pressure or cerebral edema.

sensory channels and through the thalamic nuclei, radiates to (as it were, "switching on") the whole cerebral cortex. These pathways are active in both directions. Lesions causing coma thus do so directly by damaging this alerting RAS — cortical system or the cortex.

The RAS may be damaged by any pathology involving the brainstem, or the cortex may be involved in severe generalized diseases such as terminal Alzheimer's disease or dysmetabolic states.

Indirectly, lesions may act by causing brain swelling with secondary compression of the brainstem, inducing ischemia and secondary hemorrhage (Fig. 10-2). Severe anoxia, hypoglycemia, and sedatives affect the RAS directly to reduce consciousness, to depress the cerebral cortex, or both.

Electrical events causing coma do so only when the discharge either begins in, or spreads to, deep midline structures, probably the nonspecific thalamic nuclei. From this one may deduce that epilepsy without reduction in consciousness must be focal and unilateral and that if a patient exhibits bilateral movements resembling an epileptic seizure but is not in a state of reduced consciousness, the attack cannot be epileptic in origin.

Finally, sudden traumatic lesions cause brief transient coma (concussion), but we do not know how. Possibilities include a sudden rise in intracranial pressure, shear stresses on neurons, and vibration. Brief concussion is not lethal, so the true pathology is uncertain. In more severe and long-lasting states, cerebral edema and neuronal breakage have been reported.

The brain stores enough glucose for a few seconds only. Abrupt reduction in available glucose (its only efficient metabolic substrate) or oxygen reduces cortical RAS activity suddenly, as with sudden hypotension below 50 mmHg systolic, failure of cardiac output, or acute anoxic states.

The first principle in understanding coma is that it may be produced by disorders in two areas only: a brainstem or a diffuse cortical lesion. The pathogeneses can be grouped into three categories (see Fig. 10-1):

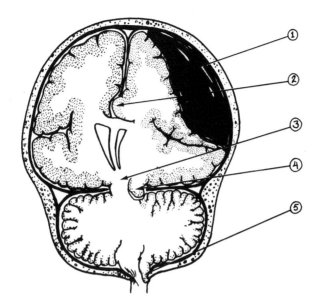

Figure 10-2   Effects of supratentorial expanding mass lesions. (1) Subdural hematoma; (2) herniation of the cingulate gyrus under the falx; (3) shift of brainstem; (4) uncal herniation; (5) cerebellar tonsillar herniation.

1. Supratentorial lesions with secondary brainstem involvement
2. Subtentorial lesions with direct brainstem involvement
3. Metabolic disorders, i.e., diffuse cortical disturbance

CLINICAL APPROACH

**Previous Brief Episodes
of Reduced Conscious Level**

You *must* get a full history from somebody other than the patient.
    The following factors suggest *epilepsy* (Chap. 15):

1. Positive family history
2. Symptoms of brain disease
3. Sudden onset and speedy recovery
4. Associated jerking or twitching of limbs, tongue biting, or incontinence
5. Occurrence during sleep or when recumbent
6. Inability to arouse the patient during the attack
7. Warning symptoms: the so-called epileptic aura
8. Focal neurological deficits occurring transiently after the attack

All of these factors suggest a form of epilepsy, which is defined as the occurrence of symptoms not under voluntary control resulting from the occasional, sudden, rapid, local, and excessive electrical discharge of gray matter neurons.
    The following factors suggest a *vascular cause* (Chap. 37).

1.   Known high blood pressure, past strokes, atherosclerotic heart or peripheral vascular disease, or valvular heart disease; hypotension; or blood disease
2.   Onset in minutes or seconds with persistent focal neurological signs or signs of meningeal irritation
3.   Severe associated headache
4.   Transient loss of vision in the recent past
5.   Association with chest pain, neck compression, or turning; palpitations, coughing, emotion, or standing up after recumbency

Narcolepsy (Chap. 18) is a condition marked by

1.   Overpowering attacks of an irresistible desire to sleep
2.   Sometimes associated with hallucinations while going to sleep or awakening
3.   Sleep paralysis
4.   Sudden loss of power in all limbs with strong emotion (cataplexy)

The following factors suggest *mechanical lesions* (Chap. 16, 18, 40).

1.   History of trauma with sudden, immediate, or (less often) slowly progressive drowsiness leading on to coma
2.   Symptoms suggesting raised intracranial pressure such as diplopia, headache, vertigo, vomiting, visual disturbance, and focal sensory or motor symptoms
3.   Rhinorrhea, otorrhea, bleeding from the ear or into the eye
4.   Fever, stiff neck, photophobia

The following factors suggest *metabolic causes* (Chap. 42, 43).

1.   History or signs of drug ingestion or alcoholism.
2.   Dyspnea, sweating; symptoms of current chest, abdominal, or blood infection.
3.   Recent febrile episodes or current fever.
4.   Slow onset over hours or days.
5.   Lack of focal neurological symptoms and signs.
6.   Symptoms to suggest past disease of liver, kidney, or lungs; thyroid or renal disease; diabetes; malnutrition or cachexia.
7.   Pupils react normally to light, both directly and consensually. The ciliospinal reflex can be obtained. The pupils are normal in size unless
     a) the patient is poisoned with opiates, when they constrict, or
     b) the patient is poisoned with gluethimide, antihistamines, anticholinergics, or ganglion-blocking agents, when they dilate.
8.   Doll's head movements are present; the response to ice-water caloric testing is either normal or there is tonic deviation of the eyes to the affected side.

Finally, remember that states of apparently altered consciousness also occur in stupor and delirious states (see Chap. 11).

Concurrently Reduced
Consciousness Not Amounting to Coma

Most of this information is given in Chapter 11. Essentially, your task is to decide whether the lesion is metabolic or structural (we will omit electrical causes for the moment), and if it is structural, whether the lesion is in the posterior fossa (below the tentorium) or if it is supratentorial.

Patients with reduced consciousness give inaccurate and brief histories, are suggestible, and are preoccupied with their experiences of the distorted present rather than with memories of the disturbed past. Therefore a history from someone else, whether it be family or friend, neighbor or employer; anyone who knows the patient will do.

When confronted with a drowsy patient, you are data-starved. Try to determine the speed of onset of the state and its current pattern. Lightening coma is not a medical emergency; deepening drowsiness is. As usual, examination of the patient only tells you *where* the trouble is; you rely on the history from all sources to tell you about its *nature*.

Your history must concentrate upon those factors mentioned previously: searching for evidence of electrical, vascular, mechanical, and metabolic disorders, and bearing in mind the possible causes of delirium; the CNS examination will be foreshortened depending upon the current state of the patient and his ability to cooperate with you.

The Patient in Coma

We have previously mentioned that the lesions that cause coma can be divided into supratentorial, subtentorial, and metabolic disorders (Table 10-1).

Supratentorial Lesions

Supratentorial diseases that can cause coma include bilateral subcortical lesions such as multiple emboli or hemorrhages, or a single mass or destructive lesion that compresses deeper diencephalic or brainstem structures.

The tentorium is a thick, hard, fibrous sheet that separates the hemispheres from the brainstem and cerebellum, dividing the supratentorial from the subtentorial area or posterior fossa. There is an opening in the tentorium through which the midbrain joins the brain to the brainstem.

Mass lesions in the brain cause pressure, first locally, all around the mass, and then downward, in a progressive manner (see Fig. 10-2). The exceptions are acute intracerebral hemorrhage and coning after lumbar puncture, in which the sudden rise in pressure can rapidly compress the brainstem. Usually however the expanding mass causes signs of focal cerebral damage, after which there is evidence of compression of the diencephalon, midbrain, pons, and medulla, in that order. This orderly progression is seen in almost all expanding lesions, and clinical examination enables one to determine the level affected at any time and to chart alterations in function as the condition worsens.

There are two forms of downward compression: *uncal compression,* in which the brainstem is pressed upon from the side and the *central syndrome.* These terms require some explanation. If an expanding mass in the temporal lobe causes it to swell, then the uncus (which is the most medial part of the temporal lobe) will be pushed medially and downward over the free edge of the tentorium. Here it will compress the third or sixth nerves (causing dilation of the pupil and extraocular palsies on that side) and also the midbrain (causing depression of consciousness). Next, the brainstem is shifted across the midline and the opposite cerebral peduncle pressed against the brainstem. This produces an upper motor neuron lesion *on the same side as the mass,* because the corticospinal fibers running in the peduncle have not yet crossed at this level.

By this stage, the opposite third nerve will also have been stretched as the brainstem is compressed and pushed down. Decerebrate rigidity and bilateral pyramidal signs also develop. All of these features appear in more or less this order: the *uncal syndrome.*

Table 10-1   Causes of Coma

Supratentorial (causing secondary mesencephalic compression)
    Large cerebral infarct with edema
    Intracerebral, subdural, extradural, subarachnoid hemorrhage
    Cerebral tumor
    Cerebral abscess
    Cerebral edema

Infratentorial
    Brainstem infarct or hemorrhage
    Brainstem tumor
    Brainstem trauma
    Cerebellar abscess
    Cerebellar hemorrhage

Metabolic

Acute onset	Hypoxia, generalized cerebral ischemia
	Hypoglycemia
	Concussion
	Poisoning
	Postepileptic
Subacute onset	Hypo- or hyperthermia
	Vitamin B deficiency (Wernicke's)
	Meningitis
	Encephalitis
	Malaria
	Organ failure: liver, lung, kidney
	Endocrinopathy: hypopituitarism
	hypothyroidism
	hypoadrenalism
	hyperparathyroidism
	Porphyria
	Acid-base disturbances
End stage of disease	Cerebral atrophies
	Lipid and other storage disease
	Nonmetastatic carcinomatous syndrome
Differentiate from	Sleep states
	Akinetic mutism
	Syncope
	Psychogenic unresponsiveness

Generalized brain swelling and masses outside the temporal lobe do not produce the same initial compression of the brainstem and third nerve, but rather press directly downward and cause herniation of the midline structures through the tentorial aperture or the foramen magnum. The first area to feel the effect of this is the diencephalon; reduced awareness, Cheyne-Stokes respirations, a loss of upward gaze, small pupils, and bilateral pyramidal signs result. Later the pons is involved;

the patient will be in coma, hyperventilating, with small reactive pupils and bilateral decerebrate rigidity. Reflex eye movements will probably be lost. Finally, with medullary involvement, coma, tachypnea or apnea, fixed dilated pupils, and a loss of brainstem reflexes are found. This progression of signs, indicating involvement of high and then of successively lower levels of the brainstem, is the *central syndrome.*

Subtentorial Lesions

The brainstem can be affected by a local destructive lesion, such as vertebrobasilar infarction or an expanding mass. In such cases, coma can be produced by

1. Compression of the brainstem RAS
2. Upward herniation of the cerebellum and midbrain through the tentorial opening
3. Downward herniation of the cerebellar tonsils or of the brainstem itself, medullary compression resulting (Fig. 10-3)

   Lesions of the brainstem often produce asymmetric signs. The coma is often sudden in onset, and the signs appear at once. Pupillary and other brainstem reflexes are abnormal or lost at an early stage, in contrast to the delay in their appearance found with supratentorial lesions.

Metabolic Coma

Metabolic coma may result from anoxia, hypoglycemia, liver or renal failure, drug ingestion, diabetes, and many other chemical or endocrine disturbances (Table 10-2); (Fig. 10-4). Although there is again a progressive involvement of the nervous system

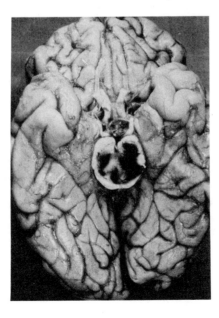

Figure 10-3   Duret hemorrhages in the brainstem secondary to its compression by the herniating uncus.

Table 10-2   Metabolic Coma[a]

With metabolic acidosis

      Diabetes
      Uremia
      Lactic acidosis
      Paraldehyde, methyl alcohol, or ethylene
       glycol ingestion (see Fig. 10-4)
      Reye's syndrome

With respiratory acidosis

      Pulmonary disease
      Neuromuscular ventilatory failure
      Central respiratory depression

With metabolic alkalosis

      Acid loss, alkali ingestion
      Conn's, Cushing's syndromes
      Diuretics

With respiratory alkalosis

      Salicylate ingestion
      Hepatic coma
      Hyperventilation

---

[a] This table demonstrates the values of blood gas analysis in the diagnosis of metabolic coma.
Adapted with permission from: Plum, F., Posner, J. *Stupor and Coma*. 3rd Ed. Philadelphia, F.A. Davis Co. 1980.

from higher to lower levels, focal or lateralized signs are less prominent than the evidence of bilateral, symmetric brain disease.

Thus the pupils usually still react to light[*] and the brainstem reflexes are retained. It is a good general rule that deep coma in the presence of equal reactive pupils indicates a metabolic lesion.

Consciousness is progressively impaired in metabolic coma. Alterations of respiration are often of specific type according to the cause of coma, e.g., hyperventilation and respiratory alkalosis in salicylate poisoning; severe respiratory depression with narcotic overdose. Focal signs, often of a temporary nature, are sometimes found but their presence does not rule out a metabolic cause for the condition. Slight involuntary movements, pyramidal signs, and tremors are often seen. Asterixis occurs in renal, hepatic, and respiratory failure. Myoclonic jerks are common in metabolic coma, especially when caused by anoxia.

---

[*] See Chapter 43 for lists of drugs affecting the eye.

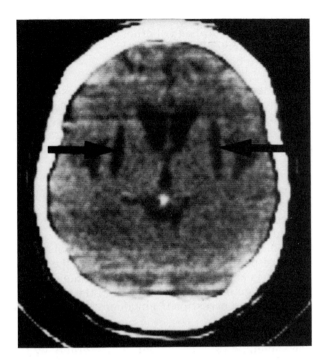

Figure 10-4 Typical CT scan findings in acute methanol poisoning. The slitlike cavities in the lateral basal nuclei are considered diagnostic of this condition.

Thus we have two areas of the brain that, when damaged, may lead to coma — the cortex as a whole and the brainstem RAS — and three types of lesion that can produce it, namely supra- and subtentorial pathologies and metabolic disorders. The type of coma, its level, and the rate of progression of the process, can all be identified by the clinical evaluation of five features: the level of consciousness, the pupils, brainstem reflexes, respiratory pattern, and motor responses as outlined in Chapter 7, (in which the immediate management also is described).

Using these tests, a decision upon which of the three pathogeneses of coma is operating should be possible. In summary, the pupils are reactive in most cases of *metabolic* coma, although with some drugs and in severe anoxia they may be fixed and dilated. Respiration is of the Cheyne-Stokes type, and all tests show more or less symmetric findings. *Supratentorial lesions* may be suspected with a third nerve palsy and asymmetric motor signs in the limbs. Caloric tests show ocular deviation to the cold-irrigated side, at least initially, later brainstem damage causes loss of these and many other reflexes. Primary *brainstem lesions* may lead to bilaterally small pupils, asymmetric or lost caloric responses and brainstem reflexes, and signs of bilateral cranial nerve and long tract involvement.

BRAIN DEATH

Nowadays, the exact definition and diagnosis of brain death is of importance not only for medical reasons. Brain death is accepted as synonymous with brainstem death and by extension, death of the person. But cortical death, with a functional brainstem (e.g., the patient breathes spontaneously), leads to a vegetative state, not death; and the question as to when (whether ?) to cease providing life-support is an ethical, not a strictly medical one.

One may diagnose brain death only when

The patient is in deep coma; all brainstem reflexes (such as pupillary, ciliospinal, corneal, cough, gag, swallowing, doll's head, and ice-water caloric tests) are absent. Strong, normally painful stimuli anywhere in the body provoke no cranial motor responses. Decerebrate rigidity is not detected. The pupils are usually not only fixed but also dilated.

No spontaneous ventilatory movements occur during a 10-min period after 100% oxygen followed by 5% CO_2 in oxygen have been given for 5 min. During the 10-min observation period, 100% oxygen at 6 L/min must be delivered by a catheter in the trachea.

Hypothermia (core temperature below 25°C), metabolic and endocrine disease, and shock can be excluded as causative factors.

Neuromuscular-blocking or sedative drugs are known *not* to be responsible for the patient's unresponsiveness, and the nature of the untreatably severe brain disease present is known. Thus after intracranial catastrophies such as intracerebral hemorrhage or severe brain injury, the diagnosis may not be hard to make, but after cardiac arrest or if any depressant drugs have been given, it is much more difficult.

The examination should be fully documented, preferably by two physicians, and depending upon the cause, a second examination at least 12 hr later should be performed; not, for example, after severe brain injury, but always if hypoxia or drug toxicity are possible or definite factors.

Spinal reflexes indicate spinal cord function; their presence is quite compatible with the diagnosis of brain death.

The EEG is of useful confirmatory value; it reflects cortical rather than brainstem activity, but does add some graphic evidence of failure of brain function. It is not however a legal necessity to perform it.

A signed opinion that (brain) death has occurred must be given before any support systems are switched off. In dealing with children aged less than 5 years, even more conservative criteria must be applied.

AKINETIC MUTISM

Another comalike state called coma vigil, or akinetic mutism, must be recognized. In this the patient retains some part of consciousness since his eyes are often open and he may appear to look around. However he is quite unable to respond to any stimuli and is incapable of voluntary movements of the trunk or limbs.

The lesion that is responsible has isolated the cortex from the RAS. It is usually situated in the posterior diencephalon and the midbrain, but bilateral extensive lesions of the cingulate gyri or frontal lobes may do the same thing.

Many of the patients have had acute cardiopulmonary arrest and enter this state at once, or they may have been deeply comatosed at first, lightening to this state. They lie immobile, at times with their eyes open, when they may seem to follow the movement of people in the room. They respond neither to painful stimuli nor to command. The prognosis for life is poor; for independent existence, hopeless.

In a similar but not identical condition, the *locked-in syndrome,* the patients do seem to be able to perceive their surroundings; great care must be taken with what is said in their presence. Some have awakened from this state to describe (to the appalled embarrassment of the staff) discussions overheard in which they were referred to as vegetables, and when the advisability of discontinuing life-support was mooted. To hear such conversations when you have no way of responding must be a terrible experience.

This condition is due to de-efferenting of the cortex, which can no longer influence the motor, effector organs. Although the patient is aware of himself and of his environment, his body makes no response to his own commands and he lies thus, "locked-in" to his body. In some cases, communication is possible with the eyes alone, such as blinking in Morse code.

Such paralysis of the body in the presence of an alert mind may occur with pontine lesions and with severe peripheral neuropathies, myasthenia, or poliomyelitis. The lesion responsible is usually in the ventral part of the pons. Some patients recover completely, but most deteriorate and die. Recovery is more likely when the cause is neuromuscular rather than pontine.

Apart from the maintenance of life-support systems and any treatment that the primary cause may require, there is no specific therapy.

In a third condition, again different from the two just described, the patient is awake but not aware. This is the *"persistent vegatative state"* which may be seen after hypoxic-ischemic coma — as following cardiac arrest. Here the patient has wakefulness without cognition, and while he may show spontaneous eye opening there is no other motor response to stimulation. The brainstem functions still and life-support measures have to be continued, without even the hope of the patient's eventual recovery.

SYNCOPE

Syncope is another word for faint, an abrupt brief period of unconsciousness resulting from diminished cerebral blood flow. This affects first the cortex and RAS which are together responsible for the maintenance of consciousness. A list of causes is given in Table 10-3.

The effect of any of the causes listed will be much magnified by a decrease in oxygen-carrying capacity of the *blood* resulting from, for example, severe anemia or carbon monoxide poisoning. If there is reduced venous return to the heart, then cardiac output must be diminished; this may occur because of pooling of blood in the periphery, in association with peripheral circulatory failure (e.g., hypovolemia from any cause), or with increased intrathoracic pressure, as during the Valsalva maneuver (disorder of the *primer*). If the cardiac *pump* is inadequate because of arrhythmias or myocardial disease, then again blood pressure or cardiac output will be diminished. If there is any obstruction to the *pathway* for the flow of blood between the heart and the brain, then selective reduction in cerebral blood flow results. This last is particularly seen during periods of exertion when the rest of the body, as it were, "steals" blood from the cerebral circulation to maintain the requirements of muscle. While postural hypotension will tend to occur when the patient is standing or, very occasionally, sitting down, disorders of the pump or of the pathway may occur at rest or during exercise.

Clinical Features

Vasovagal syncope is the common faint described by patients as a sensation of lightheadedness, "swimminess," or swaying. They may be aware of nausea and sweating;

Table 10-3   Causes of Syncope

Disorder of the primer (diminished venous return to the heart)
    Peripheral vasodilation: vasovagal attack
                                       postural hypotension
    Valsalva maneuver
    Peripheral circulatory failure: hypovolemia (diuretics,
                                                       fluid loss)

Disorders of the pump (decreased cardiac output)
    Myocardial disease: Ischemia
                               Cardiomyopathy
    Rhythm disorders: Tachyarrhythmias
                               Severe bradycardia
                               Heart block

Disorders of the pathway
    Pulmonary embolism
    Mitral, aortic, or subaortic stenosis
    Atrial mass lesions
    Cardiac cushion defects
    Subclavian steal syndrome
    Cerebrovascular disease

Disorder of the blood
    Diminished oxygen-carrying capacity

---

next their vision blurs or actually goes black, and hearing may fade. The eyes roll up in the head, sudden unconsciousness supervenes, and they fall to the floor, but quickly recover and are left only with sensations of weakness or nausea. Occasionally, if the incident lasts for more than 1 or 2 min, they will awaken in a confused state but return to normal within a few minutes. During the period of unconsciousness, they are pale, feel cold and clammy, and may be seen to give a few brief myoclonic jerks; uncommonly these may actually lead on to a grand mal seizure. Urinary or fecal incontinence is uncommon.

This type of syncope occurs when the systolic blood pressure drops below about 60 mmHg as a result of any of the causes in Table 10-3. Patients will almost invariably be standing up when the faint begins. Strong emotions often precipitate the event. People recover rapidly if allowed to lie flat and cerebral ischemia will occur if they are held up and not allowed to fall. Fainting may recur on rising quickly after the initial recovery.

Postural hypotension may occur because of instability of vasomotor reflexes (common in adolescent females, the elderly, and patients receiving hypotensive, antidepressant, or sedative drugs). The mechanism is similar to vasovagal syncope; on standing up, one's blood pressure falls because of peripheral vasodilation resulting in reduction of cerebral blood flow. This is normally compensated for as pressor reflexes induce vasoconstriction, aortic and carotid sinus reflexes induce tachycardia, and cardiorespiratory reflexes improve the venous return to the heart. Postural hypotension occurs in some normal people, particularly after prolonged bed rest and usually in the morning on rising, perhaps caused by reduced baroreceptor influence; as if the "tone" in their peripheral capacitance vessels were reduced and blood pooled within them on standing up. It is also seen after drinking alcohol, in idiopathic orthostatic hypotension, after sympathectomy, and in neuropathies affecting autonomic fibers, e.g., diabetic neuropathy.

Perhaps a quarter of the patients have a situational cause, e.g., coughing, micturition, defecation, effort, pain, apprehension, or sitting up from recumbency.

Micturition syncope is probably due to a combination of factors. Typically, the patient has been drinking alcohol during the evening; later he arises from a warm bed, peripherally vasodilated, and walks to a cold bathroom where he strains to pass urine and thus performs a Valsalva maneuver. There is also increased vagal tone during micturition. All of these factors reduce cardiac output, with consequent cerebral ischemia. In *cough syncope,* patients afflicted by a paroxysm of coughing perform a Valsalva maneuver that leads to hypoxia and increased intracranial pressure; this may actually exceed cerebral arterial perfusion pressure. Cigarette smokers with chronic bronchitis and young children with whooping cough are those usually affected.

Breath-holding attacks in children may produce sudden unconsciousness by the Valsalva maneuver; other children produce cerebral vasoconstriction by hyperventilating and then jump up from a squatting position after holding their breath for a moment (postural hypotension and Valsalva maneuver); not surprisingly a faint often follows. Unfortunately, they probably lose in neurons more than they gain in prestige.

Many *cardiac arrhythmias* reduce cardiac output and thus cause faints, usually in older female patients. Conduction defects and tachyarrhythmias of all types produce the classic Stokes-Adams attack. Even if these cannot be differentiated clinically, diagnosis may be possible with prolonged ECG monitoring. Less acutely, cardiac output may fail with acute coronary insufficiency or following *myocardial infarction.* Marked bradycardia because of *hypersensitivity of the carotid sinus* may be a problem in elderly people, in some of whom pressure on the carotid sinus during shaving or from a tight scarf or collar is enough to cause actual asystole. Overall, cardiac causes account for another 25 percent of faints.

In the presence of any obstruction to the passage of blood from the heart to the brain (such as aortic stenosis, or an intracardiac shunt), any slight reduction in cardiac output may produce transient unconsciousness and, as was mentioned earlier, the same may occur when there is any increased peripheral demand for blood, as during exercise or with a peripheral AV fistula. Again, the clinical features will be very similar to those of vasovagal syncope.

Clinical Approach

Was It Really a Faint?

This may not be an easy question to answer, since abnormal movements may occur as a result of the temporary but acute cerebral ischemia during syncope. Typical premonitory symptoms; description from others of pallor, sweating (and if you are lucky, a slow or small pulse); occurrence under strong emotion, on rising from the lying position, with coughing, or in other typical situations, all suggest syncope as the diagnosis. If the period of unconsciousness is more than a minute however, you must consider alternative diagnoses. Preceding focal weakness, speech disturbance, or abnormal movements may indicate TIA or epilepsy; palpitations may precede hemodynamically significant arrhythmias; hunger or heavy sweating point to hypoglycemia.

The differential diagnosis of syncope includes many other causes of transient episodes of neurological dysfunction. Anxious patients may *hyperventilate* acutely, which may lead to either a dissociated state resembling a true faint or may actually produce an epileptic seizure. With *vertebrobasilar insufficiency*, patients may drop to the ground with only momentary unconsciousness with neck turning or without any obvious reason; such attacks usually occur in association with other symptoms of brainstem ischemia. *Myoclonic jerks* and *cataplexy* may similarly have as their basis a transient interruption of normal RAS function; in each case the patient suddenly falls to the ground, usually without any warning symptoms. In true *petit mal epilepsy* and in certain forms of *"partial" epilepsy*, transient loss of awareness may occur, but careful history taking will usually reveal that similar attacks have occurred when the patient was lying in bed, were attended by other symptoms, or occurred when the patient was upright but produced no loss of muscle tone so that he did not necessarily fall to the ground. *Conversion hysteria* as a cause of syncope is no longer common.[*]

Basilar migraine occurs mainly among young women and rarely causes unconsciousness, patients becoming only drowsy. *Intracranial mass leisons* may produce brief episodes of loss of consciousness caused by sudden increases in intracranial pressure. They may also compress the RAS and cause seizures. Such cerebral *metabolic* disturbances as hypoglycemia, carbon monoxide poisoning, or hypoxia from any other cause, and hypertensive encephalopathy, are other less likely possibilities.

In *cryptogenic drop attacks*, women suddenly fall while walking without any evidence of even a myoclonic jerk. The cause is quite unknown and there are no other neurological abnormalities then or later. These may be examples of akinetic seizures, a diagnosis only arrived at by exclusion.

Which Mechanism Was Responsible?

The cause of 50 percent of faints is never determined, while the remainder are equally often of cardiac and noncardiac origin. In vasovagal faints, peripheral vasodilation and bradycardia combine to diminish cerebral blood flow, but some exciting cause, such as fear of joy, should be determined for confidence in that diagnosis. With chronic anxiety in young people, hyperventilation will cause peripheral vasodilation but intracranial vasoconstriction: such patients, and those with cardiac arrhythmias, may faint while lying down.

Tachycardia and vasodilatation suggest postural hypotension for physiological reasons, such as heat or alcohol ingestion, but the tachycardia will not be found in those with primary or drug-induced autonomic failure.

Particularly in elderly patients, hypovolemia (usually induced by drugs and salt restriction), myocardial disease, and cardiac arrhythmias must be considered. Obviously, drugs such as nitrites, digoxin, L-dopa, phenothiazines, and other sedatives will be of etiologic importance. Finally, cardiac symptoms, including complaints of fainting during exercise, or signs of aortic stenosis, ventricular tachycardias, conduction block, or carotid sinus hypersensitivity, and any systemic symptoms of blood disease would indicate a disorder of the pathway or of the blood.

----

[*] The ability to turn off one's RAS at will was regarded by the Victorians as evidence of the most exalted sensibility. Fortunately, times change.

Examination

If you think that diminished venous return is likely, the most important test is to measure the blood pressure (in both arms as usual) after the patient has lain down for 10 min, and then again on standing. If the pressure falls and the pulse rises, suspect physiological vasodilation or hypovolemia; if it falls but the pulse rate does *not* increase, then an autonomic lesion is present. If no change in blood pressure is found, the diagnosis may still be correct, but the circumstances are different; or the syncope may have been vasovagal. In elderly patients with likely disorders of the primer, estimate the serum sodium and chloride and obtain routine hematology values.

In the clinic you may not detect any arrhythmia, although signs of cardiac or great vessel disease or of pulmonary hypertension may be evident. If the radial pulses are unequal, a subclavian steal syndrome may be present. Since arrhythmias are common causes of syncope in older subjects, a 24- to 48-hr period of Holter monitoring would be wise. If you suspect carotid sinus hypersensitivity, massage of one sinus may be done, but only under ECG control and with the greatest of care.

Management

Management of patients with syncope depends entirely upon diagnosis, for there are no empirical treatments. From the descriptions given previously, it should be possible to achieve the diagnosis of syncope, as opposed to other conditions producing transient loss of awareness, and to determine whether the lesion is most likely to be in the primer, the pump, or the pathway.

When postural hypotension is thought to be responsible, expansion of blood volumes or restitution of autonomic function may be possible; sympatholytic drugs may be withdrawn, blood volume replaced, AV communications closed, and sodium deficiencies made up, using either salt tablets or fludrocortisone. Treatment of cough syncope is, where possible, to stop the coughing, while micturition syncope is best avoided by giving the patient a bottle to use as he sits on the side of his bed, or sometimes by removing his prostate gland. Most disorders of the pump or pathway are cardiological and we refer you to the appropriate texts.

Syncope caused by vertebrobasilar insufficiency may be regarded as a transient ischemic episode, in which case the patient may be advised to avoid neck turning or hyperextension, perhaps with the aid of a cervical collar; or one may prescribe antiplatelet drugs in case platelet emboli are responsible.

The treatment of the other conditions mentioned earlier in the differential diagnosis is covered in the appropriate section. In all cases, anemia will have an additive effect upon any other cause of syncope, and investigation to rule it out as a contributory cause is always required.

BIBLIOGRAPHY

Dougherty, J.H. et al. Hypoxic–ischemic brain injury and the vegetative state. *Neurology 31*:991–997, 1981.

Guidelines for the determination of death. *J. Am. Med. Assoc. 246*:2154–2186, 1981.

Kapoor, W.N. et al. A prospective evaluation and follow-up of patients with syncope. *N. Engl. J. Med. 309*:197–204, 1983.

Miller-Fisher, C. Syncope of obscure nature. *Can. J. Neurol. Sci.* 6:7-20, 1979.

Pallis, C. ABC of brain death. *Br. Med. J. 285:*1409-1412 et. seq., 1982.

Plum, F., Posner, J.B. *Diagnosis of Stupor and Coma.* 3rd Ed. Contemporary Neurology Series. Philadelphia, F.A. Davis, 1980.

11
Delirious States

Delirious or "confusional" states are acute, potentially reversible, or self-limiting disturbances, characterized by a reduction in conscious level, confusion, disorientation, and disorders of attention and perception. Agitation, motor hyperactivity, inattention, and hallucinations are the cardinal signs. Although caused by a wide range of etiologic factors, they all present a relatively similar clinical picture. Most often affected are the very young, the very old, and the very sick.

Delirious states are also called *acute brain syndromes* because of their abrupt onset and fulminating course and are thought to be manifestations of widespread neuronal dysfunction. All forms demonstrate a lowered level of consciousness and variable other clinical features depending upon the cause and upon constitutional factors in an individual patient. The typical form is delirium, but a number of variations are also described. We discussed the various abnormalities of mental state as well as the methods of their examination in Chapter 1.

CLINICAL FEATURES OF DELIRIUM

Prodrome

The patient is often restless, sleepless, anxious, suspicious, and irritable before other features develop; later, agitation may crescendo to terror.

Intellect and Cognition

Clouding of consciousness is invariable. This represents an intermediate point on the continuum between normal alertness and coma, a state often described as dreamlike. Thoughts may be incoherent and the patient cannot deal with abstract concepts. If delusions are present, they may be secondary to the disturbances of perception or to the underlying mood alteration. Paranoid ideas or delusions are common. Orientation is disturbed in time and place more than in person. The patient is irritable and easily fatigued and shows poor concentration and a narrow range of fleeting attention. Memory testing reveals a poor grasp of test materials and a failure of their retention. Patchy anterograde amnesia and perseveration of responses are standard.

Behavior

The patient with delirium is often negativistic or hostile and may be agitated and overactive, particularly if hallucinations or delusions are being experienced. In "occupational delirium" the patient repeatedly performs movements corresponding to a simple task that he is used to doing. His speech is rambling, muttering, incoherent, repetitive, and often slurred and hard to understand.

If the patient's condition deteriorates, all these signs become less obvious, expenditure of energy is less, and obtundation (inert delirium) develops. In states caused by an electrolyte or blood gas disorder, this hypokinetic state may be an early manifestation.

Perceptual Disturbances

It is common for the patients to experience illusions, misidentifications, and vivid hallucinations that are more often visual than auditory.

Physiological Changes

Neurological examination shows a release of primitive reflexes (e.g., grasping and sucking reflexes) and often bilateral signs of pyramidal tract involvement, but focal signs are uncommon except in hypoglycemia and when delirium complicates a preexisting brain lesion. Myoclonic jerks or seizures may be secondary to the underlying metabolic disturbance or may be the primary cause of the delirium, as with "petit mal status" and, rarely, partial complex seizures. The pupils and extraocular movements are typically normal, but that is only true if poisoning is not the cause. Asterixis is common in hepatic and uremic states and with subarachnoid hemorrhage. Respiratory patterns must be noted carefully since hyperventilation is common, suggesting a metabolic acidosis (see Chap. 10 for causes). Salicylate poisoning and hepatic failure may however cause respiratory alkalosis.

VARIATIONS FROM THE
STANDARD CLINICAL PATTERN

Neurotic Fatigue

Irritability and fatigue, with poor attention and concentration, often follow head injury, mononucleosis, or influenza. These symptoms are not accompanied by physical signs but are entirely subjective, a combination of malaise and lack of energy.

Psychosis

Symptoms resembling those of schizophrenia, depression, or manic illness may occur, either through unmasking of a preexisting psychosis or as a spontaneous event.

This situation is distinguished from an endogenous psychosis only by the evidence of impaired consciousness and the associated physical illness.

Wernicke-Korsakoff Syndrome

Classically, this consequence of thiamine deficiency is seen in alcoholics. The syndrome (described in Chap. 43) often develops when delirium ends, and it will be reversible or not depending upon how quickly you remember to give thiamine.

CAUSES OF DELIRIUM

It is unusual to find a patient delirious for a single reason. The various causes, more than one of which should be sought in every patient, are listed in Table 11-1. Thus the alcoholic with Wernicke-Korsakoff syndrome may also have a subdural hematoma, hypoglycemia, or marked dehydration. The patient with chronic respiratory disease may be in cardiac failure, may have been given sedatives, digoxin, or diuretics, or may have cerebral ischemic disease. The patient recovering from a seizure has often been given drugs and may have been anoxic during the convulsion.

Metabolic Disease

Almost any metabolic abnormality can result in delirium (Fig. 11-1), especially in children. However the most common cause in adults are in the *postoperative* and *postpartum* states, many being related to general anesthesia. *Alcoholism, sedative drugs, cocaine, marijuana, lead, hallucinogens,* and *amphetamines* commonly cause delirium, as does *withdrawal* from any of these from habituated subjects. Any reduction in cerebral *oxygen* tension, as in chronic lung disease, congestive heart failure, pulmonary edema, severe anemia, and so on, may produce this state, particularly if there is an elevation in pCO_2. *Cerebral edema* may cause a confusional state in its early stages. All the other metabolic abnormalities listed in Table 11-1 are identifiable and correctible causes.

Cerebral Trauma

Delirium after concussion normally parallels the severity of the head injury, but remember that the delirium may be caused by subdural hematoma, the likelihood of which is *not* related to the seriousness of the head injury.

Infection

Intracranial infections, such as brain abscess, encephalitis, or meningitis (particularly tuberculous) may cause delirium, as may any infection causing a high fever, especially in children and in adults with cerebral atrophy. Pneumonia, endocarditis, and other causes of septicemia caused by gram-positive organisms are other common causes. In elderly patients, delirium may be the presenting feature. Legionnaires' disease, secondary and tertiary syphilis, and rheumatic fever are less common.

Vascular Disease

A recent cerebral ischemic event may result in delirium, particularly in the elderly atherosclerotic patient. A cerebral infarct or hemorrhage (usually right-sided) or a

Table 11-1   Major Causes of Delirium

Metabolic disease

  Toxicity: Alcohol*, all sedative agents, atropine and other anticholinergic
    drugs, amphetamines, cimetidine, CO, cocaine, digoxin, hypoglycemics,
    L-dopa and receptor agonists, LSD and other hallucinogens, lead, mari-
    juana, steroids, tricyclic drugs (see Chap. 43)

  Abstinence from agents above following habituation* (e.g., delirium tremens)

  Cerebral hypoxia and hypercapnia* (cardiac failure, COPD, hypotension,
    pulmonary embolism)

  Cerebral edema (e.g., hypertensive encephalopathy)

  Hyper-or hypoglycemia: lactic acidosis, nonketotic hyperosmolar states*

  Hypo- hypernatremia, hypo- hypercalcemia*

  Dehydration or water overload; inappropriate ADH secretion

  Dialysis

  Hepatic, renal, or respiratory failure*

  Porphyria

  Hypothermia

  Hypovitaminosis B: (Wernicke's encephalopathy)

  Postpartum states: Preeclampsia

  Postoperative states*

Cerebral trauma

  Concussion*

  Subdural hematoma

  Fat embolism

Infectious causes

  High fevers from any cause, especially in children*

  Specific fevers: smallpox, typhoid, typhus, malaria, measles, pneumonia,*
    chickenpox,* Legionnaires' disease, septicemia,* urinary tract infections,*
    bacterial endocarditis,* rheumatic fever

  Brain abscess, encephalitis, meningitis

  Postinfectious encephalopathy

  Secondary syphilis, GPI

  Pancreatitis

Cerebrovascular disease

  Recent or remote cerebrovascular disease, (infarct or hemorrhage)*

  Subarachnoid hemorrhage*

---

*The more common causes.

Table 11-1 (Continued)

Cerebrovascular disease (continued)

> Vasculitides affecting brain
> Disseminated intravascular coagulation

Postepileptic

> (Delirium may also complicate seizure status.)

Neoplastic disease

> Primary and secondary brain tumors (supratentorial)
> Cachexia of carcinomatosis
> Nonmetastatic syndrome of carcinoma

Endocrinopathy

> Hypo- or hyperfunction of adrenal or thyroid glands

Degenerative brain disease (end-stage)

---

subarachnoid hemorrhage may initially manifest in this way. A brief period of confusion may be the only manifestation of a transient cerebral ischemic attack. A patient with borderline cerebral perfusion may become acutely delirious when some other minor factor (fever, mild hypoglycemia) adds its effects.

Postepileptic

Both primary generalized and partial seizures are often followed by a brief period of confusion. An EEG will be of the utmost diagnostic value in such cases. Anticonvulsant drugs may also be responsible, especially when their serum levels are too high.

Neoplasms

Delirium may be seen with primary or secondary *cerebral tumors*, in the terminal cachectic state of carcinomatosis, and as one of the *nonmetastatic syndromes* of malignancy.

Endocrine Disease

Both *Addison's* and *Cushing's diseases* are sometimes associated with a delirious state; this is also a characteristic of severe *thyrotoxicosis*. Hyperparathyroidism is a less common cause.

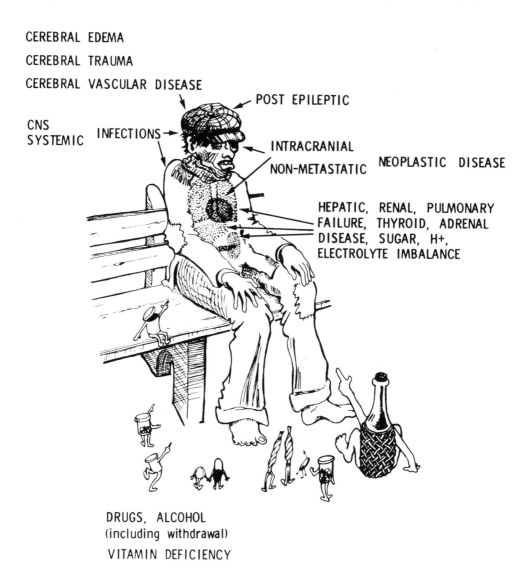

CEREBRAL EDEMA

CEREBRAL TRAUMA

CEREBRAL VASCULAR DISEASE

POST EPILEPTIC

CNS
SYSTEMIC   INFECTIONS

INTRACRANIAL
NON-METASTATIC   NEOPLASTIC DISEASE

HEPATIC, RENAL, PULMONARY
FAILURE, THYROID, ADRENAL
DISEASE, SUGAR, H+,
ELECTROLYTE IMBALANCE

DRUGS, ALCOHOL
(including withdrawal)
VITAMIN DEFICIENCY

Figure 11-1   Medical causes of delirium.

DIAGNOSIS

This depends upon an adequate history followed by a thorough general medical examination, noting all vital signs; a sound CNS evaluation; and an awareness that
in practice more than one cause is usually operating. Although you will learn little
from the patient himself, you must enquire of somebody about a history of respiratory or cardiac disease, drug or alcohol ingestion, recent changes in personality or
specific abilities, seizures, and exposure to any toxins, and other diseases.

Beware of dysphasia causing garbled speech, wrongly diagnosed as delirium.

The necessary investigations will have been suggested by the list of causes in
Table 11-1. The most productive are blood and urine cultures, chest x-ray, complete

blood count, ESR, estimation of blood sugar, electrolytes including calcium, blood gases, indices of hepatic and renal function, and a toxic screen. Blood cultures are frequently indicated, and lumbar pressure is necessary if there is any hint of meningism in adults, and always in children.

The EEG is also a most useful test in this circumstance; generalized slow activity is usually found, but some specific patterns (e.g., in hepatic coma or uremia) do occur while asymmetric abnormalities strongly suggest the presence of an intracranial lesion. Any asymmetry of neurological signs on examination will demand more sophisticated tests, such as CT scanning.

MANAGEMENT

Delirium is best treated in a general medical setting as long as one can minimize stimulation from activity around the patient. He may need to be transfered to a psychiatric unit in the acute stage if his behavior is upsetting to other patients or if the bustle of a general medical ward disturbs him; it is best if a single room on a general medical ward can be provided. This is an acute medical and metabolic emergency in most instances, but it also represents a psychiatric emergency, and the advice of a psychiatrist is often helpful, the more so since long-term care may need to be psychiatrically based.

Nursing Measures

The environment should be constant, with the lights placed high in the room to avoid shadows. Nurses should be changed as infrequently as possible and visitors restricted to one or two close relatives or friends. It may be wise to nurse a very disturbed patient on a very low bed or on a mattress on the floor. Restraints will be needed if the patient is very mobile, but only as a last resort.

Medical Measures

The first principle is that of treating the underlying condition, which obviously requires a battery of diagnostic tests in most cases. Next, one must maintain adequate fluids, electrolytes, calories, and vitamins B and C, but never give a patient a caloric load (e.g., IV glucose in water) without also administering thiamine, 50-100 mg, because the glucose might precipitate the Wernicke-Kosakoff syndrome in a thiamine-deficient patient. In delirium, barbiturates are contraindicated; for mild confusion or in drug withdrawal states use diazepam for sedation. If the condition is more severe or if there is any risk of respiratory depression, use neuroleptic drugs such as promazine, 25-100 mg, perphenazine, 1-4 mg q4h, or haloperidol, 2.5-10 mg q8h — less in elderly people. Try to avoid IM and IV injections, and never use IM paraldehyde, which is painful and induces a very reasonable paranoia.

The successful management of a patient with delirium is largely a triumph of nursing. Medical intervention aims to correct any fluid or metabolic deficiency, to prevent the patient from harming himself, and to try to find the underlying cause and treat it. There is almost always at least one delirious patient on any general ward at any one time. If you are at all concerned that a patient may be heading that way, a ward round early in the evening may show the first telltale signs; the patient messes up his food tray, picks up the bedclothes repeatedly, knocks over his water bottle, or mutters vaguely to himself. Diagnosis and early management of confusion will ensure that the other patients on the ward, and also the intern, will get a good night's sleep.

BIBLIOGRAPHY

Saper, J.R. Secondary metabolic encephalopathy. *Postgrad. Med. 69:*122, 1976.

Stengel, E. The organic confusional states and organic dementia. *Br. J. Hosp. Med. 2:*719, 1969.

12
Dementia

GENERAL FEATURES

The term dementia implies a diffuse cortical disorder affecting both hemispheres and causing a global deterioration in intellectual function. In general, a focal lesion causes specific deficits, whereas widespread involvement of the cerebral cortex causes diffuse changes in intellectual function.

The tests that are used at the bedside to assess various aspects of intellectual function are mentioned in Chapters 1 and 9. It is important to remember that the results of these tests will be meaningless unless you obtain information on the patient's prior functioning by talking to the family and employers, learning what grade in school he attained, what sort of jobs he had done, and what his interests and pursuits were in his personal life. When your bedside mental status examination has suggested dementia, quantification and exact delineation can be achieved by formal psychological testing.

Although intellect is dependent upon the normal functioning of large areas of cortex, localized disease of the brain may affect certain aspects of it more obviously than others. In association with clinical evidence of intellectual decline, such signs are dysphasia, apraxia, agnosia, epileptic seizures, and motor and sensory abnormalities may be detected, which themselves do have localizing value.

NEUROLOGICAL AND PSYCHIATRIC FINDINGS

Disorders of Intellect

The patient's *vigor, range of interests,* and ability to concentrate (his *attention span*) will be reduced in dementia as may be apparent on tests such as the reversed digit or the 100 – 7 test. The patient shows an inability to shift attention easily from one problem to another and this often results in *perseveration*. His ability to *abstract* will be affected as shown by his difficulty in explaining the moral of stories or the meaning of proverbs. It may be evident from the history of his former abilities that the patient is failing in the realm of planning and *creativity*. Thinking is often more *concrete* than abstract. Tests of *learning* and memory will show deterioration and the patient may be aware that his thinking is slow and labored. Although it comes at a later stage, *orientation* in space, time, and person may be faulty.

Motor Behavior

A history of *social withdrawal,* of disinhibited and sometimes antisocial or embarrassing behavior, of wandering, and of *restlessness* is common. Patients may cease to care for themselves properly in dress, cleanliness, or nutrition. The elderly demented patient often shows a parkinsonian picture with facial impassivity, proverty of movement, slowed shuffling gait, and a generalized flexion posture. If the bilateral lesion producing intellectual failure affects the motor areas as well, then a pseudobulbar palsy may be produced. *Perseveration* affects both speech and voluntary movement in many demented patients, and you may note that after being told to close the eyes or stick out the tongue, they continue to perform this act even when asked to do something else. When asked a question, they may give the initial answer correctly but then give that same answer repeatedly to other questions as well. Primitive release reflexes and other abnormalities described in Chapter 9 are likely to be found. Physical signs indicating cortical or subcortical disease, usually bilaterally but not symmetrically, and involving motor more than sensory functions are a late development.

Emotion

Mood tends to be *labile* and easily changed by circumstance or by suggestion. Patients are often quite *irritable* and their level of *frustration tolerance* is very low. Their affect is sometimes flat rather than labile but most commonly of all, *depression* is evident. If there is one thing that you can frequently do to improve the demented patient, it is to relieve the concomitant depression that is so often present. It is sometimes very difficult to know whether a depressed patient is also demented or just appears demented because he is depressed. Reserve judgment, treat the depression, and then reassess the patient to see if there is still evidence of an organic brain syndrome.

Personality

There is no characteristic personality type associated with brain damage or dementia. In general, the personality traits demonstrated tend to be an accentuation of those that are formerly present. Obsessional adherence to old routines may in part guard the patient against the threats of change and the confusion of the things in his environment that he does not understand. Egocentricity and demanding behavior are frequently seen.

Perceptions and Judgment

Common findings in a demented patient include a narrowed field of attention, more blunting of awareness, and impairment of time sense. The finer shade of judgment in interpersonal relationships are often altered and the patient may make serious errors of judgment in business situations. Subtle changes in judgment at an early stage in dementia may result in serious consequences, particularly before the disturbed mental state is recognized. Illusions and hallucinations are not usual features of dementia.

Physiology

There are not many specific disturbances of bodily physiology in association with dementia but urinary (and rarely fecal) *incontinence* may occur. Incontinence in dementia should be regarded as a very specific indication of bilateral medial frontal lobe involvement because it is in this area that the cortical inhibition of bladder function is localized. An early symptom may be inversion of the normal *sleep* pattern so that the patient tends to take many naps during the day but stays awake at night, puttering about the house, unwilling to go to bed. Confusion is always much worse in the evening, perhaps in part because of a lack of visual and other sensory cues from the environment. This is a point worth remembering, particularly when an elderly patient with borderline cerebral function is admitted to a hospital. One can imagine the sensory deprivation of an elderly patient with impaired vision, hearing, and peripheral sensation who is put in a plain, white, poorly lit hospital room, particularly if it is a private room. Even minor stresses, metabolic derangements, and small doses of drugs may induce a delirious state in the demented patient.

When assessing the patient suspected of having any intellectual decline, his hearing and vision should be tested carefully as should his ability to understand what is said to him. Carefully assess mood, as symptoms of depression frequently mimic those of dementia in the old. You also have to make an objective decision about the patient's degree of dementia because it may be common for wives or husbands to feel that their spouse is "failing" when he is merely hard of hearing or depressed, or else they may cover up for his failing abilities.

THE CAUSES OF DEMENTIA

Dementia results from disease within the nervous system or from general medical diseases that secondarily affect it (Fig. 12-1).

Medical Causes

In a list of general medical diseases that may present with dementia, you will see that almost all of them are treatable. To identify these problems and to give them appropriate therapy, you must first think of each possibility and carry out the appropriate investigations. This serves to emphasize the facts that dementia is a syndrome demanding etiologic diagnosis and that it does not necessarily carry with it an ominous prognosis. If the treatable causes of dementia are not considered in every case, then the result may be a tragic progression to unnecessary death.

CNS Diseases

Disorders characterized by dementia in association with specific disease of the nervous system also include many treatable conditions (Table 12-1). One must be sure that a *frontal lobe tumor* or a *chronic subdural hematoma* is not the cause of the progressive dementia with neurological signs. Since both are often "silent," almost

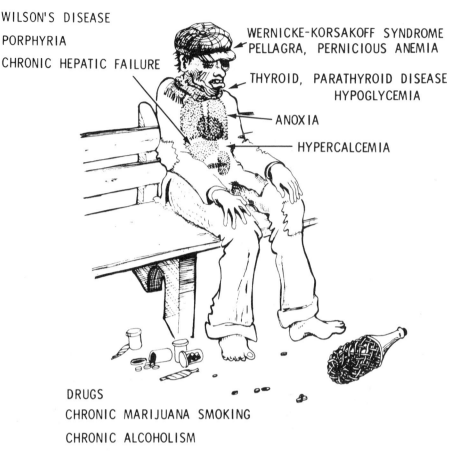

WILSON'S DISEASE

PORPHYRIA

CHRONIC HEPATIC FAILURE

WERNICKE-KORSAKOFF SYNDROME

PELLAGRA, PERNICIOUS ANEMIA

THYROID, PARATHYROID DISEASE

HYPOGLYCEMIA

ANOXIA

HYPERCALCEMIA

DRUGS

CHRONIC MARIJUANA SMOKING

CHRONIC ALCOHOLISM

Figure 12-1   Medical causes of dementia.

impossible to diagnose clinically, and yet potentially treatable, noninvasive (CT or nucleide) investigations would be defensible in all demented patients with no other clear diagnosis. Social and economic factors will probably weigh more than medical ones when this question is raised. *Multiinfarct dementia* presents with an increasing level of confusion and intellectual deficit, associated with small infarctions. There may be a stepwise progression in the disease. It is differentiated clinically from Alzheimer's disease by a past history of strokes, its relatively abrupt onset, the presence of focal symptoms and signs, and by the demonstration of focal low-density areas on CT scans. It is important to recognize because blood pressure control and treatment with antiplatelet agents or surgery may relieve or reduce the dementia. Huntington's disease is described in Chapter 46.

All the underlying CNS diseases listed are described elsewhere in this book, except for cerebral amyloid angiopathy. In this condition, heavy deposition of amyloid in the cerebral vessels leads to a combination of dementia and recurrent small cerebral hemorrhages in normotensive people. The other CNS diseases must be considered one by one when any lateralizing or localizing signs are found — Alzheimer's disease (which is the most common residual diagnosis) seldom shows such signs but rather those of *diffuse* cerebral dysfunction.

Table 12-1   Causes of Dementia

Caused by underlying medical disease

    Endocrine
        hypo- or hyperthyroidism
        hypoglycemia
        hyperparathyroidism

    Metabolic diseases
        Wilson's disease
        porphyria
        chronic hepatic failure
        hypercalcemia
        anoxia

    Deficiency states
        pernicious anemia
        Wernicke-Korsakoff syndrome
        pellagra

    Intoxication
        bromidism
        chronic alcoholism
        chronic marijuana smoking
        drugs (sedatives, tranquilizers, antihypertensives)

Due to underlying CNS diseases

    Familial
        Huntington's chorea
        leukodystrophy

    Neoplastic
        primary
        secondary
        nonmetastatic manifestations of malignancy

    Inflammatory
        subacute encephalitis
        syphilis
        kuru
        Jacob-Creutzfeldt disease
        progressive multifocal leukoencephalopathy

    Vascular
        carotid occlusion
        bilateral strokes
        hypertension
        amyloid angiopathy

    Traumatic
        chronic subdural hematoma
        posttraumatic
        punch-drunk syndrome

    Degenerative disease
        Parkinson-dementia complex
        Parkinson's disease

    Demyelinating diseases
        multiple sclerosis

Conditions of uncertain cause

    Normal pressure hydrocephalus
    Alzheimer's disease ("senile" dementia)
    Pick's disease
    Progressive supranuclear palsy

Uncertain Causes

Normal pressure hydrocephalus (NPH) (Fig. 12-2) is a syndrome of dementia with incontinence of urine and severe gait disturbance. It has been found to be a treatable cause of dementia, thus diagnosis is of great importance. In this condition there is marked dilation of the ventricles and the CSF flow pattern over the hemispheres is abnormal, as shown by the RISA cisternogram. Over half of the patients

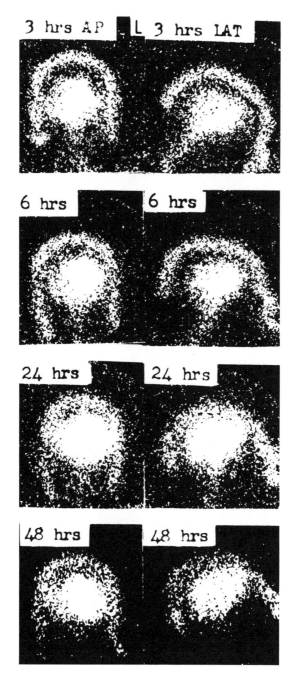

Figure 12-2   Normal pressure hydrocephalus. RISA scan showing early and persistent (48-hr) accumulation of the isotope in the ventricular system. The uptake corresponding to the position of the scalp is a marker.

with NPH will have a history of previous meningitis or of bleeding in the CSF from a subarachnoid hemorrhage or trauma.

The cerebral capillaries and choroid plexus make CSF, which leaves the ventricular system through the roof of the fourth ventricle and bathes the spinal cord and brain before passing upward over the convexity of the hemispheres to the arachnoid villi. In patients with NPH (see Fig. 12-2), the CSF appears to be absorbed mainly through the ependyma of the lateral ventricles because of failure of flow of CSF. A RISA scan will show that the CSF does not ascend over the convexity to reach the superior sagittal sinus. A CT scan (Fig. 12-3) shows large ventricles with little cortical atrophy. A shunting procedure may reverse many of the clinical features of this condition, but the long-term results have not been as good as the initial results indicated. The occurrence of a syndrome such as NPH does demand that all patients with progressive unexplained dementia be investigated for this and other treatable problems.

Other disorders for which the cause is unknown are Alzheimer's disease, Pick's disease, and progressive supranuclear palsy.

The criteria for the diagnosis of *Alzheimer's disease* include abnormalities of mental status in two or more areas of cognition, including orientation in time, place, and person; memory; language skills; praxis (such as copying tests and block design); attention; and problem solving. In addition, the intellectual change must have been slowly progressive and have occurred in later life, no disturbance

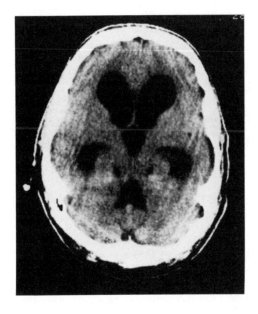

Figure 12-3 CT scan. Marked dilatation of the lateral, third and fourth ventricles but no widening of the cortical sulci, suggesting communicating hydrocephalus (NPH).

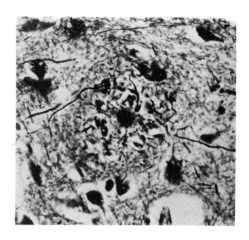

Figure 12-4   Alzheimer's disease. A senile plaque is shown centrally.

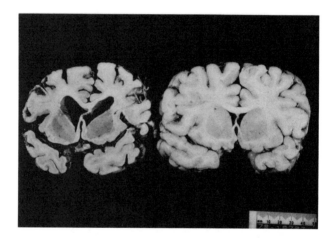

Figure 12-5   Coronal section of brain. Left-side, Alzheimer's disease. (Right side, normal.)

of consciousness may be present, and other medical/neurological causes of dementia must have been excluded.

The pathology (Fig. 12-4) is similar to that seen in the very aged brain, but there are more plaques and neurofibrillary tangles present and the progression of the illness is more rapid. Marked cortical atrophy is seen in Figures 12-5 and 12-6. Similar features are also seen in mongolism and in the punch-drunk syndrome. *Pick's disease* is rare and clinically looks exactly like Alzheimer's disease. These patients have marked atrophy of the frontal and temporal lobes, with distinctive microscopic findings.

In each case, the disease progresses insidiously, accelerating after 1 or 2 years during which minor personality changes, rigidity, loss of interest, superficiality, and so on, have exasperated the family, puzzled friends, and charmed acquaintances.

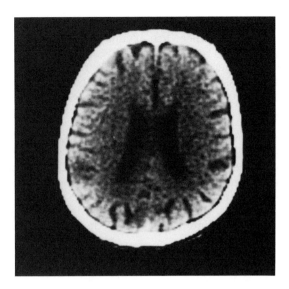

Figure 12-6   CT scan, Alzheimer's disease. The dilated ventricles and the atrophied cortex are shown.

Later, however, self-care, emotional control, and judgment and the cognitive skills listed previously obviously fail and neurological signs appear. These include minor features of parkinsonism, primitive release responses, and asymmetrically abnormal tone and reflexes. Then the accelerating tempo of the process makes the patient dependent, unreliable, and potentially harmful to himself and total care is required, until death restores that dignity compromised in life.

   Although some evidence of dementia can be uncovered in 15 percent of people over the age of 65 years, there is no place for the term "senile dementia," which is truly Alzheimer's disease.

   In *progressive supranuclear palsy* (see also Chap. 21), loss of upward and of downward gaze, rigidity of the neck and trunk muscles, dementia, dysphagia, and parkinsonian signs are the major clinical features. The condition is rare. The latter signs may respond to bromocriptine, but L-dopa is not effective.

DIAGNOSIS

The diagnosis of dementia is clinical, utilizing a history from family, friends, and/or employers, a full physical examination, and a mental status assessment. Only rarely is psychological testing necessary, and then only to quantitate and further to define the intellectual deficit or to confirm the presence of dementia in its earliest stages. These can only be done if the patient is not delirious or sleepy. After diagnosis the problem is to determine *why* the dementia is present.

   As you can see from Table 12-1, many of the diseases causing dementia are treatable, and thus it is important to identify the causative pathology. Although it would be easy to state that all tests for the listed diseases should be done, one has to show intelligent judgment in each situation. In most cases, tests will include routine hematological and biochemical screening, ESR, specific serologic testing, serum B_{12}, thyroid and liver function tests, urinary porphyrins, EEG, skull x-rays, and an isotope scan. Serum bromide and barbiturate levels may also be helpful.

If the pathology is still not determined, a CT scan may be useful (see Figs. 12-5; 12-6); it will be essential if there are asymmetric CNS signs and helpful in most cases listed under section 2 in Table 12-1. CSF examination may be needed to rule out some conditions listed there. A RISA cisternogram is probably the best test for the diagnosis of normal pressure hydrocephalus. Rarely, such tests as urinary copper or porphyrins, or enzymatic screening are indicated.

DIFFERENTIAL DIAGNOSIS

There are a number of conditions that look like dementia, where in fact intellectual status is normal. These confusing conditions include depressive and schizophrenic psychoses, some cases of Parkinson's disease, and drug intoxication. All are described elsewhere in the book. Be sure that your patient is not just deaf, is not dysphasic, and has shown a decline in intellect rather than developmental retardation.

MANAGEMENT

Needless to say, the treatment of dementia lies in the treatment of the underlying medical or neurological disease. Almost half of the causes of dementia are treatable and every case must be regarded as a problem in diagnosis rather than just a problem in disposal.

Dementia produces changes in the person that create a number of difficulties in management. The family and medical personnel may become upset and anxious about the patient's tendency to misunderstand their instructions, comments, and questions and to take their concern as a stimulus for irritability or bad temper. His limited attention and memory may produce annoying situations that may further irritate him. The families of people with damaged brains must therefore be assured about their own reasonableness and competence to maintain good interpersonal relationships, and a rational explanation for the patient's behavior should be given in terms of his brain damage. If there is an atmosphere of understanding, then tolerance and forebearance will come more readily to those who have to put up with the difficulties posed by a change in their relative, and this renewed understanding will be reflected in the patient's own return to more tolerable behavior.

The patient's home and working environments should be arranged so that he has, if possible, less opportunity to realize his decreased efficiency. Changes are likely to be tolerated badly by brain-damaged individuals; new instructions and new environments may cause great confusion. A few simple alterations in the home may make a big difference to the demented patient. A dim bedroom light at night, placed high to avoid shadows, may calm him during periods of confusion, particularly if it is difficult for him to sleep. He should be allowed to contract his life, with no unusual or difficult routines forced on him. His unconscious defenses will have established for him a set order of doing things; this pattern should be accepted, and he should be allowed the reassurance he obtains from their execution.

Financial and similar affairs always pose a tricky problem, but no more than advice can be given until the patient is no longer capable of managing his own affairs. Then the power of attorney can be vested by the patient in a member of the family or in his legal advisor.

Although drugs are commonly required in the elderly patient, it is a good general rule to use only those drugs that are absolutely necessary. Patients with dementia tolerate barbiturates very badly, becoming quite confused. If some nighttime sedation is used, then a small dose of flurazepam or diazepam is acceptable; but a tot of brandy is often just as effective. If anxiety is a problem, then diazepam may be used. Vasodilators and vitamin preparations are frequently recommended, but there is little indication that they are of any value unless a specific deficiency can be demonstrated. One must always remember that the demented patient will commonly forget to take his medication or will take incorrect doses. In most situations, it is wise to have someone else control and administer the medication. The use of precursors of acetylcholine (the main transmitter in memory pathways) has led to minor improvement in memory in some cases. Physostigmine and oral lecithin (not an approved drug but available at health food stores) have been tried, on much the same principle that leads one to give L-dopa in Parkinson's disease.

Because of a number of recurring problems in the aged, demented patient, there is a tendency for them to be placed on more and more drugs, without much attention to stopping them or reevaluating their use. Eventually many problems result from the various vasodilators, diuretics, antihypertensives, laxatives, sedatives, hypnotics, vitamins, and other drugs that were started and never discontinued.

Although some patients require a nursing home or chronic care institution to maintain them, most are better off in their own home environment with an understanding family. There are many community resources that can be marshaled to help and advise the family on how to maintain the patient successfully in the home environment, and these should be used liberally.

BIBLIOGRAPHY

Anonymous. Death of a mind. *Lancet 27:*1012-1015, 1950.

Cummings, J.L., Benson, D.F. *Dementia: A Clinical Approach.* Boston, Butterworth, 1983.

Folstein, M. et al. Mini-mental state. A practical method for grading the cognitive state of patients for the clinician. *J. Psychiatr. Res. 12:*189-198, 1975.

McKhann, G. et al. Clinical diagnosis of Alzheimer's disease. *Neurology 34:*939-944, 1984.

Myers, R.H., Martin, J.B. Huntingtons disease. *Sem. Neurol. 2:*365-372, 1982.

Ropper, A.H. A rational approach to dementia. *Can. Med. Assoc. J. 121:*1175-1190, 1979.

Strub, R.L., Black, F.L. *Organic Brain Syndromes.* Philadelphia, F.A. Davis Co., 1981.

Terry, R.D., Katzman, R. Senile dementia of the Alzheimer's type. *Ann. Neurol. 14:*497-506, 1983.

Wells, C.E. Chronic brain disease: An overview. *Am. J. Psychiatry 135:*1-12, 1978.

13
Disturbance of Memory

Memory is the capacity for retaining and making secondary use of an experience, implying a process whereby experiences are stored so that they can be retrieved later. Memory can be classified as (1) neurological, (2) genetic, or (3) immunological, but only the first will be considered here. The problem of the patient who presents with memory difficulty may be approached by first deciding if he suffers from a disorder of memory in isolation or from dementia — a diffuse intellectual impairment in which memory is just one of the faculties altered. The question is answered by doing a mental status examination that will determine whether or not other intellectual areas are involved and will give you some idea of how significant the memory impairment is. In this chapter we will discuss isolated memory loss.

THE ANATOMY OF MEMORY

The anatomical structures involved in memory include both cortical and subcortical areas. The subcortical structures involved in creating memories include the hippocampi, fornices, mammillary bodies, medial dorsal nuclei of the thalamus, and the cingulate gyri, which together form bilateral interconnected circuits. A most important area in terms of memory is the hippocampal region; bilateral hippocampal lesions result in striking memory loss, characterized by the patient's inability to form any lasting memories, information being retained only for about 30 sec. The same may be true for bilateral lesions elsewhere on the circuit.

The hippocyampal region is important in the laying down of *short-term* memory but the cerebral cortex is probably the major site of most *long-term* memory transcripts. Focal lesions do not cause generalized memory loss but rather loss of specific functions. Visual designs are more impaired with right temporal lesions than with left; memories of verbal auditory material are stored predominantly in the left temporal lobe and of music in the right. Most memories are stored in both hemispheres with interhemispheric transfer of information via the corpus callosum and other commissures. Since most memories are duplicated in the two hemispheres, cortical lesions must be bilateral to interfere with memory storage.

MECHANISMS OF REMEMBERING

A simplified concept of memory can be put forward in diagrammatic form (Fig. 13-1).

Immediate memory appears not to be RNA-dependent and is probably electrical, whereas longer-stored memories are RNA-dependent and are altered by any drugs that affect RNA synthesis. Short-term memory is a function of subcortical structures (the Papez circuit; Fig. 13-2), whereas storage is diffuse in cortical structures. Recall is an active process and it can occur from immediate, short-term, or long-term memory stores. As students know only too well, memories fade with time. It has been suggested that there is a built-in decay mechanism for memories ("physiological forgetting"). Cortical stimulation studies show that although much stored information cannot easily be recalled, it is still there. Memory is also altered by circumstances, particularly if the event to be remembered is of significance to us. Repetition and reproduction on challenge aid retention, as does a high level of motivation. Often memories are suppressed or repressed because of emotional overtones.

THEORIES OF MEMORY

Immediate and possibly short-term memories probably have an electrical basis, but it is unlikely that long-term memory is stored in such reverberating circuits. (If this were so, we would expect a grand mal seizure to wipe them out, which it does not.) An intriguing suggestion has been made that selective synapses are set up by a pattern of central neuronal stimulation and that there may be formation of specific membrane proteins at the synaptic sites. This would result in the formation of "favored" synapses.

CLINICAL ASSESSMENT OF MEMORY

General observations during the interview of a patient have great value. One can get some idea of the patient's perceptions, his mood and emotion, his speech pattern, and his level of attention by observing his answers during history taking.

Specific tests of memory that can be performed at the bedside were described in Chapter 1. Having decided whether a patient with a memory problem has a specific memory disorder or a memory disorder as part of a more diffuse dementia, you must then decide what the cause of the problem might be. The causes of memory loss are shown in Table 13-1.

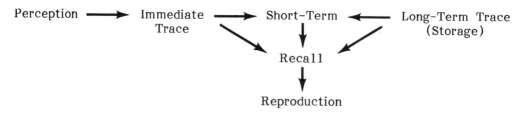

Figure 13-1

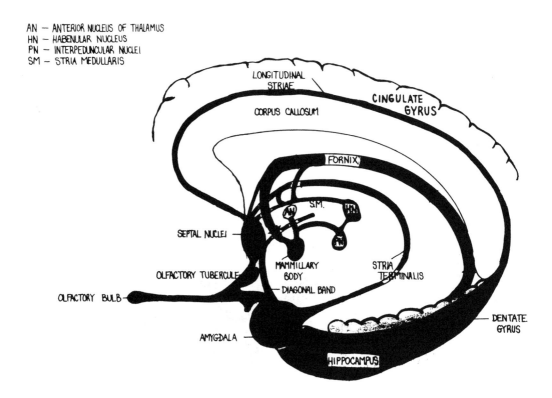

Figure 13-2   Diagram of the structures the limbic circuit comprises (hippocampus, fornix, mammillary bodies, mammillothalamic tract, anterior nucleus of thalamus, cingulate gyrus). In the late 1930s, Dr. James Papez first defined this circuit as the anatomical substrate of emotion; but it is equally important in memory processes.

Table 13-1   Classification and Causes of Memory Disorders

Acute onset but of brief duration

Any cause of delirium
Temporal lobe seizures
Transient global amnesia
Head injury
Electroconvulsive therapy (ECT)
Hysterical amnesia
Alcoholic "blackout"

Acute or subacute with residual effects

Wernicke-Korsakoff syndrome
Herpes simplex encephalitis
Tuberculous meningitis
Vertebrobasilar ischemia
Anoxia
Temporal lobe surgery
Severe head injury

Slowly progressive

Depression
Tumors of the third ventricle
Progressive dementia
Chronic sedative ingestion

Specific memory disorders (agnosias)

CAUSES OF MEMORY LOSS

Memory Disorders of Acute
Onset but of Brief Duration

During any confusional state, memories will not be laid down normally, if at all; as a result, the patient will be more or less amnesic for that period.

Temporal lobe *seizures* may cause complete loss of memory for the episode, or the patient may remember the initial aura but lose memory for subsequent parts of the seizures. In this situation the loss of memory is usually brief unless the seizure is followed by a period of automatism; the patient usually does not remember this period, which can last for hours. If temporal lobe seizures result from a left-sided focus, there may be specific defects in verbal memories, but if the lesion is on the right side, there may be more effect on the patient's graphic and nonverbal memories.

Transient global amnesia is a very interesting form of memory loss that occurs suddenly, persists for a number of hours, and ends as suddenly as it appeared. The patient during this episode lays down no memories and may appear to be acting in a peculiar or dazed fashion. During this period of confusion he may ask the same questions repeatedly but does not retain the answers. When the episode is over, there is no residual deficit but he recalls something of the amnesic period and the problem seldom recurs. A temporal lobe seizure or vertebrobasilar ischemia could account for the syndrome but there is increasing evidence that it is actually ischemic in origin.

Head injury may cause a brief period of amnesia for the moment of the trauma or, if more severe, will cause a *retrograde amnesia* for prior events and an *anterograde amnesia* ("posttraumatic") for subsequent ones. The retrograde amnesia is usually brief if the injury is not severe, but the anterograde amnesia is often longer. For a minor head injury, the amnesia lasts for minutes; a longer period suggests a much more severe concussion.

Electroconvulsive therapy (ECT) may cause retrograde and anterograde amnesia similar to that of a head injury. Repetitive ECT may induce more long-lasting memory disturbance, especially when the treatments are given closely spaced.

Hysterical amnesia usually has a sudden onset, and is total for all memories, for years back. The patients may complain that they cannot remember anything in their previous life or of the sudden onset of memory loss which is total for the period involved. This latter type of hysterical amnesia resembles transient global amnesia. The patient is usually repressing stressful conflicts and cannot "afford" to remember any events during this period; thus memory loss appears to be total. Most true amnestic syndromes have patchy areas of retained memory. The patient who strolls into the local police department stating he does not know who he is or where he came from is almost invariably suffering a conversion reaction. The television programs about people wandering the countryside searching for their past identity also depict hysterical amnesia.

Alcoholic blackouts are described in Chapter 43.

Memory Disorders of Acute or Subacute Onset with Residual Effects

The *Wernicke-Korsakoff syndrome* includes both an impaired ability to recall events and other information that had been well established before the illness (retrograde amnesia) and an impaired ability to acquire new information (anterograde amnesia). These patients may otherwise have relatively normal intellectual function. Confabulation may or may not be present and is a much overrated component of this syndrome, which is fully described in Chapter 43.

Herpes simplex encephalitis frequently involves both temporal lobes and in those patients who recover, the same disturbance of memory may be seen. This syndrome is discussed further in Chapter 40. Tuberculous meningitis tends to affect basal regions most severely but can also damage the temporal lobes, resulting in severe memory disturbances.

Because the inferior aspect of both temporal lobes is supplied by the vertebrobasilar circulation, memory disturbance may occur from *ischemia* in this area. *Anoxia* and *carbon monoxide* poisoning may also selectively involve the hippocampi, which are particularly susceptible to hypoxia. Such lesions will produce a global anterograde amnesia.

Memory may be affected by *temporal lobe surgery,* but if a normal temporal lobe remains on the other side, the defect is minimal. If the left temporal lobe is removed, the patient may experience some difficulty with auditory stimuli and with right temporal lobectomy, some difficulty with visual figures.

Severe *head trauma* may cause prolonged retrograde and anterograde amnesia. The memory loss for this period will be permanent despite otherwise full recovery. Depending upon the amount of destruction of brain tissue from the injury, a variable degree of disturbance in retaining new memories may continue.

Slowly Progressive Memory
Disorders with Associated Symptoms

Patients with a rare *tumor of the third ventricle* have been noted to have a progressive disturbance of memory. This may be due to involvement of the circuitry involved in the laying down of memories, particularly the medial dorsal nuclei of the thalamus and the other structures involved in Papez' circuit. Much more common causes of progressive memory disturbance are the *dementias,* especially the premature cerebral atrophy of Alzheimer's disease. These are discussed fully in Chapter 12.

Most, if not all people, complaining of memory disorders really have a failure of concentration only, not memory. During periods of anxiety or depression these patients do not make a permanent memory trace because of preoccupation, emotional upset, or overstimulation. Therefore a careful inquiry into their emotional state and concentration is important too.

Specific Defects of Memory

Visual, auditory, and spatial *agnosias,* as well as asterognosis, might be defined as specific memory defects in that the patient appears not to remember information relating to these functions. In agnosias, the patient seems to "forget" how to recognize what he sees, hears, or feels. This is really a disorder of recognition, and this aspect of memory is localized to the cortex. This is not surprising since recognition depends upon cortical perception of a new stimulus and cortical matching of that stimulus with similar ones perceived in the past. In the same way, apraxia (Chap. 9) may be regarded as an inability to recall how to perform some motor act, evidencing damage to a specific cortical area.

TESTS OF MEMORY

Some patients will complain of their memory loss, and thus testing will naturally follow. The memory disturbance may be indicated by the family in other circumstances; but sometimes the disturbance of memory may only be apparent by your observations during the interview and should lead you to carry out careful tests of memory and intellectual function as outlined in Chapter 1. These will include digit retention, story recall, and the repeating of three named objects a few minutes later. Other questions, such as what the patient had for breakfast, how long he has been in the hospital, and the names of his doctors and nurses, are only useful if you know the correct answers.

Treatment

The only treatment of amnesic syndromes is that of the cause in most instances. Thus seizure control, antiplatelet therapy, or psychiatric intervention for alcoholism, depression, and hysterical illness may be appropriate in specific cases. As mentioned in Chapter 12, the use of precursors of the transmitters involved may produce some symptomatic benefit, but such therapy is not standard. Hyperbaric oxygen improves retention and recall, but just for a few hours. Vitamins are only of value in the Wernicke-Korsakoff syndrome. Vasodilators are of no help.

SOME PRACTICAL ADVICE ABOUT LEARNING

Most of us learn poorly because we do not learn properly. To make the most of your time spent in attempting to acquire new data you might use the following aids.

1. Overlearn: Set a criterion of being able to repeat to yourself the whole matter to be learned not once, but more than once.
2. Challenge yourself by occasionally retesting your learning.
3. Avoid similar subjects for study. Do not learn the causes of motor neuropathy and the causes of sensory neuropathy one after the other, or these will become blurred together. Add a "filler" between the two, such as the causes of headache or a discussion of sleep disturbance, or have a nap.
4. Do not try to learn anything by rote without understanding *how* the process or condition operates, and how a patient might present who is affected by the problem. Only commit to memory those things that you know you might use in understanding or practicing medicine; just remember where the list is to be found for everything else. What you don't use, you lose.
5. If possible, learn in a quiet atmosphere, memtally relaxed, and for short periods only.
6. Recall that distortions and loss of memories occur with all succeeding stimuli, not just with new and similar learning tasks. The best time to learn by rote is before you go to bed (and to sleep).

BIBLIOGRAPHY

Slade, W.R. *Geriatric Neurology.* New York, Futura Publishing Co., 1981.

Whitty, C.W.M., Zangwill, O.L. *Amnesia.* 2nd Ed. London, Butterworths, 1977.

14
Disorders of Speech

Speech is communication by language. The language may convey an idea, a feeling, or a command. The same thoughts may also be expressed in writing or by gesture (pantomime), so language may be regarded as a means of communication by the spoken word, writing, or gesture. For this communication to be meaningful, you have to receive and interpret these sounds when they are spoken by others; speech depends upon the interpretation as well as upon the expression of thoughts. Speech is thus a product of the mind, a psychological as well as a physiological function. Words can be regarded as an instrument of the mind whereby we may most efficiently communicate our thoughts to others.

LOCALIZATION OF SPEECH FUNCTIONS

Certain functions, of which speech is the best known example, are localized chiefly or exclusively in one hemisphere. It is thought that in early life either hemisphere can function for speech if the other is damaged. However there is an hereditary tendency for speech to be established on the left side, irrespective of whether one is right- or left-handed. Although virtually all right-handed people have left hemisphere dominance for speech, half of all left-handed people do also. One means of determining the dominant hemisphere is Wada's test in which amobarbital (Amytal Sodium) is injected into the internal carotid artery while the patient counts and moves the contralateral hand. If the injection is into the nondominant side, the patient stops counting for about 30 sec and develops a contralateral hemiparesis. This disappears in about 5 min and the patient denies that he had had any weakness at all. If the dominant hemisphere has been injected, then there is a speechless period of 1 to 2 min with a resumption of confused counting and the patient is well aware that he had been paralyzed on the opposite side.

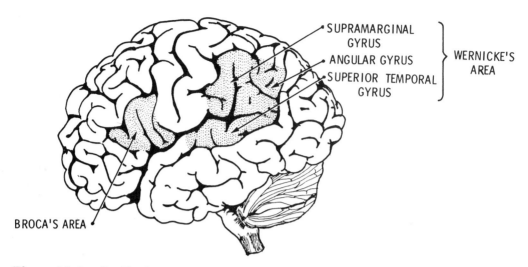

Figure 14-1   Cortical speech areas.

Another difficulty has been to decide whether speech is localized to a small area of the dominant hemisphere or whether it relies upon the integration of many areas and can therefore be lost by a lesion that disconnects them.

A simplified concept of speech localization is shown in Figure 14-1. When a lesion disrupts speech, it usually does so by affecting the area for reception (posterior temporal area) or for expression (Broca's area). Thus a lesion in the receptive or sensory area causes the patient to have difficulty understanding what is said to him or even what he is saying himself; whereas a lesion in the motor or expressive cortex causes the patient to have difficulty formulating or expressing what he want to say.

Phonation, the production of vocal sounds, is a function of the larynx; the current of expired air causes the vocal cords to vibrate, producing sound waves. These sound waves are amplified in the chest, nasopharynx, and mouth. The timbre of the voice depends upon the size and shape of the glottis and the thickness of the vocal cords. Pitch depends upon the tension of the cords: in states of tension or excitement the vocal cords contract and the voice becomes higher pitched.

Articulation is the modification of the vibrations in the currents of air as they pass through the nasopharynx and mouth, the shape of which are varied by movements of the lips, palate, and tongue. The soft palate moves to open or close the nasal airways so that the expired air passes either through the nose or through the mouth. The tongue takes a number of positions to shape vowels and consonants, and the lips help a little in vowel production but mainly shape the labial sounds, *P,* *B,* and *M.*

The complex mechanisms of articulation involving the lips, jaws, tongue, palate, larynx, and respiratory muscles are integrated and coordinated by both hemispheres but with dominant control from one, usually the left.

Disorders of speech can be classified as follows:

1.   Dysarthria: difficulty in articulation
2.   Dysphonia: disturbance in the production of sound
3.   Mutism: a complete loss of speech
4.   Aphasia (same as dysphasia): a disturbance of communication involving language

DYSARTHRIA

Neurons in each hemisphere exert control over the nuclei of the brainstem on both sides, whence the cranial nerves innervate the various muscles involved in articulation. Dysarthria can occur from a lesion at any of the levels mentioned, but may also be the result of local oral disorders such as cleft palate, tonsillitis, lingual ulcers, and ill-fitting (or lost) dentures.

A lesion in one hemisphere seldom causes significant dysarthria because the bulbar nuclei are bilaterally innervated and thus get some input from the normal hemisphere. Occasionally, one can detect dysarthria for a short time after a cerebral infarction, but this disappears unless facial paralysis or dysphasia are prominant.

Bilateral cerebral lesions however may cause a *pseudobulbar palsy* with a spastic dysarthria. These patients have slow speech and also difficulty in swallowing and coughing and labile or incontinent emotions.

The most common causes of bilateral lesions are strokes, multiple sclerosis, trauma, and motor neuron disease. The speech sounds are tight-lipped and almost spat out as the patient obviously has difficulty in modulating his speech sounds.

A brainstem lesion produces a *bulbar palsy* with flaccid paralysis of the muscles of articulation. Formerly, the most common causes were poliomyelitis and diphtheria, but now they are probably motor neuron disease and brainstem strokes. If the seventh nerve is involved, there will be slurring of the labial sounds so that the patient has trouble pronouncing *B* and *M*. If the ninth nerve is involved, the speech will be nasal and a loss of gutturals will cause particular difficulty in pronouncing *G, K,* and *Q*. With damage to the tenth nerve, again there is nasality and difficulty in phonating because of weakness or paralysis of at least part of the larynx, a dysphonia (see below). With twelfth nerve involvement, the dentals will be slurred, giving rise to difficulty in pronouncing *D* and *T*.

Lesions involving the *cerebellum* and its pathways may result in ataxic or scanning dysarthria because of incoordination of the muscles of articulation. This can be seen in multiple sclerosis, hereditary ataxias, and malignancy, or it may be due to alcohol or drug (e.g., phenytoin) toxicity. In these cases, the speech sounds staccato, disjointed, perhaps abnormally regular, with an obvious tendency for syllables to be separated, rather as children do when they read a difficult poem.

Disorders of the *extrapyramidal system* such as Parkinson's disease or phenothiazine toxicity cause a slow, quiet, monotonous dysarthria. A disorder of the *myoneural junction* (myasthenia gravis) results in progressive weakness and fatiguing of the muscles of respiration and articulation. Thus the patient's voice may fade away as he continues to speak. Primary disorders of the *muscles* of articulation, such as polymyositis and some dystrophies, result in a constantly weak and indistinct voice.

DYSPHONIA

Dysphonia is an abnormality in the production of sound for speech. The most common cause is a simple laryngitis caused by edema of the vocal cords, but it may also result from paralysis of one or both of them. It is possible to distinguish disturbances of articulation from those of phonation by asking the patient to whisper and hum. If a patient can whisper normally, articulation is intact, and if he can hum with his mouth open, phonation is normal.

MUTISM

Mutism is rare and usually has a psychological basis. However it may occur in some
patients with mental retardation, severe psychiatric withdrawal states, akinetic
mutism (Chap. 10), in strokes producing severe expressive dysphasia (see the following discussion), and in severe bulbar palsy, including myasthenia gravis.

DYSPHASIAS

Speech consists of the expression of internal thoughts, using visual or auditory symbols so that others may comprehend these thoughts. The thoughts themselves may
be formulated as a form of internal speech using words (a form of shorthand whereby thoughts are symbolized) or may remain as wordless impressions, decisions, or
feelings. Words themselves are the only symbols that we normally use to delineate
our thoughts.

Rarely are single words enough to convey to others our mental content; combinations of words are more usually needed, and these we combine using the rules
of grammar and syntax to convey to others propositions, descriptions, feelings, and
so forth. It is easiest to speak words, and although they are symbols themselves,
they may also give rise to further symbols, in this case letters; thus writing is the
creation of graphic symbols of auditory symbols.

Because with any disorder of the brain, the higher functions are lost or affected before the lower, one may arrange the levels of speech output in order.

1. Perfect ability to communicate abstract as well as concrete propositions, feelings, and descriptions using language
2. Reduction in the ability to use complex or compoumd sentences in communication, usually with bad grammar and difficulty with abstract ideas
3. Difficulty in finding words, circumlocution, anomia
4. Use of jargon and abnormal pressure of speech
5. Slowness and stumbling speech with impaired fluency and syntax
6. Use of emotional words, expletives, single words or phrases, or *Yes* and *No*
   only
7. Total inability to communicate using language symbols

With a progressive lesion, it may be expected that evidence of disease will be
detectable in this order.

Despite the failure of a patient to communicate using language, this is not to
say that his ability to think in words and sentences is necessarily impaired; internal speech may be unaffected despite gross impairment of his powers of communication.

It is unfortunate that so often more than one word is used for the same concept
in neurology. The terms *aphasia* and *dysphasia* are interchangeable. Dysphasias
may affect mainly the comprehension of language (when they are called *receptive
dysphasias*) or the verbal expression of ideas (when they are called *expressive
dysphasias*). Spoken or written speech may be involved more or less in any form,
but because writing (involving the use *of* symbols *for* symbols) adds another level
of complexity, it is usually more affected than spoken speech.

The concept of dysphasia implies that there is a block between the conversion
of internal thought, whether or not expressed in words, into language symbols (expressive dysphasia), or between the conversion of language symbols (speech or writing produced by other people) into internal thought (receptive dysphasia). In

practice the two forms almost always occur together because brain lesions are seldom so discrete that they affect only a very small area. Also the cortical areas subserving language are functionally and anatomically interconnected, not only with each other, but also with the various cortical areas concerned with auditory and visual reception and with those concerned with the initiation of voluntary movements or those body parts used to communicate by using language.

The lesions responsible for dysphasias are situated both anterior and posterior to the Rolandic fissure. Broca's and transcortical motor dysphasias are due to lesions in the posterior part of the inferior frontal gyrus and slightly above that, respectively. These areas are most intimately concerned with speech production. These two forms are known as *anterior* dysphasias, in contradistinction to *posterior* dysphasias in which the lesion is in the parietotemporal region (see Fig. 14-1). The angular gyrus is thought to be responsible for processing written language. Wernicke's is the prototype; the others are far less common.

There are many classifications of dysphasias, most of them complex, and all, but for perhaps one, wrong. That in Table 14-1 has only the merit of being understandable and workable; it is incomplete, indeed oversimplified.

Examination of the Patient with Dysphasia

Spontaneous Speech

One of the characteristics of normal spontaneous speech is that it is relatively *fluent.* Patients with posterior dysphasias retain that fluency, whereas those with anterior forms struggle to express speech.

Their *rate* of speech output is slow and labored. The normal *inflection, rhythm,* and sentence *structure* are lost, causing abnormal emphases, irregularities, and alterations in the prosody (inflection and rhythm) of speech. Patients with anterior lesions also articulate badly. Sentences are short and agrammatical, although the actual words used may be normal. Small, grammatical ("filler") words such as if,

Table 14-1   Classification of Dysphasias

Anterior, nonfluent ("expressive")

    Broca's

    Transcortical motor

Posterior, fluent ("receptive")

    Wernicke's

    Pure word deafness

    Transcortical sensory

    Conduction

Pure word blindness (pure alexia)

---

but, then, what, how, and so on, may be left out so that only important words are
said. Thus the speech has a *"high substantive content"* and may sound rather like a
telegram being read aloud.

Contrast this with the fluent speech of the patient with a posterior dysphasia;
here there is a much higher rate of output, even pressure of speech, which spews
out effortlessly with normal articulation, rhythm, and inflection. The sentences
tend to be long and contain many short words which mean little. Some of them
may be abnormal either because a syllable (a "phoneme") is changed ("God save the
been"); because of phonemic paraphasia or changing of a word, ("God teacup the
Queen"); or because an abnormal word (a neologism) is introduced ("Vooping save
the Purkot"). The difference between fluent and nonfluent spontaneous speech is
easy to identify. The best test is, of course, to take a history from the patient, during which he will be more concerned with the content than with the form of his
utterances. To test it more formally, ask the patient to describe the room he is in,
or his home, or a drawing that you show him, listening to the speech patterns used
in his answers.

Comprehension

Next, test the patient's comprehension of spoken language. Again, the history will
let you determine this, but make sure that the patient is not deaf, if he seems to
be having difficulty. To test for failure of comprehension of speech, give simple
but progressively more difficult commands to perform certain actions or get him
to point to objects that you name in the room.

Repetition

Repetition of spoken language is almost always abnormal in dysphasias, except in
the transcortical forms. Start by getting the patient to repeat digits after you,
then shorter and longer words, phrases and then sentences. Those with many short
words, for instance, "There are no ifs, ands, nor buts about it," or "If he were not
here I would go away," are the hardest to manage.

Word Finding (Naming)

Word finding may be tested by asking the patient to name objects shown or body
parts pointed out to him. Things he hears or touches may also be used to test naming ability in other than the visual modality. With visual agnosia however, tactile
naming will be preserved.

Overlearned Sequences

Finally, the ability to repeat overlearned series such as the days of the week, months
of the year, numbers, or the alphabet may be tested (see Table 14-2).

Reading

Tests of reading ability are really exactly the same as those used for comprehension
of spoken language, but they test the visual rather than the auditory modality. A
simple way is to give the patient a list of objects in the room asking him to point to
them, or show him a card with written commands that he is to carry out. However,
he should not read these aloud or else one is not testing purely visual reception.

Table 14-2   Form for the Examination of Dysphasias[*]

Spontaneous speech

    Test: Note speech during the interview
    Assess: Rate, rhythm, articulation, effort required, pressure of speech, phrase length, paraphasias, substantive content

Comprehension

    Test: Spoken directions: Point to . . . Is this . . . ? Do . . .
           Written directions, as above
           Read prose (e.g., newspaper headlines)
           Interpret the prose read

Word finding (naming)

    Test: Visual: objects, body parts, colors
           Auditory: coins, paper, keys, tapped glass, etc.
           Tactile: objects placed in right or left hand

Repetition

    Test: "There are no ifs, ands, or buts about it at all"
           "If he were not here, I would go away"

Series speech

    Test: Alphabet, days of week, months, count to 20

Writing

    Test: Signature, address, description of room or weather
           Writing to dictation

---

[*]N.B. In all these tests, record the patients' verbal responses exactly as they were uttered and describe any nonverbal responses made.

Writing

Tests for writing include (starting with the simplest), requests for the patient to write his signature, to write a description of the objects of the room around him, to write all or part of a letter to his family or friends then to write to dictation simpler, then more difficult words or sentences. Patients with anterior dysphasias make large, messy, poorly formed letters, and their grammar is bad. The writing of those with posterior types is much better formed but contains spelling errors. If a patient has an anterior left-sided cerebral lesion however, he probably has a right hemiparesis so make allowances if he is writing with his left hand.

    Patients who have major motor weakness may be unable to carry out your directions, even though they understand them, so only ask them to do only things that you know they can do spontaneously.

**Characteristics of the
Clinical Forms of Dysphasias**

Anterior Dysphasias

Broca's: In this syndrome, spontaneous speech is ungrammatical and is not fluent; repetition of spoken and written speech is poor; and word-finding is impaired, although some series speech may remain. Writing is large, messy, scrawling and ungrammatical. Some receptive element will probably be present too, especially for syntactically complex sentences. "Pure" motor aphasia (also called verbal apraxia) is characterized by poor fluency and errors in articulation, but the grammar employed is correct and comprehension is normal (see Table 14-3).

Transcortical Motor: This form closely resembles Broca's dysphasia, but repetition is preserved.

Posterior Dysphasias

Wernicke's: Here spontaneous speech is fluent but contains a high proportion of filler words and abnormal words. (Confusingly, the substitution of an abnormal word, or a wrong word, or a syllable is termed *paraphasia.*) In severe cases, the patient produces a string of neologistic jargon, as when under pressure.[*] Comprehension of both spoken and written language is usually profoundly disturbed, so the patient has the greatest difficulty in reproducing spoken or written speech. Writing is well formed but, like speech, contains spelling errors or wrong words. Series speech and word-finding are variably impaired.

Pure Word Deafness: The lesions here are sited in one or both temporal lobes. The clinical picture is that of a patient who can comprehend only written, not spoken, language so he can easily read to himself but cannot make sense of what he hears. Spontaneous speech is quite good but the patient cannot repeat what is said to him. The condition is uncommon.

Pure Word Blindness: This is also known as *alexia without agraphia.* A left occipital lobe infarct produces a right homoymous hemianopia, so nothing is seen to the right. Our right occipital lobes cannot comprehend words presented to our left visual field; these have to be processed in the left angular gyrus region. Unfortunately, the splenium is also damaged by this stroke so the impulses from the right visual cortex cannot reach the left side. Therefore only written language cannot be understood.

Conduction Dysphasia: Although the spontaneous speech of patients with conduction dysphasia will resemble the fluent paraphasia of those with other posterior dysphasias, their comprehension of spoken and written speech will be rather good. They have however a marked difficulty in *repeating* spoken and written speech. This dramatic difference between their failure with repetition but retained comprehension is diagnostic. One such patient, who was asked to repeat the word "president" said "Presidum-dum-dum, Presidum-dum; dammit, I mean Kennedy." Word-finding may be much impaired and reading aloud impossible, although the patients can read silently and with understanding.

The responsible lesion is thought to affect the arcuate fasciculus, which connects Broca's and Wernicke's areas; when damaged, conduction of impulses along this pathway is not possible. Hence its name.

---

[*] If the patient does not have a hemiparesis, his speech may be interpreted as psychotic.

Table 14-3   Summary of Major Findings in Dysphasias

	Spontaneous Speech Fluency	Naming	Repetition	Comprehension
Broca's	Nonfluent	Poor	Poor	Good
Wernicke's	Fluent	Poor	Poor	Poor
Conduction	Fluent	Fair	Poor	Good
Transcortical motor type	Poor	Poor	Normal	Good
Transcortical sensory type	Fluent	Poor	Normal	Poor

Transcortical Sensory Dysphasia: One clinical feature common to all of the varieties of dysphasia previously described is difficulty in repeating spoken language. In the transcortical dysphasias however repetition is near normal. The patient is silent unless spoken to, when he responds by repeating back to the examiner, quite fluently, exactly what was just said to him (echolalia) or with irrelevant semantic jargon. He has absolutely no comprehension of what is said: in fact he will fail badly in all the other tests of language function, except repetition.

In the two forms of transcortical dysphasia, the lesion is the border zone between the territories of the middle and posterior or anterior cerebral arteries, respectively.

Although even the preceding classification is hardly simple, and the differences between the types may appear sophisticated, the complex nature of the subject may be less vexing if one remembers that aphasias are no more than disorders of communication involving language; hence all the tests described are just variations on the theme of examining the patient's ability to comprehend and to communicate using spoken or written speech. Bear in mind that the most difficult tast is to recognize that the patient is dysphasic. When you have done that, you have already localized the lesion to the dominant hemisphere and will probably be considering neurological referral.

Treatment of Dysphasic States

Because in most instances, it will have been a stroke that caused the dysphasia (although tumors, subdural hematomas, local trauma, and encephalitis are other possible causes), one will be busy treating that in the earliest stages. When the patient's neurological condition is stable, attention should be paid to the management of the language disturbance. Confusion, severe motor deficits, the presence of other speech problems, and denial or inattention syndromes lessen the chance of good results from speech therapy. Moreover, the evidence that speech therapy is truly more effective than the patient's everyday interaction with his family or even with volunteers, is inconclusive.

Traditional methods tried to get the patient to relearn the words and grammar he formerly used. New approaches include the teaching of sign language based on that used by the American Indians (Amerind) for those with maximal impairment of language comprehension; and teaching the nonfluent patient to speak rhythmically, as if to music (melodic intonation therapy). Both of these methods are still under trial but seem to offer more than plain efforts at reeducation. The physician is still responsible for the psychological support of his dysphasic patient, and for the detection of the moment when untreatable frustration leads on to treatable depression, so common with left-sided strokes.

BIBLIOGRAPHY

Kertesz, A. *Aphasia and Associated Disorders.* New York, Grune & Stratton, 1979.

15
Epileptic Seizures

Epilepsy is a tendency to recurring epileptic seizures; the latter, through a brilliant insight, were recognized by Hughlings Jackson as being the result of occasional, sudden, rapid, local, and excessive discharges of gray matter — and this half a century before Hans Berger invented the EEG.

There are two major types of epileptic seizures. The first (type I), is also known as primary generalized or idiopathic epilepsy. The second (type II), is also known as partial or focal epilepsy.

Unfortunately, the terms most often used are confusing. *Generalized* is a term used for a specific class of epilepsy, but it is also used as a descriptive term for seizures that are "generalized" in their appearance. Similarly *grand mal* is another term used for the class of generalized seizures, but also for a tonic-clonic seizure that begins as a focal discharge, which brings it into another class. An international committee has wrestled with the nomenclature for years but the results have not been entirely satisfactory nor fully accepted.[*]

---

[*]We were going to use the terms type I and type II for the two major types of epilepsy because we feel that the recent attempts to use the international classification terminology *generalized seizures, partial seizures, partial complex seizures,* etc., have added nothing to understanding and continue to confuse pathophysiology with description. We doubt if the International Classification will survive in its present form, and feel no regret. Or are we tilting at windmills?

In type I epilepsy, no pathological or structural cause is found for the attacks, and they appear to be due to an inherent genetic lowering of threshold for convulsions. Anyone can be made to have a convulsion under certain circumstances, but in patients with idiopathic epilepsy, thresholds are set so low that seizures occur spontaneously. The epileptic discharge originates in a deep midline area of the brain and upper brainstem and spreads to both hemispheres causing a sudden seizure without warning (Figs. 15-1, 15-2).

In type II epilepsy however, a focal brain lesion is the cause of the abnormal epileptic discharge, even if a structural lesion cannot be found on full clinical investigation. The type of seizure resulting probably indicates the area of the brain where the abnormal electrical discharge begins. However it may then spread to other areas along fiber tracts. The clinical manifestations may therefore be due to the localized discharge initially but then reflect its spread elsewhere. The former causes the so-called aura that is often present in focally originating seizures. Sometimes the spread is rapid, causing a generalized seizure without a preceding aura, and this must be differentiated from type-I or idiopathic generalized epilepsy.

Patients should be questioned very carefully to determine their type of seizure and also for circumstances that may have precipitated it. It should be remembered that half of the patients with epilepsy have more than one form of seizure pattern.

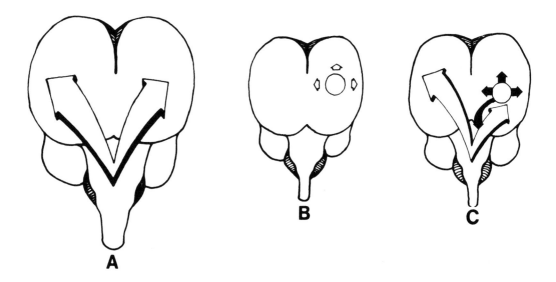

Figure 15-1   (A) Type I (generalized) seizures. The abnormal electrical discharge may be hypothesized as originating in deep central brain regions, spreading simultaneously to all cortical areas; (B) Type II (focal) seizures. The abnormal electrical discharge activates local neurons only; (C) Secondary "subcortical" seizures. An abnormal cortical electrical discharge activates local neurons initially but also, presumably by spreading centrally, triggers a generalized discharge.

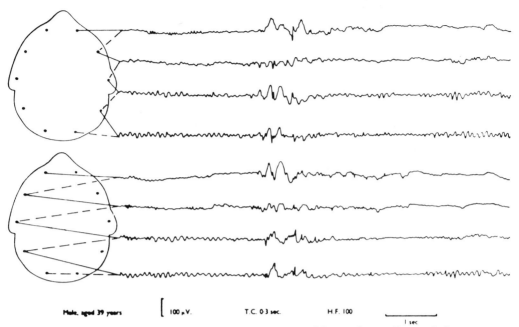

Male, aged 39 years.   100 μV.   T.C. 0.3 sec.   H.F. 100   1 sec

Figure 15-2   Type I grand mal seizure. A burst of irregular spike and slow-wave activity is seen bilaterally, unaccompanied by any clinical signs.

TYPE I SEIZURES

In this class of epilepsy the abnormal discharge appears to arise in deep central structures of the brain, a genetic factor is present so the family history is often positive for epilepsy, seizures do not begin before the age of 3 years and seldom after 20, there is no pathological abnormality of the brain, and there are no physical signs in between seizures. All investigations (apart from the EEG) are normal. The patient is not aware that any seizure is about to start and has no knowledge of the events that occur during it. He has no memory of having had the attack except for its effects, such as incontinence, tongue biting, sore muscles, or of finding himself on the floor.

Grand Mal

The first sign in a *grand mal seizure* may be a sudden cry followed by the patient suddenly falling to the ground with every voluntary muscle contracting tonically. This lasts for 30 sec or less. Then, periods of relaxation interrupt the tonic spasms, producing a clonic phase again for about 30 sec. The spasms of contraction get briefer and less intense toward the end of the seizure, and the patient lapses into a state of flaccid paralysis for another 30 sec or so while breathing is slowly reestablished. Because of the interference with respiration during the tonic and clonic phases, the patient is often cyanotic by this time. If the bladder is full, he is often incontinent in the tonic phase, and may bite his tongue in the clonic phase. The patient usually awakes after a few minutes, is confused briefly, then feels drowsy and falls asleep for an hour or more. The only sequelae are a mild headache, some muscle aching, and perhaps a sore tongue.

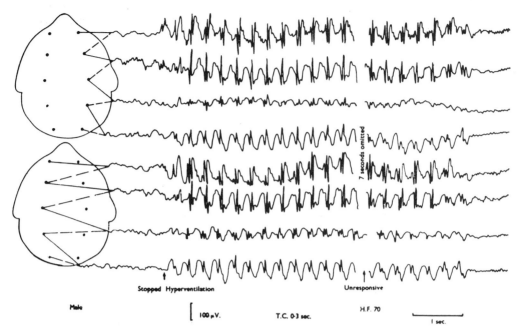

Figure 15-3   Type I petit mal epilepsy. Twelve seconds of regular 3-Hz spike-and-wave activity during which the patient ceased hyperventilating and was unresponsive to command.

Petit Mal

Petit mal seizures consist of brief lapses of attention and awareness lasting 15 sec or less (Fig. 15-3). They are much more common in childhood. This is worth remembering because "little seizures" in adults are usually of temporal lobe origin and not petit mal. Petit mal seizures do not begin in adulthood, but childhood petit mal occasionally persists into adult life.

Such attacks may occur many times a day and are similar each time. The child may suddenly stare, his eyes turn upward or to the side, and the eyelids flutter at about three contractions per second. The episode is always brief, after which the patient returns to his former activity as if nothing has happened. Occasionally as many as 500 a day may occur. They can often be precipitated by hyperventilation and occasionally by photic stimulation, such as sunlight seen through a picket fence or a TV with vertical flip-flop.

An unusual form of type I epilepsy is the *akinetic attack* in which the child will suddenly drop to the floor and then get right up again.

Myoclonus

These brief jerky movements may be physiological — we all get them on falling asleep in bed at night — and may occur during the day in otherwise normal people or in those with grand mal seizures. A sinister form accompanies infantile spasms (West's syndrome of progressive motor and intellectual deterioration in small children who have lightning spasms, nodding, or extensor spasms. The EEG trace shows chaotic disorganization. Many of these children die of the disease).

Symptomatic myoclonus occurs in Alzheimer's and Jacob-Creutzfeldt diseases, in cerebral lipid storage disorders, and in viral encephalitis, including subacute sclerosing panencephalitis (SSPE) (Chap. 40). Toxic agents (see Chap. 43) are other causes. Following cardiac arrest with severe brain hypoxia, myoclonic jerks may interrupt voluntary movements to a severe degree — action myoclonus — and this may also occur rarely as a familial disorder. When myoclonic jerks occur segmentally, in one limb for example, a spinal cord lesion such as MS or a local tumor may be the cause.

Febrile convulsion is the term used for a single seizure of any type occurring in a child aged between 3 months and 5 years during the phase of rising temperature during an infection. Perhaps 5 percent of all children in this age group experience them and in 30 to 40 percent of cases they recur. About 10 percent of these children will later have nonfebrile epilepsy. Those who go on to have recurrent nonfebrile seizures have had two or more of the following factors when first seen: a family history of epilepsy, abnormal neurological or developmental status, or an atypical (focal or prolonged) seizure.

TYPE II SEIZURES

The manifestations of type II or focal seizures depend upon the area involved by the spreading epileptic discharge (Figs. 15-4, 15-5). The most "epileptogenic" region of the brain is the temporal lobe, and thus the most common form of focal seizure is of temporal lobe origin. However if the focus is in a motor area, the manifestations will be motor, or sensory if the lesion is in the area of the parietal lobe sensory strip. Because the temporal lobe is involved in emotion, memory, olfaction, hearing, and many other functions, seizures generated from this area are often colorful in their diversity and complexity. However the discharge may

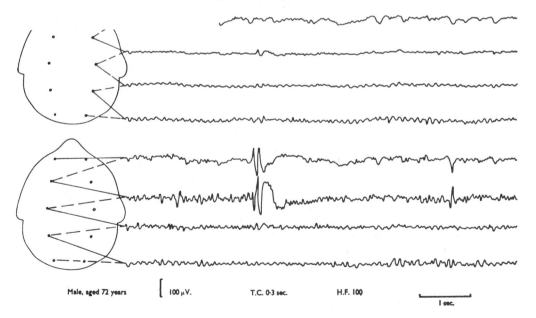

Male, aged 72 years   100 μV.   T.C. 0·3 sec.   H.F. 100   1 sec.

Figure 15-4   Type II focal epilepsy. Left frontal spike discharges, occurring in a patient with a left frontal meningioma.

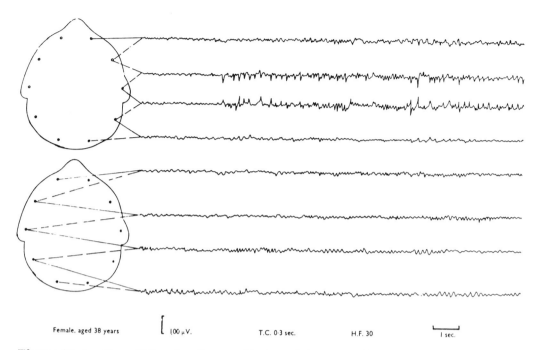

Female, aged 38 years   [100 μV.   T.C. 0·3 sec.   H.F. 30   1 sec.

Figure 15-5   Type II focal epilepsy. Fast activity and spikes arising from the right temporal lobe.

spread rapidly to other areas causing a grand mal seizure as described under type I without any of the prior focal manifestations.

Although these seizures arise from a focus somewhere in the cortex, less than 40 percent of cases show abnormalities on the CT scan, suggesting that the responsible area of abnormal brain may be very small, even microscopic.

Motor

A *motor seizure* often results from a lesion in or around the motor strip and may result in unilateral *tonic* muscle contraction in the face, trunk, arm, or leg. The seizure may cause adduction of the shoulder; flexion of the elbow, wrist, and fingers; and extension of the hip and knee. More commonly, the motor contractions are repetitive *(clonic)* and occur in one localized area, such as the hand. When one part of the body is initially affected followed by spread to other areas (e.g., fingers, to hands, to arm, to face), the condition is known as a *jacksonian march* or *jacksonian seizure*. Most last about 1 to 2 min. *Adversive attacks* are those in which the patient's head or eyes are turned forcibly to one side. The lesion here is usually in the opposite posteroinferior frontal region. *Visceromotor* signs in focal seizures include piloerection, defecation, urinary incontinence, sweating, salivation, and miosis.

During seizures, most patients are pale but some occasionally flush. *Automatisms* are patterns of activity that look purposeful but may include chewing movements, smacking of lips, repetitive but complicated movements of the arms or legs, or even walking. The patient may move about in a dazed, confused manner carrying out repetitive, semipurposeful acts such as opening and closing a window. An unusual motor seizure pattern is that of *infantile spasms* of children, known as *salaam* attacks (Fig. 15-6), which occur with severe degenerative brain disease. These children make sudden major movements, frequently of the trunk, including bending of the waist, without apparent loss of balance (West's syndrome, p. 224).

Sensory

Special sensory symptoms in epilepsy include unformed hallucinations of color, shapes, zigzags, flashes of light, and other visual phenomena. Patients may also hear sounds such as rushing water in both ears. (Hearing is represented bilaterally). *Somatosensory* symptoms include sensations of heat and cold, heaviness or light-ness, the feeling of a limb becoming larger or smaller or seeming to move, and other internal sensations. The patient may experience numbness or tingling or more unusual sensations on one side of the body. Some of these sensory changes, particularly the visceral ones, are experienced bilaterally. *Viscerosensory* symp-toms are common as an aura, especially the so-called epigastric aura in which the patient feels an indefinable sensation from the epigastrium rising through the chest to his head. This is often followed by loss of consciousness.

An unusual form of seizure is *reflex epilepsy*, a seizure induced by specific sensory input. Recurrent seizures have been reported in patients from listening to music, or only certain types of music; from reading; from touching certain fabrics; from certain visual shapes and forms; and from startle. These can be treated with deconditioning as well as with anticonvulsants.

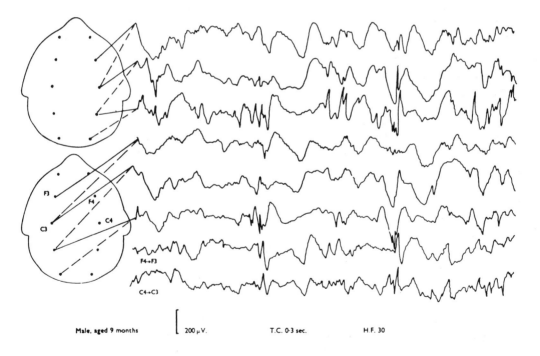

Male, aged 9 months   200 μV.   T.C. 0·3 sec.   H.F. 30

Figure 15-6 Type II epilepsy. Severely disorganized, high-voltage, irregular delta activity and spikes recorded from a child with salaam attacks. This pattern is known as *hypsarrhythmia*. The EEG tracings shown are from Bayliss, S.G. In *Epilepsy*. W.E.M. Pryse-Phillips. Bristol, John Wright & Sons, 1969. Courtesy of the author and publishers.

Psychological

Complex and formed *hallucinations* of sight or hearing may occur, very much as if a film or tape recording of an experience in the patient's past were being replayed before him. He is usually able to recognize the events portrayed as being from his past. Unlike a schizophrenic, the epileptic patient with hallucinations recognizes the unreality of the phenomena. Probably the most characteristically localizing type is the olfactory hallucinations that is produced by a focal epileptic discharge in the medial temporal lobe (uncus), giving rise to the term *uncal seizure.*

Epileptic illusions are usually visual, the patient having the sensation that objects are getting larger or smaller, changing their shape, size, or color, or appearing to come nearer or go further away. Illusions of memory produce the well-known experiences of *déjà vu* and *jamais vu* in which incorrect feelings of recognition or of strangeness occur. In the first case, the patient knows he has never been in this particular situation before, nevertheless there is the overpowering sensation that it is all familiar and he has seen it all happen previously. In *jamais vu,* he may recognize his family and home or surroundings but feels that they are invested with an aura of strangeness or unfamiliarity. Most people have experienced brief *déjà vu* phenomena on occasion, but patients with temporal lobe epilepsy may have them frequently.

Affective change consists of an emotional upsurge without any exogenous reason. About 60 percent of patients with temporal lobe seizures experience anxiety or fear as part of their seizure; and anger, depression, and occasionally happiness may be the emotion experienced. Only rarely are seizures pleasurable, but the Russian novelist Dostoyevski described these well, as he had them, and once stated that he would give the rest of his life for another seizure. It is of interest that in each of his novels an epileptic person appears. When psychological symptoms are present as part of the seizure, the focus is usually in the temporal lobe. Other unusual seizure forms include those characterized by bizarre activity or by crying, laughing, or running.

After the seizure is over and the electrical activity of the brain has returned to a more normal state, *motor or sensory deficits* may remain *(Todd's palsy),* or the patient's *level of consciousness* may be still somewhat reduced so that he manifests a confusional state, automatic behavior, or an acute psychotic disturbance.

ICTAL ANALYSIS

When a patient who may have had a seizure is first seen the family and, if possible, other observers should be questioned in detail about a history of epilepsy in the family and about any circumstances that may have precipitated the episode, such as emotional stress, depression, insomnia, alcohol ingestion or withdrawal, overhydration, hunger, or flashing lights. You should determine if the attacks tend to occur at certain times of the day or of the month. If the patient is already known to have epilepsy, you must determine what his control has been like in the past and whether he is faithful in taking his medication. Information about birth trauma and febrile convulsions should be sought, and any history of head injuries, past neurological diseases, or other serious illnesses will also be important. You must also find out if he is taking other drugs of any type. In addition to all of these background factors, a minute analysis of the nature of the episode, including everything that the patient and observers can remember about it, is absolutely essential. Leading questions may be necessary to aid the patient in recalling any of the symptoms and signs just outlined.

After the ictal analysis is complete, you will be in a good position to know whether the patient has type I or type II attacks, and if type II, where the lesion is. Neurologists will usually have made up their mind from the history about the type of epilepsy and often about the site of any focal discharge before they start the physical examination.

CAUSES

A list of causes of seizures would be so long as to be useless; every CNS disease damaging the gray matter can be responsible, and we will not attempt to cite them. However, type I seizures have a genetic basis, although no structural cause in the brain that we can detect. Indeed, the detection of any physical signs or test result suggesting a localized area of abnormality makes the diagnosis untenable. People with no past history of epilepsy may lower their threshold by hyperventilation (cerebral ischemia resulting), alcohol excess or withdrawal, fluid overload, hypoglycemia, or stresses such as chronic sleep deprivation. Lowering of thresholds may also make a formerly nonepileptogenic lesion now spark off a seizure.

Type II seizures complicate a host of CNS problems; congenital, inflammatory, traumatic, neoplastic, metabolic-toxic, vascular, and degenerative. In the first 24 hr after birth, hypoxia and intracerebral hemorrhage and low magnesium, calcium, or sugar levels, are the most common causes. In the subsequent week, developmental defects, kernicterus, pyridoxine deficiency, and acute infections should be considered first. To these causes one must add febrile convulsions and infantile spasms in the next 6 months, while all of these, inborn metabolic errors and postinfective encephalopathies are common causes up to the age of 3. After that, the primary generalized (type I) epilepsies may be manifested, usually before the age of 20. However seizures without localizing characteristics by any means of investigation may occur at any time of life. The concern is always whether or not one is missing a neoplasm in epilepsy of late (after 25 years) onset, for which reason full investigation is required for both biochemical and structural disorders.

MANAGEMENT

The diagnosis of epilepsy is basically a clinical decision. Frequently, the information required to make it comes not from the patient, but from relatives or workmates who can describe the pattern of seizure activity. When illustrating the instruments used in neurological diagnosis in Figure 2-1, we included the telephone because of its great importance in aiding diagnosis in just such situations as this. From the description one can also determine whether the seizure is, for example, of grand mal type, a focal motor seizure, or an absence attack. Between seizures there are no physical signs diagnostic of epilepsy itself, only of any pathology that may be causing it. Almost by definition, type I or generalized seizures cannot be diagnosed if abnormal neurological signs are detected, and in such cases further investigation is required.

In the absence of any physical signs, one is probably justified however in closely observing the patient as an outpatient in four circumstances.

1. Patients with the range of 3 to 15 years, who have had one grand mal or any number of true petit mal seizures without focal signs. If they had not had seizures before the age of 3, it is likely that their present seizures represent type I epilepsy, and an EEG can be performed as a baseline without other tests, unless it suggests a focal lesion.

2. Febrile convulsions do not require investigation unless the seizures are focal, prolonged, or associated with neurological abnormalities, but the cause of the fever must be determined (it could be meningitis or cerebral abscess). Admission to hospital is wise on the first occasion, but thereafter the child who convulses during a fever, but has no signs of a serious underlying infection, should be manageable at home with symptomatic remedies. If the seizure was focal, prolonged, or associated with neurological abnormalities, or if there is a history of nonfebrile epilepsy in the family, treatment is indicated. Febrile seizures are relatively benign as only 2 percent of these children will be epileptic by age 7, and the parents should be reassured about the situation, as they are often scared and overprotective.

3. Minor epileptic attacks occurring infrequently over years and without accompanying neurological abnormality will require simple outpatient tests (EEG and isotope or CT scan). Such patients do not need inpatient investigation, but neurological consultation is wise.

4. A person who has had a single seizure without focal features, and who has no abnormal physical signs, can be investigated similarly. If these tests show no focal lesion, long-term outpatient follow-up is all that is required. Further investigation will be required if the character of the seizure alters or if any abnormal signs develop. Extensive initial investigation is not always required if one is planning to observe the patient in the future. After all, continued observation *is* an investigation.

If a clinical diagnosis of type II (focal or "partial") epilepsy is made, the next problem is to determine the pathology. This often requires assessment in a neurological center. After the EEG and CT scan have been performed, one may have some idea of the localization of the lesion and sometimes also of its nature.

When a patient goes home after he has been investigated in the hospital, further management must be on three major fronts: psychological, social, and pharmacological.

Psychological Management

The psychological management of patients with epilepsy really is that of any attendant personality changes, depression, or psychosis. If brain damage is found, it is usually the cause of the seizure, rather than *vice versa,* and management consists of a scaling-down of the patient's activities and responsibilities so that he can cope with his restricted life without frustration. Drug therapy is of value only if the patient would benefit from mild tranquilizers. Patients with epilepsy do not often develop signs of brain damage caused by their disorder, but if they do, the cause is probably toxic levels of anticonvulsants. Careful monitoring of serum levels will prevent this.

Patients with focal seizures frequently become depressed to the extent that they would benefit from tricyclic drug therapy. There is also a tendency for seizures to become more frequent when the patient is in a depressive state, and although tricyclics themselves may increase seizure frequency, their overall effect in depressed epileptic subjects is beneficial. Often the depression may be reactive, related to the patient's attitude about his epilepsy and the social repercussions of the disorder. Explanation, reassurance, and social management may be the most effective remedies in this situation.

Social Management

To get the patient's full cooperation in managing his problem, and to help him deal with its effects on his life, it is absolutely essential to explain about seizures and their therapy. It is always useful to direct his attention to an epilepsy association, and practitioners should obtain for themselves information about epilepsy to pass on to the patient and make sure there is ample opportunity later for questions based on his reading of such material. It is important to discuss openly some of the ideas and concepts that the patient and his family may have about epilepsy. Reassurance is essential; he must understand that this is not a mystifying illness, but quite explicable. All of us are potentially epileptic, and the problem is based purely on our threshold for having seizures. The epileptic patient is only at one end of a continuum, part of that 1 percent of the population subject to spontaneous epileptic seizures because of their low threshold or a focal area of brain damage. The patient must understand that he is not at the end of his effective life; only small life alterations need to be made in most cases, and a vast proportion of patients achieve total seizure control while remaining at work without any problems.

Couples should understand the genetic risks of the various seizures, the potential problems in pregnancy, and the risks of taking anticonvulsants (and of not taking them), so that they can make informed, intelligent decisions about having children. Most children with seizures do not have brain damage, and when they have achieved reasonable seizure control, they can continue in school and learn normally. Intelligence is not diminished by having seizures, although it may be affected by anticonvulsants at toxic levels and, of course, by any underlying brain pathology causing the seizures. There are few forms of employment that are not open to adults with epilepsy, although it is not legal for them to drive in most countries until the seizures have been controlled for at least 1 year, unless they occur only during sleep.

For a patient with a chronic disability, work is not only economically necessary, but it is also therapeutic. If there is any difficulty obtaining employment, then retraining should be arranged by the appropriate local agency, and the doctor should make a point of contacting a prospective employer to reassure him about hiring persons with epilepsy, explaining the condition and its effects on the employee in question. All of this, needless to say, is with the employee's knowledge and consent. The work record of patients with epilepsy is extremely good and their competence and industry are often rated better than those of other workers; they have, after all, had more difficulty than others in getting jobs and probably try harder than others to keep them.

Pharmacological Therapy

The patient must be told *why* he is being given drugs, *what* the drugs are, and their likely *side effects.* He must understand, too, that they are not curative but suppressive agents and that the benefit to be gained is entirely dependent upon careful adherence to treatment schedules. Irregular or intermittent medication will not only result in poor control but may lead the physician to increase the dosage or vary the drugs when they have not been given a fair trial.

Those chosen will vary with the type of epilepsy. Four main groups of agents will be described: most patients will be controlled on one or a combination of these. There is no fixed dosage for these agents, because their therapeutic effect depends upon their blood levels; the serum monitoring of anticonvulsant levels is extremely helpful and allows one to check that a patient is taking his medication regularly and that he is being prescribed the correct dosage (Table 15-1). Signs of toxicity are dose-dependent.

Table 15-1   Drugs Commonly Used in Epilepsy

Drug	Adult Dosage	Ideal Serum Level
Phenobarbital	1.5-3 mg/kg p.o. once daily	70-170 μmol/L
Phenytoin	5 mg/kg p.o. once daily	30-80 μmol/L
Carbamazepine	7-10 mg/kg/day in three doses p.o.	17-42 μmol/L
Primidone	10-20 mg/kg/day in three doses p.o.	25-45 μmol/L
Ethosuximide	15-30 mg/kg/day in three doses p.o.	280-570 μmol/L
Valproic acid	15-30 mg/kg/day in three doses p.o.	350-700 μmol/L

If there is no urgency, anticonvulsants can be increased slowly over a few weeks until a good therapeutic effect is obtained and blood levels are adequate. Both phenytoin and phenobarbital can be started at the normal maintenance dosage, when therapeutic levels will probably be reached within a week. Other anticonvulsant drugs should be increased to maintenance levels over 1 to 2 weeks to avoid side effects (carbamazepine, primidone, valproic acid, clonazepam, and most others). In an emergency, effective levels of phenytoin can be achieved within minutes with IV dosage. Toxic side effects are particularly common in the early stages of anticonvulsant therapy, and the patient should understand that most will clear over a few days or weeks.

Drug therapy should be continued for at least 2 years, and usually 5 years, after the last seizure, and then, after discussion with the patient, a decision can be made about whether or not they should be discontinued. About half the patients will get a recurrence of seizures when drugs are stopped. The decision, to a great extent, depends upon the patient's attitude about the risk of having a further seizure. He must understand that the possible recurrence of seizures might endanger him, might cause him to lose his job, or cause a great deal of social embarrassment. If he is willing to risk that, to see if he can get along without medications, then this is acceptable, but if he feels the recurrence of seizures would be too upsetting, then the drugs should be continued. It is not acceptable to reduce the dosage of the drug as an alternative. If the patient is to be on anticonvulsants, then the dosage must be at full therapeutic levels.

The following is a brief description of the more important groups of anticonvulsant drugs. The list of possible drugs is long, but only the more important ones will be discussed.

Phenytoin

Phenytoin (Dilantin) has been used since its introduction by Merritt and Putnam in 1938, and still remains one of the most widely used and effective anticonvulsants available. Phenytoin tends to decrease posttetanic potentiation, which is the enhancement of synaptic transmission that follows rapid, repetitive neuronal stimulation. Thus phenytoin will decrease the spread of the discharge around an epileptic focus and along axons to distant sites. This effect apparently is due to its influence upon the uptake of calcium and sodium by the neurons. It is this ability to stabilize excitable membranes that also makes phenytoin of value in treating cardiac arrhythmias.

When taken orally, phenytoin is completely absorbed and is distributed throughout the body, metabolized in the liver, and excreted in the bile. It is then reabsorbed and eliminated mainly in the urine.

Phenytoin is a drug of choice in the management of type I grand mal seizures. It is also effective in type II partial seizures of motor, sensory, or temporal lobe type. It is *not* useful in petit mal seizures and may actually worsen them. It may be effective in the treatment of status epilepticus when given in very high dosages IV (1000 mg over 1/2 to 2 hr) following the use of intravenous diazepam. Phenytoin is usually given orally for long-term maintenance, intravenously for acute epileptic emergencies, but *not* intramuscularly, where it forms crystals in the tissues, is erratically absorbed, and achieves unpredictable blood levels.

A wide range of blood levels is possible in different individuals taking the same dosage of phenytoin. Both the therapeutic and the toxic effects parallel the blood level and not the amount taken by mouth. Always a problem in clinical medicine is the difficulty of getting patients to take their medication as prescribed. This is particularly so in a long-term disorder like epilepsy in which the patient usually feels quite well. Poor compliance can be detected by measuring blood levels periodically.

Blood levels are achieved and the drug is eliminated slowly (half-life 24 to 40 hr), producing relatively stable levels that are affected little by sudden changes in dosage (Fig. 15-7). Patients were usually given 100 mg three times a day, but it has been found to be just as effective to give the total daily dosage at one time if this is more convenient. For instance, a fisherman or forest worker might find it more convenient to take his total daily dosage at breakfast. Because a large dose given at once may cause some gastric irritation, it is usually taken with an antacid or after a meal. The once-a-day dosage is usually begun after 2 to 4 weeks of divided dosage so that the blood level is stable.

If a patient is taking 300 mg of phenytoin each day, you can expect a blood level ranging anywhere from 10-80 µmol/L with an average of 60 µmol/L. It may take up to 15 days to achieve this level, but it will then remain stable if the dosage is maintained. The effective therapeutic level in the treatment of epilepsy is 30-80 µmol/L.

There is a clear relationship between the early neurological complications and the blood level. In most patients nystagmus occurs at about 80 µmol/L, ataxia and incoordination at 100 µmol/L, and lethargy and drowsiness at 125 µmol/L. Confusion and irritability are usually noticed and occasionally patients have hallucinations, delusions, and psychotic reactions with heavy overdosages. Cerebellar signs are also common, but transient; actual cerebellar atrophy has rarely been observed in human taking excessive phenytoin.

Gum hypertrophy is common and may be prevented by good dental hygiene, but surgical resection of the hypertrophied gum tissue is occasionally necessary. Gum hypertrophy is not necessarily dose related and may persist despite decreasing the dosage.

A measleslike rash occurs in about 5 percent of patients, usually disappearing rapidly on discontinuing the drug, but rash, fever, hepatitis, and lymphadenopathy indicate a hypersensitivity reaction, requiring discontinuation of the drug. Lupus

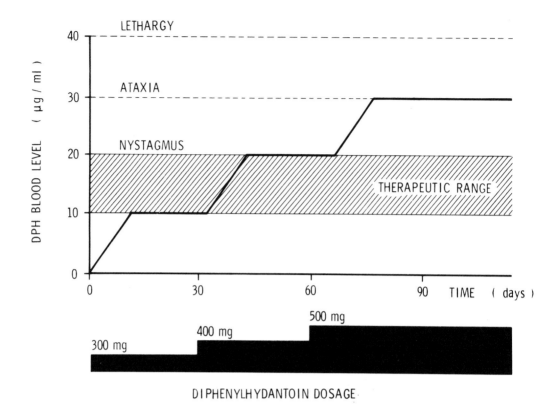

Figure 15-7 Diagram of the various phenytoin blood levels occurring with different dosages. The side effects of phenytoin are dose dependent.

erythematosus may occur, but this is rare; prompt withdrawal of the drug usually results in complete recovery. There is a family history of lupus in 20 percent of the patients who develop lupus while taking phenytoin, suggesting that it may just precipitate a latent tendency to collagen-vascular disease.

Facial hirsutism occurs in most of the patients and may be due to a stimulant action on steroid production. For this reason, and because up to 15 percent of children born to women taking the drug have dysmorphic facial appearance, it may be advisable to select another anticonvulsant in children, adolescents, and women.

Megaloblastic anemia occurs only rarely and is due to an interference with folic acid metabolism. This can be prevented by giving 0.1 mg of folic acid daily. Because of this complication one should probably do a hemogram occasionally in patients on long-term phenytoin to look for megaloblastic changes. The addition of folic acid to therapy does not interfere with seizure control. This effect upon folic acid metabolism may also explain the neuropathy that occasionally occurs. Rickets or osteomalacia may complicate long-term therapy because of induction of hepatic microsomal enzymes. A reversible syndrome resembling a lymphoma is also described.

Valproic Acid

Valproic acid is most useful in the management of petit mal seizures of the absence type, but it may also be helpful in grand mal and myoclonic seizures. It is now regarded as the drug of choice for petit mal seizures. The usual adult dosage rises from 15 up to 40 mg/kg daily in divided doses. Its main unwanted effects are gastric irritation, hair loss, weight gain, drowsiness, and tremor. Thrombocytopenia and hepatic dysfunction are less common but more serious and require estimation of bleeding time, platelet counts, and liver function tests for the first few weeks of treatment.

Barbiturates

The barbiturate most commonly used for type II seizure is phenobarbital. Patients can usually take this medication in a single daily dose after blood levels have been achieved because of the very slow buildup of phenobarbitone in the nervous system and its extremely slow excretion. The usual adult dosage is 60–100 mg/day orally. The drug can also be given intramuscularly if required (usual dose, 100 mg).

Unwanted side effects include drowsiness, altered sleep patterns, behavioral and intellectual change in children, dizziness, blurred vision, dysarthria, ataxia, and depression. These symptoms usually result from overdosage although they may occur at low or normal dosage. Skin rashes, including the Stevens–Johnson syndrome, are hypersensitivity reactions. Long-term side effects include folate deficiency with megaloblastic anemia, a syndrome resembling rickets caused by enzyme induction, and artifically low antidiuretic hormone (ADH) and protein-bound iodine (PBI) levels. Because of their slow absorption and accumulation in the nervous system, barbiturates are of little value in treating status epilepticus.

Primidone (Mysoline) is chemically related to the barbiturates and is of value in the same conditions, although it is suggested that it is more effective in focal epilepsy. Tablets (250 mg) are prescribed in divided dosages up to a maximum of 2 g/day. Most patients require 750–1000 mg/day. The unwanted side effects are similar to those produced by barbiturates but there is a greater frequency of irritability and personality change.

Succinimides

Succinimides are drugs of choice in the treatment of pure petit mal epilepsy. Ethosuximide (Zarontoin) is the agent most frequently used in a dosage of 250 mg three times a day. The effects of overdosage include vomiting, dizziness, drowsiness, ataxia, hiccups, headaches, and photophobia. Hypersensitivity reactions again include skin rashes, perhaps of the Stevens–Johnson type, blood dyscrasias, and a lupuslike syndrome.

Carbamazepine

Carbamazepine (Tegretol) is an excellent drug in type I and type II grand mal and all forms of focal epilepsy, and it is usually prescribed (in adults) up to a maximum of 400 mg three times a day. Overdosage produces drowsiness, dizziness, ataxia, blurred vision, and confusion. Hypersensitivity reactions result in skin rashes, liver and bone damage, and a lupus syndrome. Bone marrow damage and other serious side effects are not common with this drug, but the other annoying side effects are common, and about 15 percent of patients cannot tolerate it. This drug is becoming the drug of choice in grand mal and focal seizures and has fewer long-term side effects than phenytoin. One minor drawback is the slowly increasing dosage required to reach therapeutic blood levels over the first 1 to 2 weeks.

Other Anticonvulsant Therapy

In some forms of childhood epilepsy, and occasionally in women who have attacks premenstrually, *diuretics* may be of value, particularly spironolactone and acetazolamide.

An old form of therapy, the *ketogenic diet* may be useful in children who have uncontrolled seizures. It is based on the fact that metabolic acidosis (as is produced by this diet) has an anticonvulsant effect. It is not very practical because it is very unpalatable.

Methsuximide (Celontin) is not a particularly useful anticonvulsant alone, but it has found a place in the management of intractable seizures when added to a major anticonvulsant such as phenytoin or carbamazepine. The usual maintenance dosage is 300 mg four times a day to achieve serum levels of 10-40 µmol/L. A personality change and drowsiness are the major side effects.

Chlorazepate (Tranxene-R) has also been found useful as an "add-on" anticonvulsant in type II seizure states; dosages of up to 30 mg t.i.d. may be used.

Corticotropin (ACTH) may be of value in the control of some seizures, particularly myoclonic seizures. *Amphetamines* have been used in cases of refractory epilepsy with good results, but their problems and hazards are well known. A number of new drugs on the market promise to be effective but await further evaluation.

Diazepam is of little or no value when given orally unless the seizures are a result of tension and anxiety, which may induce hyperventilation and respiratory alkalosis. Intravenously however, it is the drug of choice in all forms of status epilepticus no matter what the cause. Other oral benzodiazepines can be given with effect in epilepsy; they include nitrazepam and clonazepam. These agents are particularly useful in reducing myoclonic seizures.

Although the leading therapy in epilepsy may be anticonvulsant drugs, it is important to identify the factors precipitating seizures because steps may be taken to manage them. Stress, alcohol, hyperventilation, hypoglycemia, and lack of sleep may be important precipitants and can all be treated, primarily by patient education.

Management of Attacks

Status Epilepticus

Status epilepticus is a medical emergency that occurs when the patient has two or more seizures without regaining consciousness between them. An altered state of consciousness appearing as a fuguelike state, confusion, or lethargy, with no motor movements may also appear to be continuous or almost so *(petit mal status)*. Myoclonic status can occur when the patient has frequent repetitive jerky movements, usually affecting the whole body, and focal motor seizures may also be continuous and demand emergency management.

Five percent of all patients with epilepsy have status at some time. Most of them have focal seizures. The condition is an emergency because of the effect of repetitive grand mal seizures upon ventilation, resulting in anoxia, cerebral ischemia, and cerebral edema. The longer the status lasts, the greater the mortality. Management depends upon maintaining a good airway, stopping the seizure, attending to the body's metabolic needs, and identifying the cause.

Guard the Airway: The patient should be removed from any place of danger and his chin held up so that the neck is extended. When the seizure has stopped, a pharyngeal airway may be inserted. If there are recurrent attacks at short intervals, the patient may have an endotracheal tube passed when he is relaxed between seizures to maintain the airway and to prevent aspiration.

Do *not* attempt to put anything in the mouth when there is ongoing muscular contraction; this is usually impossible, and any attempt to force objects into the mouth results in broken teeth, which may be inhaled into the bronchi. The old advice to put a spoon or similar objects into the mouth should be vigorously discarded. Because of the common erroneous idea that something must be put between the teeth, one woman in the heat of the moment put her fingers in the patient's mouth during a grand mal seizure and thus lost the ends of two of them. The nursing tradition of putting a padded tongue depressor at the head of the patient's bed has only one benefit — it enables one to determine at a glance which patients in hospital have seizures.[*]

Stop the Seizure: The drug of choice is diazepam, 10 mg intravenously. This should be repeated every 10 to 15 min, as required, up to a maximum of 40 mg, although rarely as much as 100 mg may be necessary over 24 hr. In case of respiratory depression, have an Ambu bag available. Lorazepam 1 to 4 mg may be as good, and has an even longer action.

Because diazepam precipitates on the plastic tubing of an IV set, only about 15 percent will get into the patient if it is put in an IV bottle or high up the tube. Diazepam should be injected directly into the vein or right at the IV site by a bolus method, with the IV briefly clamped to prevent backflow on injection.

A patient with any form of status epilepticus should be hospitalized as soon as possible, maintaining the airway at all times. If IV diazepam is ineffective in controlling seizures, the patient will have to be anesthetized and an endotracheal tube inserted to allow adequate ventilation and cerebral oxygenation.

Although seizures are usually stopped by IV diazepam, they may begin again if the underlying process is ongoing (intracerebral hemorrhage, brain trauma, drug toxicity or withdrawal, or infection). In such cases, other anticonvulsants, such as phenobarbital or phenytoin, should be given for a more prolonged effect. Phenytoin 1000 mg IV over 1/2 to 2 hr is usually effective; or it can be given slowly IV in dosages of 50 mg/min for 5 min, which dosage may be repeated at hourly intervals, if necessary, up to a maximum of 1 g in a patient who has not received it before. The patient is given 300 to 400 mg daily from then on by oral or IV routes. Cardiac irregularities and hypotension may occur with IV injections and the patient must be watched carefully for these complications. Alternatively intravenous *lidocaine* may dramatically stop seizures without excessive sedation. A 10 to 30 mg bolus is given IV and an IV drip at 200-300 mg/hr is begun and continued for 12 to 48 hr.

Intravenous phenobarbital can be given in a dosage of 200 mg in 50 ml of normal saline over 10 min, but there is a delay of at least 20 min before it attains tissue levels that are adequate to stop the seizure acitivty. If phenobarbital is given in repeated doses until the seizures stop, then toxic levels undoubtedly will be eventually reached.

Pentobarbital however has a GABA-like CNS depressant action, and given as an IV infusion in dosages of 100-150 mg/hr may be of value in refractory status epilepticus.

---

[*]The idea is firmly embedded in nursing folklore, but is slowly being eroded. Attorneys, conscious of the damages awarded for lung abscess caused by inhaled teeth, do a better job of stopping the mischief than we do.

Petit mal status may be diagnosed when a prolonged period of altered levels of consciousness (confusion, memory loss) occurs in a patient with petit mal. In patients who are not known to have petit mal epilepsy, the condition will probably not be clinically diagnosed because the patient just appears to be very confused, although the diagnosis may be made on inspection of an EEG. Intravenous diazepam, as suggested previously, or IV trimethiadone, 100 mg, usually abort the attack.

Many other drugs have been recommended for status in the past, but today a good general rule is to use diazepam IV as recommended earlier with added phenytoin or phenobarbital for a more lasting effect. If such measures are inadequate (after 40 to 100 mg diazepam have been given without a permanent effect), then an anesthetist should be called. It is not worth risking cerebral anoxia by trying all sorts of other medications and waiting to see if they work. If diazepam in these dosages over a short time does not stop the seizures, *call an anesthetist immediately.*

Attend to the Body's Metabolic Needs: Patients in status epilepticus may well be in metabolic imbalance with deficiency of magnesium, calcium, vitamins, sugar, or oxygen. Their blood pressure may be abnormally high, or they may be in renal failure. Blood gas estimation with determination of serum electrolyte and sugar levels is essential, and IV fluids should be given unless the patient awakens and is able to swallow.

Attend the Cause of the Status: The most common cause of status epilepticus is probably sudden anticonvulsant withdrawal or the administration of convulsant drugs or chemicals to a patient with epilepsy. The most common convulsant agent ingested is alcohol, but alcohol *withdrawal* may also provoke status. Most patients who have a focal lesion causing status epilepticus have frontal lobe disease, such as subdural hematoma, brain laceration, frontal neoplasm, or occlusive vascular disease. Status may be an early sign of encephalitis, cerebral abscess, and septicemia.

A full neurological examination is required as soon as the seizures are stopped, and all information possible should be obtained from relatives, bystanders, and so on. An EEG and CT scan should be done. Lumbar puncture may be done later if indicated by signs of meningeal infection. Anticonvulsant drugs should be continued, and one should determine what the blood levels of their current drugs are, particularly since these patients often have gone into status because of poor compliance.

The Single Seizure

If you are sure that the patient has had a seizure and have identified precipitating factors, then further evidence should be obtained from bystanders to help determine the type of seizure, whether type I (generalized) or type II (focal). If the patient remembers *anything at all* about the onset or course of the seizure, then he undoubtedly has type II epilepsy and requires further investigation. Meanwhile, a search should be made for other CNS symptoms, and the examination should attempt to demonstrate a site of brain dysfunction that may be the site of a epileptic focus.

Investigations have been mentioned previously. The whole purpose of investigation is to demonstrate a lesion that may need surgical removal, but it must be admitted that only a small percentage of patients with epilepsy have such a lesion.

Children with febrile convulsions with a positive family history need little else done if one EEG is within normal limits. A child with one grand mal or a few petit mal attacks needs no more than a baseline EEG, provided there are no neurological findings on examination, but he should be followed carefully. Any patient with focal seizures requires referral to a neurologist, except possibly elderly people who have had brief minor attacks for years before diagnosis and in whom investigation may do more harm than good.

Noninvasive outpatient procedures such as EEG, skull x-rays, and isotope or CT scans are perfectly safe, and if all are negative, an operable lesion is most unlikely. Adults with one or more attacks should have these tests performed. If their neurological examination is negative and the seizure is thought to be of type l rather than type ll, it is unlikely that further investigation will be required. If there is any doubt however, neurological referral is advisable. If you are not sure that a "seizure" was truly epileptic, a serum prolactin level may help, because high levels are found immediately after a seizure but not with hysterical attack.

Repeated Seizures

The management of recurrent epileptic seizures depends upon the type of seizures and the age of the patient. The management of febrile seizures and the indications for prophylactic therapy were mentioned earlier in the chapter.

For most adults phenytoin, 300 mg/day, is effective as a starting dosage for recurrent seizures. Many neurologists however now begin with carbamazepine because of fewer long-term side effects. Treatment is begun with 100 mg twice daily and increased by 100 mg every 2 days to a maintenance of 800-1200 mg/day in divided doses. Two weeks after this dosage has been commenced the patient should have blood levels estimated and the dosage modified according to the results. The therapeutic range for both of these drugs is given in Table 15-1. As time goes on, one must balance the anticonvulsant dosage to keep it within the therapeutic range of these drugs, then other medications may have to be added.

Patients with type ll seizures are usually treated with phenytoin, carbamazepine, or primidone. Aim to use one single drug, monitoring compliance and metabolism with repeated blood levels.[*] More combinations of drugs are possible but are best handled by a neurologist. Surgery can be contemplated in patients with a well-localized focus if drug therapy fails — a small proportion.

The drug of choice for petit mal seizures is valproic acid, 500 mg t.i.d.

Patients with myoclonic epilepsy of any type may respond to clonazepam 2-6 mg/day, nitrazepam (2-60 mg/day), or ACTH.

Children with infantile spasms (salaam attacks), usually with progressive neurological deficit, may respond to ACTH. Even though the eventual outcome may not be altered, the ACTH does diminish the severity and frequency of the attacks.

Eighty-five percent of patients with epilepsy will have almost complete seizure control with proper management and can live perfectly normal lives with the exception of driving a vehicle on the public highway. There are also commonsense prohibitions, such as not working on ladders or scaffolding, and it would be unwise for a patient with epilepsy to take up a profession such as a tightrope walker or steeplejack. Patients should be advised to avoid situations in which loss of control, even momentarily, might be of danger to themselves or others. With that provision in mind, epileptic patients can be assured that they can live an almost normal life in every way as long as the precipitants of seizures are avoided, medications are taken regularly, and follow-up appointments are kept. Most Canadian provinces allow patients to return to driving a motor vehicle when they have been seizure-free for 2 years, whether or not they are on anticonvulsant medication.

---

[*]Do not change medication dosage until the current dosage has had time to produce a steady state, elimination balancing ingestion: this takes at least five half-lives.

Febrile Seizures

Febrile seizures occur in about 5 percent of children and are essentially benign.
Treatment of the acute episode is to cool the child but it is possible to prevent
the seizure with 0.2 mg/kg diazepam by rectum when the temperature starts to
rise. The usual intravenous dose can be injected by a tuberculin syringe (without
the needle) into the rectum. It is possible to give the same dose intravenously,
but by the time a vein is entered, an effective therapeutic level could have been
obtained from the rectal route.

An alternative is to use oral nitrazepam 0.5 mg/kg/day in three divided
doses. Continuous prophylaxis using valproate may be considered when there are
evident developmental abnormalities, evidence of significant CNS damage, or for
very prolonged or repeated seizures. This group would comprise only 10 percent
of the total. Only about 10 percent of this group will eventually become epileptic.
It is important to avoid "fever phobia" in the parents of children and to explain
carefully how to manage a fever using acetaminophen and nitrazepam as discussed
previously.

When first seen, the child has had the seizure and is usually well again. No
investigations are required in this situation, but the child should be carefully
examined and the parents reassured. Because 1 in 10 will have another seizure
within the next 12 to 24 hr, the diazepam or nitrazepam can be given anyway.
It is disconcerting for everyone if a lot of reassurance and explanation is given
but the child has a recurrent convulsion on the way home. Admission is only indicated on the first occasion. The child should be carefully examined for evidence
of bacterial sepsis or meningitis and a CBC should be done. Only a few will require a lumbar puncture, and this is not necessary if the child at that point appears to be alert and otherwise well. Meningitis is frequently sought in this situation but rarely found.

BIBLIOGRAPHY

Delgado-Esqueta, A. et al. The treatable epilepties. *N. Engl. J. Med. 308*:1576–
1584, 1983.

Gomez, M.R., Kloss, D.W. Epilepsies of infancy and childhood. *Ann. Neurol. 13:*
113–124, 1983.

Klawans, H.L. Status epilepticus. In *Clinical Neuropharmacology,* Vol. 3, New
York, Raven Press, 1978.

Laidlaw, J., Richens, A. (eds.). *A Textbook of Epilepsy.* 2nd Ed. Edinburgh,
Churchill-Livingstone, 1982.

Pryse-Phillips, W.E.M. *Epilepsy.* Bristol, John Wright & Sons, 1969.

Sands, H., Minters, F.C. *The Epilepsy Fact Book.* New York, Scribner's, 1979.

16
Raised Intracranial Pressure

The brain, its covering membranes, and the cerebrospinal fluid (CSF) are enclosed within containers, the skull and spine, which are almost rigid and allow for very little expansion. *Hydrocephalus* is an abnormal increase in the amount and pressure of CSF present within this confined space. It almost always implies a reduction in brain volume, either because of ventricular enlargement or because of cortical atrophy. *Raised intracranial pressure* denotes a rise in the pressure of CSF above 180 mm of CSF measured by lumbar puncture with the patient lying on his side. The pressure is taken to be the same as true intracranial pressure, although this is not necessarily so. The intraventricular pressure when measured directly at operation in the sitting position is between 20 and 40 mm of CSF. Since there is very little venting possible, a persisting increase in volume of any of the intracranial or intraspinal contents quickly leads to a rise in pressure and ultimately to hydrocephalus.

Raised intracranial pressure (ICP) associated with hydrocephalus can be caused by: (1) excess production of CSF or a failure in its drainage, or (2) obstruction to CSF flow. Such obstruction may occur either between its site of production in the choroid plexus of the lateral, third, or fourth ventricles and its outflow into the subarachnoid space (*noncommunicating* or *obstructive* form); or within the subarachnoid space between the fourth ventricular roof foramina and the arachnoid granulations around the dural venous sinuses (*communicating* hydrocephalus). Raised ICP without an abnormal amount of CSF present occurs in cerebral edema from any cause and in association with expanding lesions.

PATHOGENESIS

Excessive Production of Cerebrospinal Fluid

Excessive production of CSF is rare. A papilloma of the choroid plexus is an uncommon but widely quoted cause. An increase in pCO_2 and vitamin A toxicity can both increase the amount of CSF produced by the choroid plexus and may produce symptoms (benign intracranial hypertension; discussed later).

Intracerebral Obstruction

An intraventricular cyst or compression of the third ventricle by neoplasms such as pituitary tumors or pinealomas may be responsible for obstruction of CSF flow (Fig. 16-1). In children aqueduct stenosis as a congenital defect or caused by a previous infection may obstruct the flow of CSF from the third to the fourth ventricle. In the posterior fossa obstruction may occur because of a neoplasm, the Arnold-Chiari malformation (Chap. 50), or chronic basal meningitis. Obstruction to CSF flow is present in many infants born with neural tube disorders, e.g., meningomyelocele (Fig. 16-2).

Extracerebral Obstruction

Obstruction to the flow of CSF over the convexity of the hemispheres toward the absorption site at the arachnoid granulations around the venous sinuses may occur from any chronic inflammation of the meninges. Blood in the CSF from any cause, such as a subarachnoid hemorrhage or trauma, can obstruct the CSF pathways over the hemispheres and result in the syndrome of "normal"-pressure hydrocephalus, (although raised ICP is likely to have been a factor in the pathogenesis of this condition).

Decreased Absorption

If venous pressure is markedly increased, then the hydrostatic pressure within the superior sagittal sinus offsets the active transport mechanism of the arachnoid granulations, and CSF may not be filtered. In a superior sagittal sinus thrombosis or occlusion of the dominant transverse sinus (which may occur in association with otitis media), the same picture is seen. Although it is usually an acute process,

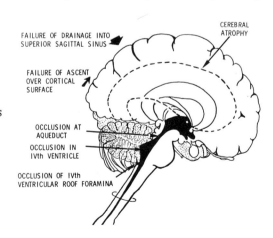

Figure 16-1 Sites of lesions producing hydrocephalus.

FAILURE OF DRAINAGE INTO SUPERIOR SAGITTAL SINUS

CEREBRAL ATROPHY

FAILURE OF ASCENT OVER CORTICAL SURFACE

OCCLUSION AT AQUEDUCT

OCCLUSION IN IVth VENTRICLE

OCCLUSION OF IVth VENTRICULAR ROOF FORAMINA

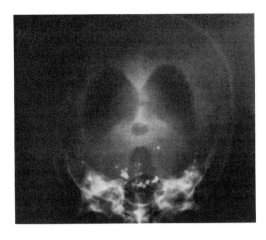

Figure 16-2 Huge ventricular dilatation shown by ventriculography. Chronic obstructive hydrocephalus caused by Arnold-Chiari malformation.

chronic venous obstruction can produce a picture similar to benign intracranial hypertension.

Cerebral Edema

An increase in the water content of the brain can occur for many reasons (Table 16-1). With *vasogenic* edema, damage to the blood-brain barrier allows fluid to leave the capillaries and to enter the brain's extracellular space, mainly in the gray matter. This occurs focally around brain tumors, abscesses and hematomas, and in the contused brain, and expands the brain tissue locally. The effect of any mass lesion (see following section) is magnified. Inflammatory swelling of the brain is also due to vasogenic edema and is seen in the encephalitis, meningitis, and other infections or parainfectious encephalopathies (see Chap. 40).

Table 16-1   Causes of Cerebral Edema

Vasogenic
      Malignant tumors
      Abscess, meningitis
      Postinfectious states
      Hematoma
      Cerebral contusion

Cytotoxic
      Ischemic infarction
      Hypoxia (e.g., post cardiac arrest)
      Hypertensive encephalopathy
      Dysequilibrium syndrome
      Acute organ rejection
      Lead and tin poisoning
      Hepatic failure

Hydrostatic
      Obstructive hydrocephalus

With *cytotoxic* edema, the water is mainly within astrocytes in both gray and white matter. A severe episode of cerebral anoxia is the most common cause, but some toxins also are occasionally responsible.

A marked rise in intravascular pressure (acute hypertension), hypoxemia, and hypercapnia also lead to a generalized increase in extracellular fluid volume. Ischemia caused by vasospasm further damages the brain tissue. During acute rejection of a transplanted organ, seizures, hypertension, headache, and confusion witness the development of edema in the white matter — rejection encephalopathy.

In cases of high-pressure hydrocephalus, fluid crosses the ependyma into the periventricular space (*hydrostatic* edema). This is shown well on CT scans.

In all cases, as a result of the increased amount of intracranial fluid retained, pressure rises and blood flow falls, and if the edema is vasogenic, the edematous brain acts as an expanding mass lesion. In either instance, further damage to the brain ensues.

Mass Lesions

Mass lesions include neoplasms, subdural and extradural hematomas of any type, and cerebral abscesses. The rise in pressure produced causes symptoms directly in proportion to the lesion's speed of increase. Thus the patient with a very slowly growing tumor, such as a frontal meningioma, may show no signs of raised intracranial pressure, although the tumor when removed may be extremely large. On the other hand, a fast-growing metastatic tumor of much smaller size may quickly produce a marked rise in ICP with distortion of intracranial structures, an uncal or central syndrome, and perhaps death if the expanding mass is not removed or the increased ICP somehow reduced.

Skull Lesions

In some children, premature fusion of the cranial sutures (*craniosynostosis*) prevents the head from expanding as the brain grows (Fig. 16-3). This gives rise to an abnormally long, wide, or high skull. If a number of sutures are prematurely closed, the cranium cannot expand as the brain grows in size.

CLINICAL FEATURES

Among children, obstruction to the normal passage of CSF out of the ventricular system (noncommunicating hydrocephalus) is most common, although craniosynostosis and failure of CSF absorption because of sinus thrombophlebitis are also important causes. Adults are more likely to suffer from the effects of mass lesions or from cerebral edema. While clinical examination may enable identification of the pathogenesis and even the site of the lesion, it should be clear that the clinical picture may have three components:

> The effect of the initial lesion, if there is one. Thus a secondary hematoma may produce a contralateral hemiparesis or a focal motor seizure by compression of the cortex beneath it.
> The effects of raised intracranial pressure, e.g., headache and papilledema.
> Secondary effects of the raised intracranial pressure. These include drowsiness from pressure on the reticular activating system in the brainstem and sometimes a sixth nerve palsy, a nonspecific pressure effect that can be a false localizing sign because it occurs on either side. Compression of the

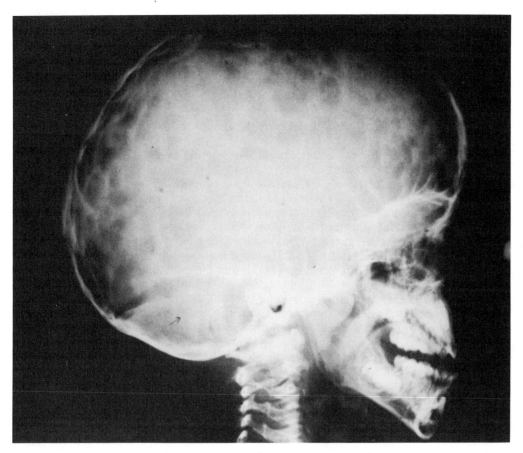

Figure 16-3 Craniosynostosis. No cranial sutures are visible. The head could not expand to accommodate the developing brain and intracranial pressure increased; "copper-beating" of the calvarium results.

fourth ventricle floor causes vomiting, slowing of the pulse rate, and a rise in blood pressure. Other effects may be due to uncal herniation (Chap. 10), posterior cerebral artery occlusion (contralateral hemiparesis and sensory loss; homonymous hemianopia), and pressure of the brainstem against the opposite edge of the tentorium (Kernohan's notch syndrome). This latter syndrome can give rise to the false localizing sign of a hemiparesis ipsilateral to the mass lesion (false localizing signs are further discussed in Chap. 9).

In infants, the head circumference may rise abnormally fast (see Fig. 4-1), the fontanels may be open and bulging, percussion of the skull may give rise to a "cracked pot" sound when tapped, and transillumination of the skull may show excessive light shining through. Listlessness, failure to thrive, and vomiting are other common signs in infants. Sometimes a murmur can be heard over the scalp. The eyes are pushed forward and slightly downward (sunset sign). In adults, these signs should not be expected because the sutures have fused. In children whose heads can still expand before the skull sutures are firmly closed, many of the signs seen in adults may be missing.

When compensation for the raised intracranial pressure fails, major neurological features occur both in the child and adult. These include

1. Headache, worse in the morning
2. A reduced level of consciousness
3. Nausea, vomiting, and vertigo
4. Double vision resulting from a sixth nerve palsy
5. Grand mal seizures
6. Brief obscurations of vision caused by papilledema

On examination the patient may be drowsy, or the level of consciousness may be decreased even to the point of coma. Apart from the signs produced by the lesion causing the raised ICP (e.g., visual field abnormalities, focal seizures, or localizing motor or sensory signs), other signs often found are absence of pulsations of the retinal veins, blurring of the disk margins or papilledema, and retinal hemorrhages, and later, secondary optic atrophy. Signs of meningeal irritation (meningism) are due to traction on the larger vessels and meninges at the base of the brain causing reflex neck stiffness. Late signs include evidence of an upper motor neuron lesion on one or both sides, a reduction in pulse rate, and a rise in the systolic blood pressure, probably caused by damage to the medullary centers.

Rarely, with long-standing hydrocephalus, the enlarged third ventricle may press downward and forward upon the pituitary. This gives rise to hypopituitarism with evidence of growth failure, hypothyroidism, or sometimes obesity and genital atrophy. Pressure in this region may also damage the optic nerves or chiasm producing constricted visual fields, particularly on the temporal sides.

An abnormally large head is not always a result of raised intracranial pressure. In certain *storage* diseases the brain and head may be excessive in size. Brain *cysts* (which may be bilateral and symmetric) can also expand the head. Overgrowth of the skull, as in *Paget's disease,* may be associated with a cranial circumference greater than normal in the adult.

MAJOR CAUSES

Among adults, the lesions that cause a rise of ICP present in three major ways: acute, subacute, and chronic.

Acute

With an acute rise in ICP, various combinations of false localizing signs, the uncal or central syndromes (Chap. 7), and signs resulting from the expansion of the mass itself will all be present. In *acute extradural hemorrhage* caused by traumatic skull fracture and bleeding from the middle meningeal artery, there will be local brain compression, signs of raised intracranial pressure, and eventually a central syndrome. Trauma and anoxia both give rise to generalized *cerebral edema* (Fig. 16-4), accompanied over the course of hours by signs of raised ICP and a central syndrome. Cerebral edema in *herpes simplex encephalitis* may cause the uncal syndrome.

Hypertensive encephalopathy may be diagnosed in the presence of severe hypertension, seizures, papilledema, and a decreased level of consciousness.

Intracerebral hemorrhage occurs in hypertensive patients because of the rupture of a small vessel in the deepest part of the brain. Bleeding in the posterior fossa (pons or cerebellum) is described in Chapter 37; it causes acute neurological

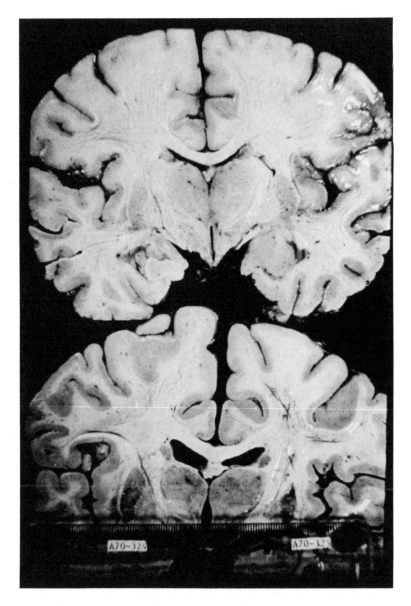

Figure 16-4   Diffuse brain swelling because of cerebral edema. The ventricles of the upper brain are compressed and the gyri flattened. The lower brain is normal, for comparison.

localizing signs, such as cranial nerve palsies, and headache, neck stiffness, vomiting, vertigo, and often loss of consciousness. With hemorrhage in the basal ganglia or putamen, the lateralizing deficits (hemiparesis, hemianopia, gaze palsies, etc.) are more obvious. Headache, stiff neck, seizures, and inital loss of consciousness are also common. *Subarachnoid hemorrhage* may present in a similar manner; although in such patients the sudden onset of severe headache and meningism should enable a clinical diagnosis to be made. *Sinus thrombosis* tends to occur in children with dehydration, otitis, or sickle-cell disease and in adults with the same conditions or with frontal sinusitis, septicemia, or bacterial endocarditis. These conditions should be picked up on general physical examination. Seizures in association with evidence of raised ICP, fever, and focal signs are diagnostic pointers. In all such cases, emergency referral to a neurological center is mandatory.

Subacute

Subacutely evolving increased ICP may occur with a *cerebral abscess.* The patient may show evidence of an infection, headache, and focal signs and symptoms usually pointing to a frontal, temporal, or cerebellar lesion. Some forms of *meningitis* present in a similar way (Chap. 40). *Subdural hematoma* may occur without a definite history of trauma and should be considered, particularly in the very young, the very old, and those with any degree of cerebral atrophy or with a history of chronic alcoholism. Focal and false localizing signs, personality change, and alterations in the level of consciousness may be expected.

Rapidly growing malignant intracerebral *tumors* may give rise to the same history and findings. Other masses that grow slowly but attain a large size can distort the CSF drainage system gradually or prevent reabsorption, but they may produce the classic symptoms of raised ICP with focal signs and symptoms only at a late stage. Seizures are not uncommon and are frequently focal. *Increased venous pressure* caused by compression of the superior vena cava should be evident on general clinical examination and is another cause of this syndrome.

Chronic

The terms *benign intracranial hypertension* and *pseudotumor cerebri* refer to a condition of raised ICP not caused by an expanding mass lesion or to obstruction to CSF flow. In this condition, the ventricles are of normal size or may be small. The mental status and formal neurological examinations and the CSF constituents all are normal. The syndrome is rare in males. The diagnosis *must* be confirmed by lumbar puncture with pressure measurement as described in Chapter 8. Because tumors (gliomatosis cerebri, gliomas, metastases, AV malformations) and chronic encephalitis all may present this way, CT scanning has to be done before the CSF is taken.

Many causes have been reported, but the mechanisms by which they act are uncertain. They include

1. Obesity (the cause in 90% of the patients, almost invariably female)
2. Administration of the birth-control pill, nalidixic acid, tetracycline, or excess vitamin A
3. Chronic respiratory insufficiency
4. Acute iron deficiency anemia
5. Cushing's syndrome, Addison's disease, steroid administration or withdrawal (especially in children)
6. Hypoparathyroidism
7. Pregnancy

The patient will have complained of symptoms suggesting raised ICP, such as headache, diplopia, visual blurring, and obscurations, but no localizing neurological abnormalities will be found. Examination may show papilledema and perhaps sixth nerve palsy but little else except for obesity, endocrinopathy, or signs of CO_2 retention. The history is really all-important in determining the likely cause. If the

EEG and CT scans are normal in a patient with raised pressure but no localizing signs, pseudotumor is the most likely diagnosis.

Treatment is of the cause, where this can be demonstrated. In most cases strict weight reduction will relieve the problem. Drugs such as acetazolamide, furosemide, chlorthalidone, and steroids may be selected for long-term treatment of unresponsive cases. Follow-up must be rigorously undertaken, with repeated examination of the fundi, visual acuity, and perimetry. It often takes months before symptoms completely resolve and years until pressures fall. It is unusual for the condition to require surgical shunting, but in some unresponsive patients, chronic papilledema leads to optic atrophy and visual impairment, in which case such procedures may be necessary.

INVESTIGATION

When the patient arrives in the hospital, the following investigations may be of value in the diagnosis of the cause of raised ICP.

Skull X-Ray

A calcified pineal gland may be seen to shift across the midline away from an expanding mass. If the ICP has been present at some time, decalcification of the posterior clinoid process may be apparent. A "beaten copper" appearance of the upper part of the cranial vault may be seen with long-standing ICP (see Fig. 16-3). Similar findings occur in the lower two-thirds of the skull in many normal people, but it is only significant when present over the superior aspect.

Craniosynostosis may be diagnosed by x-rays that show fusion of the coronal, sagittal, or lambdoidal sutures. The pituitary fossa may be expanded and its floor eroded or "doubled" by an intrasellar mass lesion. Abnormal calcification may be seen, allowing diagnosis of tumors, AV malformations, etc. (see Chap. 8).

CT Scan

The CT scan is the procedure of greatest value among all those mentioned. The site of any intracerebral obstruction should be demarcated (Figs. 16-5, 16-6) as when, for instance, the lateral and third ventricles are dilated but the fourth ventricles are small (aqueductal lesion), displaced (posterior fossa mass), or occluded (ependymoma or other local tumor). If the fourth ventricle is also enlarged, then the obstruction is in its roof foramina, or else the condition is a communicating hydrocephalus.

Abscess, tumor, intracerebral hemorrhage, and extracerebral fluid collections should also be well shown, if the technique of enhancement is used.

Generalized brain swelling will be implicated if the ventricles are small as in pseudotumor cerebri. Midline shift and other evidence of "mass effect" and localized hypodense areas occur with cerebral edema, infarct, and some tumors.

Electroencephalogram (EEG)

The EEG may show marked abnormalities when either cerebral abscesses or herpes encephalitis are present. Abnormalities may well be seen in the case of a tumor or vascular accident when one may see features characteristic of a destructive lesion, although the EEG is not effective in differentiating between vascular and neoplastic diseases. A normal EEG in the presence of definite increased intracranial pressure probably excludes a cerebral although not necessarily a cerebellar abscess.

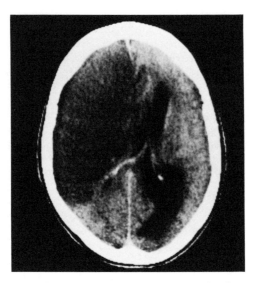

Figure 16-5 CT scan. Left anterior and middle cerebral artery occlusions have caused huge local brain swelling, midline shift to the right, compression of the left and dilatation of the right lateral ventricle. The patient was coning at this stage.

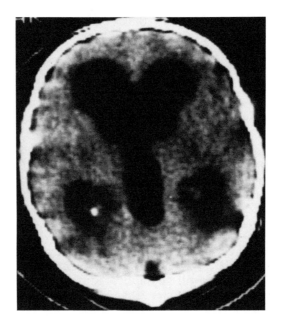

Figure 16-6 CT scan. Acute increase of intracranial pressure caused by a large, ultimately fatal, cerebellar hematoma.

Isotope Scan

Cerebral tumors, vascular accidents, subdural hematomas, and abscesses all alter the blood-brain barrier and may give rise to a positive isotope scan. A negative scan however does not absolutely exclude any pathology.

Other Studies

Angiography or ventriculography may be selected in unusual cases, but these are not often required if a CT scan can be performed. Other investigations may be directed toward finding any extracerebral cause of increased intracranial pressure such as primary carcinoma of the lung, parathyroid gland dysfunction, endocrine disease, or local mastoid infections.

TREATMENT

The definitive treatment of raised intracranial pressure is always the treatment of its cause, e.g., removal of a tumor or hematoma or drainage of an abscess. There follows a discussion of measures that are directed toward the problem of the relief of abnormally high ICP; but *all* cases demand full neurological assessment, and for continued care, ICP monitoring may be required in a neurosurgical unit.

Steroids have therapeutic effect only if cerebral edema is of the vasogenic type. Dexamethasone, 10-20 mg IM or IV initially and henceforward 4 mg q6h is used, the dosage being reduced progressively after 4 days. If the cause can be remedied however, reduction to, e.g., 1 mg q6h may proceed faster.

Raised ICP resulting from cytotoxic or hydrostatic edema responds poorly to steroid therapy. The patient whose pressure rise is due to cerebral edema not of the vasogenic type may be hyperventilated and given mannitol while being transferred to a neurological center. Drainage of CSF with an intraventricular catheter, therapy with barbiturates, powerful diuretics, and hypertonic solutions, and hypothermia are available there, where also the cause may be directly susceptible to treatment.

If mannitol (1-1.5 g/kg body weight given as IV infusion over 15 min) is going to be used, dexamethasone should be given intramuscularly, or otherwise it will be washed out in the urine. As in the case of "coning" during lumbar puncture, the patient may be hyperventilated by facial mask or after intubation. If vomiting is a problem, a nasogastric tube should be passed, and intubation should probably be carried out anyway. In all patients with cerebral edema, blood gases, blood pressure, and body temperature must be restored to normal and volatile anesthetics avoided.

In patients who have long-standing rise in intracranial pressure, the most important treatment is again directed at the cause of the condition. In most patients with pseudotumor cerebri a cause is present that is treatable, e.g., weight reduction. Dexamethasone effectively reduces the pressure and may be given initially in a high dosage if continuing visual obscurations suggest a permanent threat to sight. Acetazolamide and chlorthalidone have a weak effect in reducing ICP, but they are of value as long-term measures in symptomatic patients.

Sudden obstruction to CSF flow may occur if a lumbar puncture is performed in a patient with a posterior fossa mass lesion because the cerebellar tonsils may then descend into the foramen magnum, causing immediate compression of the medulla with cessation of vital functions (coning). In such cases the following steps are indicated until the neurosurgeon can put in an emergency ventricular tube.

1. Tilt the patient's head down as far as possible.
2. Reinject 5-10 ml of sterile saline, if this is immediately available. If not, close the lumbar puncture needle with a stylette and inject the saline as soon as possible, withdrawing the needle immediately after injection.
3. Call for an Ambu bag or an anesthetic trolley and begin hyperventilating the patient. Hyperventilation lowers the carbon dioxide level and thus causes marked vasoconstriction, diminishing the volume of the intracranial circulation and reducing pressure temporarily. This is however no more than a holding measure that may protect the patient for a time until definite treatment of the pressure rise can be instituted.
4. Inject dexamethasone 20 mg IM and set up an intravenous infusion of mannitol 20% giving 1-1.5 g/kg in 10 min. Insert a catheter into the bladder.

If the patient has been tipped head down, it is possible that the medulla and cerebellar tonsils will disimpart; if this occurs, treatment can be continued with further dexamethasone every 6 hr orally or intramuscularly. The cause of the catastrophe must be diagnosed and treated definitively as soon as possible.

BIBLIOGRAPHY

Corbett, J.J. Problems in the diagnosis and treatment of pseudotumor cerebri. *Can. J. Neurol. Sci. 10:*221-229, 1983.

Cutler, R.W.P., Spertell, R.B. Cerebrospinal fluid: A selective review. *Ann. Neurol. 11:*1-10, 1982.

Fishman, R.A. Cerebrospinal fluid. In *Diseases of the Nervous System.* Philadelphia, W.B. Saunders Co., 1980.

Miller, J.D. The management of cerebral edema. *Br. J. Hosp. Med. 22:*152-165, 1979.

17
Headache

Headache is one of the most common symptoms encountered by both the family practitioner and the neurologist. It is a symptom and not a disease. The patient who complains of headache is best approached with a knowledge of the varieties that can occur and of the characteristics of each (Table 17-1). Diagnosis is achieved by history taking, rather than by physical examination and investigations. Almost all patients who seek help because of long-standing, chronic recurring headache have migraine, or muscle contraction headache, or both.

MECHANISMS OF HEAD PAIN

Headache can result from inflammation or distortion (traction or compression) of any of the pain-sensitive structures inside the head. These include the large sinuses and veins, the large and medium-sized arteries at the base of the brain, the basal dura, and those nerves that convey pain impulses from the face and head (the fifth, seventh intermedius, ninth, and tenth nerves), as well as the roots of C2 and C3. Extracranial pain-sensitive structures include the skin, scalp, fascia, muscles, and arteries. The mucosa of the sinuses, mouth, pharynx, and nose are pain sensitive too, but the brain parenchyma is not; nor are the dura over the convexity of the brain, the pia-arachnoid, the ependyma, nor the skull (although the periosteum is slightly sensitive).

The mechanism of pain in migraine is unclear. It is generally accepted that the initial stage is vasoconstriction of the intra- and extracranial vessels, followed by vasodilation. The initial vasoconstriction may cause local or generalized cerebral ischemia, and the following vasodilation of extracranial vessels may distort the free nerve endings subserving pain in the arterial walls and release pain-producing substances into the surrounding tissues, resulting in the throbbing headache.

253

Table 17-1   Classification of Headache

Migraine (vascular)

    Common
    Classic
    Complicated
        vertebrobasilar
        retinal
        hemiplegic
        ophthalmoplegic
    Cluster

Muscle contraction

Combined (vascular and muscle contraction)

Nonmigrainous vascular

    Fever
    Hypoxia
    Hangover
    Hypoglycemia
    Severe hypertension
    Following concussion or seizures
    Vasodilating drugs

Traction

    Expanding masses
    Brain swelling
    Obstruction to CSF flow
    Postlumbar puncture

Cranial inflammation

    Intracranial (infection, arteritis, bleeding)
    Extracranial (cranial arteritis, cellulitis)

Disease of nearby structures

    Eyes, ENT, sinuses, teeth, skull, and neck

There are many factors that seem to influence the appearance of the headache: overtiredness, alcohol ingestion, noise, bright lights, pain elsewhere, certain foods, oversleeping, fasting, vasodilating drugs, the oral contraceptive pill, and hormonal changes of the menstrual cycle, pregnancy, and menopause. Some of these factors tend to precipitate headaches, while a few, such as pregnancy and menopause, tend to improve them. The foods that are associated with migraine usually contain a lot of tyramine, nitrates, serotonin, or their precursors. No final common pathway whereby all of these mechanisms may act has yet been determined, but it is likely to involve the prostaglandin fractions, which are extremely vasoactive.

Although it is useful to separate headaches that are primarily vascular (migraine) or muscle contraction, it should be remembered these are probably part of a spectrum, and many patients have a mixture of both forms of physiological change and overlap of symptoms.

DESCRIPTION OF HEADACHE TYPES

Migraine (Vascular) Headache

Migraine headaches occur in about 10 to 20 percent of the population, affecting children as well as adults. Of the types of migraine, *common migraine* is indeed the most common. This is a throbbing vascular headache, often bilateral and associated with nausea. In *classic migraine*, an aura precedes the pain, which is usually unilateral, whereas *complicated migraine* signifies an accompanying transient but distressing neurological deficit. *Cluster migraine* may or may not be a primary vascular headache, but it is normally so described and shares some features in common with the others (Fig. 17-1).

Figure 17-1   Usual sites of pain in four varieties of headache.

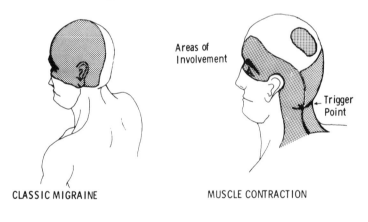

CLASSIC MIGRAINE   MUSCLE CONTRACTION

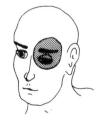

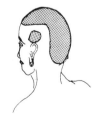

CLUSTER MIGRAINE   VASCULAR HEADACHE

A positive family history of migraine is found in 60 percent of patients. Although migraine is said to be much more common in women, population studies show only a slight increase of women over men. It seems that more women with migraine seek medical advice, and this heavily weights information coming from the clinical experience of hospitals, doctors offices, or headaches clinics.

Migraine often occurs in childhood, but is sometimes unrecognized because the child complains more of recurrent abdominal upset and vomiting and motion sickness rather than headache. Periodic vomiting in childhood and recurrent sleepwalking are common childhood manifestations of headache. When children reach puberty, 50 to 75 percent will stop having migraine, but paradoxically this is the age when most adult migraineurs begin to develop headache.

The migraineur probably inherits a pattern of vascular responsivity that results in an exaggerated vascular change to internal and external noxious or threatening stimuli — thus an exaggerated protective response.

The clinical features of any one patient's migraine may change over the years, with periods of remission, the headaches returning again in association with physical, physiological, or psychological stress. It has been said that migrainous patients are intelligent, tense, meticulous, and obsessional, but this personality pattern more correctly reflects the patient who gets headaches and seeks medical attention than the relaxed, easy-going migraineur.

Common Migraine

This headache is characteristically throbbing or pounding, with a background of continuous aching. It is of any degree of severity, may be uni- or bilateral, and is poorly localized. The pain may refer to the face or eyes and occasionally to the neck. The headache usually lasts for hours and is relieved by sleep. If there is a psychological precipitant, the patient often notes his headaches during periods of stress or tension, but it is not uncommon for patients to have "letdown" headaches *after* stress. In this situation the headaches tend to occur on weekends, in the evenings, or on vacations. Noise, bright lights, and concentration make the headache worse, and the scalp often feels tender when the hair is brushed or the head lies on a pillow. Associated symptoms may be anorexia and nausea, slight blurring of vision, mild dizziness, photophobia, hyperacusis, and irritability.

Although migraine headaches of various types are characteristically throbbing and aching, these patients may also complain at times of sharp, shooting, or "ice-pick" pains in the head, lasting seconds only.

Classic Migraine

In this form, an *aura* precedes the throbbing headache. This may consist of flashing lights, showers of sparks or spots, or areas of blotting out of the visual field (scotomata). Rarely, more formed visual hallucinations occur. Other symptoms before the headache might include speech difficulty or numbness around the mouth, in a hand, or on one side of the body. Motor weakness may also occur on one side, usually in the hand. All of these premonitory symptoms and signs usually disappear as the headache develops, but they may occur with the headache.

The headache is usually unilateral, severe, and throbbing. The duration is seldom longer than 3 to 4 hr and more prolonged migraine usually means that the patient is developing a muscle contraction headache in association with the vascular one, particularly if it lasts for days. The times of occurrence are similar to common migraine and the precipitating factors are the same. Associated symptoms include autonomic abnormalities such as diarrhea, nausea and vomiting, anorexia, flushing or pallor of the face and body, and nasal congestion. Irritability, depression, and drowsiness are also commonly associated. The frequency of migraine attacks varies from a rare headache every few months to daily headaches for 1 or 2 hr at a time.

Complicated Migraine

If we accept that the initial occurrence in the pathophysiology of migraine is constriction of intracranial vessels, then it is easy to understand how the resulting cerebral ischemia might produce a long-lasting effect. Complicated migraine is little more than classic migraine with a more pronounced neurological deficit. This might include protracted blindness because of retinal ischemia, ophthalmoplegia, hemiparesis, or hemianesthesia, or persistent dysphasia. Such syndromes may outlast the headache, and the ophthalmoplegia may last for 2 to 3 days.

Ophthalmoplegic migraine is an unusual type for the paralysis of ocular muscles and the diplopia may persist for many days following the headache.

It should not be forgotten that patients will occasionally develop permanent neurological deficit from migraine, and strokelike syndromes are being increasingly recognized as migraine complications. Although we have seen only a few permanent hemiparetic syndromes, more commonly we have recognized homonymous hemianopia as a permanent sequel of migraine with occipital infarction evident on the CT scan.

Cluster Migraine

This unusual form of severe craniofacial pain goes by many other names, including periodic migrainous neuralgia, histamine cephalgia, ciliary neuralgia, and Horton's headache. Although one of the most characteristic and stereotyped syndromes in medicine, it is often missed or at least misdiagnosed. It is most common in men who suddenly develop a localized unilateral retro-orbital or temporal pain (it is one of the few headaches that the patient will point to with one finger). The attacks can occur at any time but often awaken the patient from sleep in the early hours of the morning. They occur in clusters, headaches occurring daily for a few weeks before disappearing for months or years. In some cases, they later become continuous with no remission. Alcohol is a frequent precipitant of the headache. This is one of the worst pains one can experience, with relief often being obtained only by one or more doses of a narcotic.

Associated with the severe pain, profuse lacrimation and nasal discharge on the same side are characteristic. Perhaps a quarter of the patients develop a Horner's syndrome with intense miosis and ptosis on the same side as the pain, and a few show flushing and puffiness of the face.

Migraine Variants

In young women, vertebrobasilar involvement may occur rather than carotid vasoconstriction *(vertebrobasilar migraine)*. This results in an occipital headache with associated brainstem symptoms such as vertigo, diplopia, bilateral motor or sensory symptoms, slurred speech, and excessive drowsiness. Cortical ischemia may cause temporary blindness.

Carotidynia is a syndrome of tenderness over the carotid artery in the neck, with an added aching pain spreading up the neck to the lower jaw and face. The cause is unknown. It may be relieved by steroids or by antimigraine agents but usually clears in a week or two if left alone.

Severe, pounding migrainelike headaches occur rarely during sexual intercourse in both sexes. These *orgasmic headaches* probably represent migraines precipitated by physiological stress and muscle tension in the neck during intercourse. Other variants are the childhood manifestations of periodic or cyclic vomiting, sleepwalking, and motion sickness.

Migraine acompagnée is a term used for symptoms such as visual scintillations, paresthesias, or dysphasia, that mainly occurs in older people because of cerebral vasospasm, i.e., migraine. They progress in an orderly march and usually last longer than the normal 20 to 60 min of TIAs, which they otherwise closely resemble. Patients with this "late-life migraine" do not always have any headache with the neurological deficits, but they usually do give a past history of migraine or else develop headaches later. Management does not differ from that of migraine in other age groups; it is the diagnosis that is difficult.

Muscle Contraction Headache

Muscle contraction headaches are usually due to muscle spasm in the posterior or lateral cervical muscles. The pain will radiate to the top of the head or the bitemporal and bifrontal regions (Fig. 17-2). It is experienced as a tight, bandlike pressure, usually of moderate severity. The patient's personality frequently contains traits of anxiety, emotional overexpression, or rigid self-control. The headache is usually bilateral. Frequency, duration, and special times of occurrence are variable in each patient. Aggravating factors are psychological tension, noise, concentration, and cervical muscle strain. Although often called "tension" headache, tension is only the most common cause of this problem and the most common aggravating factor when other causes are present. The same muscle contraction and pain may occur from other causes of cervical muscle spasm, including cervical spondylosis, concussion, "whiplash" injuries, and rarely a posterior fossa tumor. The headache is often long-lasting and some patients say it never goes away. This is probably the only headache that will continue for weeks or even months without relief. One can see the tension in the patient's muscles as the whole body seems to be more rigid. The spasm occurs not only in the neck but also in the paraspinal muscles, causing poor posture, and in the arms. (In a reversed way, musculoskeletal causes of painful spasm may produce referred neck and head pains of this type.) The subject may persistently clench the teeth, causing aching in the temporomandibular region; sit in rigid stiff positions, and grip a steering wheel so hard that the arms ache.

Combined Headaches

These headaches are a combination of the vascular and muscle contraction headaches just discussed. It is very common for patients with long-standing migraine to develop muscle contraction (tension) headaches, as well as it is for patients with severe muscle contraction headaches to develop a vascular component when the headaches are at a peak. The headaches may be uni- or bilateral, are poorly localized, and vary from mild to severe. They are often said to be constant, lasting days, weeks, or months, and although the patient takes quantities of analgesics, these are seldom effective. A few autonomic symptoms may be associated, but not as frequently nor as severely as in common or classic migraine. The scalp is often tender and the pain may be somewhat relieved by compression of the superficial temporal arteries, only to return when the pressure is removed.

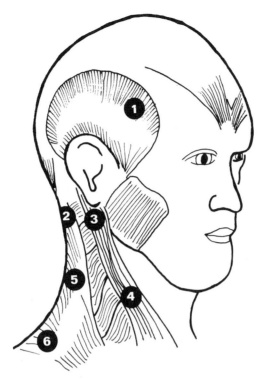

Figure 17-2 Some trigger points in muscles of the head and neck. Muscle spasm (myofascial pain) can induce severe local and radiating pains. (1) Temporalis; (2) Splenius capitis; (3,4) Sternomastoid; (5,6) Trapezius.

Nonmigrainous Vascular Headaches

These have all the features of a vascular headache but are due to some underlying disorder such as a hangover, hypoxia, concussion, hypoglycemia, fever, or hypertensive crisis. Hypertension as a cause of headache is overrated; hypertensive patients do not have any more headaches than the rest of the population. However there is a definite *pressor headache* associated with sudden *severe* elevations of blood pressure.

Traction Headache

Although it is not often that a patient consulting his physician for headache will turn out to have a brain tumor, the traction headache is the one that all physicians worry about. It is also the reason why we tend to analyze all headaches with great care so that we do not miss an intracranial mass lesion. The pain is not quite as typical as we would like and is often characterized just as a steady, bursting, or pressure sensation, dull in nature, and felt deep within the head. Patients with other headaches will use the same words occasionally, so the description is not diagnostic. The headache is usually not rhythmic, and it seldom throbs. It is continuous in only about 10 percent of patients and is rarely as intense as migraine.

It is often relieved by aspirin or cold packs applied to the skull, which may give the physician a mistaken sense of security. It is poorly localized and may be referred to the eyes or neck. Special times of occurrence include the early morning, some relief being obtained from the upright posture as the day goes on. Any added increase in intracranial pressure, as with stooping, coughing, or bending, makes the headache worse, but this again is not a point that differentiates it clearly from other forms. Possibly more suggestive of an expanding intracranial lesion is the *abrupt onset* of head pain with these maneuvers.

The associated symptoms depend upon the *rate of expansion* of the intracranial mass and its *site* more than upon its size. Vertigo, nausea, vomiting, drowsiness, pain on ocular movement, and irritability are often present, and if there is any herniation of intracranial contents, then such specific signs as sixth or third nerve palsy may appear.

The site of the headache may have some diagnostic value because two-thirds of the subjects with brain tumors complain of pain over or near the region of the mass. Those with posterior fossa lesions often complain of occipital headache; unfortunately, associated nuchal muscle tension and neck stiffness or tenderness may lead one to diagnose a typical muscle contraction headache unless the other characteristics are noted.

Another danger is that this headache is often not particularly severe in the early stages, and the patient's description may not be precise, again leading to a false sense of security. Some growing tumors merely accentuate the patient's usual headache, e.g., of muscle contraction or of migrainous type; here the diagnosis is indeed difficult, and this situation points up the need for a careful neurological examination in all patients with head pain.

Headache of Cranial Inflammation

The headaches of meningitis and subarachnoid hemorrhage are rapid in onset, severe, and associated with evidence of meningeal inflammation. Inflammation of extracranial structures (cellulitis, local abscess) is usually easily diagnosed, but the headache to watch for is that of cranial (temporal) arteritis, a giant-cell arteritis that characteristically involves the temporal and ophthalmic vessels and will cause blindness in half the patients if untreated. The unilateral temporal pain is associated with local tenderness and redness over the scalp, and the temporal arteries are tender, cordlike, and pulseless (see Chap. 42).

This syndrome is associated with polymyalgia rheumatica; 50 percent of the patients with this latter syndrome have position biopsies of their temporal artery. Cranial arteritis must be considered in any patient in the older age group who presents with a unilateral headache because of the danger of blindness if the diagnosis is missed and the patient does not receive high-dosage steroids. A high ESR, often over 100, is confirmatory, but a temporal artery biopsy must be done, because treatment requires steroids for 1 to 2 years. It is tragic to incur all the serious long-term effects of steroids in an elderly patient who may only have cervical osteoarthritis.

Headache Caused by Disease
of Nearby Structures

Except for glaucoma and iritis, diseases of the *eye* seldom cause headache. *Glaucoma* presents with pain in the eyes radiating frontally and sometimes to the temporal regions with a red eye, misty vision, a hazy cornea, and a dilated, sluggishly reacting pupil. *Iritis* also presents with a red eye but this time the pupil is *not* dilated, although again cloudiness of the media, and ocular and frontal pain may be present. Most patients who come to the physician with headache have already had their eyes tested because of the common belief that it is often due to eye strain. Headache in children may be the only manifestation of an *otitis media*. *Nasal sinus* disease is a common cause but the patient usually makes this diagnosis on his own and treats it according to the recommendations on television.

Nasal vasomotor reactions are associated with congestion of the nasal and paranasal mucosa; a moderate steady retro-orbital or bifrontal headache is common, often precipitated by upper respiratory infections and allergies. *Dental caries* and dental abscesses may present as headache, but more commonly a patient with headache mistakenlv feels that his teeth are the cause and has them removed unnecessarily. The *temporomandibular joints* are a common origin of head or facial pain (Costen's syndrome) among tense patients who irritate their TM joints by excessive clenching of the teeth. Pain from the TM joint is commonly referred to the face and may present much like trigeminal neuralgia. It is important to remember that the chronic tension state is the underlying problem, and overzealous and expensive treatment aimed at the TM joint is often unsuccessful in the long term.

DIAGNOSTIC STRATEGY IN HEADACHES

Every patient who presents with a headache needs a full history taken to determine the characteristics and the background circumstances leading to the appearance of the headache, and physical and neurological examinations must be done. Such full evaluation takes a significant amount of time. If a busy physician does not have that amount of time, then he must reschedule the patient for an occasion when he *can* devote proper attention to the history and examination. Only with this approach will both the patient and physician feel confident about the assessment.

Tension headache, some forms of migraine, and headache in association with a systemic or local infection are the most common causes, by far.

When seeing a patient with headache, first decide whether the headache falls under the general heading of vascular, muscle contraction, or traction by having the patient describe all of its aspects. These include its character, severity, site, paths of reference, frequency, duration, times of occurrence, associated symptoms, and aggravating and relieving factors. Inquire what the patient does about the headache and how effective these measures are. His description of what he does often gives you the best estimate of its severity. Determine whether this is a new phenomenon, the reappearance of an old one, or an alteration in an old pattern. Ask why the patient is consulting you about it now. Ask also about events that precede the headache, such as auras, psychological stresses, the consumption of certain foods or drugs (especially the birth-control pill), hunger, loss of sleep, and so forth. Ask about other symptoms that occur at the same time, such as visual disorders, nausea or vomiting, faintness, or other focal neurological problems.

Inquire also about the patient's mood and about the presence of any of the somatic symptoms of depression (see Chap. 51), because an increase in the frequency or severity of headaches may be due to a depressive illness. If you have to use leading questions, interpret the replies with care.

During the physical examination, pay close attention to the skull and the cervical muscles, looking in particular for tenderness, meningism, and a decreased range of neck mobility. Some headaches with a vascular component improve when the superficial vessels are compressed, but this may also occur in traction headaches. Look carefully for papilledema, always examine the visual fields and acuity, and then proceed with the standard neurological examination. Take the blood pressure and examine the ears, nose, throat, and teeth. Further diagnostic procedures will depend upon whether or not you have made a confident clinical diagnosis. If you have not, and feel that the headache is a complex or serious problem, it is best to refer the patient early for a second opinion and further investigation.

In a patient with no past history of headache who now develops a severe headache, serious enough to bring him to seek your help, look carefully for neck stiffness and other signs of meningism. Half of all cases of subarachnoid hemorrhage start with a warning leak, which produces a "sentinel headache" out of the blue. Other neurological signs will not be detected, however. If you have any doubt about this, refer quickly for advice about the need for CT scanning or lumbar puncture.

Traction headaches require rapid referral to a neurological center for evaluation for an intracranial mass lesion. Tension and vascular headaches are probably best managed with a minimum of investigation, unless, as in the middle-aged patient who develops such symptoms for the first time, you are concerned about an underlying but clinically silent lesion. An isotope scan or a CT scan is probably all that is required to make sure that a significant intracranial mass lesion (big enough to cause headache) is not present, but if there is any evidence to suggest an intracranial lesion as a cause of the headache, a CT scan should be done. Every patient whose headache began after the age of 55 needs an ESR done as part of the workup for cranial arteritis.

The yield from skull x-rays and EEG examinations in the investigation of patients with headache, but without physical signs, is extremely low, and if negative they may provide false reassurance. The EEG generates enough confusing and irrelevant information to suggest this test should not be done to assess headache. As long as a scan is normal, further tests are seldom requested, but the patient naturally should remain under clinical observation.

MANAGEMENT OF HEADACHES

Although the history can diagnose most headaches, this part of the interview has another function; it is therapeutic. Because the treatment of vascular and tension headaches of psychogenic or stress-induced illnesses is only fairly successful, a careful, detailed history and examination is a vital therapeutic tool. In its absence, if the patient retains any lingering doubt about his doctor's diagnosis, even the most favored psychoactive drugs are of little help.

Migraine Headaches

From the history, precipitating or related factors should be learned including missed meals, specific foods, menstruation, ingestion of the birth-control pill and physical or psychological stresses. A family history is often positive, but it is not necessary for diagnosis. Unless the patient is recovering from an episode of complicated or cluster migraine, examination will show no CNS abnormality.

Only now is one ready to advise prophylaxis.* First, employ simple measures to counteract any of the factors mentioned that have been identified as of possible relevance. Even if the patient has not noted a clear association of some factors we advise them to obey all the rules for migraine to gain control of the headaches.

---

*Cerebral edema and even small infarcts have been demonstrated in migrainous subjects, so prevention of attacks is more than just a convenience.

Table 17-2   Foods That May Induce Vascular Headaches

Cheese: all forms except cottage cheese
Chocolate
Citrus fruits and juices
Alcohol: beer, red wine
Nuts
Smoked and pickled fish and meat
Pork products
Beef concentrates: stock cubes, bouillon cubes
Chicken livers
Mushrooms
Onions
Monosodium glutamate: Soy Sauce
Nitrites

Meals should not be missed, and all patients in whom this may be a precipitant should be warned not to go hungry for a prolonged period. All patients with migraine should be tried on an exclusion diet. The foods in Table 17-2 should be completely avoided; all contain tyramine, serotonin, or phenylethylamine, substances that are capable of inducing headache in a high proportion of migraine sufferers. Chinese foods in restaurants contain monosodium glutamate, a vasodilator that can also cause headaches. Women with migraine taking the birth-control pill should be withdrawn from it and alternative measures adopted. It is seldom possible to treat stressful situations except by learning new coping techniques. Tranquilization is not particularly effective. In some subjects a long course of psychotherapy is required, which may not be acceptable to many as they often see their problem as headache, not the underlying stress, tension, and overreaction to life situations.

One schedule of prophylactic therapy runs as follows and may be used if the listed measures, particularly including diet, are not effective (Table 17-3).

1. Aspirin, 600 mg, each morning, whether there is headache or not, and a further 600 mg at onset of headache. If this causes gastric irritation, add metoclopramide, 10 mg, before the aspirin dose.
2. Propranolol, 20 mg four times a day up to 30 mg or even 40 mg four times a day, given in 3 month courses.
3. Amitriptyline, 25 to 50 mg at bedtime for 2 months.
4. Pizotyline, 0.5 mg daily (one tablet), increasing to three a day in 1 week. If unsuccessful after a month, slowly increase to a total of 5-6 mg/day, decreasing to a maintenance of 2 mg/day when headache is controlled.

If the patient still has headaches after these measures have been tried sequentially, and the precipitating factors have been managed, the patient should be referred to a neurologist.

At the onset of the first symptoms of headache the patient may be able to abort the headache by using simple analgesics such as aspirin or acetominophen taken 20 min after metoclopramide 10 mg, and then resting or lying down in a dark room. Measures taken at the onset are much more effective than those used during the attack.

Table 17-3   Treatments for Migraine

---

1. Diet and removal of precipitating factors

2. Treatment of attacks
    a) Minor analgesics
       Aspirin 600 mg or acetaminophen 325 mg, 2-3 every 4 hr
       To increase absorption add metoclopramide 10 mg with the aspirin dose
    b) Antiemetics
       Dimenhydrinate (Gravol) tabs 50 mg 1:2 q6h
                                   inj. 50 mg q6h
    c) Ergot preparations
       Ergotamine tartrate tabs 1 mg, 1-3 at start of headache and repeated in
          4 hr if needed[a]
       Ergotamine compound tabs. Megral, Cafergot, Gravergol. etc.

3. Prophylactic medication
    Propranolol tabs 10-40 mg q.i.d.[b]
    Amitriptyline tabs 25-100 q.h.s. for 2-3 month courses
    Pizotyline (Sandomigran) tabs 0.5 mg 2-4 daily
    Minor tranquilizers
    Carbamazepine tabs 100-200 mg t.i.d.
    Cyproheptadine tabs 4 mg, 2-6 daily
    Methysergide tabs 2 mg, 1-6 daily in 4 month courses[c]
    Lithium carbonate to attain serum level 0.6-1.6 mg/dl (cluster migraine only)
    Indomethacin tabs 25-50 mg b.i.d. (cluster migraine only)

---

[a] Sublingual tablets, inhalations, and suppositories are also available, and may act faster and be more effective.

[b] Contraindicated in patients with bronchospasm, cardiac failure, or cardiac conduction defects.

[c] Serum creatinine and IVP required every 6 months because of risk of retroperitoneal fibrosis.

In the stage of the classical migraine prodrome (paresthesias, visual symptoms, etc.), intracranial vasodilatation may abort both these symptoms and the succeeding headache; the easiest way to achieve this is to have the patient rebreathe into a paper bag, thus raising $PaCO_2$ levels. During the headache phase, inhaled pure O_2 may also be effective within 5 min. This is also useful for the severe pain of cluster migraine; the patient can have the O_2 cylinder at home with him.

During the attack, oral medications may be vomited. Oral ergotamine has been the mainstay of treatment for years, but we doubt if it is very effective. When given sublingually (one tablet at once and another 1 to 2 hr later, if needed), by suppository, or by inhalation it still has less effect than when given by injection (ergotamine tartrate 0.25-0.5 mg IM). To this one may add cyclizine hydrochloride, 50 mg, as an antiemetic.

If any single, severe headache persists longer than 2 days, reassess the diagnosis considering the presence of major psychological stresses. If migraine still seems most likely, a 3-day course of steroids (e.g., prednisone 60 mg, then 40 mg, then 30 mg) may be tried. Alternatively, as long as you are sure of the diagnosis, 4-10 mg of dexamethasone IV in one dose or sodium amobarbital (up to 500 mg every 8 hr IV with fluids) may abort the attack. Whatever methods are chosen, severe and prolonged migraine warrants hospital admission for observation.

Patients with *cluster migraine* may be given a course of methysergide (2 mg three or four times daily) starting after the first headache of a new cluster and continuing for 1 or 2 weeks longer than the usual bout lasts, up to a maximum of 5 months. If the attacks have a regular periodicity in the year, then administration can be tailored to this, so that the drug is only given for 4 to 8 weeks at a time. Alternate-day steroids, ergot, and the dietary measures mentioned previously have all been found useful in prophylaxis of some patients.

During the acute phase of a cluster headache, the patient is in agony and meperidine 50-100 mg may be needed and repeated as necessary. Inhalation of 100% O_2 is often helpful. Intravenous atropine has also been used with good effect; 1.8-2.4 mg, a full atropinizing dose, is used. Morphine is not indicated because the patient is vomiting and already has severe ciliary muscle spasm. Chronic cluster migraine responds well to lithium, if other drugs have failed. A variant, paroxysmal hemicrania, may respond to indomethacin.

Muscle Contraction Headache

Headache of this type, resulting from prolonged tension in the cervical, temporal, and occipitofrontalis muscles, often has a basis in psychological stress. Prolonged close work may cause frontal head pain secondary to frontalis muscle contraction rather than to any ocular lesion, but the association is usually clear to the patient.

Tension headaches require psychological exploration so that underlying factors are made evident, after which explanation (the essential basis of reassurance) will be acceptable and even therapeutic. Whether you do this is depth yourself or arrange psychiatric referral, explanation must precede drugs and psychotherapy. Drugs are not particularly helpful in this headache but are needed if the headaches are severe and frequent. The drugs employed are analgesics, the minor tranquilizers such as diazepam 2-10 mg t.i.d., or chlordiapepoxide 5-25 mg t.i.d., for 1 or 2 weeks at a time. Major tranquilizers such as thioridazine 10-50 mg or promazine 25-100 mg may also be used if the others fail but should be short-term. Marked anxiety, especially in older patients, may actually be symptomatic of brain disease or of depression. In all such patients, the results of a full clinical examination are negative, one may well go back, sit down again and search more carefully for evidence of a depressive disease (see Chap. 51).

Overall, the drug therapy of this form of headache is not particularly successful, especially if that is the extent of your therapeutic measures. Techniques that are more successful in reducing pain and in reminding the patient that tension and muscle contraction is the basis of their distress, include muscle relaxation exercises, neck exercises, local heat, and massage. Pressure on any trigger points identified, or their injection with local anesthetic, is often helpful. An outline of therapy in muscle contraction headache is in Table 17-4.

Combined Headaches

If the headaches do not occur frequently, simple analgesia using aspirin or acetaminophen with metoclopramide, for example, is likely to be all that is necessary. Patients who come to their physician complaining of such headaches probably require more specific measures than this, and those measures outlined previously in the discussion on the prophylaxis of migraine and of tension headaches will be required. This is probably one of the most common headache types seen in clinical practice. Time spent with the patient defining its exact qualities, the circumstances in which it occurs, and learning about his life-style is time well spent. In all forms of headache, the physician's demonstration of interest and concern is a powerful factor in reducing anxiety and will reinforce the effect of any drug treatment prescribed.

Nonmigrainous Vascular Headaches

Any marked rise in blood pressure should of course be treated if it is the cause of headaches such as this. Fever, hypoglycemia, and drug ingestion should be excluded as causes. If toxic agents, e.g., products of alcohol metabolism, are thought to be relevant, specific measures may be available, but if they are not, the condition is usually self-relieving as the toxin is metabolized or excreted. Simple analgesics such as acetylsalicylic acid, 300 or 600 mg, or acetaminophen, 500-1000 mg, may be used, but a better treatment for this form of headache is treatment of its cause.

Traction Headache

Traction or distortion of the pain-sensitive structures at the base of the brain by an expanding mass lesion such as a tumor, abscess, blockage to CSF pathways, or hematomas may cause the type of pain described in the first part of this chapter. Relief must be obtained by either removing the cause or reducing the intracranial pressure, as is described in Chapter 16. Pain should not be treated by narcotic analgesics, such as morphia, because of the danger of respiratory depression. Urgent referral is mandatory.

Table 17-4   Treatment of Muscle Contraction (Tension) Headaches[*]

Phase I	Explanation and reassurance Aspirin, 600 mg, at onset of headache Neck exercise and postural correction General exercise program Local heat or ice packs Pressure to trigger points Muscle massage
Phase II	Continue above measures Amitriptyline 20-50 mg q.h.s. Local injection of trigger points with lidocaine (Xylocaine) 1%
Phase III	Continue above measures Physiotherapy

[*]If combined headaches are present (muscle contraction plus vascular symptoms) then institution of migraine therapy along with these measures may be necessary.

Exertional Headache

A headache with similar symptoms to traction headache is the *benign exertional headache,* characterized by sharp head pain with any exertion. Lifting, coughing, sneezing, or bending may produce sudden pain that disappears when the exertion is stopped. Although such patients deserve careful assessment, the underlying cause is uncertain and the problem often clears eventually by itself.

Headache Caused By Overt Cranial Inflammation

There is no place for treatment with analgesics before the cause of an inflammatory headache is diagnosed. The warnings about the depressant qualities of analgesic drugs apply here as in the last section.

Treatment must be that of the cause. The inflammatory end-products and cerebral edema accompanying meningitis and the occasional hypertension and irritative effects of the blood with subarachnoid hemorrhage are in each case responsible for severe headaches of traction, vascular, *and* inflammatory type. If more powerful analgesics than codeine are necessary because of the patient's distress, then the patient must be monitored carefully in a unit with full nursing and respiratory support facilities.

Although biopsy of a temporal artery may temporarily relieve the pain of *cranial arteritis,* this is in no way a therapeutic measure, and all patients must be treated *immediately* upon clinical diagnosis with high dosages of steroids, e.g., prednisone, 100 mg/day, reducing over 7 to 10 days to a maintenance dosage of 30-40 mg on alternate days according to the fall in the ESR and to the improvement of the patient's condition. Steroid therapy will probably be required in these patients for at least a year; otherwise a recurrence of the acute disorder is likely. Their clinical status and ESR should still be followed carefully for another 2 years at least.

Headaches Caused By Disease of Nearby Structures

Dental pain is usually referred to the face rather than to the head, but sometimes diseased upper molars may cause pain radiating up to the temples, the diagnosis of primary dental disease being made by the effect of hot or cold substances held in the mouth, by tapping on the tooth, and, if necessary, by dental x-rays. Patients with acute *glaucoma* may be treated initially with acetazolamide, 250-500 mg t.i.d., and if the diagnosis is sure and an ophthalmologist is not available, then physostigmine 1% may be given as eye drops repeatedly until a skilled opinion is available.

Local heat in the form of warm packs, 1% homatropine eye drops, and local steroids are the mainstay of treatment of *iritis* but again, such measures are only advised if an ophthalmologist is not available. Otherwise, immediate referral is mandatory on an emergency basis.

Upper respiratory infections producing *sinusitis* and occlusion of the ostia may cause severe frontal pain, and this will be suggested by the history of a recent upper respiratory infection with continued nasal discharge, perhaps nosebleeds and local pain, and tenderness over the involved sinus. Figure 17-3 shows the CT scan of a young man who developed an abscess in the frontal lobe from frontal sinusitis and presented with severe frontal headache of weeks duration. Local decongestant drugs and a course of broad-spectrum antibiotics may be prescribed, but the diagnosis should be first confirmed by sinus x-rays, and if there is any suggestion of osteitis complicating sinusitis (as may well happen in a case of frontal sinus infection), urgent ENT referral is required. Temporal pain caused by disease of the

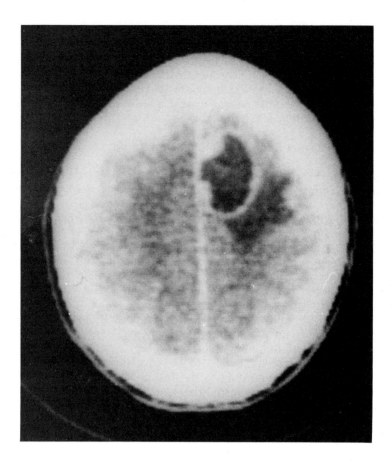

Figure 17-3   CT scan, enhanced. A large right frontal abscess with surrounding edema is seen. This patient had had chronic symptoms of frontal sinusitis; the abscess was presumably secondary to that.

temporomandicular joint may be relieved for a short time by the patient biting on a wooden spatula placed between the back teeth. Chronic muscle tension, dental malocclusion, and distortions of the joint surfaces are probably responsible for the pain. The treatment is essentially a combination of relaxation therapy and dental and orthodontic treatments, but the condition also requires the therapy discussed under muscle contraction headache.

BIBLIOGRAPHY

Dalessio, D.J. (ed.). *Wolff's Headache and Other Head Pain,* 4th Ed. New York, Oxford University Press, 1980.

Lance, J.W. Headache. *Ann. Neurol. 10:*1-10, 1981.

Lance, J.W. *Mechanisms and Measures of Headache,* 4th Ed. London, Butters-worth, 1982.

Travell, J.G., Simons, D.G. *Myofascial Pain and Dysfunction: The Trigger Point Manual.* Baltimore, Williams & Wilkins, 1983.

18
Sleep and Related Disorders

Research on sleep over the last few decades has opened up one of the most fascinating areas of medicine. Such research has also enabled us to understand (and so to treat more rationally) disorders of sleep, which are among the most common complaints that patients bring to physicians. Because this is an area of particular importance in present-day medicine, the student will be amply rewarded if motivated to read in more depth on the physiology of sleep.

PHYSIOLOGY OF SLEEP

Sleep may be divided into two types. *Nonrapid eye movement sleep* (NREM sleep) is divided into stages I, II, III, and IV, according to its depth. *Rapid eye movement sleep* (REM sleep) is characterized by alterations of blood pressure, respiration, and pulse and accompanied by darting eye movements. If awakened at this time, the subject will relate a vivid dream.

When falling asleep, one passes from a state of alertness to drowsiness and then into stage I sleep, characterized by muscle relaxation and by the appearance on the EEG of low-amplitude, fast-frequency waves. During this stage the person often denies having been asleep if spoken to. As the subject falls asleep he enters stage II with spindles of 12- to 16-Hz waves on the EEG, and then in turn stages II and IV sleep, which are characterized by higher-amplitude slow waves. In these stages there is profound muscle relaxation and the person is difficult to arouse.

A healthy young adult going to bed at night rapidly passes through drowsiness with mental fantasies into stages I and II and then into longer periods of stages III and IV sleep. After about 90 min of NREM sleep, the first episode of REM sleep occurs. This initial dream lasts 5 to 10 min but during the night four to five further REM periods occur, each becoming progressively longer as the night continues. After the first REM period the subject again drops down through the deeper stages of sleep and oscillates about every 90 min between one type of sleep and the other.

Infants spend much of their time in stages III or IV sleep but 50 percent of their sleep is of the REM type. By the age of 5, REM sleep takes up about a quarter of sleep time, which is comparable to a young adult's pattern. Five to ten percent of sleep is in stage I, 50 percent in stage II, and 20 percent in stages III and IV. The REM sleep decreases somewhat after age 50.

Despite tremendous advances in understanding the physiology of sleep, our interpretation of the meaning of dreams has not advanced much since Joseph, son of Jacob, counseled the Pharoah (see Genesis 41.25).

INSOMNIA

Insomnia is the most common sleep complaint. Because of a general lack of understanding of sleep physiology and of the drugs that affect sleep by many practicing physicians, it is also one of the most commonly mismanaged problems in medicine. Insomnia is the inability to get to sleep or to stay asleep for the time expected by the individual. It is only an abnormality when the patient complains about it, as a person who sleeps for only 3 hours a night may accept this as his normal pattern and be delighted that he has time to do other things while the rest of the world dozes.

In most cases of insomnia there is an underlying psychological disturbance. Over 85 percent of insomniacs have one or more major pathological scores on the Minnesota Multiphasic Personality Test (MMPI), particularly on the scales for depression, sociopathy, obsessive-compulsive features, and "schizophrenia." It is common for patients to concentrate on their sleep disturbance and ignore or deny the underlying emotional problem.

We all hear references to "good sleepers" and "poor sleepers." Poor sleepers have been found to spend less time in REM sleep and more time in NREM stages I and II. They also have an increased heart rate, peripheral vasoconstriction, and a higher body temperature during sleep, suggesting a higher level of physiological arousal, which demonstrates that their sleep is different not only in quantity but also in quality from that of normal persons.

The management of insomnia consists of treating the underlying emotional problems. Most drugs, e.g., barbiturates, used for insomnia lose their effect after a week. Unfortunately, the patient's sleep may be further disturbed when he stops the medication, because of rebound effects, and he may then begin taking it again. Flurazepam however has been shown to induce normal patterns of sleep, and it maintains its effectiveness in the long-term. Flurazepam, 15 mg, may be used nightly and increased only if still required after the first week because its effectiveness may not be apparent in the first few nights. Diazepam is also an acceptable medication to help manage insomnia, but you should never depend upon drugs alone in handling this problem. Such drugs are also best used intermittently, because active metabolites accumulate to give constant blood levels.

SOMNAMBULISM

Sleepwalking is a common phenomenon in children but tends to disappear spontaneously as they get older. There is often a family history of sleepwalking and of other disorders, such as night terrors, enuresis, and nightmares, which often affect the sleepwalker as well.

During sleepwalking the person may carry out quite complex acts but the episode is usually brief and there is amnesia for the event. Although one might expect sleepwalking to occur during dreaming, it does not; it occurs almost entirely during stage IV NREM sleep. The person is able to perceive the world around him to some extent because he walks around people and furniture. Sleepwalking can sometimes be induced by lifting a subject to his feet during NREM sleep.

Although there is little evidence of psychological disturbance in children who sleepwalk, there is some evidence that adults with this problem do have some underlying psychopathology.

The management of sleepwalking includes protection of the sleepwalker from injury, because he may wander into areas of danger or fall downstairs. A nightly dose of amitriptyline has helped our adult sleepwalkers, although the patients sometimes return to their sleepwalking patterns after 3 to 6 months despite the medication.

ENURESIS

About one out of every six children are bedwetters at age 5, but up to 3 percent of healthy young adults still wet the bed occasionally.

Primary enuresis refers to enuresis that continues after infancy, without any prolonged dry periods occurring. This has a genetic basis in some cases but otherwise results from organic disease such as urethral obstruction, ectopic ureter, diverticulum of the anterior urethra, epispadias, or chronic urinary tract infection.

Secondary enuresis is the recurrence of enuresis after a prolonged period of dryness and may be due to psychological disturbance or to organic disease such as infection or diabetes.

Enuresis occurs in NREM sleep, often in the first third of the night. Electroencephalographic studies have shown that the episode begins in stage IV sleep and is associated with a burst of rhythmic delta waves, after which the sleep pattern switches to stage II or I and micturition occurs.

It is important to determine whether enuresis is primary or secondary. If primary, then reassurance and explanation are helpful, particularly because many other family members may have had, and outgrown, the same problem. One must look for organic problems in both primary and secondary cases. Careful attention must also be paid to psychological factors. An understanding and empathetic approach must be taken with the children or they may see the encounter as a form of punishment. It is important to recognize not only psychological cases of enuresis but also the psychological trauma and lowered self-image that can result. Parents often take a punitive attitude toward the child. Not only is this ineffective but it may augment the psychological factors that worsen secondary enuresis.

Therapy of primary enuresis begins with a reassuring explanation to the parents and the child based on your interview and examinations. The child is advised to restrict fluids after supper, and on weekends and after school to see how long he can hold urine in his full bladder. A parent should awaken the child late at night, usually when retiring, to have the child void again.

Imipramine, a tricyclic drug, is a moderately effective treatment, but children are often made irritable by this drug. Its effect could be through decreasing stage IV sleep, or there may be a more direct effect on bladder innervation. An alternative method of therapy is the conditioning approach using a mild electric shock pad, which awakens the child at the first drop of urine. The Mozes detector has shown excellent results in clearing enuresis in 80 percent of children within 3 months. One has to be aware of the psychological effect of this type of machine, and it has to be explained to the child with understanding and encouragement.

NIGHT TERRORS AND NIGHTMARES

A night terror ("pavor nocturnus"; "incubus") is characterized by sudden awakening from sleep with intense anxiety, autonomic overstimulation, movement, and crying out. Despite the appearance of terror, there is no memory for the event, except for the feeling that something strange has just happened. The child with night terrors may also have enuresis or sleepwalking. Night terrors arise during stage IV NREM sleep, often within the first hour, and the child shows an impaired arousal response but a waking alpha EEG pattern, extreme motility, sleepwalking, and vocalization in the form of terrified screams or moaning. Pulse and respiratory rates increase but the episode is over within a minute or two. The person then has a feeling of intense fear and anxiety, respiratory restriction (thus the medieval image of a devil on the chest), and an overwhelming sensation of doom. Night terrors, like sleepwalking and other disorders of sleep, may be primarily disorders of arousal.

A nightmare is a normal but frightening dream, and the subject often has good recall of the episode initially if it is due to arousal from REM sleep. It may be induced by the REM rebound that occurs after stopping a course of drugs, such as barbiturates, that suppress REM sleep. Nightmares however are more common in childhood. Persistent nightmares in adults suggest some underlying psychopathology.

The first step in management consists of determining the exact characteristic of the sleep disturbance. Children with night terrors seldom require psychotherapy or medication. In adult cases, nightmares require only explanation and reassurance, but it is important to recognize that many medications used at bedtime may actually increase nightmares. L-dopa and propranolol may increase dreaming; if treatment is required (when these drugs must be continued), then diazepam or flurazepam should be used, not barbiturates.

HYPERSOMNIA

Hypersomnia is characterized by a tendency to sleep for prolonged periods. Unlike in narcolepsy, the tendency to sleep is not irresistible, and the person may feel that this is his normal pattern. Characteristically, patients with hypersomnia feel confused on awakening and have difficulty becoming completely alert.

In *idiopathic hypersomnia* patients sleep long and deeply at night and have daytime somnolence and sleep spells. Many are confused on waking ("sleep drunkenness"). The cause is not known.

The *Kleine-Levin syndrome* is associated with bulimia (a tendency to eat excessively), hypersexuality, and periods during which sleep is prolonged. The patients are usually young men who sleep excessively for a number of weeks, awakening only to eat voraciously any food put in front of them. They also have a tendency to act out sexually during this state. The disorder often clear spontaneously after a few years.

The pickwickian syndrome* of periodic ventilatory insufficiency caused by gross obesity is characterized by chronic sleepiness and a tendency to fall asleep easily when at rest.

---

*Named after the Fat Boy, in Dickens' *The Pickwick Papers*, who was usually asleep.

Excessive daytime sleepiness is usually a symptom of chronic sleep loss, the sleep apnea syndrome, or a psychological disorder such as depression, in which excessive sleep provides an escape from the stresses of everyday life. However medical disorders such as hyper- or hypothyroidism, hypoglycemia, anemia, and pulmonary, hepatic, or renal failure, should also be considered in patients with this complaint. Causes in the CNS include any pathology in or around the third ventricle, hypothalamus, or midbrain (encephalitis, tumor, posttraumatic, etc.).

Diagnosis is achieved in most cases by asking about symptoms of cataplexy (indicating the narcolepsy syndrome), excessive snoring (sleep apnea), and chronic use of stimulants or sedatives.

Like the patients who describe themselves as "poor sleepers," hypersomniacs show a sleep pattern suggesting a more aroused or light type of sleep. Fatigue, lethargy, and impaired motor and intellectual performance by day result. While treatment is normally of the cause, tricyclics may be of value when none is found.

The *sleep apnea syndrome* is characterized by prolonged and recurrent periods of apnea at night and symptoms of chronic fatigue and sleepiness during the day. Two main forms occur, obstructive and central.

In the obstructive form, chronic upper airway obstruction occurs because of obesity, micrognathia, chronic upper respiratory diseases, hypothyroidism, or myotonic dystrophy, etc. During the night the patient snores loud and long, but repeated apneic spells occur as the pharyngeal walls collapse, and despite intense inspiratory effort, airflow is impossible. At such times the arterial PO_2 levels fall, the PCO_2 levels rise, and there is a risk of hypertension, cardiac arrhythmias or infarction, and sudden death.

The patient is unaware of these spells and of the "snorting" snoring that punctuates the beginning of the respiratory phase, so a history from the spouse is needed to confirm your suspicions based on the patient's complaint of prolonged daytime drowsiness. Many are obese males who smoke and drink alcohol excessively. They may respond to weight loss, stopping smoking and drinking, and to the drug protriptyline. If these measures are not adequate, a permanent tracheostomy or surgical procedure to widen the pharynx or larynx are recommended.

In the central form of sleep apnea, the spells are not preceded by noisy breathing but occur repeatedly in silence, not wakening the patient. In most cases no cause is found, but previous encephalitis, autonomic failure, and excessive alcohol intake have all been associated. This may be a cause of the sudden infant death syndrome. Therapy is with protriptyline and the careful avoidance of all forms of central depressant drugs, including alcohol.

NARCOLEPSY

Narcolepsy, a common syndrome probably with a genetic basis, consists of a tetrad of symptoms: sleep attacks, cataplexy, sleep paralysis, and hypnagogic hallucinations (waking dreams).

The *sleep attacks* begin before the age of 30. They are characterized by irresistible, brief (5 to 10 min), REM sleep episodes occurring at times of decreased sensory stimulation. The patients may fall alseep at their desks, in movies, in front of television, or in front of their house guests, later awakening refreshed. Some patients feel perpetually drowsy and have superimposed sudden sleep attacks. Although these may occur many times a day, there is usually a refractory period of a number of hours after each one. Sleep laboratory studies usually show that there is only a 10 min latency before a REM period occurs after going to sleep, while normal people seldom have REM sleep until they have slept an hour or more.

Cataplexy is a sudden relaxation of muscle tone because of generalized motor inhibition. It is usually precipitated by emotion, which causes the patient to slump, often falling on the floor but remaining conscious during this brief period. Narcoleptics often learn to steel themselves against extreme emotion, particularly laughing, to avoid these episodes. Some patients get only a partial weakness, as shown by the sudden sagging of their jaw, face and head, or their arms may drop to the sides. Rarely a patient will show slowing of speech or of all movements for a brief period.

Sleep paralysis may occur in normal subjects in the interval between sleep and wakening, e.g., on awakening in the morning when the person finds that he is completely unable to move. In some older Western cultures this is known as the "Old Hag." Even though it may have occurred many times before, it is frightening, but seldom lasts longer than 60 seconds. Even a gentle touch terminates an attack.[*] In narcolepsy, attacks occur at the onset of sleep too.

Hypnagogic hallucinations[†] are vivid auditory or visual hallucinations or illusions that occur, like sleep paralysis, when the patient is in the state between wakefulness and sleep. He is aware of what is going on around him but also experiences a vivid hallucination, e.g., the sight, sound, or voice of a long-dead parent, at the same time.

Although narcolepsy is classically a tetrad of symptoms some patients also manifest symptoms of *sleep drunkenness* and of *periodic confusion.* Narcoleptic symptoms reflect normal components of REM sleep occurring at abnormal times. The sleep attacks represent fragments of REM sleep in people who have the other components of the tetrad; but patients who have *only* sleep attacks may have NREM sleep during the episodes. Both cataplexy and sleep paralysis represent the motor inhibition that characterizes REM sleep. Hypnagogic hallucinations represent a vivid dream, such as would be normal during REM sleep but now occurring in the drowsy state.

Narcoleptic patients are a great risk on the highway as 77 percent report being drowsy when driving, 40 percent have fallen asleep at the wheel, and 16 percent have actually had accidents because of this.

Infrared pupillography may become a more objective test for narcolepsy because the pupil is large when the patient is alert, small when asleep, and intermediate when drowsy. Also, characteristic pupillary waves can be recorded during the period between alertness and sleep.

Narcolepsy must be differentiated from the other causes of hypersomnia noted previously and from vertebrobasilar ischemia, multiple sclerosis, myasthenia gravis, familial periodic paralysis, and epilepsy. While these differentiations can be made by history, the EEG will be useful in characterizing the type of narcolepsy and should be requested in all cases. (See Table 18-1.)

After a definite diagnosis of narcolepsy has been made, the situation should be explained fully to the patient, to his family, and often to his employer. The patient should not drive until therapy has been proved successful. This may begin with methylphenidate, 10 mg daily, increased as required. The average patient needs 20-60 mg/day to control sleep attacks. Cataplexy, sleep paralysis, and hypnagogic hallucinations may not be helped by methylphenidate, but imipramine or clomipramine can be used for these symptoms. Begin with 25 mg of clomipramine daily, increasing to 25 mg t.i.d., if required. Protriptyline or propranolol can be used

---

[*]The fable of the Sleeping Beauty may have been based upon this syndrome, the touch of the Prince's kiss unlocking her immobility. Mundane stimuli however are equally effective.

[†]Hypnopompic hallucinations are the same thing on waking up. The term is quite unnecessary.

Table 18-1   Causes of Paroxysmal Somnolence

Narcolepsy

Chronic alveolar hypoventilation

Hypothalamic disease: Kleine-Levin, tumor

Hypokalemia

Depressive illness

Sleep apnea

Drugs: sedatives, tranquilizers, amphetamines

---

if the response to these drugs is not satisfactory. Amphetamines, once the mainstay of therapy, are not often used because of the addiction, tolerance, and medicolegal complexities associated with long-term use. Gamma-hydroxybutyrate promises to be a major advance in the treatment of narcolepsy but it is still an experimental drug.

MEDICAL CONDITIONS ASSOCIATED WITH SLEEP

Myocardial infarction and episodes of *angina* commonly occur at night. There may be some relationship to the physiological changes of REM sleep, but this has not been a consistent finding in all studies. However it is now recognized that sleep is not a quiet state of suspended animation, but a period with variable and often increased electrophysiological, biochemical, physiological, and psychological activity; almost an "autonomic storm." Such stresses may induce episodes of angina, myocardial infarction, or *cerebrovascular accidents*.

Patients with *duodenal ulcers* secrete much more gastric acid at night than normal subjects, primarily during REM sleep. This probably explains the common nocturnal pain and discomfort of patients with ulcers.

Asthmatic attacks commonly occur at night, particularly in the early morning during stage II, rarely in stage IV periods.

Pregnant women spend less time in the deeper stages of sleep. There may be increased sleeping and drowsiness during the first trimester of pregnancy but increased wakening as pregnancy continues.

Sleep disturbance in *mental illness* is well known. Depressed patients may have oversleeping, difficulty getting to sleep because of superimposed anxiety, and early morning awakening. They take longer to get to sleep and spend twice as much time in light stages, often claiming they are not asleep at all. A disturbance in sleep patterns may predict deterioration in some mental illnesses; thus in schizophrenia, acute episodes are often preceded by increasing insomnia, restlessness, and excessive eye movements during REM sleep, suggesting overstimulation of the arousal system. In chronic organic brain syndromes some patients have excessive REM sleep while others show little.

In encephalitis, delirious states, and dementing illnesses, *reversal* of the normal sleep pattern may occur, with periods of sleep during the day and alertness during the night.

Nocturnal seizures are common, especially in type II epilepsy. Both random and regular discharges within the pyramidal system may be recorded because of a decrease of inhibition. These cause the jerking, twitching, or myoclonic movements that may be seen at the onset of sleep and they may also initiate focal or generalized seizure activity.

Vascular headaches commonly *begin* between the hours of 6 and 8 A.M., but the cluster headache appears earlier, usually between midnight and 3 A.M. Arm or hand pain and paresthesiae occurring at night or on waking are typical of carpal tunnel syndrome.

BIBLIOGRAPHY

Cherniak, N.S. Respiratory dysthythmias during sleep. *N. Engl. J. Med. 305:*325-330, 1981.

Guilleminault, C., Lugaresi, E. *Sleep/Wake Disorders: Natural History, Epidemiology, and Long-Term Evolution.* New York, Raven Press, 1983.

Orr, W.C., Altshuler, K.Z., Stahl, M.L. *Managing Sleep Complaints.* Chicago, Yearbook Medical Publishers, 1982.

Roth, B. *Narcolepsy and Hypersomnia.* New York, Karger, 1980.

19
Disorders of Smell and Taste

Disorders of smell are uncommon but are of occasional diagnostic value. Anosmia (loss of the sense), parosmia (distortion of the sense, illusions of smell), and hallucinations will be described.

ANOSMIA

Usual with infective and chronic allergic disease of the upper respiratory tract, anosmia may also be a focal sign of neurologic disease if the first nerve is damaged on the floor of the anterior cranial fossa or if the postganglionic fibers are ruptured as they penetrate the cribriform plate. This is quite common after relatively mild head injuries, usually to the back of the head; the former occurs because of pressure down upon the nerve in cases of olfactory groove meningioma, glioma of the orbital surface of the frontal lobe, or anterior cerebral artery aneurysm. Chronic basal meningitis constricting the nerve is a possible but uncommon cause.

PAROSMIA

Parosmia signifies a distortion of the usual sense of smell, an odor being perceived at normal or reduced thresholds but having a different quality (usually unpleasant) from the usual and expected one. It may occur with any of the causes that later go on to produce anosmia or during recovery from it; it also occurs with the use of nasal drops, following influenza, and in association with temporal lobe damage on either side. It is occasionally a symptom of depressive illness.

HALLUCINATIONS OF SMELL

Hallucinations of smell may be subdivided between those interpreted as of part of the body — sweat, fetor oris, or feces, for example — and those of external objects, such as gas, food, or perfume. In the former case, the subject is invariably suffering a biochemical depressive illness whether or not he admits to being unhappy. In the latter, symptoms usually precede other characteristics of temporal lobe epilepsy, accompany the classic signs of schizophrenia, or occur during delirious states from any cause.

LOSS OF TASTE

Loss of taste for sweet, bitter, salt, and sour is found with damage to the chorda tympani or its central connections (and theoretically with ninth nerve damage, also if the posterior third of the tongue is tested, which it hardly ever is). Strict lateralization is present peripherally and thus must be respected in testing, but representation is probably bilateral in the brainstem and temporal lobe.

Causes of unilateral loss of taste are identical to those listed under facial palsy (Chap. 23) with the exception of those lesions of the nerve situated distal to the point where the chorda tympani leaves it. The chorda tympani may also be damaged during middle-ear surgery. Bilateral loss occurs with thin-fiber neuropathies (e.g., diabetes), in vitamin B deficiency, sometimes following head trauma, and in hypothyroid, hypogonadal, and hypoadrenal states. It has also been recorded in the setting of collagen-vascular diseases such as Sjögren's syndrome and as a side effect of some drugs.

BIBLIOGRAPHY

Douek, E. *The Sense of Smell and Its Abnormalities.* London, Churchill-Livingstone, 1974.

20
Visual Disorders

SUDDEN LOSS OF VISION

About 44,000 people go blind each year in North America. Sixty percent of them are over 70 years of age, and five times more women are affected than men. Senile macular degeneration (35 percent), diabetic retinopathy (12 percent), cataracts (5 percent), glaucoma (8 percent), and myopia (3 percent) are the chief causes, while acquired optic atrophy, congenital abnormalities, and other ocular diseases such as detached retina rank next. Most of these have one common characteristic: they are of *slow* onset; perhaps weeks, months, or years of failing vision preceded the final loss of sight. Only a few of them are curable, unlike most of the causes of *sudden* visual loss to be considered here that arise over minutes or hours out of a state of normal vision and are in many cases only transient.

Sudden visual loss may be uni- or bilateral, may involve all or a sector of the sight of one or both eyes, and may be either transient or permanent. Obviously, the first things to establish are the extent and severity of the visual defect, its cause, and its permanence.

Therefore try to find out whether the loss is in *one* eye (has the patient closed the other eye and thus become quite unseeing?) or *both*. Is vision affected patchily (a scotoma,* visual field constriction, or hemianopia) or *totally*?

Patients with hemianopia may complain that they brush into objects on the hemianopic side; histories of traffic accidents, bruising, broken objects, and

---

*A scotoma is an island of visual loss within the remainder of the intact visual field.

reading difficulties (seeing only half a word or a sentence on the page) are common. Some patients with hemianopia recognize that they can only see one-half of their visual field, but others do not. Commonly, they say that they cannot see out of one eye, when it is really the visual field of both eyes toward that side that is affected.

Macular damage is localized to a small area of the retina but creates a major visual defect, a large central scotoma, described by patients as though blindness had occurred. On careful testing of the visual field, you can determine that it is central vision that is lost, some sight remaining peripherally. The pinhole test is useful here, because through a 1-mm hole light falls only on the macula; hence in this situation nothing will be seen.

Obstruction of CSF flow around the optic nerve cuts off venous return and increases pressure on the outer optic fibers causing papilledema. Visual field constriction and an enlarged blind spot are the usual field defects resulting.

Primary damage to the optic nerve, such as occurs in multiple sclerosis, mostly affects the thickly myelinated fibers. The papillomacular bundle, which carries impulses from the macula, is especially involved, and damage to it produces a central scotoma or centrocecal scotoma (the visual field defect appears like a very enlarged blind spot which extends outside central vision). Glaucoma reduces retinal blood flow, increases pressure upon the optic nerves and causes corneal edema, thus reducing vision in three ways.

Finally, a reminder: to examine the fundus adequately, if the pupil is not already quite dilated, you must dilate the pupil yourself. Test the visual fields first and ensure that the patient does not have glaucoma and is not sensitive to tropicamide. These parasympatholytic drops take about 20 min to work; their effects are reversible with pilocarpine. The patient should not drive for the remainder of the day. Precipitation of glaucoma is possible but unlikely, and adrenergic side effects are common only in people also taking tricyclic or monoamine oxidase-inhibiting drugs.

TYPES OF ACUTE VISUAL LOSS

Loss of the Whole Field

Bilaterally

Bilateral, whole-field loss occurs only when there are lesions in two sites; either in both retinas, both optic nerves, both optic tracts or radiations, or both occipital lobes (Fig. 20-1). In the latter however, a single vascular lesion, such as a basilar occlusion, might be responsible (Table 20-1).

One should first examine the retinas for evidence of bilateral disease. This might occur from decreased retinal artery flow resulting from *hypertension,* particularly in preeclampsia or uremia, or it might occur with acute *hypotension,* causes of which range from a severe gastrointestinal hemorrhage to a simple faint (see Chap. 10). Bilateral retinal lesions can also occur with *retinal burns* caused by exposure to flash, bright lights such as sunlight, or any source of ultraviolet light.

Bilateral disease of the optic nerve may occur in demyelinating lesions, such as *neuromyelitis optica* (a form of multiple sclerosis), *Leber's optic atrophy,* and acute *disseminated encephalomyelitis.* Certain *toxins* produce severe bilateral optic nerve damage (see Chap. 43).

Lesions of the optic radiations or occipital cortex bilaterally can result from diffuse *cerebral edema* following trauma or lead intoxication. *Basilar occlusion*

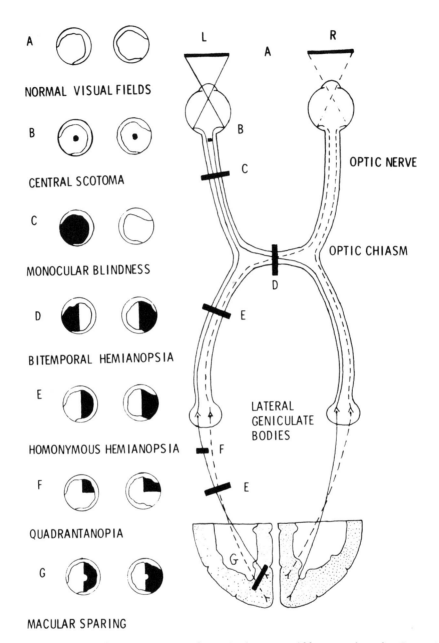

Figure 20-1   Field defects resulting from lesions at different sites in the optic pathways.

may produce bilateral occipital cortex ischemia and resultant cortical blindness. Some such patients may not be aware that they are blind (Anton's syndrome). Posterior cerebral artery flow may be reduced bilaterally in *severe cardiac failure* or with any other condition reducing cardiac output, in *hypertension,* in vertebrobasilar *migraine,* or in spasm associated with a posterior cerebral artery *aneurysm, porphyria,* or *paroxysmal hypertension.* The visual cortex is very sensitive

Table 20-1   Causes of Acute Visual Loss

Bilateral whole field loss

Lesions of both retinas
  hypertension
  hypotension
  retinal burn (flash, UV light, sun)

Lesions of both optic nerves

  multiple sclerosis (neuromyelitis optica)
  Leber's optic atrophy
  acute encephalitis
  toxins (methyl alcohol, quinine, tobacco, ect.)

Lesions of both optic radiations or central cortex

  cerebrak edena (trauma, toxic)
  cerebral ischemia (hypertension, vertebrobasilar emboli, migraine, severe
    hypotension)

Unilateral whole field loss

With eye pain

  glaucoma
  optic neuritis (demyelinating, idiopathic)
  iridocyclitis
  vitreous hemorrhage

Without eye pain

  occlusion of the central retinal artery
  embolism
  ischemic optic neuropathy (idiopathic, cranial arteritis)
  macular or vitreous hemorrhage

Bilateral partial field loss

  Optic chiasm or tract: compressive
  Optic radiation: infarct, tumor, subdural, encephalitis
  Occipital cortex: ischemia, edema

Unilateral partial field loss

  Intraocular bleeding
  Local retinal lesions, e.g., detachment
  Optic nerve damage, e.g., compression
  Central serous retinopathy
  "Tunnel vision"

to ischemia from any cause. In cases of cortical blindness, the pupillary light reflexes will be present because their pathways do not include the occipital lobes.

Hysterical blindness (see Chap. 6) can be considered in younger patients when the onset is sudden, the eye examination normal, the pupils reactive, and the patient's psychological state suggestive. *Tunnel vision* may be another psychologically determined problem if not caused by glaucoma, pigmentary retinopathy, occipital ischemia, or severe optic atrophy. The size of the field seen by the patient will not increase as gaze is moved further away as it would in normal "funnel" vision.

Unilaterally

Unilateral Whole Field Loss: Because any lesion situated behind the chiasm would produce a hemianopia, the lesion here must be at or anterior to it, e.g., in the optic nerve, the retina, or the refractive media. If a refractive error or ocular disease is not the cause of the monocular visual loss, then the patient's field defect will almost certainly be a central scotoma. If the eye is painful, causes include *glaucoma, retrobulbar neuritis, acute iridocyclitis,* or *vitreous hemorrhage.*

If there is no eye pain, causes include *retinal detachment, occlusion* of the central retinal artery, and compressive or ischemic optic *neuropathy,* in most of which the loss is permanent (see later discussion). A swollen disk with retinal hemorrhages and acute loss of vision strongly suggests disk infarction or inflammation, not raised intracranial pressure. *Amaurosis fugax* is an acute unilateral visual loss, usually transient, in most instances caused by platelet emboli from internal carotid stenotic lesions. Patients with *papilledema* may complain of transient obscurations of vision, perhaps because of intermittent increases in intracranial pressure. An unusual condition, *central serous retinopathy,* affects young males who suddenly develop scotomas associated with retinal edema for unknown reasons. Fortunately, they tend to recover.

Loss of Part of the Field

Bilaterally

To understand the problem of bilateral partial field loss, we must determine exactly what the form of visual loss is. Diplopia, hemianopia, monocular blindness, and blurred vision may all lead to the complaint of partial loss of vision in both eyes. Many people seem to consider that the left eye is responsible for the left visual field and the right eye for the right field; so when a patient says he cannot see out of his right eye, you must examine him for a right homonymous hemianopia. Although central scotomas and homonymous hemianopias may be diagnosed by history, bitemporal hemianopias are often not noted by patients.

Homonymous hemianopia is due to a unilateral lesion between the optic chiasm and the occipital cortex. This might be a transient ischemic attack or an infarct, migraine, or hypertensive encephalopathy. Occipital lobe tumors or AV malformations, posterior subdural hematomas, and acute toxic encephalopathy in association with fevers are less likely causes.

If the homonymous defect is exactly similar in the two eyes, it is termed congruous. This suggests a posterior lesion, probably in the occipital lobe. The more anterior the lesion, up to the optic chiasm, the more incongruous are the defects produced. Homonymous defects may "split" the macula with no change in visual acuity; thus a unilateral lesion producing even complete homonymous hemianopia does not explain a decrease in visual acuity.

Bitemporal hemianopias are due to pressure on the chiasm (Table 20-2), usually from below. Pituitary insufficiency or syndromes of excessive hormonal production may be expected in the case of a *tumor* rising up out of the pituitary fossa. Midline *aneurysms,* local *arachnoiditis,* or *tumors* such as meningiomas, may also press on the chiasm.

Visual field constriction is usually due to papilledema or second nerve compression, or occurs as a dissociative (hysterical) phenomenon as mentioned earlier.

Table 20-2   Major Causes of Chiasmal Compression

Pituitary adenoma

Craniopharyngioma

Suprasellar meningioma

ICA aneurysm

Basal arachnoiditis

Bilateral optic neuritis (discussed later) may produce central scotomas. Toxic and genetic causes are most common, but it also occurs in a form of multiple sclerosis.

Unilaterally

Unilateral partial field loss indicates that there is a scotoma or a sector defect. The likely mechanism is damage to the optic nerve in or behind the orbit, but in front of the optic chiasm, because retinal and optic nerve lesions produce defects only in the ipsilateral eye. Pressure from a tumor or edema are the most likely causes in the orbit.

Trauma to the globe with bleeding into the vitreous and acute uveitis will markedly reduce vision overall, or will produce a focal field defect. Following diabetic coma or any severe electrolyte disturbance, hydration of the lens may be abnormal, with the same result.

At the retinal level, platelet, air, or fat emboli may produce large central scotomas (Fig. 20-2). Migraine is a common cause of apparent unilateral partial field defects; retinal detachment and occlusion of the central artery of the retina in collagen diseases, polycythemia, hypertension, diabetes, or embolization are other causes. Optic nerve damage occurs in retrobulbar neuritis and papillitis, which have many causes (see the following).

A centrocecal scotoma (in which the field defect runs between the macula and the blind spot) may be detected on perimetry, but seldom clinically. Deficiency of vitamins B_1 and B_{12} in "tobacco-alcohol amblyopia" is a well-recognized cause. Glaucoma and toxic agents are others.

OPTIC NEURITIS

The term *retrobulbar neuritis* refers to inflammation of the optic nerve behind the optic nerve head; hence no abnormality is seen on inspection of the fundus with the ophthalmoscope. True bulbar neuritis or *papillitis* usually occurs in children. The term is used for neuritis that has spread more anteriorly and gives rise to a swollen, red, engorged disk, which looks remarkably like papilledema. The differentiation is made by testing visual acuity, for in retrobulbar neuritis and papillitis, the major damage to the maculopapillar fibers results in a large central scotoma. With papilledema there will be much less damage to the fibers coming from the

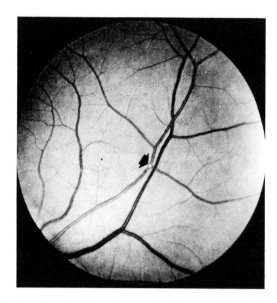

Figure 20-2   Cholesterol embolism in a retinal arteriole during an episode of amaurosis fugax. The patient had a large internal carotid artery ulcer and plaques on that side.

macula and elsewhere and the visual defect will consist of an enlarged blind spot with or without constriction of the fields.*

Optic neuritis is more common in women, usually between the ages of 20 and 50 years. They complain of unilateral vision loss, eye tenderness, and pain especially on movement, all increasing over a few days. Apart from a central scotoma with diminished visual acuity (especially for color vision), a sluggish pupil with an afferent defect and a normal disk are the main findings. Months or years later, primary optic atrophy supervenes. The most common single cause is a plaque of demyelination in the retrobulbar region. Such patients need a full neurological examination and skull series, the latter to detect evidence of expansion of the pituitary fossa, ethmoiditis, or optic nerve compression. A lumbar puncture is not necessary. Follow-up by a neurologist or ophthalmologist is wise. Steroid therapy rids the patient of pain, but it does not affect the ultimate prognosis. Almost all patients regain sight in the eye, but with repeated attacks, vision does decline. Perhaps half of all cases eventually develop signs of multiple sclerosis.

In patients over the age of 50, *ischemic optic neuropathy* is more likely. This presents suddenly as painless visual loss in one eye (the other being affected months or years later in about a third of the cases). The disk is swollen, but the retina is normal. The visual defect is altitudinal, with or without a central scotoma. This finding must make one consider cranial arteritis as a cause, requiring emergency ESR and steroid prescription (see Chap. 42), but ischemic infarction of the optic nerve of nonarteritic type is actually more common. Here the ESR

---

*You may find the following a useful mnemonic: If the patient sees nothing and you see nothing; retrobulbar neuritis. If the patient sees nothing and you see something; papillitis. If the patient sees something and you see something; papilledema.

is normal and temporal artery biopsy is negative. The cause is unknown but carotid stenosis is often found. Diabetes and hypertension are not closely associated. Investigations are unrewarding and treatment nonexistent.

Many other conditions cause optic neuritis, which may be bilateral. Toxins (see Chap. 43), syphilis and orbital infections, postinfectious encephalopathy, vitamin B_{12} deficiency, and Leber's optic atrophy are examples, but all are less common than the two conditions described.

It is wise to refer all cases for expert evaluation because compression of the optic nerve may produce identical signs that will be improved with steroid treatment. However with optic nerve compression, visual fields commonly show a temporal field defect rather than a central scotoma; optic atrophy is commonly seen, with other evidence of an anterior intracranial lesion (such as headache, anosmia, exophthalmos, or endocrinopathy) and skull films may be abnormal. Because treatment is probably available for such cases, all must be carefully investigated.

OPTIC ATROPHY

Slowly progressive visual loss may occur because of neurological disease, although ocular problems such as refractive error, macular degeneration, cataracts, and diabetic and other retinopathies are much more common causes. You can diagnose a refractive error by the pinhole test: if a patient looks through a card pierced by a pin, the effect of faulty refraction is abolished and vision should improve. If the lesion is of the macula, where most, if not all, of the light entering through the pinhole impinges on the retina, he will see nothing. The other conditions should be obvious on general ocular examination. Most of the neurological causes of slowly increasing blindness present with the sign of optic atrophy. Other signs include a slowly reactive pupil and a temporal field defect or scotoma.

As mentioned in Chapter 2, there are two kinds of optic atrophy: primary and secondary or consecutive (consecutive, that is, upon previous papilledema). In the former, the disk appears as "a stark white moon in a deep red sky," with normal vessels and no evidence of hemorrhages or exudates, although pigmentary retinopathy may be present. In the latter, the previous papilledema has caused the disk to take on a pink or yellow tinge, and its edge is less well outlined against the retina, which may still show the ravages of the former condition. The causes of secondary (or consecutive) optic atrophy are those of papilledema (see Chap. 16). The primary form has a number of apparently unrelated causes (Table 20-3).

Familial Conditions

These include almost all of the spinocerebellar degenerations, lipid storage diseases, certain familial neuropathies, and the sex-linked recessive condition associated with bilateral optic atrophy called Leber's disease.

Demyelinating Diseases

In multiple sclerosis, the atrophy is usually unilateral, or at least one side is much more affected than the other, until a late stage. Here there is early involvement of the temporal side of the disk because the heavily myelinated maculopapillar bundle runs from the macula to that side of the disk and bears the brunt of the demyelinating process. The resulting gliosis (not fibrosis) is responsible for the pallor. In pernicious anemia and in tabes dorsalis primary optic atrophy also may be seen.

Table 20-3   Causes of Optic Atrophy

Papilledema (consecutive)

Familial disorders (bilateral signs)
    Spinocerebellar degenerations
    Lipid storage diseases
    Familial neuropathies
    Leber's disease

Demyelinating disorders
    Multiple sclerosis
    Pernicious anemia

Tabes dorsalis

Ischemic optic neuropathy

Pressure on optic nerves or chiasm
    Glaucoma
    Orbital lesions
    Pituitary and parasellar lesions

Drugs and toxins
    (see Chap. 43)

Ischemic

Atrophy will follow ischemic optic neuritis within months or years (see preceding discussion and Chap. 42).

Pressure

Pressure on the optic nerves may lead to atrophy of the disc (see Table 20-3). This pressure may arise inside the eye, as with glaucoma; from behind the globe, as with orbital neoplasms or other causes of orbital swelling; or it may occur at the optic foramen because of periostitis, bone tumor, or Paget's disease. Pressure on the chiasm also might be responsible, as with a pituitary tumor, suprasellar meningioma, or giant aneurysm of the internal carotid. Long-standing, high intracranial pressure may produce atrophy, but papilledema usually precedes it, therefore it is not of the primary type. Slowly progressive visual failure results from compression of the optic nerve and is not a feature of optic neuritis caused by, for example, multiple sclerosis.

Drugs and Toxins

There are a host of toxic agents that may damage the optic nerves, and they usually lead to bilateral disk pallor. They are listed in Chapter 43.

    Therefore when optic atrophy of this primary type is seen, a full examination of the nervous system is required, in addition to careful inspection for other evidence of congenital or of ocular disorders. The family history will be important here, as always, to allow diagnosis of one of the hereditary disorders (although a negative family history will not exclude them). One must inquire about the consumption of drugs of all types over the preceding years. Particular attention must be paid to visual acuity, to the general ocular examination, and to the external ocular movements. Optic atrophy leads to a diminution in color vision, and its detection is an indication for color tests.

Ophthalmologic or neurological referral is wise in all cases, although there is not always an opportunity to treat the cause. Nevertheless, some forms of atrophy that are dependent upon high circulating levels of cyanide (tobacco amblyopia, Leber's atrophy) may be treated by hydroxycobalamin, and of course, pressure on the optic nerves, tabes dorsalis, and pernicious anemia are definitely treatable.

PAPILLEDEMA

Swelling of one or both optic nerve heads demands urgent etiologic diagnosis. If caused by optic neuritis, a central scotoma with markedly impaired visual acuity and a slow or absent direct pupillary response may be expected. If caused by compression of the optic nerve or by some systemic cause (see benign intracranial hypertension, Chap. 16), the field defect will be little more than an enlarged blind spot, the acuity will be unimpaired and the pupils normal, at least in the early stages. However spontaneous pulsations of the retinal veins will not be present, and both specific (headache, vomiting, hemiparesis) and nonspecific (sixth nerve palsy) features may be detected. In long-standing or acute cases, retinal hemorrhages, transient obscurations of vision, and peripheral constriction of the visual fields are added.

The list of causes of papilledema is long (see Glaser, 1978). Apart from expanding intracranial mass lesions of all types, a host of infectious, toxic, metabolic-endocrine, hematologic, circulatory, and other neurologic conditions might be responsible. Because however any patient seen with papilledema must be presumed to have a mass lesion until proved otherwise, and must therefore be referred for expert assessment, the various conditions will not be discussed in detail here. In *pseudopapilledema,* the optic nerve head is elevated and the physiologic cup is absnet, but spontaneous venous pulsations are present. Referral to an ophthalmologist is advised as a precaution in all cases because other local and treatable causes of a swollen disk do exist.

PHOTOPHOBIA

Unusual discomfort felt in the eyes caused by light is known as photophobia. Its best-known cause is meningeal irritation in meningitis or encephalitis, but subarachnoid blood, migraine, raised intracranial pressure, syphilitic iritis, and glaucoma are other causes, and it complicates the use of the "dione" drugs in epilepsy.

BIBLIOGRAPHY

Glaser, J.S. *Neuro-Ophthalmology.* Hagerstown, Harper & Row, 1978.

Jamieson, M. Loss of vision. *Br. Med. J. 288:*1523-1526, 1984.

Perkins, E.S., Hansell, P. *An Atlas of Diseases of the Eye,* 2nd Ed. Edinburgh, Churchill Livingston, 1971.

21
Ocular Problems

ABNORMALITIES OF THE PUPILS

When Hollywood wants to show that a doctor is indeed doing the things a doctor should do, particularly in an emergency, they have him shine a light in the patient's eyes. In part, this reflects the fact that the pupillary response as a clinical sign has been recognized for hundreds of years; yet it remains one of the most important signs in clinical medicine.

The pupillary reflex pathway (Fig. 21-1) runs from the retina through the optic nerve to the lateral geniculate body and thence to the superior colliculus and the Edinger-Westphal nucleus in the mesencephalon. From here, efferent parasympathetic fibers run with the third nerve to the pupil, relaying in the ciliary ganglion. A light shone in one eye causes constriction of both pupils, the ipsilateral *directly* and the contralateral *consensually*. A weak light stimulus may produce initial constriction followed by dilation of the pupil. A tendency for the pupil to constrict and dilate rhythmically to a light stimulus is known as *hippus,* a common finding of no clinical significance.

It is a common observation that the pupil of the eye closer to a window appears to be smaller than the other, but this is an optical illusion.

When the patient is asked to look at a near object, the pupils constrict (accommodation), dilating again when he looks at a distant object. This is useful to remember when examing the fundus, because the pupil will be larger if a patient is asked to look into the distance.

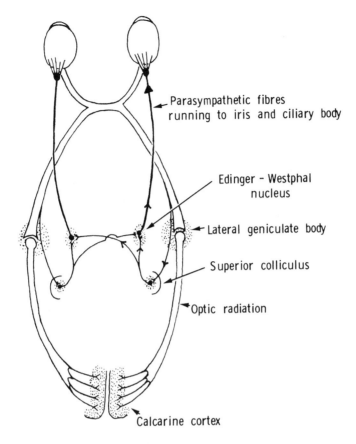

Figure 21-1 Pathway of the pupillary reflex.

The pupil size should be measured in millimeters for accurate comparison and to follow changes occurring in comatose states, for example.[*]

Third Nerve Lesions

A unilateral dilated pupil may indicate paralysis of its parasympathetic supply. Causes include compression of the nerve, by a posterior communicating artery aneurysm, tumor, or herniating uncus; ophthalmoplegic migraine; and Adie's pupil, described later. Among patients in the hospital the use of mydriatic drops may be confusing unless a note is made in the chart that they have been instilled. If you are in doubt, one drop of 1% pilocarpine in the eye will constrict the pupil dilated because of third nerve compression but *not* a pupil paralyzed by mydriatics. The dilated pupil of a third nerve lesion is usually accompanied by ptosis and lateral deviation of the eye. If the patient is conscious, he will complain of diplopia.

---

[*]The pupillometer is an ingenious method of accurately recording pupillary change by measurement of pupillary size of the dark, using infrared light. The pupil can then be tested with light, dark, accommodation, and other stimuli and a continuous recording of pupil size made.

The term *mydriasis* is applied to pupillary dilation greater than 6 mm. When bilateral, drugs and fear are the most common causes, although bilateral uncal compression can do this too. Transient mydriasis is usually caused by migraine or the presence of Adie's pupil (discussed later).

Miosis

Pupils less than 3 mm in diameter are described as miotic. This is not always abnormal because in very young or old people, in those with pupillary-constricting drops in the eyes, and in those treated with morphia, small pupils are to be expected. A light reaction will be present however if one looks very carefully.

Miosis also occurs with damage to the sympathetic pathway anywhere along its course; as part of the presentation of the Argyll Robertson pupil; and with pontine lesions that damage the sympathetic paths bilaterally, e.g., hypertensive hemorrhage. Local eye conditions producing miosis include healing iritis and old trauma.

Horner's Syndrome

Horner's syndrome (Table 21-1) indicates a lesion somewhere in the long three-neuron sympathetic pathway running from the hypothalamus through the brainstem and cervical cord to the sympathetic ganglia in the neck, and subsequently to the eye along the carotid and ophthalmic arteries (Fig. 21-2A,B). Associated with the small pupil will be mild ptosis and decreased sweating on the same side of the face. The localization of the lesion to the first, second, or third neuron can be done by pharmacological testing, if this is important in diagnosis.[*]

Argyll Robertson Pupil

Argyll Robertson pupils are small, irregular, and unequal, unresponsive to light, but reactive on accommodation. They are characteristically associated with syphilis, and in this situation are almost always bilateral. If unilateral, diabetes or a midbrain lesion (multiple sclerosis, encephalitis, neoplasm, trauma) are the most common causes (Table 21-2). It is difficult to explain this abnormality anatomically, but lesions of the periaqueductal gray matter probably produce the pupillary changes, while syphilitic iritis may explain the smallness, irregularity, and inequality. This type of pupil has been likened to a high-class prostitute who accommodates but does not react.

Loss of the light reflex may be due on the afferent side to second nerve lesions, centrally to those in the midbrain, and on the efferent side to third nerve compression, ophthalmoplegic migraine, lesions of the ciliary body, or neuropathies (but usually not in diabetic neuropathies). Botulism is a rare cause, but important because it may be the clue to the nature of an otherwise inexplicable paralytic state.

[*]Site of Neuronal Damage	Cocaine 5%	Paredrine 1%
First	Full dilatation	Pupil dilates
Second	No effect	Pupil dilates
Third	No effect	No effect

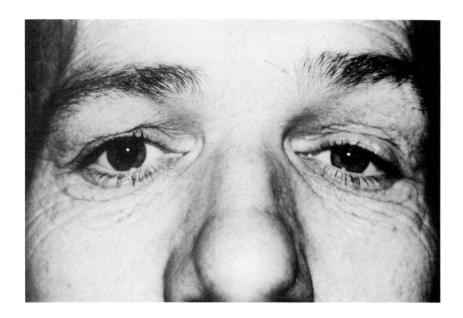

Figure 21-2A   Ptosis and miosis in Horner's syndrome.

The Myotonic (Adie's) Pupil

The myotonic pupil is dilated and seems not to react to light. However it *will* react slowly to a constant bright light, dilating again if the patient is kept in a dark
room for 10 min. It will also respond with a slow constriction if convergence is
maintained for 30 to 45 sec; looking at a distant object will then cause slow dilation. Because of denervation hypersensitivity, the pupil will constrict if a drop of
pilocarpine 1/8% is instilled into the eye. This pupillary abnormality is usually unilateral and seen in young women; it is often associated with absent deep tendon
reflexes (Holmes-Adie syndrome). The condition is benign but important to recognize to prevent subjecting the patient to unnecessary investigation.

Marcus Gunn Pupil

Disease of one optic nerve may result in a different light response in each eye.
This can be demonstrated by alternating the light source back and forth from one
eye to the other ("swinging flashlight test"). A difference in the rapidity of the
pupillary response may be evident; the abnormal pupil shows an initial paradoxic
dilation as the light is quickly moved across to it from the normal eye. This may
be the only sign that indicates an afferent (optic nerve) lesion, such as retrobulbar
neuritis. The other pupil dilates too because it is the afferent stimulus that is
weak, while the efferent pathways are unaffected, but usually you are not looking
at it; the pupils are actually equal in size. This is not true with an efferent lesion,
which causes pupillary inequality (anisocoria).

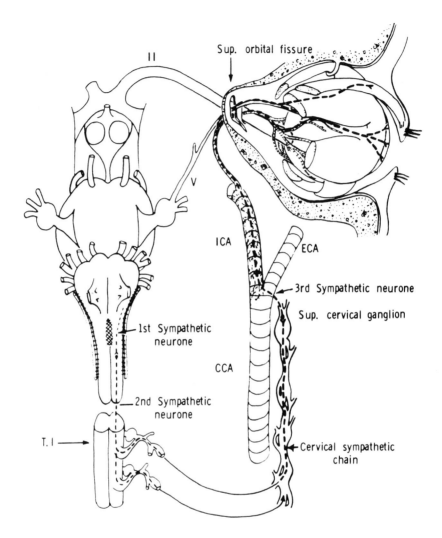

Figure 21-2B   Sympathetic pathway from the brainstem to the eye.

DIPLOPIA

Diplopia refers to the subjective awareness of two images when only one object is present. Binocular diplopia occurs because the image falling on the retina of the deviating (abnormal) eye lands away from the macula. Thus the image is interpreted by the patient as lying in a position peripheral to the point of fixation. Because the image does fall on the macula of the normal eye, the patient appreciates two images.

There are three useful rules governing the relationship of the images.

1. Displacement of the false image may be horizontal, vertical, or oblique; this image is less precise than that from the normal eye.
2. The separation of the images is greatest in the direction in which the weak muscle has its purest action.

Table 21-1   Causes of Horner's Syndrome

First neuron

    Hypothalamic lesions
    Third ventricle tumor
    Pituitary tumor
    Basal meningitis
    Brainstem or cervical cord disease: infarct,
        syrinx, tumor, multiple sclerosis

Second neuron

    Cervical rib
    Pancoast tumor
    Aortic aneurysm
    Supraclavicular or cervical lymphadenopathy
    Klumpke's palsy
    Thyroid mass lesion

Third neuron

    ICA occlusion, arteritis, aneurysm, trauma
    Cavernous sinus lesion
    Paratrigeminal syndrome (Raeder's)
    Orbital tumor or infection

Table 21-2   Differential Diagnosis of Argyll Robertson Pupils

Neurosyphilis

Multiple sclerosis

Diabetes mellitus

Pineal tumor

Wernicke-Korsakoff syndrome

Midbrain encephalitis

3. The false image is maximally displaced in the direction in which the weak muscle should normally move the eye, i.e., it is always the peripheral image.

A few other general rules are also helpful.

1. If the eye cannot move outward, there is a sixth nerve lesion.
2. If the eye, when deviated *inward,* will not move *down,* there is a fourth nerve lesion.

3.   All other defects in eye movements are due to third nerve lesions. Of course, failure of the eye to move in any direction might be due to muscle paralysis rather than to a specific nerve lesion. The clinical setting often serves to differentiate a myopathic process from a neuropathic one.

Analysis of the Abnormality of Eye Movement

First you should determine which muscle pair is involved. If the maximal displacement is on lateral gaze to the right, then the pair to be considered are the left medial and the right lateral recti, which turn the eyes in that direction. If it is with the eyes deviated to the right and upward, then the right superior rectus and the left inferior oblique are the muscle pair to consider, and so on (see Chap. 2). The next step is to determine which individual muscle of the pair is the one involved. The patient must indicate which of the two images is displaced peripherally, which is easier to do if a red glass is placed over one eye. Because a third nerve lesion causes multiple faults, it is often easier to work out which muscles are acting normally.

Fourth nerve palsies are hard to characterize clinically, but a helpful test is to hold a reflex hammer horizontally in front of the patient; if two images are seen, with one angled upward, then the fourth palsy is one the side to which the "arrow" points.

A hint about the nature of the problem may also come from observing the patient's compensating head position — turned to the side of a sixth nerve palsy, and tilted away from the side of a fourth palsy with the chin depressed.

Causes of Diplopia

There are many causes of diplopia, but the history will often indicate the correct one before the eyes are examined. There are four major classes of cause (Fig. 21-3).

Failure of Accommodation

Failure of accommodation occurs in normal people when they become drowsy, and is also common in patients with narcolepsy, who are prone to episodic drowsiness and sleep attacks. Patients on cholinergic drugs and anxious people may also have difficulty in accommodation.

Displacement of the Eyeball

Displacement of the eyeball has to be fairly marked before compensatory mechanisms fail and diplopia results. Proptosis may be due to a primary tumor of the orbit (such as a lymphoma, hemangioma, meningioma, neurofibroma, or optic nerve glioma), or to a secondary tumor. When it occurs in hyperthyroidism, either the retro-orbital swelling or the myopathy of the extraocular muscles may be responsible. Traumatic and inflammatory lesions are other causes, e.g., mucocele or orbital pseudotumor (see Chap. 42).

Intrinsic Muscle Weakness

Muscle weakness can cause diplopia, because of a myopathy (polymyositis, myotonic dystrophy, ocular myopathy) or an abnormality of the myoneural junction (myasthenia gravis). These abnormalities are usually bilateral, although not always symmetric, and tend to affect eye movements in all directions. Expect to find ptosis and evidence of muscle disease elsewhere.

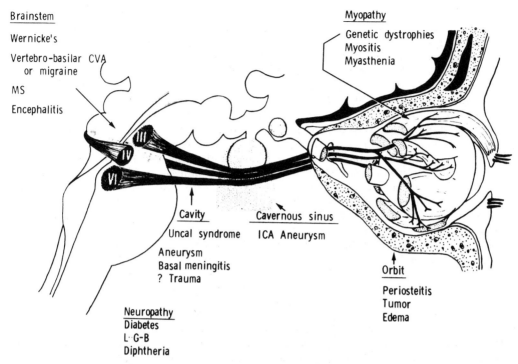

Figure 21-3   Sites of some lesions that can cause diplopia.

Nerve Lesions

Isolated Third Nerve Palsy: The appearance is characteristic: the eyelid droops down over the eye that is deviated outward and moves only sluggishly back into the midline on attempted gaze to the other side. The pupil may or may not be dilated and pain is sometimes present.

If the pupil is dilated and unresponsive and the eye is painful, an ICA or posterior communicating artery aneurysm, or a parasellar mass lesion are most likely. As causes of a painless complete third nerve palsy, consider ophthalmoplegic migraine (a headache precedes or follows the palsy), head injury (history), pressure from a nasopharyngeal or parasellar tumor, or the uncal syndrome. Vascular disease is another common cause.

If the pupil is spared but the eye is painful, diabetic (ischemic) neuropathy is likely, although mass lesions can do this as well; often no cause is found. If pain is absent, multiple sclerosis and myasthenia gravis must be considered, as well as these last.

Partial third nerve palsies, in which some of the muscles supplied by the nerve still function, occur in myasthenia, orbital lesions including hyperthyroidism, and cranial arteritis. Bilateral third nerve palsies occur in the Landry-Guillain-Barré syndrome, myasthenia, Wernicke's encephalopathy, hyperthyroidism, diphtheria, and some rare muscle dystrophies. It is sometimes hard to differentiate them from supranuclear gaze palsies.

Complicated Third Nerve Palsies: When the fourth, fifth, and sixth nerves, or other parts of the nervous system, are involved simultaneously, localization is rather easier. A parasellar lesion may involve all three oculomotor nerves, the first two divisions of the fifth nerve and the sympathetic supply, as well as causing proptosis. Tumors, aneurysms, and local inflammatory disease are most likely at this site. Most of these also cause eye pain. At the superior orbital fissure and in the orbit, infection, edema and primary, secondary, or invasive nasopharyngeal tumors cause variable involvement of all three nerves, with proptosis and pain.

Isolated Fourth Nerve Palsy: Isolated fourth nerve palsy is uncommon. A recent head injury is the most likely cause; MS, diabetes, hypertension and pressure from a tumor are less likely. Many cases are unexplained.

Isolated Sixth Nerve Palsy: Here the eye is adducted and cannot abduct much past the midline. The sixth nerve has a long course and is the one most commonly affected by local pathologies. About 30 percent of cases are due to tumor, 20 percent are unexplained, perhaps caused by vascular disease, and the remainder are due to lesions at sites along the nerve. The more common problems include brainstem lesions (MS, Wernicke's, tumor) and damage to the nerve in the cranial cavity (trauma, raised intracranial pressure, meningitis, tumor); at the tip of the petrous temporal bone (periostitis); in the cavernous sinus (aneurysm, caroticocavernous fistula, parasellar tumor, inflammatory disease; see Fig. 21-4); in the superior orbital fissure or orbit (inflammation, Paget's disease, edema, tumor); anywhere along the nerve (diabetes, Landry-Guillain-Barré syndrome, diphtheria); at the myoneural junction (myasthenia, botulism); or in the muscle, as part of a myopathy. Isolated sixth nerve palsy is a well-known "false-localizing sign" of raised intracranial pressure, being stretched across the tentorial edge as the brainstem is pushed downward as a result of a mass lesion above it. It also complicates otherwise benign infections in children; the site of the lesion in these cases is not known.

All patients with diplopia caused by an oculomotor palsy need specialist evaluation, but routine office examination will frequently allow an etiologic diagnosis to be made, as long as you first determine which nerve or nerves are involved and next look carefully for other signs to suggest the site of the damage. Skull films with good visualization of the superior orbital fissure and sella turcica; a glucose tolerance test and ESR, specific serology, and routine hematology and biochemistry are always needed. An ENT examination and CT scanning are often required (Fig. 21-5). Never forget myasthenia as a cause of an apparent oculomotor nerve palsy but do not rely completely on the edrophonium (Tensilon) test; if myasthenia is clinically a possible diagnosis, get an EMG.

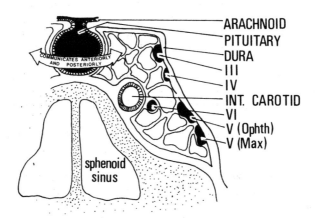

Figure 21-4   Diagram of the anatomy of the cavernous sinus.

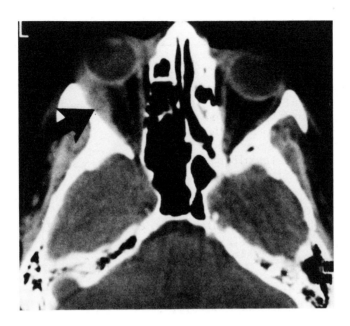

Figure 21-5   Retro-orbital tumor causing exophthalmos and diplopia.

PTOSIS

Ptosis (drooping of the upper eyelid) can be partial or complete, unilateral or bilateral. There is a wide variation in the normal appearance of the eyelids and one has to accept a certain amount of eyelid drooping as normal in many individuals.[*]

It is difficult to define exactly what constitutes pathological ptosis, but it is probably reasonable to accept as abnormal any more than 2 mm of difference in the eyelid positions when measured in relation to the corneal margin or pupil. Deciding on normal variation with bilateral, equal eyelid drooping is more difficult.

Having identified ptosis, one has to determine the structures that are involved and the pathological process that caused it (Table 21-3). The structures concerned in keeping the upper lid elevated are the third nerve and sympathetic supply, the levator palpebrae superioris and Muller's muscle, and the myoneural junctions.

The Eyelid

Pseudoptosis may be a congenital anomaly with unequal palpebral fissures. Early photographs, if available, may show this to be a long-standing developmental abnormality. A number of these youngsters will have *jaw-winking* associated with it. This is an embarrassing tendency for the eye to blink each time the jaw is opened.

Blepharospasm in the anxious or hysterical patient may resemble ptosis, but the fact that the lids flutter is characteristic.

---

[*] . . . with one auspicious and one drooping eye . . ." *Hamlet* 1.ii. 11.

Table 21-3   Causes of Ptosis

Unilateral

      Voluntary suppression of diplopia
      Local abnormality of the lid
      Horner's syndrome
      Congenital ophthalmoplegia*
      Third nerve lesions*
      Ophthalmoplegic migraine*

Bilateral

      Constitutional or normal variation
      Myopathies; ocular forms and myotonic dystrophy*
      Myasthenia gravis*
      Tabes dorsalis
      Bilateral third* or sympathetic lesions

---

* Ophthalmoplegia is usually present too.

The Muscles

Some forms of myopathy involve the eyes and make the patient tilt his head back to see from under his drooping lids. It is worth noting that the muscle of the lower lid is involved as well and it will rest at a higher level when weak. Except in those myopathies that selectively involve the eyes (ocular myopathies), weakness of proximal limb muscles will usually be obvious. Other diseases of muscle affecting the eyes include thyrotoxicosis, myotonic dystrophy, and myositis.

The Third Nerve

Ptosis is often the first manifestation of a third nerve lesion in the conscious patient and may precede the pupillary and extraocular muscle involvement. In third nerve lesions, the eye may be completely shut, but with lesser degrees of involvement, the patient has a furrowed forehead on that side from attempts to open the eyelid. The nerve can be involved at the nucleus in the midbrain (stroke, Wernicke's, tumor), as it crosses the edge of the tentorium (the uncal syndrome, Chap. 10), or in its course along the base of the brain (diabetic vascular lesion, cavernous sinus thrombosis, sphenoid ridge meningioma, superior orbital fissure syndrome). In diabetic third nerve palsy, the pupillary fibers may be spared because they are peripherally situated in the nerve and the ischemia tends to affect central regions more severely.

Sympathetic Supply

The sympathetic nerves supply the tarsal muscles. When they are damaged a mild ptosis results, associated with a small pupil, lack of sweating on the same side of the face, and occasionally the appearance of enophthalmos (Horner's syndrome, see Table 21-1).

Sympathetic fibers leave the hypothalamus and travel down through the brainstem to the cervical area. A second neuron runs out in the C8-T1 roots to the cervical sympathetic ganglia in the neck and a third travels from the ganglia along the walls of the common and later the internal and external carotid arteries and their branches such as the ophthalmic artery (see Fig. 21-2A, B).

Horner's syndrome can result from a lesion of the first neuron caused by any pathology in the brainstem or cervical cord such as a stroke, tumor or syrinx. The second neuron in the neck can be damaged by a carcinoma at the apex of the lung (Pancoast tumor) or by neck trauma. A lesion of the third neuron running along the carotid vessels may occur with carotid inflammation or occlusion or trauma, e.g., an arteriogram performed by directly puncturing the carotid vessels.

Gaze Palsies

When the two eyes, "yoked" together so that they move in parallel, fail to move in any particular direction, this is known as a gaze palsy. Normally, four major mechanisms govern such movements.

The saccadic system is used to switch gaze voluntarily from one object to another; the cortical origin of the commands is the frontal eye field in the other hemisphere (the right side controls gaze to the left), but the paramedian pontine reticular formation is the origin of the final common pathway.

Smooth pursuit of a moving visual target depends upon input from the occipital cortex, but brainstem and cerebellar lesions also impair such movements.

It is important to maintain fixation of the eyes, e.g., on the road ahead when riding a cycle on a rough track; the vestibular system governs their position and makes instant corrections as the head moves to maintain a constant image on the retinas.

Fourth, when one scrutinizes a close object, the eyes converge: a pathway including the occipital cortex and the tectum of the brainstem governs this.

Thus lesions in a number of sites causes impairment of gaze mechanisms. The most common disorders causing gaze palsy are sited in the frontal cortex; as a result, deviation of the eyes to the other side is impossible and they look *toward* the side of the cortical lesion and thus away from the paralyzed side of the body. With brainstem damage, the eyes look *away* from the side of the lesion and toward the paretic side of the body.

Vertical gaze palsies suggest either bilateral or midline brainstem damage. With upgaze paresis, suspect a problem in the tectum of the midbrain; with downgaze problems, bilateral ventral lesions at the same level may be responsible. In some patients with brainstem damage (at various sites) the eyes are vertically divergent — *skew deviation.*

Progressive External Ophthalmoplegia (PEO)

In this condition of increasing weakness of voluntary conjugate eye movements, the reflex, e.g., doll's head movements, may still be elicited. Upward gaze is first affected, after which all eye movements are progressively limited. Although at first this was thought to be a myopathy, the maintained parallelism of the ocular axes and the demonstration that nuclear and nerve lesions may produce changes in the eye muscle biopsy resembling myopathy, have suggested that it has a supranuclear (i.e., upper motor neuron) origin.

PEO is often associated with other neurological syndromes, including progressive supranuclear palsy (see Chap. 12), muscular dystrophies, retinitis pigmentosa, damage to the corticospinal tracts or posterior columns, basal ganglion involvement, hereditary neuropathies, and spinocerebellar degenerations. In hyperthyroid stages and in other probable autoallergic conditions associated with orbital inflammation, (pseudotumor orbiti, discussed later), there is again a failure of gaze, initially upward. Proptosis, chemosis, and restriction of gaze in all directions appear later.

Myoneural Junction

Ptosis is a common sign in myasthenia gravis, in which the ocular muscles show characteristic fatigue if the eyes are held in the elevated position without blinking. When the patient is asked to look down again, the lids will droop. This may improve with only a few blinks, so make sure that the patient keeps his eyes wide open during this test. There may be temporary improvement with IV edrophonium (Tensilon), 10 mg.

A pretty test to show myasthenic ptosis is as follows: ask the patient to look upward while you hold up one of his eyelids with your thumb. After about 30 sec let it go and let the patient's gaze return to the horizontal. Ptosis will now be asymmetric, showing most or only in the eyelid not held up by you. Twitching or fluttering of the eyelids in myasthenia is also described and is almost pathognomonic.

Such patients will probably have evidence of muscle fatigue in the extraocular muscles, causing diplopia; in the bulbar muscles, causing dysphagia; and in the proximal limb muscles, causing weakness, e.g., on walking or elevating the arms. Ocular myasthenia may be more resistant to treatment than myasthenia involving the limb muscles. Occasionally it occurs alone without skeletal muscle involvement. In many cases however the patient with ocular myasthenia will later develop limb weakness too.

Muscle

Ocular, oculopharyngeal, myotonic, and advanced facioscapulohumeral dystrophies and polymyositis may also produce weakness and ptosis. Ptosis and proptosis occur together in pseudotumor orbiti.

NYSTAGMUS

Nystagmus is a disturbance of ocular posture and usually consists of a slow drift of the eyes in one direction followed by a quick correction for this drift. The continuous repetition of these drift-correction movements is significant, but one or two drifts only may not be.

The eyes receive tonic innervation from various structures, and nystagmus may result from any imbalance in this system. Thus it may result from a lesion in the retina, labyrinth, brainstem, cerebellum, or cerebral hemisphere. Although it would seem that because nystagmus may reflect damage to so many structures, it can have but little localizing value, that is not true because the most common sites of the disease causing it are the peripheral labyrinth, brainstem, and cerebellum. Moreover, the type of nystagmus that occurs from each site may be characteristic.

In noting and describing nystagmus you should observe (1) the position(s) of the eyes in which nystagmus occurs, (2) the direction of gaze in which the amplitude is greatest, and (3) the direction of the fast component, which is taken, by convention, as the direction of the nystagmus, only because it is the most obvious. In fact, the quick phase is the correction and the physiological or pathological aspect of nystagmus is the slow drift. Nystagmus may be of various types (see Tables 21-4 and 21-5).

Table 21-4   Classification of Nystagmus

Pendular
Jerk
    Horizontal: peripheral
                 central
    Vertical
    Rotatory
    Retraction
    Ataxic
    "See-saw"

Table 21-5   Causes of Nystagmus

Pendular forms
    Congenital
    Imperfect ocular fixation
        miner's nystagmus
        long-standing amblyopia
        macular degeneration
        optic atrophy
        cataracts

Jerk nystagmus
    Peripheral (labyrinthine)
        any inner ear disease
    Central (brainstem, vestibular nuclei, or cerebellar)
        multiple sclerosis
        brainstem ischemia
        syringobulbia
        encephalitis
        hereditary ataxias, cerebellar lesions

Ataxic nystagmus (medial longitudinal fasciculus)
    Brainstem lesions
        multiple sclerosis
        encephalitis
        ischemia
        tumors

See-saw nystagmus (brainstem)

Latent nystagmus (uncertain causes)

Optokinetic nystagmus (physiological)

Pendular Nystagmus

Horizontal nystagmus of equal amplitude in each direction of gaze, and thus with *no* fast component may be caused by an absence or decrease of central vision, particularly before the age of 6 years. The common congenital nystagmus is similar. Pendular nystagmus may also be due to degeneration in the macula or retina, longstanding amblyopia, optic atrophy, cataracts, or cerebellar plaques of multiple sclerosis. It can also occur due to poor lighting and was commonly seen in miners before there was adequate lighting down in the mines.

Jerk Nystagmus

Horizontal

Horizontal jerk nystagmus is due to a lesion in the vestibular system; thus the lesion could be in the labyrinth, the vestibular nerve, the vestibular nuclei, the medial longitudinal bundle, the vestibulocerebellar connections, or in even the high cervical cord. Slight unsustained horizontal nystagmus may also be seen in normal individuals when looking more than 30° to the side.

Depending on whether the lesion is central or peripheral, the appearance of a horizontal jerk nystagmus alters.

Peripheral Lesions: Peripheral types result from a lesion in the labyrinth. They have their greatest amplitude *away* from the side of the lesion (Fig. 21-6A, B). A unilateral labyrinthine lesion will cause a *direction-fixed* nystagmus, in which the fast component is always in the same direction, whichever way the patient is looking. The amplitude is normally greatest when he looks away from the side of the affected labyrinth.

Central Lesions: A central vestibular lesion (one involving the brainstem connections) causes a nystagmus with its greatest amplitude *toward* the lesion. The fast component is in the direction of gaze; thus the slow movement is always toward the position of rest and the fast movement is always toward the periphery.

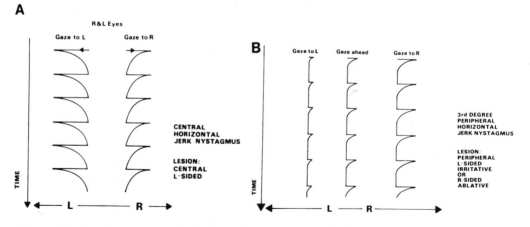

Figure 21-6   Nystagmus. (A) Direction-changing; (B) Direction-fixed.

This form of nystagmus occurs in both directions of gaze, even though the lesion may be unilateral. Thus it will have its fast component toward the right when looking to the right, but toward the left when looking to the left. This is referred to as a *direction-changing* nystagmus. Nystagmus persisting for more than 3 weeks is usually of central origin.

The most common causes of a central horizontal jerk nystagmus are multiple sclerosis, drugs affecting the cerebellum, brainstem ischemia or infarction, or encephalitis. Nystagmus is common in hereditary ataxias because of the degeneration in the cerebellar system.

Vertical

Vertical nystagmus indicates that the eye movements are up and down — with the fast component in either direction but usually upward. The lesion causing upbeat nystagmus is usually in the mesencephalon or upper pons; with downbeating nystagmus it is in the low brainstem, as with multiple sclerosis, Chiari's malformation, or local infarction.

Rotatory

Rotatory nystagmus occurs with brainstem lesions, but occasionally labyrinthine disorders cause it too.

Retraction and Convergence

These forms indicate that the lesion is in the region of the mesencephalon. Pineal tumors in young men are classic causes.

Ataxic Nystagmus (Internuclear Ophthalmoplegia)

Ataxic nystagmus consists of defective *adduction* of one eye associated with a coarse, irregular, jerk nystagmus of the other, *abducting* eye. In almost all other forms of nystagmus, the movement of the eyes is in parallel but here it is only seen in the abducting eye.

It indicates a lesion in the medial longitudinal fasciculus in the brainstem and multiple sclerosis is a common cause, especially if it is bilateral. Brainstem ischemia, tumors, or encephalitis and cervical cord injuries are also described as causes.

See-Saw Nystagmus

See-saw nystagmus is a rare spontaneous dissociation of movement of the two eyes, seen with high brainstem lesions. One eye may look up and the other down; their movements are in phase but in different directions.

Latent Nystagmus

Latent nystagmus is brought on when one eye is covered, as during ophthalmoscopy. It is of no diagnostic significance.

Optokinetic Nystagmus (OKN)

OKN is physiological and is induced by having the subject watch a moving object such as a rotating striped drum or a moving striped tape. It is normally present. When absent in one or other direction, it is an abnormality, ascribable to a lesion in the posterior part of the visual pathways or in the brainstem. Uncertainty about the precise localization of such lesions reduces its diagnostic value.

PAIN IN THE EYES

Pain-sensitive structures in the eye include the cornea, conjuctiva, and sclera, iris, ciliary body, and choroid. Pain may occur because of inflammation and distortion from without or from within. Ischemic pain may also occur, rarely. Pain caused by spasm of the external ocular muscles is uncommon.

The most common emergency disorders presenting with eye pain are (apart from *trauma,* which will be self-evident), closed-angle *glaucoma* and *corneal damage;* one an internal, the other a surface lesion, but both associated with visual loss. The visual loss however provides the clue to the nature of the painful process. With corneal lesions, such as ulcers or keratitis, blurring of vision occurs with excessive tear formation and pain on eye closure; with internal lesions such as temporal arteritis, glaucoma, or retrobulbar neuritis, the loss is not just blurring, but a constriction, segmental loss or total loss of vision with stages running from imprecise vision, to grayness, to blackness. *Iridocyclitis* may produce only mistiness of vision. Redness of the eye occurs with both surface lesions (e.g., *scleritis, keratitis,* and conjunctivitis) and internal ones, including *glaucoma* and *iridocyclitis.*

The type of pain felt is of value in diagnosis. Pain on ocular movement strongly suggests traction of an inflamed optic nerve and its surrounding pain-sensitive pia-arachnoid. Pain in the eye is usually accompanied by *photophobia,* but not always. Iridocyclitis, glaucoma, optic neuritis, cluster migraine, and trauma may produce constant pain throughout the whole eye. Try to obtain a history of similar past attacks or of drug ingestion, particularly of drugs with anticholinergic effects because a history of ocular trauma, of excessive eyestrain, or of being in the dark (as in movie houses) just before the onset of pain may suggest *glaucoma.*

Other neurological conditions may cause eye pain, usually with accompanying pareses of eye muscles. Third nerve compression, diabetic third nerve palsy, and certain probably autoallergic, conditions are examples.

Orbital pseudotumor is characterized by the onset in middle age of conjunctival injection, eye pain, visual loss, proptosis, and unilateral ocular palsy. The ESR is usually greatly raised. As in the similar *Tolosa-Hunt syndrome* (recurrent ocular pain and extraocular palsy), response to steroids is good.

The pain of a surface lesion is well localized and less likely to radiate to the head. It is invariably associated with blurred vision and excessive tear formation (unless the lacrimal glands are diseased), and it is known to all who have had sand or an eyelash in the eye. Photophobia and blepharospasm are frequently present. The pain is made much worse by eye closure. In all cases, eye tenderness may be expected, which is not therefore a useful diagnostic point.

Pain of *sudden* onset suggests trauma, closed-angle glaucoma, or cluster migraine, while a *gradual* onset of pain is more common with optic neuritis, migraine, and iridocyclitis.

BIBLIOGRAPHY

Glaser, J.S. *Neuro-Ophthalmology.* Hagerstown, Harper & Row, 1978.

Hollenhorst, R.W. The pupil in neurologic diagnosis. *Med. Clin. N. Am. 52:*871, 1968.

Leigh, R.J., Zee, D.S. *The Neurology of Eye Movements. Contemporary Neurology Series No. 23.* Philadelphia, F.A. Davis Co., 1983.

22
Facial Pain and Numbness

FACIAL PAIN

Of the many pain syndromes in neurology, pain in the face is of particular importance. One can sometimes be dispassionate about pain in a limb or a seemingly distant portion of our bodies, but our face has strong significance in our concept of "self." It is a mirror to the world and a sounding board for ourselves. Disorders around the area of the face have much greater personal significance than many disorders that occur elsewhere.

The pain-sensitive structures of the face and the anterior part of the head are mostly innervated by the fifth or ninth cranial nerves, although referred pain from other areas may also be felt in the lower part of the face.

The major causes of facial pain may be conveniently subdivided under four headings as in Table 22-1.

1. Caused by local structural changes in craniofacial tissues
2. Caused by irritation of nerves: the neuralgias
3. Referred pain
4. Atypical facial pain

CLINICAL APPROACH

Quality of Pain

The pains in facial neuralgias are brief, knifelike, or lancinating, whereas the post-herpetic neuralgias are classically described as burning. Pain described with an exuberance of phraseology, marked anguish, and with great intensity may be

308

Table 22-1   Causes of Facial Pain

Local pain syndromes

Facial pain from local pathology, e.g., tumor of CP angle or skull base, or
brainstem lesions
Migraine headaches (especially cluster migraine; carotidynia)
Temporal arteritis

The craniofacial neuralgias

Major neuralgias
trigeminal neuralgia
glossopharyngeal neuralgia
Minor neuralgias
occipital neuralgia
geniculate neuralgia
vagal neuralgia
Postherpetic neuralgias
Ramsay Hunt syndrome
postherpetic neuralgia

Referred or reflex facial pain

Dental, ocular, ENT disease
Temporomandibular arthralgia (Costen's syndrome)
Muscle contraction headache (tension, cervical spondylosis, posttrauma)
Angina pectoris

Atypical facial pain

---

associated with depression (*atypical facial pain*). Severe boring pain felt unilaterally behind the eye and radiating into the face occurs in cluster migraine. Toothache,
ocular disease, and sinusitis produce crescendos of pain or continuous aching, frequently with a throbbing component. Constant pains may also be felt in association
with an infiltrating carcinoma at the case of the skull, usually arising in the nasopharynx, and also with brainstem vascular disease. Central irritation of the fifth
nerve fibers by, for example, demyelination, produces a pain indistinguishable from
that of trigeminal neuralgia, but other neurological signs may be present.

Site

Trigeminal neuralgia is felt in the fifth nerve territory, usually the second or third
divisions and very seldom in the first. Glossopharyngeal neuralgia is felt in the
back of the throat, lower jaw, gums, and neck on the involved side. Postherpetic
neuralgia is usually the first division of the nerve, whereas cluster headache is felt
largely in or just posterior to the eye, the pain also extending up into the frontotemporal area and occasionally more diffusely below the eye. Referred pain is usually felt in the lower part of the face, often bilaterally, and the same is true of
atypical facial pain. Trigger zones on the cheek or in the mouth are characteristic
of the classic neuralgias.

Timing

The classic neuralgias are brief knifelike stabs of pain described as lancinating and lasting only seconds, with no pain between the jabs; pain of much longer duration, perhaps even continuous, occurs in all the other types. With cluster migraine, 40 to 60 min of acute pain occurs at night, waking the patient from sleep, unlike the classic neuralgias, which hardly ever do so. Constant or long-lasting pains occur with infiltration or irritation of the fifth nerve by, for example, nasopharyngeal tumors, aneurysms of the posterior communicating artery, or chronic basal meningitis. Atypical facial pain tends to be constant.

Cluster migraine occurs in bouts lasting a few weeks (hence the name), with months of freedom in between (see Chap. 17).

There is also a periodicity with the classic neuralgias, often with repeated paroxysms of pain over the space of 1 or 2 weeks, followed by a remission lasting up to months. Postherpetic pain usually goes away within 2 years, but it is almost constant while it is present. Such spontaneous complete remission seldom occurs with the classic neuralgias. Chewing and recent dental work may produce pain from the temporomandibular joint, usually associated with overclosure of the bite, and it is susceptible to dental treatment. Chewing and the presence of hot or cold fluids in the mouth may produce glossopharyngeal neuralgia and accentuate the pain of toothache. Touching the skin may intensify the continuous background pain of postherpetic neuralgia and may trigger neuralgia.

Associated Symptoms

These are of great importance. Mucosal and periosteal lesions producing primary facial pain may be associated with symptoms of sinusitis (nasal discharge, sometimes bloody; postnasal discharge; a history of recent upper respiratory infection). Cluster headaches are often associated with a small pupil, conjunctival engorgement, and severe lacrimation and nasal congestion, with an outpouring of sweat on the same side of the face and of clear fluid from the nostril, the whole episode looking rather like an intense, localized parasympathetic discharge. Central lesions producing a picture of trigeminal neuralgia include vascular disease, neoplasm, syringobulbia, and multiple sclerosis. Other clinical signs of these conditions will probably be found and almost always will be associated with a loss of the corneal reflex and perhaps subjective or objective alteration in sensation in the territory of the affected nerve. Peripheral infiltrating or compressive lesions of the nerve are also associated with sensory change, which rules out the diagnosis of trigeminal neuralgia. Posterior communicating artery aneurysm, nasopharyngeal carcinoma, cerebellopontine angle tumor, and chronic basal meningitis may all be expected to produce at least some signs in other cranial nerve territories. Evidence of depressive illness should be seen in patients with atypical facial pain.

In the classic neuralgias (trigeminal and glossopharyngeal), in cluster migraine, and in atypical facial pain, there are no physical signs on examination of the cranial nerves (although unilateral ptosis and miosis are seen in 25 percent of cases of cluster migraine). With dental, sinus, or jaw lesions, at least local signs will be available, while with irritation of the fifth or ninth nerves, postherpetic neuralgia, and brainstem disease, neurologic signs may be expected.

In the absence of physical signs, referred pain from heart, jaw, or other structures, atypical or depressive pain, or classic neuralgias will be most likely. In the presence of *any* physical signs however, full investigation is required, which may include x-ray studies of the nasopharynx and of the skull including the internal auditory meatus, lumbar puncture, and in many cases contrast radiography or CT scanning.

CLINICAL PRESENTATIONS

Local Pain Syndromes

Facial Pain Caused by Local Pathology

Any infection or tumor in the facial region or in the nose, pharynx, or ear may cause pain in the face. Common causes are toothache, nasopharyngeal tumors, or trauma to the face and vascular lesions, probably the most important of which is cranial arteritis, a local inflammation in the temporal vessels that is felt as a pain over the temporal region and posterior facial area. The arteries are reddened, pulseless, and tender. Half of these patients may go blind if the diagnosis is not made and the condition treated quickly with steroids (see Chap. 42).

Vascular Causes of Facial Pain

Cluster migraine is a very severe eye and head pain. It originates in the ocular, frontal, or frontotemporal regions and often spreads over the side of the head and face. The pain is associated with watering of the eye and nasal discharge on the same side, conjunctival suffusion, and sometimes ptosis and miosis (Horner's syndrome) which often remain after the acute pain is gone.

The condition is most commonly seen in males and its timing is peculiar, frequently waking the patient from sleep in the early hours of the morning, often at the same time each day. These pains occur daily over the course of a few weeks before disappearing, only to return weeks or months later for another bout. Treatment is with prophylactic drugs for migraine as describec in Chapter 17. Lithium is also of value in prophylaxis. If one is called to a patient in this severe pain, one should probably give a narcotic analgesic or parenteral ergotamine. Intravenous atropine may occasionally give excellent relief. Whether this is a neuralgia or a form of migraine is not clear.

Classic and common *migraine* headaches are usually experienced in the side of the head but sometimes the patients feel the headache in the facial region as well. The differential diagnosis is not difficult because of the throbbing, aching quality of a vascular headache, as opposed to the sharp, lancinating, or burning sensation characteristic of most types of neuralgia.

The Neuralgias

Major Neuralgias

Trigeminal Neuralgia: Trigeminal neuralgia is characterized by recurrent paroxysms of sharp, stabbing pain in one or more branches of the nerve on one side of the face, occurring in people over aged 50 who show no physical signs of fifth nerve dysfunction.

The cause is uncertain; the disorder has often been referred to as idiopathic trigeminal neuralgia or tic doloureux. However careful examination of the trigeminal nerve and ganglia has disclosed microneuromas and vascular compression. Other fifth nerve lesions that may result in pain in trigeminal distribution include compression by an aneurysm or tumor, trauma, and multiple sclerosis, but these are truly idiopathic trigeminal neuralgia. Because trigeminal neuralgia tends to occur only in the elderly age group, one should suspect multiple sclerosis if it develops in a younger person. There is an association between trigeminal neuralgia and diabetes. Finally, a redundant loop of the anterior–inferior cerebellar artery may touch the fifth nerve, causing electrical "chatter," felt as pain. The proportion of patients with "idiopathic" trigeminal neuralgia in whom this occurs is not known.

Trigeminal neuralgia is the most common of the classic neuralgias. It usually develops after the age of 50 and is more common in women and, for some reason, on the right side of the face. The pain comes on in paroxysms; individual jabs of pain last only seconds, but a paroxysm may last for up to 15 or 20 min. These attacks of "lightning" pain may recur daily or several times a month, but the patient often has pain-free periods between bouts. The term *tic douloureux* alludes to the grimace that is often made with each jab of pain. Patients usually have trigger points, stimulation of which will precipitate the pain, commonly over the malar area, at the base of the nose, or along the gums. Because of aggravation of the pain with eating or chewing, many patients begin to fast when a bout develops. The facial pain rarely occurs on both sides and *never* affects both at the same time, a useful point in differentiating it from other types of pain which *may* spread to the other side of the face; any pain that crosses the midline warrants a different diagnosis.

The differential diagnosis includes a number of disorders that cause sudden jabbing pain in the side of the face, but these can usually be eliminated by a careful history and examination. There may be confusion over pain from *dental* problems or from those arising from the *nasal sinuses*. *Costen's syndrome,* caused by a disorder of the temporomandibular joint, often causes jabbing pain that radiates into the face but this can be differentiated by the tenderness in the TM joint and by the dull aching pain remaining in the background when the jabs have gone. In trigeminal neuralgia there are paroxysmal jabs of lightning pain but no pain at all between them. Another confusing disorder is *cluster migraine,* not because it is very similar but because this very severe vascular headache is often unrecognized while everybody knows that trigeminal neuralgia exists, and physicians tend to make the more familiar diagnosis. *Herpes zoster* will show the typical vesicles, and one can establish the diagnosis of *glossopharyngeal neuralgia* by spraying the tonsillar region with local anesthetic which should abolish the pain for a brief period. If one does find neurological signs among the cranial nerves, such as loss of sensation over the face or weakness of the masseter or temporalis muscles, one must consider a compressive lesion simulating trigeminal neuralgia. The *muscle contraction* headaches that refer from the occipital region are often felt as a pressing ache behind the eyes; these may be unilateral. This referral to the trigeminal region often draws attention away from the cervical muscles where the problem originates. The distribution of *atypical facial pain* is often over the central part of the face, quite unlike that seen with trigeminal neuralgia.

Treatment of all the classic neuralgias is first with oral carbamazepine (Tegretol), a drug that gives excellent results in most patients in a dosage slowly increasing from 100 mg twice a day to a maximum of 200 mg four times a day. The most common side effects of this drug are ataxia, drowsiness, and confusion; marrow depression has been recorded rarely. Before carbamazepine was available, about half the patients responded to oral diphenylhydantoin. If the patient does not respond to carbamazepine, then baclofen is often helpful in controlling the pain.

The condition responds well to alcohol injection or radiofrequency destruction of the gasserian ganglion. These techniques are about 90 percent effective although they may have to be repeated. A few patients still complain of pain in a totally anesthetic area even after nerve block or surgical section ("anesthesia dolorosa"). Trigeminal root section was the usual operation performed, but nowadays, more selective lesions can be placed using, for example, cryotherapy, and these may be warranted in patients who do not respond to drugs.

Based on the observation that many patients have fifth nerve irritation from the pulsation of an artery abutting the nerve, a very successful surgical treatment in recent years has been to separate the two by a small sponge. The drawback is that this involves an operation to expose the posterior fossa region.

The therapeutic results from carbamazepine however are often so dramatic that this can be used as a diagnostic test in uncertain situations, for the patient's pain sometimes disappears within hours after the first few doses. Results as good as this are rarely seen with other causes of facial pain.

Glossopharyngeal Neuralgia: This major neuralgia is characterized by paroxysmal bursts of sharp, stabbing pain localized to the region of the ear, throat, tongue, and jaw. It is much less common than trigeminal neuralgia and may be bilateral. It also has trigger zones, which are usually in the tonsillar area, tongue, or external auditory meatus. Thus the patient may precipitate the pain by swallowing or by talking, yawning, or placing a finger in his ear. There is no neurological deficit on examination.

That is the only neuralgia that is a significant hazard to the life of the patient. Because the glossopharyngeal nerve innervates the carotid sinus, patients may have syncope, convulsions, or even cardiac arrest when a paroxysmal discharge occurs. Atropine will prevent the bradycardia and hypotension, but it does not affect the pain. Dehydration and wasting are also significant problems in the patient who is unwilling to swallow because he knows that it will cause a stab of pain.

Spraying a local anesthetic onto the tonsillar region and the posterior pharynx is a useful test to differentiate this disorder from trigeminal neuralgia affecting the mandibular division. Only rarely will glossopharyngeal neuralgia result from secondary causes such as tumors, aneurysms, or systemic inflammatory disease. The treatment is again with carbamazepine or baclofen; if this fails, intracranial section of the nerve proximal to the ganglion is required.

Minor Neuralgias

Occipital Neuralgia: There is some confusion between this syndrome and muscle contraction headaches caused by tension or cervical spondylosis. The latter produces long-lasting pain over the back of the neck and occiput with radiation bifrontally, but in occipital neuralgia, sharp lancinating pains occur in the occipital region only and have a trigger point in that area. Relief can be obtained by injecting the area with procaine and hydrocortisone; if this is only effective for a short time, then an alcohol block can be done or the nerve can be sectioned.

Geniculate Neuralgia: This is a neuralgia of the sensory portion of the seventh nerve which results in lancinating pain around the ear. The pain may radiate to the external ear, the mastoid region, the soft palate, or the neck. The explanation for the area of radiation is probably based upon central connections between the fifth, sixth, and ninth nerves in the spinal nucleus and tract.

Vagal Neuralgia: A vagal neuralgia may occur in the territory of the superior laryngeal nerve. The patient has unilateral neck pain aggravated by movements of the neck and by swallowing or speaking. The paroxysmal pain radiates from the side of the larynx up behind the ear, to the gums, or even down over the shoulder and breast. Most patients are female and middle-aged or older. Many have a trigger point near the pyriform fossa. Massage of the neck may relieve the neuralgia temporarily but carbamazepine is of more lasting value.

Postherpetic Neuralgias

Herpes zoster may cause two painful facial syndromes. The first is the *Ramsay Hunt syndrome,* characterized by pain in or behind the ear associated with herpetic vesicles in the external auditory meatus. There may be weakness or paralysis of the masseter or facial muscles and decreased salivation on that side. Vesicles can sometimes be seen over the eardrum, tongue, uvula, external ear, or in the auditory canal.

A second herpetic syndrome is *herpes zoster ophthalmicus* with supraorbital
neuralgia. This results in a severe, burning, aching, or stabbing pain around and
above the eye; often it becomes a long-lasting pain syndrome. One often sees
cutaneous scarring, redness, or edema around the eye, and there is often hyperesthesia in that area. Corneal ulceration with infection can result in blindness.
Only 2 percent of patients with ophthalmic herpes get this type of neuralgia, but
the incidence increases with age. Treatment is unsatisfactory, but the pain spontaneously improves after 2 years. Recently, acyclovir has been found effective
for the acute-stage pain and it hastens healing, but it has no effect on the incidence
of postherpetic neuralgia. Spraying ethylchloride locally may be effective, particularly if it is done frequently to start with and then daily, protecting the eye while
spraying. Avulsion of the supraorbital nerve or local alcohol block is sometimes
helpful, and undercutting of the skin of the area may give relief. However if therapy fails, time heals.

Referred or Reflex Facial Pain

Facial pain may originate from the eye, ear, nose, throat, teeth, sinuses, temporomandibular joint, heart, or muscles of the head and neck. Patients often feel that
any pain in the face originates in their teeth or sinuses. If it is around their eyes,
they will initially have their eyes tested, and it is all too common for patients presenting with specific facial pain syndromes to have bought an expensive pain of
glasses, had their sinuses drained and a few teeth removed, and invested in a new
set of dentures. The cosmetic results are excellent but the analgesic results poor.

One common form of referred facial pain is that resulting from temporomandibular (TM) joint disorders. Pain from the joint caused by excessive biting, malocclusion, or arthritis is referred to the frontal and parietal areas of the skull and
to the face. The patient may relate the pain to the ear and often experiences sharp
pain radiating toward the jaw and tongue. The mechanism in most patients is that
of chronic jaw-clenching because of tension and anxiety, and often a self-perpetu-
ating spasm of the muscles of mastication occurs. Many of them have bruxism
(nocturnal tooth-grinding) suggestive of an underlying chronic tension state or personality disorder. On examination, there is tenderness anterior to the ear over the
TM joint and one may feel crepitus. Jaw opening is often limited, and the discomfort can be relieved by putting a tongue depressor between the back teeth and asking the patient to bite gently upon it; this removes pressure from the joint. The
existence of this syndrome has been questioned; it has been suggested that it represents a watered-down version of atypical facial pain (discussed next), and certainly
it often responds gratifyingly to tricyclic drugs.

The eyes are not a common source of pain in the face despite the commonly
held myth in the general populace that much eye pain and headache are due to
visual disturbances. An exception is probably glaucoma, which can cause severe
pain around the eye and should be recognized and treated appropraitely. Sinusitis
as a cause of facial pain is well known to anyone watching TV commercials. Otitis
is another cause, particularly in the young.

Angina pectoris is an unusual cause of facial pain. Cardiac pain is usually referred from the chest to the jaw region, but we have seen some patients with angina complaining of pain in the anterior face or posteriorly as far as the ear.

Atypical Facial Pain

This is a common facial pain syndrome characterized by a constant aching, throbbing, or burning in the facial region. It may be mild or severe and is often

experienced bilaterally. The pain may spread over the scalp, neck, and even to the shoulder or arm. It is often worse at night. There are usually no trigger zones, and examination shows no sensory loss nor any neurolgoical abnormalities.

The syndrome is usually seen in middle-aged women and is aggravated or precipitated by illness, surgical procedures, social problems, or depression of mood. By the time such patients reach the neurologist, they are usually truly depressed and it is important to recognize this emotional component of the disease. Psychiatric evaluation and social assessment are both important.

Treatment consists of tricyclic drugs and supportive psychotherapy. A recent report indicates there may be benefit from dothiepin in 70% of cases, initially with 80% pain free after a year. Carbamazepine is not of value, and surgery is mischievous. The late Dr. Henry Miller commented that ". . . every new generation of neurosurgeons has to learn all over again the futility of aggressive therapy . . ."

FACIAL NUMBNESS

Episodic brief facial numbness commonly occurs in migraine.

The complaint of continuous numbness of the face is always a serious symptom. Although patients who are depressed may have this symptom, most such complaints point to an underlying organic disease process. The lesion is usually situated in the brainstem or in the fifth nerve itself (Fig. 22-1); it is less often cortical. The major differentiation between brainstem and fifth nerve lesion is difficult, but if all three modalities (pain, temperature, and touch) are involved, this suggests a

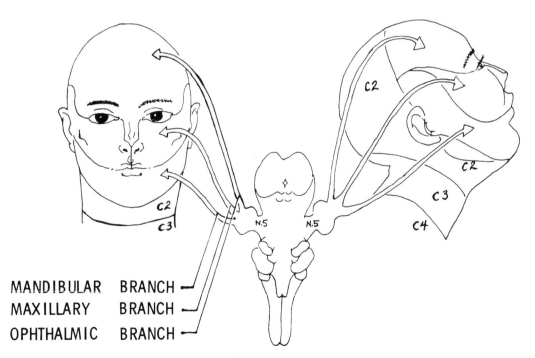

Figure 22-1   Sensory distribution of the trigeminal nerve.

Table 22-2   Causes of Isolated Facial Numbness

Central lesions

> Multiple sclerosis
> Syringobulbia
> Brainstem vascular disease
> Migraine

Peripheral lesions

> Cerebellopontine angle tumor
> Nasopharyngeal tumor
> Chronic basal meningitis
> Trigeminal neuroma
> Poisoning with hydroxystilbamidine,
>   trichloroethylene (Trilene)
> Arnold-Chiari malformation
> Dental and facial trauma; surgery
>   to fifth nerve
> Raeder's paratrigeminal syndrome

No cause detected

> "Benign" trigeminal sensory
> neuropathy

---

nerve lesion, while if there is dissociation of sensation, a brainstem lesion may be suspected. If all three divisions of the nerve are involved, again the lesion is likely to be either in the cranial cavity as the nerve leaves the brainstem and runs toward the gasserian ganglion or in the ganglion itself. A lesion that is more distal will affect only one of its three divisions (see Table 22-1).

This is usually at the cerebellopontine angle but may be a primary or secondary tumor at the base of the skull or, rarely, a pontine glioma. In basal skull tumors, the mandibular division may also be involved, causing weakness of the masseter, temporalis, and pterygoids on that side.

Cerebellopontine (CP) angle tumors usually cause complaints of sensorineural hearing loss and tinnitus. Headache, vertigo, balance and gait disturbance, facial numbness, pain, or weakness are less common symptoms. Examination reveals involvement of the auditory or cochlear branches of the eighth nerve and a decreased corneal reflex. Other evidence of fifth or seventh nerve damage occurs in about half the cases seen, and cerebellar signs occur in over half. Evidence of raised intracranial pressure, corticospinal tract involvement, and sixth cranial nerve involvement are less commonly found. It is interesting that facial pain is an unusual finding with compression of the fifth nerve by a tumor or aneurysm.

In perhaps a fifth of the patients, no cause is ever found. Such patients are described as having *trigeminal sensory neuropathy of benign type,* because it may clear spontaneously. Pain is sometimes felt by these patients but is seldom, if ever, an initial symptom. The corneal reflex is frequently retained and they do not have motor weakness.

Perhaps 10 percent of patients with facial numbness have *multiple sclerosis,* diagnosed on the basis of the later appearance of signs of involvement of other areas of the nervous system. A number of other conditions also produce facial numbness, accounting, in all, for some 20 percent of cases seen. These include viral *encephalitis* of the brainstem presenting as an acute illness with involvement of the fifth and often also of the sixth and seventh nerves and signs of meningeal irritation, *dental* and *facial trauma, chronic pansinusitis,* and rarely, *collagen-vascular disease,* and the rare *neuroma of the gasserian ganglion.*

Therefore a patient who is seen with clinical evidence of fifth nerve sensory involvement must be examined carefully to see whether or not he has dissociated sensory loss, and whether one, two, or three divisions of the nerve are involved (with or without additional motor involvement). The corneal reflex must be tested with great care.

Investigation should include x-rays of the skull base, nasopharynx, and internal auditory meatus and CT scan of the posterior fossa. Serological tests for syphilis and lumbar puncture (with or without posterior fossa myelogram) may be necessary to demonstrate a raised level of protein, IgG, or cells in the CSF. An EMG study of brainstem reflexes may confirm involvement of the ophthalmic division of the fifth nerve and may also indicate damage to the seventh. Audiometry will probably be of value in CP angle tumors and, if there is any doubt about the diagnosis, an ENT specialist should be asked to carry out further testing and to examine the posterior nasal space, perhaps assisted by tomography of that region. Only if all of these investigations are negative can an exclusion diagnosis of benign trigeminal neuropathy be made and the patient observed for recovery over the course of the ensuing months or years.

BIBLIOGRAPHY

Dalessio, D.J. Evaluation of the patient with chronic facial pain. *Am. Fam. Physician 16:*84-92, 1977.

Feinmann, C., Harris, M., Cawley, R. Psychogenic facial pain: Presentation and treatment. *Br. Med. J. 288:*436-438, 1984.

Fromm, G.H. et al. Baclofen in the treatment of trigeminal neuralgia. *Ann. Neurol. 15:*241-244, 1984.

Horenstein, S.H. Isolated facial numbness. *Ann. Intern. Med. 80:*49-53, 1974.

23
Facial Palsy

The muscles of the *upper* part of the face obtain innervation from the motor cortex on each side. Thus the right frontalis and orbicularis oculi are supplied by motor fibers running in the seventh nerve, whose nuclear anterior horn cells receive cortico-pontine fibers from the left and also from the right motor area. The nerve supply to the muscles of the *lower* right face however comes from other anterior horn cells in the seventh nerve nucleus, which receive impulses only from the opposite (left) cerebral cortex.

With a unilateral left cortical lesion therefore the frontalis and orbicularis oculi on the right will still function, but the orbicularis oris and platysma will not. A unilateral *upper* motor neuron lesion produces only a *lower* facial weakness. If the nerve is damaged at the nucleus, in the cerebellopontine angle, within the facial canal, or immediately upon leaving the canal, *all* the muscles, both upper and lower, on that side of the face will be paralyzed.

Therefore one can decide whether the cause of weakness is an upper or lower motor neuron lesion by seeing whether the frontalis and orbicularis oculi muscles are involved (lower) or if they are not (upper). If the lesion is of the upper motor neuron, then weakness of the corresponding hand and arm are likely.

LOCALIZATION OF LESIONS

Supranuclear

Cortical Lesions

Paresis of the lower half of the face can result from a contralateral *cortical lesion* in the motor area controlling facial movement. Usually, such a lesion will give rise to typical upper motor neuron weakness in the arm as well.

Corticopontine Tract Lesions

These may occur anywhere between the cortex and the facial nuclei, and although cerebral *infarction* is the most common cause, this type of paresis can result from a *tumor* or from other compressive lesions, from *multiple sclerosis,* or from *amyotrophic lateral sclerosis.*

Nuclear

If the lesion involves the facial nucleus in the pons, other signs may indicate involvement of local brainstem structures including the medial lemniscus and the nuclei and fibers of the fifth, sixth, or eighth (vestibular) nerves. Lesions within the pons include a *tumor, multiple sclerosis,* and *infarction.* Congenital absence of the facial nuclei or nerves is also described in *Mobius' syndrome* which is characterized by bilateral facial paralysis from birth and also by palsy of the sixth nerves and sometimes deafness.

Infranuclear

In the Cavity

When the seventh nerve leaves the brainstem it crosses the cranial cavity at the cerebellopontine angle and enters the internal auditory meatus in company with the eighth nerve and the nervus intermedius (Fig. 23-1). In the cavity, it is adjacent to the nerves and also to the fifth and sixth cranial nerves and to the middle cerebellar peduncle. Lesions here may affect all or any of these, with complaints of vertigo, tinnitus, or deafness; reduction in facial sensation and loss or diminution of the corneal reflex; and a sixth nerve palsy and facial weakness, or cerebellar signs on the same side. In the internal auditory meatus and the facial canal, the site of damage to the nerve may be determined as follows.

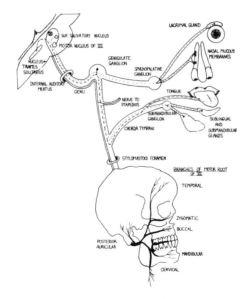

Figure 23-1   Course, relations, and distribution of the seventh nerve.

In the Meatus

There will be associated damage to the

1. Greater superficial petrosal nerve (loss of tear formation in that eye)
2. Eighth nerve (tinnitus, deafness, vertigo)
3. Nerve to stapedius (hyperacusis in that ear)
4. Chorda tympani (diminution of taste in the anterior two-thirds of the tongue)

The most common lesion here is a *tumor* or *fracture* of the petrous temporal bone
following trauma.

At the Genu

There will be associated damage to the eighth nerve fibers and also to the nerve to
the stapedius and to the chorda tympani. Signs will be as suggested previously.
    The most common causes here are *trauma, mastoiditis,* the presence of a *neo-
plasm* which is usually benign, and *herpes zoster.* The face is often painful with
this latter disorder (Ramsay Hunt syndrome) and the patient will sometimes complain of deafness or vertigo caused by involvement of the eighth nerve as well.

In the Facial Canal

Only the chorda tympani will be involved with the facial nerve at this site, and if
the lesion is very low down in the canal, even that will be spared. The most common causes here include *infections* of the middle ear and mastoid area which involve the nerve because of local extension of the inflammation. Facial paralysis
sometimes occurs also in diphtheria, mumps, measles, chickenpox, and tetanus.
Sarcoidosis causes facial paralysis, often bilaterally because of involvement of the
nerve in the canal and not in the parotid gland (although this may also be affected).
The *Guillain-Barré* syndrome may produce bilateral facial weakness and, in these
cases, the lesion probably affects all or any part of the nerve.[*]
    Trauma (e.g., skull fracture) may damage the nerve either as it runs in the
petrous bone or facial canal or after the nerve has left the stylomastoid foramen,
when direct stab, surgical, or gunshot wounds to the face, ear, or parotid gland
may produce facial paralysis.
    Less common causes of facial paralysis include lead poisoning, thiamine de-
ficiency, and polyarteritis nodosa, but the most common cause of all (three in four)
is *Bell's palsy.* Herpes zoster and trauma are next most frequent causes.
    In the assessment of the patient with apparent facial palsy therefore, the first
question to ask is whether or not both the upper and the lower face are involved.
If they are, then it is a lower motor neuron lesion. If the pathology involves the
seventh nerve nucleus, full examination will almost always show other signs of a
brainstem lesion, but usually the site of damage is distal. Assessment of tear formation, hearing, and taste, as well as general neurological examination and blood
pressure recording will be essential.

----

[*]Muscle diseases such as facioscapulohumeral muscular dystrophy, myotonic dystrophies, ocular myopathy, and myasthenia gravis may also cause bilateral but
   partial facial weakness, the upper part of the face often being affected more
   than the lower.

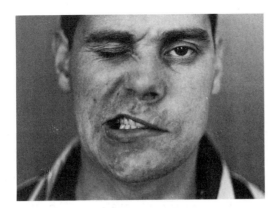

Figure 23-2   Left Bell's palsy. The patient is trying to close his eyes tightly.

BELL'S PALSY

This is a common peripheral facial paralysis of unknown cause that affects perhaps 20 out of 100,000 people per year (Fig. 23-2). The onset is always sudden, never progressive, and the paralysis is almost always unilateral. Although most causes will recover spontaneously, the severity of the cosmetic effects, the complications during the course of the illness, and the dangers of incomplete recovery warrant some form of therapy. Many patients relate the onset to exposure to the cold or wind. It has been suggested that it is more common in taxi drivers, and during World War II it was seen in Army personnel driving trucks with the windows open. Hereditary factors may play a role, because 30 percent of the patients have a positive family history of Bell's palsy. Because the disease sometimes occurs in epidemics, a viral cause has been suggested, and recently, the herpes group of viruses has been implicated in some cases (herpes simplex, Epstein-Barr). It is suggested that Bell's palsy is only part of a viral inflammatory disease.

Whatever the initiating cause however, the nerve becomes further damaged by edema and ischemia because it is entrapped within the bony facial canal. The site of the lesion is usually below the geniculate ganglion.

Clinical Features

At the onset, the acute, unilateral, lower motor neuron flaccid paralysis of one side of the face is accompanied or preceded in half the cases by pain behind the ear, which reaches a peak within 2 or 3 hr. There may be associated fever, dizziness, tinnitus, decreased hearing, or a mildly stiff neck. All the functions of the facial nerve may be affected producing motor weakness of all the facial muscles on that side and frequently loss of taste on the anterior two-thirds of the tongue. There will be inability to wrinkle the forehead and close the eye because of weakness of the frontalis and orbicularis oculi. Eversion of the lower eyelid, loss of the nasolabial fold, and dropping of the corner of the mouth with drooling of saliva are usual. In some cases, there is only partial palsy, which may make the diagnosis more difficult. Hyperacusis resulting from paralysis of the stapedius muscle, and reduced lacrimation and salivation, indicate a lesion proximal to the end of the canal, sometimes even proximal to the geniculate ganglion, but these are uncommon in Bell's palsy.

Bell's palsy usually involves only the seventh nerve. Evidence of other neurological deficits suggests some other disorder such as a stroke, tumor, infection, or multiple sclerosis. Recent studies have shown that the fifth and other cranial nerves can be involved, usually subclinically, and the disorder can be a manifestation of a more generalized but mild peripheral neuropathy. It is a good rule however to suspect a more sinister CNS disorder if more than the seventh nerve lesion is evident.

Treatment

General supportive measures such as mild analgesics and warm coverings for the face and ear can be started immediately. The eyelid should be taped shut; artificial tears may be instilled twice daily to prevent drying of the conjunctiva.

Medical therapy for Bell's palsy has in the past included a variety of treatments from reassurance to vasodilators. Most are useless; only steroid therapy started early reduces the chance of some residual paralysis. The suggested course of therapy for an adult consists of 60 mg/day of prednisone for 5 days, tapering to zero over a further 6 days. The patient should be evaluated weekly for the first 2 weeks and then again in 4 weeks.

If the symptoms worsen when the steroids are reduced or if the postauricular pain returns, then therapy with prednisone 60 mg/day may be restarted and the course repeated. Surgical decompression of the nerve has fallen from favor because it has been shown that such patients do worse than if they had no therapy at all. The only surgical procedure that may be of benefit in these patients is surgical autografting of the hypoglossal to the seventh nerve if spontaneous recovery does not take place.

Complications and Prognosis

Although at least 90 percent of patients with Bell's palsy will recover spontaneously, the physical and social disability of those who do not warrant the use of immediate prednisone therapy in all cases, even though this may not be of much value if started after the third day. Patients more likely to be left with some paresis are those with hyperacusis or decreased tear formation, those with diabetes or hypertension, and those over 60 years of age. In most cases however recovery starts within 2 weeks of onset, the upper facial muscles recovering first. Complete restoration of function may not be completed for over a year. If there is no improvement by the 18th day, some permanent disfigurement may be expected.

The occurrence of *crocodile tears* a month or so after the initial palsy is due to aberrant regenerating fibers that grow to the lacrimal instead of the salivary gland. If other regenerating fibers reach the wrong muscles, then abnormal associated movements may be seen, such as winking when the jaw is open. If recovery is slow, contractures of the facial muscles can occur, and incomplete recovery may lead to *clonic facial spasms.* Another cause of these abnormal movements is a long loop of the anterior inferior cerebellar artery impinging on the seventh nerve in the posterior fossa and producing electrical "chatter."

BIBLIOGRAPHY

Adour, K.K. Diagnosis and management of facial paralysis. *N. Engl. J. Med. 307:* 348-351, 1982.

The treatment of Bell's palsy. In *Recent Advances in Clinical Neurology,* Vol. 3, Chap. 12. W.N. Matthews and G.H. Glaser (eds.), New York, 1982.

24

Deafness, Vertigo, and Tinnitus

DEAFNESS

Although the person who is blind evokes universal sympathy, the deaf person is often only regarded as a source of irritation. This is unfortunate because deafness has major social implications at all ages and is a source of much distress to the sufferer.

Because many causes of deafness can be treated, early diagnosis is important. Even minor degrees of deafness in children may lead to secondary learning disabilities and a reduction in language skills that may affect the child throughout life unless steps are taken early to treat or compensate for the hearing defect.

Symptoms

As stated in Chapter 2, deafness may be of two types. The first is *conductive* (or middle-ear) deafness, characterized by decreased perception especially of low-pitched sounds, with relatively preserved bone conduction by Rinne's test (Fig. 24-1). The second type is *nerve* (or sensorineural) deafness, which is characterized by decreased perception of *high*-pitched sounds and relatively decreased bone conduction on Rinne's test. (The word *conduction* in this context refers to the conduction of sound impulses through the vibration of the tympanum and ossicles to the middle ear). In nerve deafness there may be damage to the cochlear apparatus or to the eighth nerve itself in any part of its course from the cochlear apparatus to the brainstem.

The auditory threshold of patients with conductive deafness is high, but they will be able to hear, for example, speech, if its volume is sufficiently loud. Sensorineural (nerve) deafness leads to not only a rise in threshold but also often distortion of sounds, so speech discrimination may be especially poor.

323

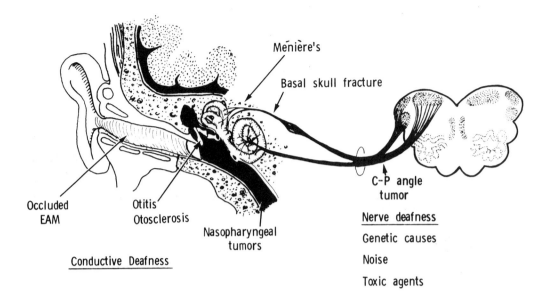

Ménière's

Basal skull fracture

C-P angle
tumor

Occluded   Otitis
EAM   Otosclerosis

Nerve deafness

Nasopharyngeal   Genetic causes
tumors

Conductive Deafness   Noise

Toxic agents

Figure 24-1   Sites of eighth nerve damage.

Poor hearing in an infant may be suspected if a sudden loud sound does not evoke eye blinking. A startle reflex should be present in the newborn and by 4 months the head and eyes should turn toward a loud sound. A hearing problem should be suspected if the child is not saying any words at 1-1/2 years. A school child may be regarded as dull, unintelligent, or uncooperative if a reduction in hearing is not noticed, and the child's school performance will fail. Adults may complain of associated symptoms such as tinnitus, vertigo, ear pain, or discharge and will be able to describe their hearing deficit quite accurately. Failure to hear a telephone conversation in one ear is a common early symptom of any type of deafness; difficulty understanding conversations with background noise suggests a cochlear or auditory nerve lesion ("cocktail-party deafness").

Sudden hearing loss is usually unilateral. It must be treated as an emergency if permanent deafness is to be avoided. The more common causes are listed in Table 24-1.

Hearing Loss with Rapid Onset

Middle-Ear Deafness (Conductive Deafness)

As usual, the diagnosis is frequently made by history. Earache, discharge, and fever point to a peripheral infective cause. Association with other evidence of systemic infection sometimes incriminates viruses as the cause of sudden deafness. Recent scuba diving, flying, or sudden exertion may rupture the round window, producing sudden deafness and vertigo because of the sudden pressure change. Direct trauma can traumatize the end-organ or nerve, often caused by bleeding.

Table 24-1   More Common Causes of Acute Hearing Loss*

Location	Cause	Approximate Frequency (%)
Middle ear	Trauma, blast injury, and sudden pressure change	10
	Otitis media	
Cochlear and labyrinth	Ménière's	10
	Tertiary syphilis	7
	Acute labyrinthitis	2
	Viral illness (mumps, measles, influenza)	9
Eighth nerve	Compression (e.g., CP angle mass, basal meningitis, traumatic edema	14
	Vascular and blood dyscrasias (anemia, leukemia, hyperviscosity)	5
	Ototoxic drugs	4
	Herpes zoster	
CNS	Psychogenic	5
	Multiple sclerosis	2
Idiopathic	(? Autoallergic)	25

Rare causes constitute the remainder

*Figures adapted from Morrison, A.W., 1978 (see Bibliography).

Nerve Deafness

Ménières disease will be suggested by a past history of previous similar episodes. Tinnitus and vertigo are usual other complaints, both strongly suggesting the cochlea as the site of the lesion causing the deafness, which is usually bilateral. The drugs causing deafness are listed in Chapter 43; aspirin and aminoglycosides are the most common offenders.*

    Multiple sclerosis, tertiary syphilis and eighth nerve compression by a cerebel-lopontine angle tumor or basal meningitis, occasionally present with sudden deafness; a full CNS examination is therefore obligatory in all cases. Other causes

*To avoid the danger of toxicity it has been recommended that streptomycin levels should be kept below 25 μg/ml and gentamicin levels below 6 μg/ml 2 hr after the last injection. The next dose should not be given unless the levels are below 2 μg/ml.

are encephalitis and such specific viral infections as measles, mumps, and herpes zoster. Hematological causes include anemia, leukemia, macroglobulinemia, and polycythemia. Vascular disease affecting the vertebrobasilar circulation has never actually been proved as a cause, but everyone knows that it is one, occurring mainly in people with past symptoms suggestive of vertebrobasilar insufficiency but who now present with sudden deafness (or vertigo) with no other sign to suggest brainstem infarction.

Head trauma with a basal skull fracture may cause direct damage to the middle or inner ear or cause eighth nerve damage, deafness resulting, but positional vertigo is a more common sequela of basal fractures.

Hearing Loss with Slow Onset

Middle-Ear Deafness

Wax or inflammatory products in the external meatus will reduce acuity gradually but not strikingly. In the middle ear, chronic infections that may have been smouldering since childhood, effusions, and otosclerosis should be considered. In the latter a positive family history is often found.

Locally invasive tumors, such as cholesteatomas, nasopharyngeal carcinomas, epidermoids, and the rare glomus tumors (which also cause pulsating tinnitus), are less common causes. Facial pain, nasal blockage, and discharge and dysfunction of other cranial nerves are their usual manifestations.

Nerve Deafness

Because of the loss of hair cells on the organ of Corti that increases in some people as they grow older, bilateral high-tone hearing loss occurs; this represents the most common single cause in the elderly. Aspirin, neomycin, and kanamycin, as well as other drugs (see Chap. 43) may lead to deafness slowly, not just suddenly. A history of past attacks of deafness with fullness in the ears, vertigo, and tinnitus suggests Ménière's disease, while past meningitis, direct trauma, local infections or syphilis (especially congenital syphilis) may also lead to progressive loss of hearing.

With prolonged exposure to loud noise, as in industrial situations, gradually increasing deafness of the nerve type may be expected. "Pop" music is often in a decibel range that damages hearing, and as the musicians develop impaired hearing they tend to play louder.*

Cerebellopontine angle tumors also typically present with slowly progressive loss of hearing; eighth nerve schwannomas are the most common.

Subacute loss of hearing also occurs in some patients with spinocerebellar degenerations and Refsum's syndrome, but it is an incidental rather than a presenting feature. Certain metabolic and endocrine disorders, including hypothyroidism, diabetes, and chronic renal disease, also induce deafness. Discussion of the many genetic and perinatal influence causing congenital deafness is beyond the scope of this book.

All these conditions should be considered when the history is taken, most of them (if not most of the patients) being susceptible to treatment. Examination must include otoscopy, with tuning-fork tests and clinical evaluation of auditory acuity to indicate the likely site of the lesion. If there is any suggestion of a

_____

*And worse.

sensorineural type of hearing loss, the CNS should be examined carefully, and in addition, examination and investigation may be directed toward metabolic or endocrine disease as indicated previously. Because progressive deafness is such a crippling complaint, all patients merit specialist referral. The formal auditometry which will almost invariably be ordered can usually determine both the degree of hearing loss and its anatomic site of origin with great accuracy. Other investigations include evoked potential studies, skull x-rays with tomography of the internal and auditory meati, and frequently CT scanning, which is the best method of demonstrating posterior fossa lesions, particularly in the region of the cerebellopontine angle (Fig. 24-2 A-D). Examination of thyroid or renal function or of glucose tolerance may also be indicated according to the findings on general medical examination.

There is a common popular feeling that hearing aids will correct all types of hearing loss, but this is not so. It is important to determine exactly what type of hearing loss is present before a patient commits himself to an expensive hearing aid, and advice on this matter should come from the ENT consultant. If a specific treatable cause for deafness can be found, then all efforts should be directed at this cause. Remember, too, that a hearing aid indicates bilateral deafness.

VERTIGO

Vertigo is an illusion of movement based upon sensory misinformation, which may derive from abnormalities in the peripheral or in the central nervous system. The disturbance will involve those structures that normally make us correctly aware of our position in space, including vision, proprioceptive pathways from joint and tendon organs, the labyrinthine system and its connections, and the neck muscles. Vertigo may result when any of these structures increase or decrease their input into the system for controlling position in space.

To define vertigo as essentially rotational, as is commonly done, ignores the input from labyrinthine structures functioning to inform about nonrotational acceleration. Probably hallucinations of movement up and down, forward and backward, or sideways, have just the same significance as the sensation of personal rotation in the environment or of the environment rotating around ourselves.

Clinical Approach

Is This Vertigo?

Obviously this is the vital question. You must determine that a patient experiences some illusion of his movement in space or of the environment around him. Make him describe just what it was that he was experiencing which he calls dizziness or vertigo, for many other sensations are subsumed under that term. These include a sensation of impending faint or loss of consciousness that may be associated with visual blacking out, palpitations, sweating, or actual fainting and may have definite emotional precipitants or postural changes related to its onset.

A feeling of dysequilibrium or loss of balance with an illusion of movement but without true vertiginous sensations may also be termed vertigo or dizziness by the patient. This sensation may occur from disturbances in the peripheral sensory system involving proprioceptive input and from disturbances of the motor and cerebellar systems. Elderly patients often have some degeneration in the eighth nerves, poor vision, and mildly decreased proprioceptive sensations. Put together, these give a patient a poor sense of his position in space, and he has a sensation of swaying which he may describe as dizziness. This was termed the *multisensory* or *earthbound astronaut* syndrome by Drachmann.

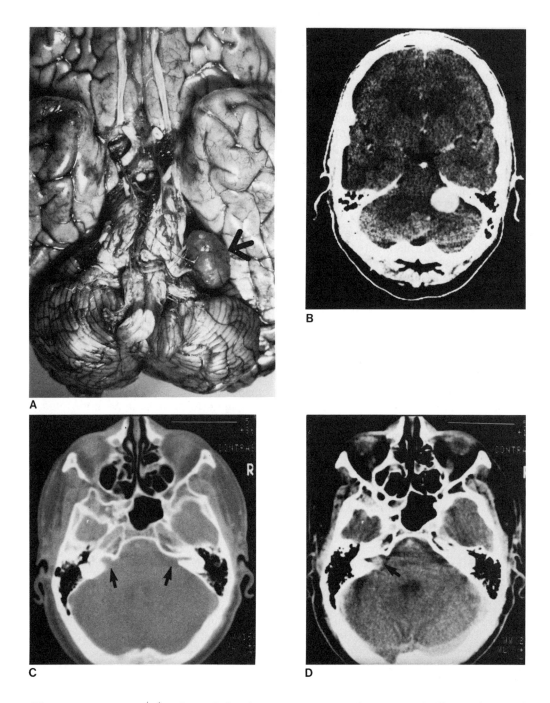

Figure 24-2A-D   (A) A large left-sided schwannoma in the cerebellopontine angle causing local compression but found incidentally at autopsy. (B) Enhanced CT scan showing large acoustic neuroma. (C) CT scan showing enlarged left auditory meatus. (D) CT scan showing tumor in the canal.

Ill-defined "lightheadedness" is often psychogenic in origin but a careful assessment of the patient is required before the symptom can be regarded as functional rather than caused by some serious underlying disease. Anxiety, depression, drug ingestion, and postural hypotension are common causes.

Many other sensations, weakness, visual blurring, or dimming, and anxiety, for example, may lead the patient to complain of dizziness. If you are in doubt, then try spinning him around on a stool or do a cold caloric test. These normally produce vertigo; let the patient compare his sensations after those stimuli with his presenting symptoms.

Which System is Responsible for the Problem?

Physiological vertigo occurs with bending down or when the neck is hyperextended. When visual cues are missing (as at great heights, following lens extraction, or with marked diplopia or refractive errors), vertigo may have an ocular origin. Lack of other sensory inputs causing vertigo were mentioned before; thus posterior column disease and peripheral neuropathies may lead to the complaint of dizziness. Finally, a number of systemic disorders may do the same. Thus aminoglycosides, sedatives, alcohol, antihypertensives, and so forth (see Chap. 43) may cause acute or chronic symptoms, and systemic infections, hypothyroidism, collagen-vascular diseases, and hypoglycemia may induce dizziness, although usually only as a secondary complaint.

The presentations of depression are discussed in Chapter 51. Dizziness (not true vertigo) is a common complaint of depressed people. Anxiety — not always admitted as such by patients who only complain of *bad nerves, tension,* or *worries* — may lead to acute or chronic hyperventilation. Numbness of the hands, visual blurring, dyspnea, constriction of the chest, and nausea often accompany the symptom, and stress factors should be definable. Since "dizziness" includes a feeling of being about to faint, one might question the patient about chest pains, dyspnea, rapid heart action, and symptoms of postural hypotension. Syncope is considered in Chapter 10.

Thus the history and examination must be directed toward systemic, otologic, cardiac, visual, and psychiatric etiologies as well as to the central nervous system.

Is the Vertigo of Central or Peripheral Origin?

Vertigo may be due to a lesion of the labyrinthine structures or first sensory neuron, or it may arise as a result of CNS disease, usually at brainstem level. In the former, jerk nystagmus is almost always associated, but in the latter, nystagmus may be only slight or indeed absent. Table 24-2 lists the main differences between the presentations. A good general rule is that peripheral vertigo is usually associated with direction-fixed horizontal jerk nystagmus with few other signs added; central lesions cause milder vertigo and direction-changing nystagmus and are usually accompanied by obvious evidence of a CNS lesion.

By now it should be obvious that the history is all-important in making the diagnosis, but examination still adds much. Assuming that you have ruled out cardiac and vascular causes (postural hypotension, Stokes-Adams attacks, carotid sinus syndrome, valvular lesions, and subclavian steal syndrome), ocular lesions, and psychiatric causes (these last by history and examination of mental state, perhaps coupled with 2 min of hyperventilation to see if the symptoms are reproduced), you must examine the CNS and the ears, nose, and throat with great care as described in Chapter 2. Pay special attention to the examination of all the cranial nerves, to Romberg's test, and observations of the patient's gait and turning. Carry out

Table 24-2   Usual Presentations of Central and Peripheral Causes of Vertigo

	Peripheral	Central
Incidence	Common	Uncommon
Direction of vertigo	Same as fast component of nystagmus	Variable
Severity	Marked	Mild
Latency after, e.g., head movement	5-30 sec	Immediate
Fatigability with time	Present	Absent
Romberg's test and gait	Patient falls/sways to side of slow component of nystagmus	Variable
Nystagmus	Horizontal jerk-type, direction-fixed	Jerk-type, direction-changing; may be vertical; pendular forms also possible
Common associated symptoms and signs	Hearing loss, tinnitus, frequently no other signs	Visual dimming, drop attacks, cranial nerve, long tract, cerebellar signs may be found
Ice caloric tests	Reduced response on affected side	Responses often hard to interpret
More common causes	Benign positional vertigo Ménière's syndrome Peripheral vestibulopathy	VBI Multiple sclerosis Posterior fossa mass lesions

positional testing, ice-water caloric testing, inspection of the external auditory meatus and tympanic membranes, and tuning-fork tests of hearing.

The purpose of all these tests is to try to reproduce exactly what the patient was experiencing in his former attacks. If that can be done, the diagnosis is often quite plain. Drachmann was able to determine the cause of dizziness in 91 percent of the patients referred to a special clinic, with a careful history and examination including neuro-otological examination and the preceding procedures (Table 24-3). His findings provide a good outline of the problems to consider in patients with vertigo and show the relative importance of different causes. Many patients had

Table 24-3   Major Causes of Dizziness[*]

Pathology	% of Cases
Peripheral vestibular disorders	38
Hyperventilation syndrome	23
Multiple sensory deficits	13
Psychiatric disorders	9
Brainstem CVA	5
Cardiovascular disease	4
Multiple sclerosis	2
Visual disturbances	2
Other causes or undiagnosed	15

[*]Some patients had more than one diagnosis. Results of
Drachmann, D.A., Hart, C.W. An approach to the dizzy
patient. *Neurology* 22:323, 1972.

been previously undiagnosed, mainly because the importance of hyperventilation caused by anxiety was not recognized and because the concept of multiple sensory deficits was not thought to be relevant.

Numerous investigations are available to localize and to characterize the cause of the complaint. If you need more than routine hematology and biochemistry, ESR, thyroid function tests, and specific serology, then the patient will probably merit specialist referral. Audiology, electronystagmography, skull x-rays with tomograms, evoked responses, and CT scanning are preeminent among the tests used.

Common Conditions

Some of the more common conditions will now be described.

Benign Positional Vertigo (BPV)

Acute severe vertigo, often with nausea and vomiting, occurs a few seconds after the head obtains a certain position, e.g., on sitting up in bed or bending down. If the head is moved to the same position a second time, the vertigo may not recur. Direction-fixed jerk nystagmus, which seldom lasts more than 60 sec, is noted during the spell. Recent head injury or systemic infections are occasional causes, but usually the syndrome strikes a healthy adult without preceding disease. Repeated episodes may occur, but the condition finally goes away in less than 6 months. No CNS findings should be present, but positional testing should precipitate an episode. Rarely, a central lesion can show itself in this manner. Full examination is therefore necessary in all cases. The pathogenesis is thought to be displacement of small calcareous chips within the semicircular canals, called otoconia, which sink freely in the endolymph as the head adopts a different position and cause excessive and unwanted stimulation of the receptors, producing the hallucination of rotational movement.

Peripheral Vestibulopathy

Also known as *vestibular neuronitis* or *acute labyrinthitis,* this condition resembles BVP in almost everything except its much longer duration — hours or days in each single attack, with nausea, vomiting, and incapacitation. A recent or current otitis or upper respiratory infection occasionally seems to be casual. Measles, mumps, and mononucleosis have been incriminated. Some hearing loss may accompany this syndrome. The examination findings of a "peripheral" type of nystagmus unaccompanied by cochlear or CNS signs, resemble those in BPV.

Ménière's Disease

This condition is characterized by the occurrence in older patients of repeated acute and severe attacks of vertigo, nausea, and vomiting lasting up to a day and made much worse by head movement. The accompanying nystagmus is of peripheral type. Chronic tinnitus, progressive (usually bilateral) deafness, subjective distortion of sounds, and a sense of pressure in the ear are other important features. The disease is caused by an excess of endolymph in the semicircular canals. A chronic state of imbalance may also occur with these patients in addition to the acute attacks. Patients with Ménière's disease have been shown to manifest abnormal glucose tolerance, hypothyroidism and hypoadrenalism with unusual frequency. If the diagnosis is suggested clinically, screening tests might be of value. As the attack begins, the patient should be instructed to get into a comfortable position and stay there, and to take nicotinic acid 100 mg every half hour for three doses. Proprietary antiemetic drugs such as dimenhydrinate, 50 mg, may be taken by mouth or intramuscularly if the patient is vomiting.

Between attacks, oral betahistine (Serc) may be employed. However if drug therapy cannot be tolerated or is ineffective, some new surgical techniques are available, and we believe that all patients with Ménière's disease should be referred for ENT assessment.

The triad of recurrent vertigo with tinnitus and deafness should be present before the diagnosis of Ménière's syndrome can be assumed. Other less common causes of this syndrome must also be considered in the differential diagnosis. These include acute ischemia, secondary to occlusion of the anterior inferior cerebellar artery; skull trauma, with a basal fracture; blast or noise trauma; and toxicity, which is mainly caused by aminoglycoside antibiotics.

Central Causes of Vertigo

If the features of vertigo and accompanying nystagmus given in Table 24-2 suggest a central cause, then expect to find other signs indicating brainstem disease. All such patients require referral to a neurologic or otologic center. Evidence of involvement of the fifth, seventh, and cerebellar structures, with deafness, tinnitus, and mild vertigo, would suggest a cerebellopontine angle tumor, enlarging to compress the brainstem. In older patients unequal radial pulses, evidence of generalized atherosclerosis by history or examination, occurrence of vertigo with neck turning or extension, and symptoms to suggest transient brainstem disorders (such as diplopia, bilateral visual dimming, loss of consciousness, drop attacks, ataxia, or motor or sensory signs) all suggest vertebrobasilar insufficiency. Multiple sclerosis will be suggested if examination shows evidence of multifocal CNS involvement in a younger patient. If the signs point to a brainstem lesion in isolation, a posterior fossa tumor must be excluded.

Vertigo occurs as a comparatively minor symptom in some patients with temporal lobe epilepsy and CNS system degeneration. In the lateral medullary syndrome, it is severe, but the clinical picture should allow rapid diagnosis.

TINNITUS

Tinnitus is a sensation of noise, usually described as hissing, whistling, or humming caused by degeneration of the organ of Corti in the inner ear. Clinicians often ask about "ringing in the ears," but hissing and rushing noises are more common. The sound may be loud and may interfere with hearing; it is often constant, which is extremely disturbing to patients who may become annoyed and resentful and, in due course, depressed. Even the brief constant sound we all hear from time to time, probably caused by unequal pressures in the middle ear, is annoying.

Sensorineural deafness is very frequently accompanied by intermittent tinnitus. If a deaf patient has not had at least some degree of tinnitus in the past, his deafness is probably of the conductive type.

The causes are to be found in damage to any part of the auditory system and are similar to those of deafness. Thus it may be physiological (as previously explained or after a very loud noise) or pathological, caused by any acute or chronic middle-ear disease, such as otosclerosis, otitis, and so forth. Wax in the ears is seldom a cause.

When caused by lesions of the cochlea or of the eighth nerve, tinnitus has essentially the same causes as sensorineural deafness; thus presbycusis is probably the most common cause, at least in older people. It also affects patients who are severely anemic, and it is an early symptom of Ménière's syndrome. Ischemia of the cochlea, use of salicylates, alcohol, amyl nitrate, quinine, or the aminoglycoside antibiotics, nerve compression, and trauma are other possibilities, whereas more centrally at the level of the cerebellopontine angle, chronic basal meningitis, tumor, or aneurysm may be responsible. More central lesions seldom produce tinnitus, although a rushing sound may be heard in the first stage of a focal seizure because of involvement of temporal lobe structures. Unfortunately most cases have no demonstrable cause, but the symptom is too unpleasant to allow a diagnosis of idiopathic tinnitus to stand without a full otologic examination.

Pulsating tinnitus, or bruits, may be heard in the ears quite normally, particularly in anxious patients with hyperactive circulations. Stenosis in the homolateral carotid system, a tumor of the glomus jugulare, or arteriovenous communications in the region of the ear or cavernous sinus may also produce this complaint.

Except for those patients in whom depression is a primary factor, the therapy of tinnitus is disappointing. If a local abnormality is found it should, of course, be corrected, but unfortunately, most of the elderly patients who are disturbed by continuous or paroxysmal tinnitus do not have any demonstrable cause. For them, one can offer a mild tranquilizer and reassurance that the severity of the symptom is not necessarily correlated with the likely degree of deafness. Recently intravenous lidocaine and nafronyl have been given in daily dosages for a week with good results in about half the patients so treated. If this therapy is only partially successful, oral carbamazepine or phenytoin may have a good effect in those cases. Otherwise portable masking devices worn like a hearing aid are available and these seem to relieve about one in three sufferers.

BIBLIOGRAPHY

Baloh, R.W. *Dizziness, Hearing Loss and Tinnitus: The Essentials of Neuro-Otology.* Philadelphia, F.A. Davis Co., 1983.

Drachmann, D.A., Hart, C.W. An approach to the dizzy patient. *Neurology 22:* 323, 1972.

Hazell, J.W.P. Tinnitus. *Br. J. Hosp. Med. 13:*468-471, 1979.

Morrison, A.W. Acute deafness. *Br. J. Hosp. Med. 12:*237-249, 1978.

Rudge, P. *Clinical Neuro-Otology. Clin. Neurol. Neurosurg. Monogr. Ser.* Vol. 4, Edinburgh, Churchill-Livingstone, 1984.

Troost, B.T. Dizziness and vertigo. *Stroke 11:*301-303; 413-415, 1980.

Wolfson, R.J. et al. Vertigo. *Clin. Symposia* (Ciba-Geigy) 34:1-32, 1982.

25
Bulbar and Pseudobulbar Palsy

The term *bulbar palsy* refers to a *lower* motor neuron lesion in the pons or medulla affecting the lower cranial nerves. *Pseudobulbar palsy* refers to an *upper* motor neuron lesion affecting the same structures; apart from the absence of wasting and fasciculations, the clinical features may be very similar.

BULBAR PALSY

Bulbar palsy may be mild or complete, unilateral or bilateral, and may involve one or many cranial nerves. Trigeminal motor nuclear involvement leads to weakness with atrophy and perhaps fasciculations of the temporalis and masseter muscles. There is consequent difficulty in biting and jaw protrusion. Involvement of the seventh nerve produces facial weakness, sometimes with fasciculations and involving both the upper and lower parts of the face. Weakness of the orbicularis oris produces some difficulty in pronouncing the letters *M* and *B,* the labial consonants. Involvement of the ninth, tenth, and eleventh nerve nuclei produces the classic triad of dysphonia, dysarthria, and dysphagia, although dysarthria may also be produced by facial or by tongue weakness. The dysphonia is usually a nasal speech with difficulty in pronouncing *Ks.* The patient may regurgitate fluids through the nose, being unable to close off the nasopharynx with his soft palate. Unilateral laryngeal weakness produces little in the way of symptoms or signs but if there is bilateral weakness, the cords are fixed in the cadaveric position resulting in dyspnea, stridor, and inability to cough.

Because of the difficulty with swallowing and lip movements, drooling of saliva may occur. Although palatal and pharyngeal sensation may be intact, the gag reflex is likely to be lost. Unilateral lesions cause the palate to be drawn to the *normal* side on attempted phonation. Involvement of the twelfth nerve gives rise

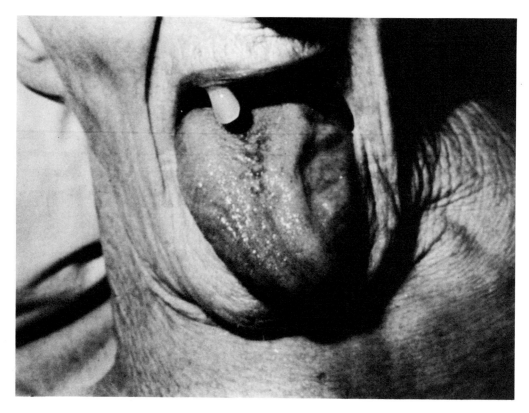

Figure 25-1 Left twelfth nerve palsy caused by compression by a huge cervical mass (goiter).

to weakness with atrophy and fasciculations of the tongue, which deviates toward the *weak* side when the patient attempts to protrude it (Fig. 25-1).

Long-tract signs, both sensory and motor, may be expected with intrinsic brainstem disease or with pressure upon the pons or medulla. There are important regulatory centers for blood pressure, respiratory rate and depth, and vomiting in the medulla, which may be stimulated or depressed by a local lesion. Particularly with a pontine lesion, sudden downward jerks of the eyes with slow upward restitution of their position occurs, aptly termed *ocular bobbing.* A fluttering movement of the soft palate is described as *palatal myoclonus* and this, like *hiccup* (discussed later) and generalized or whole-body *myoclonus,* is another sign of brainstem disease in a small number of patients.

The diseases producing true *bulbar palsy* may be *intrinsic* (that is, actually inside the brainstem) or *extrinsic,* involving the cranial nerves after they have left the brainstem and are crossing through the cavity between it and the exit foramina or passing through the foramina or soft tissues outside the skull. Examples of intrinsic lesions are syringomyelia, brainstem tumors, poliomyelitis, and a form of motor neuron disease called progressive bulbar palsy.

Extrinsic lesions involve the nerves directly, e.g., resulting from direct trauma, or from pressure from glands enlarged by tumor, reticulosis, or infection. Diphtheria, the Guillain-Barré syndrome, and botulism are other peripheral neuropathies affecting the lower cranial nerves. Myasthenia gravis may produce marked weakness of the bulbar as well as of the spinal and ocular muscles, and chronic basal meningitis (secondary carcinoma, reticulosis, sarcoidosis, tuberculosis, syphilis) may involve any of the cranial nerves. Polymyositis and myotonic dystrophy are myopathic causes.

PSEUDOBULBAR PALSY

Pseudobulbar palsy implies a lesion of the corticobulbar fibers above the relevant neuronal cell bodies; thus it must be sited above the pons. Because many of the lower cranial nerves receive innervation from the motor cortex on both sides of the brain, lesions usually have to be bilateral to produce the syndrome. This is seen in motor neuron disease, in multiple sclerosis, with bilateral cerebrovascular accidents (usually hypertensive), and also in Parkinson's disease. As mentioned before, there will not be any wasting or fasciculations in such cases, and the jaw jerk is increased. *Pathologic emotionality,* in which the patient expresses emotions without necessarily feeling them, so that laughter or crying may occur without any external stimulus, is yet another symptom of brainstem disease.

The pattern of bilateral weakness gives rise to the usual picture of dysphagia, dysarthria, and dysphonia, which is not always easily distinguishable from that caused by a lower motor neuron lesion, unless a careful search for atrophy is made. Long-tract signs elsewhere in the body may be expected; for example, bilateral corticospinal signs in the limbs in patients who have had hypertensive lacunar strokes. Although bilateral lesions cause pseudobulbar palsy, an acute unilateral cerebral lesion may *seem* to be responsible when a lesion on the opposite side has occurred in the past with apparent good recovery.

HICCUPS

This symptom needs no description. Although usually caused by diaphragmatic irritation by local gastric causes (distension, bleeding, ileus, subphrenic abscess), basal pneumonia or pleurisy, and occasionally with myocardial infarction, a number of brainstem lesions cause prolonged hiccuping. These include stroke, (the lateral medullary syndrome); brainstem tumor or encephalitis; or multiple sclerosis. Treatment regimens include

1. Putting dry sugar on the back of the tongue.
2. Stimulating the posterior pharynx with a nasogastric tube.
3. Chlorpromazine, 25-50 mg IV.
4. Metoclopramide, 10 mg IV q4h.
5. Various other drugs have been found useful including methylphenidate, anticonvulsants, and quinidine. If all fail, left phrenic nerve block (and later crush) may be needed because the repetitive contractions are exhausting.

BIBLIOGRAPHY

Currier, R.D. *Syndromes of the medulla oblongata.* In *Handbook of Clinical Neurology,* Vol. 2. Vincken, P.J. and Bruyn, G.W. (eds.), New York, Elsevier, 1969.

26
Weakness

One of the most common symptoms heard by physicians is that of feeling weak. The word *weakness* has many meanings and one must define precisely which one the patient intends when he uses it.

The possible causes include the *psychological,* when the patient is perhaps complaining more of lack of drive and of energy to carry out tasks than of actual failure of strength. Disorders of the *upper motor neuron* will give rise to weakness, varying from minimal reduction in power to complete hemiplegia. Disturbances of *cerebellar* function may cause mild homolateral weakness, and disorders of the *basal ganglia,* resulting in both difficulty in starting a movement and in increased activity in antagonistic muscles, will do so contralaterally.

Disorders of the *lower motor neuron* cause weakness because of involvement of the anterior horn cell, the motor fiber, the end-plate, or the muscle. Patients who have *pain* in their joints or periarticular *stiffness* may not want to make a full range of movement because of the discomfort; this may be expressed as weakness.

Severe *proprioceptive* disorders may give the impression of loss of strength because adequate feedback information about the power of the movement being made cannot be received by the patient.

It is therefore essential to define the nature of the patient's weakness, and having done so, to go on to characterize the particular movements that are affected, the duration and progress of the symptom, and the presence or absence of associated pain or stiffness. The pattern of involvement may also be diagnostically helpful; different conditions affect the eyes, bulbar muscles, neck, shoulder or pelvic girdles, or all or part of a limb, or may produce hemiplegia or paraplegia.

The speed of onset of weakness was briefly considered in Chapter 9. Further pointers are given in Table 26-1. Sometimes a patient will be unable to localize his weakness, finding the whole body more or less affected, while another may be

Table 26-1   Weakness of Rapid Onset

Minutes	Cerebrovascular disease
	Postepileptic (Todd's paresis)
	Compression of peripheral nerves
	Drug effects
Hours	Encephalitis, myelitis
	Familial periodic paralysis
	Myasthenic crisis
	Botulism, diphtheria, poliomyelitis, organophosphate poisoning
Days	Guillain-Barré syndrome
	Polyarthritis
	Polymyositis
	Tick-bite paralysis
	Myasthenia gravis
	Acute thyrotoxic myopathy

able to point out particular movements that are involved. Although we have chosen to discuss proximal and distal weakness as the main object of this chapter, some discussion on other patterns of weakness and pain is also necessary.

GENERALIZED WEAKNESS

Painless

The patient who complains of weakness all over may be unable to distinguish local from generalized loss of power or may have any one of a number of possible disorders.

The main psychiatric syndromes causing generalized weakness are depression, chronic anxiety, and hysterical conversion reactions. The cardinal signs of depression and anxiety are noted in Chapter 51. *Neurasthenia* (irritable fatigue) is common in patients with inadequate personalities and in normal people following traumatic, infective, or neurologic diseases. Inquire carefully whether it is *energy* or *power* that is lost and whether or not the patient *fatigues* easily. In *myasthenia gravis,* fatigability is the cardinal sign and must be differentiated from lack of energy or lack of persistence occurring in psychiatric disorders; ocular or bulbar involvement is usual in myasthenia, not in functional states.

Fatigue and anergia are both common complaints of patients with multiple sclerosis; the precise lesion causing them is still uncertain. Interestingly, they are greatly relieved by amantadine, an antiviral agent also of value in the management of Parkinson's disease.

Cardiorespiratory disorders may be responsible for this generalized weakness, but they are seldom a diagnostic problem. *Genetic, metabolic,* and *endocrine* muscle diseases produce weakness that is sometimes generalized, although a proximal distribution is the most common pattern (Chap. 45).

Malnutrition and cachectic diseases may produce weakness without pain, with or without an associated peripheral neuropathy. Bilateral disorders of the upper motor neuron, of the basal ganglia, or of the cerebellum again produce weakness, but that weakness is associated with other complaints such as abnormal movements, incoordination, and so forth.

Painful

When the patient complains of ill-localized or generalized weakness and *pain,* a number of other conditions must be considered. Muscle pain is sometimes a feature of *polymyositis* and of other causes of muscle inflammation such as *viral myositis* or *alcoholic myopathy*. In *polymyalgia rheumatica,* muscle stiffness and pain are leading symptoms, and affected patients may complain of weakness that is not actually present when one tests power in a formal manner. The same is true in rheumatoid arthritis and in other joint diseases. Muscle discomfort may occur in *myotonic disorders* (which also generate the symptom of weakness), in patients who are anxious or *depressed,* and in association with abnormal movements in *basal ganglion disorders*. In all of these however, other symptoms usually overshadow pain as a presenting symptom.

LOCALIZED WEAKNESS

If the patient can delineate a pattern of weakness, the localization and the pathological diagnosis of the lesion may be easy, as with disorders of the upper motor neuron, cord, or peripheral nerves. However myotonic, ocular, and FSH dystrophies and myasthenia gravis may cause only localized weakness in their early stages. If the patient has no pain and can point to part of one limb as being weak, a nerve lesion, such as a cubital tunnel syndrome, is most likely. Bulbar palsy is considered in Chapter 25.

Painful localized weakness is perhaps more common. *Cramps,* including occupational cramps (Chap. 27), *joint diseases,* and *ischemia,* e.g., intermittent claudication, are possible causes. If these can be excluded, a few *neurogenic disorders* can also cause pain in the weak part. Neuralgic amyotophy, diabetic femoral neuropathy, and the carpal tunnel syndrome are examples of this. Poliomyelitis and the early stages of the Guillain-Barré syndrome may be painful at the onset. Muscle pain from other causes is also considered in Chapter 27.

The term *hemiparesis* (or hemiplegia) indicates weakness of one side of the body. Strokes, tumors, subdural hematomas, and migraine are examples or causes. *Quadriparesis* means weakness of the four limbs and of the trunk; *paraparesis,* of the legs. The former is usually caused by a high spinal cord or brainstem lesion or to severe peripheral neuropathy or myopathy. Paraparesis suggests a cord lesion below T1, or a problem affecting the cauda equina or peripheral nerves. Table 26-2 lists some intracranial and peripheral pathologies that can be responsible.

PROXIMAL WEAKNESS AND WASTING

Complaints of difficulty in rising from a bed, for a chair, or from a squatting position; in climbing stairs; or in any task requiring one to raise the arms above the head, such as brushing the hair, hanging the wash, or stacking plates or books on

Table 26-2   Common Causes of Paraparesis*

Acute onset (hours or days)	
Spinal trauma	Fracture-dislocation with compression ischemia, laceration, contusion, or hematoma of the cord
Cord compression	Prolapsed disk Vertebral collapse (malignancy, infective, traumatic)
Acute myelitis	Viral Postinfective Demyelinating disease Ischemia
Cauda equina lesions	Disk herniation, spinal stenosis Tumor
Lower motor neuron lesions	Poliomyelitis Guillain-Barré syndrome Tick paralysis
Slow onset	
Spinal cord compression	Cervical spondylosis Spinal tumor Lesions at foramen magnum
Intracranial	Bilateral lacunar strokes Parasagittal meningioma
Systemic diseases	Subacute combined degeneration
Multiple sclerosis	
Spinocerebellar degenerations	
Motor neuron disease	

*Paraparesis is the term used for weakness, and paraplegia for paralysis of the legs.

shelves, all suggest weakness in the pelvic or shoulder girdle muscles. The causes may lie in the muscles themselves or in the appropriate nerves or nerve roots.

Most of the factors that might differentiate between these are unfortunately not specific, but the history may help to some extent. The family history, for example, is a vital factor in the diagnosis of some neuropathies and of all dystrophies. Duchenne's dystrophy and its variants are sex-linked recessive traits, whereas limb-girdle forms (congenital, childhood, and adult types) are autosomal-recessive. Most other dystrophies are autosomal-dominant traits. If there is no family history, recall that wrong diagnoses made in family members may have been "polio," "stroke," or "arthritis," and that siblings may have died at an early age with more severe forms of neuromuscular disease. Drug and alcohol ingestion is another factor in the history of obvious importance (see Chap. 43), whereas specific questions directed toward endocrine (adrenal, thyroid, and parathyroid) and autoallergic functions (rash, Raynaud's phenomenon, hematuria, joint pain and swelling) are also of value because myopathies may complicate these conditions.

An *onset* in infancy or childhood suggests an inherited muscle disease. Among adults, polymyositis, endocrine/metabolic myopathies, myasthenia, or nerve lesions all are more likely. *Muscle tenderness* appears in polymyositis but seldom in other myopathies; *cramps* are more common in neurogenic disease (see Chap. 27). Symmetry may be found with myopathies and diffuse neuropathies, but it is seldom seen in isolated nerve lesions. It is much more common for symmetric neuropathies to occur in the distal rather than the proximal muscles.

Weakness of the *ocular muscles* occurs with some dystrophies, especially the myotonic form, in myasthenia, and in hyperthyroidism; but also with progressive external ophthalmoplegia (see Chap. 21). *Facial involvement* is seen in some dystrophies, myasthenia gravis, and the Guillain-Barré syndrome; thus it is not very helpful in determining the site of the pathology. *Bulbar involvement* causing dysphonia, dysphagia, and dysarthria can be caused by both neurogenic and myopathic processes such as motor neuron disease, poliomyelitis, diphtheria, botulism, myasthenia, polymyositis, and muscular dystrophies. If the *neck* is very weak, consider polymyositis, myasthenia, myotonic and facioscapulohumeral dystrophies, or hyperthyroidism. In Table 26-3, causes of severe *respiratory muscle* weakness are listed.

Muscle twitching *(fasciculations)* suggests anterior horn cell disease, but it is occasionally seen in polymyositis and with root lesions. Patients may ignore their wasting but will often note fasciculations. Associated *long-tract signs* naturally exclude any primary muscle disease. *Reflex loss* suggests either neuropathy or chronic and severe myopathy. Proximal *sensory symptoms* such as numbness or paresthesia should make one consider cord or root lesions in the cervical or lumbosacral areas, or else peripheral neuropathy.

Fatigability is classic in myasthenia but an uncommon complaint in other types of proximal muscle weakness. *Intermittent weakness* may occur in periodic paralysis and in myasthenia. Improvement of stiffness and weakness with exercise is seen in some myotonic disorders. *Weakness without wasting* occurs in some patients with myasthenia, polymyositis, and some metabolic myopathies, but usually the two occur together. The muscles may be unusually large: in Duchenne's dystrophy, hypothyroidism, and some storage diseases, the calves or tongue may show this apparent *hypertrophy*. Wasting with surprisingly good power may occur with generalized cachexia.

In summary, diffuse proximal weakness usually indicates a myopathic process. Rarely, a neuropathy may be primarily proximal as in some cases of the Guillain-Barré syndrome and the spinal muscular atrophies. The list of possible causes of proximal muscle weakness given in Table 26-4 should be considered as for reference only. The most useful and basic approach is first to decide whether the weakness is nonspecific or is due to muscle or nerve disease. Having made that decision, one can then approach such a diagnostic list for more specific possibilities.

Table 26-3   Neurological Causes of Acute Respiratory Failure

Cord	Spinal cord lesion above C4
Nerve	Guillain-Barré syndrome
	Porphyria
	Poliomyelitis
	Diphtheria
	Tetanus
	Motor neuron disease (terminal)
End-plate	Myasthenic crisis
	Cholinergic crisis
	Poisoning

Table 26-4   Causes of Proximal Weakness*

Neuronal disorders

    Guillain-Barré syndrome
    Spinal muscular atrophies (hereditary motor neuropathies)
    Cord or nerve root lesions, e.g., C5,6; L1,2,3
    Neuralgic amyotrophy
    Diabetic proximal motor neuropathies

Muscle diseases

    Inherited dystrophies
    Periodic paralyses
    Acquired myopathies (e.g., hypokalemic, polymyositis,
      collagen-vascular diseases, chemical and drug-
      induced disease, hyperthyroidism, etc.)

*Most of these conditions are described in Chapters 44 and
45.

DISTAL WEAKNESS

Distal muscle weakness is almost invariably a result of damage to motor neurons
at the anterior horn cell, motor root, spinal nerve, plexus, peripheral nerve, or
motor end-plate level. Primary diseases of muscle are rarely the cause.

Clinical Approach

Distal muscle wasting and weakness affecting the arms produces weakness of fine
movements of the fingers, so that while weights may be lifted or the arms raised
above the head, small tasks such as threading a needle, writing, playing a musical

instrument, or doing up buttons, will be particularly affected. Patients are usually aware of the wasting of muscles in the hands because they can see them, unlike their shoulder or pelvic girdles, for example. They may also be aware of fasciculations or of deformity in the hands. In the legs, weakness of the feet may give rise to complaints of discomfort or foot pain toward the end of the day or after any exercise, and of difficulty standing on tip-toe. Patients may catch their feet in rugs and on steps. The likely causes of distal muscle weakness and wasting may be classified according to the site of the lesion producing them.

Acute Cord Lesions

Pyramidal signs may be expected below the level of the lesion, as well as long-tract sensory loss with a well-defined upper level. Radicular pain may occur and dysesthesia or anesthesia may be found in a segmental distribution corresponding to the level of the cord affected. Such lesions may be due to *transverse myelitis, bleeding into the cord, compression* due to trauma, *poliomyelitis,* and *cord ischemia,* either because of pressure from a *prolapsed disk* or in association with *dissecting aneurysm* of the aorta.

Chronic Cord Lesions

Here again pyramidal signs and long-tract sensory loss should be sought below the level of the lesion. With *syringomyelia,* dissociated anesthesia (Chap. 9), a pyramidal syndrome and anterior horn cell damage occur. In *motor neuron disease,* the anterior horn cell and corticospinal tract damage produce both upper and lower motor neuron lesions. *Cord ischemia,* pressure from a local *disk,* or *neoplasm,* and the chronic *spinal muscular atrophies* are other causes of anterior horn cell disease, with or without long tract signs.

A prolapsed cervical disk and cervical spondylosis may compress the anterior roots causing atrophy of arm or hand muscles. Less common root lesions are extradural *tumors, arachnoiditis,* and *chronic meningitis.* If the posterior roots are also involved, sensory changes and radicular pain will be further complaints.

Lower lumbar root lesions, caused by, for example, *prolapsed disks, myelodysplasia,* or *arachnoiditis* can lead to wasting of those muscles innervated by L4, L5, and S1. The bulk of the calf or anterior tibial muscles may be visibly reduced, but wasting of the intrinsic muscles of the foot is hard to identify clinically.

Brachial or Lumbosacral Plexus Lesions

The peripheral bronchogenic carcinoma that spreads from the apex of the lung into the lower part of the brachial plexus *(Pancoast tumor)* usually causes severe pain with weakness and atrophy of the small muscles of the hands. Sensory change accompanies this, in the distribution of the lower trunk of the brachial plexus, which carries fibers distined for the median, ulnar, and medial cutaneous nerves of the arm and forearm. Sensory diminution thus will occur on the ulnar side of the hand and on the medial side of the forearm and arm up to the axilla, and perhaps in median nerve territory too. Weakness and wasting will be exclusively located in the median and ulnar territories.

Pressure from lymphadenopathy may produce a similar picture as may, rarely, cervical ribs, which usually only cause Raynaud's phenomenon in the hands. If an infant is found to have wasting of the small hand muscles, there may have been *traction* on the lower part of the brachial plexus at birth, particularly in a breech delivery with aftercoming arms.

Lumbosacral plexus lesions are less common; diabetic motor neuropathies are most common, but psoas muscle and other retroperitoneal masses can involve the fibers destined for the quadriceps or adductors. More distal lesions, because of direct or indirect trauma (e.g., compression by the fetal head, misplaced injections, or pelvic fractures), may lead to peripheral weakness through direct damage to the sciatric nerve.

Median, Ulnar, and Peroneal Nerve Lesions

The most common causes of these are continued chronic pressure upon the ulnar nerve at the elbow where it lies in the olecranon groove behind the medial epicondyle, or upon the median nerve at the wrist where it crosses underneath the flexor retinaculum. The former produces the cubital tunnel syndrome, the latter the carpal tunnel syndrome (Chap. 44). With a median nerve lesion, the thenar musculature will be wasted and weak, while with an ulnar lesion there will be weakness of the thumb adductor, long flexors of the fifth and fourth fingers, and of the interossei. Root lesions of C8 and T1 or generalized *peripheral* neuropathies are otherwise likely causes if both thenar *and* hypothenar muscles are involved as well as the interossei.

Common peroneal palsy is indeed common, usually as a result of compression but sometimes as part of a multiple mononeuropathy. Posterior tibial nerve lesions are unusual. Almost any cause of a generalized peripheral neuropathy can lead to weakness and wasting of distal leg muscles, often long before the hands are similarly involved. Patients who have a hemiparesis are particularly prone to develop a common peroneal palsy on that side (Maloney's sign). This probably is due to the continued immobility of their externally rotated leg as it lies on the mattress.

Primary Muscle Disease

Distal muscles share in the wasting process of any severe, long-standing myopathy, but only at a late stage. Proximal wasting will have antedated wasting in the hands or feet. In the earlier stages of *myotonic dystrophy,* small hand-muscle wasting may be seen, but one should also look for diminution of the bulk of the sternomastoids and for facial weakness (Chap. 45). Rare *distal myopathies* are described.

Local Causes

With *rheumatoid arthritis, Raynaud's phenomenon, vascular insufficiency* from any cause, *prolonged immobilization,* or *disuse,* wasting of all distal muscles is often found in association with trophic changes such as atrophy of the fingertips and nails, loss of hair, and thickening or swelling of the skin.

27
Muscle Cramps, Stiffness, and Pain

Muscle contraction results from the sliding of the actin and myosin filaments between each other as a result of electrical excitation. The action potential is transferred across the synaptic cleft by chemical means, causing depolarization of the end-plate and inducing a spreading action potential throughout the muscle. The release of calcium from the sarcoplasmic reticulum initiates the contraction. The sliding-filament theory of muscle contraction holds that filaments of actin and myosin are interdigitated and that these filaments slide between each other during contraction because of the movement of crossbridges between them. In the presence of ATP, Mg^{2+}, and Ca^{2+} (now released by the arriving action potential), enough energy is produced to initiate the sliding of the actin and myosin filaments together. The resultant tension is the contraction.

Relaxation is also a process requiring energy for the active reaccumulation of calcium by the sarcoplasmic reticulum. The system seems at first sight to be fairly simple, but there are complexities. The main one is that the muscle contains at any time only enough ATP (which must be recreated by a number of metabolic processes), for a few contractions. This "recharging" is slower than the rate of destruction of ATP.

The chemical disorders that may give rise to cramps because of failure of muscle relaxation include abnormalities of muscle glycogen metabolism, abnormal interaction of actin and myosin causing a persistent contraction in the absence of initiating action potentials, and failure of the sarcoplasmic reticulum to reaccumulate calcium.

MUSCLE CRAMPS

Origin in Nerve

The condition known as *ordinary muscle cramps* may occur at any age. The calves are usually affected, and the muscle is felt by the patient as hard and partly contracted so that the ankle cannot be dorsiflexed voluntarily and pain is felt deeply in the muscle. This symptom is particularly common in elderly people at night and is a frequent cause of loss of sleep and great discomfort. The precise causes are not known, but the site of the abnormality is thought to be in the spinal cord or motor nerves rather than in the muscle itself. Medication taken at night may prevent the cramps: quinine sulfate, 200-400 mg; calcium lactate, 600 mg; or phenytoin (Dilantin), 200 mg are all effective.

The most common cause of cramps in young women is *pregnancy*. Other causes at any age include *dehydration* and partial *denervation of muscle* from any cause. Motor neuron disease is one important example. In such cases the symptom is invariably associated with activity and ceases when the patient relaxes. *Prolonged* contraction of muscles can also cause cramping physiologically, which may be the cause of abdominal or leg cramps during swimming in cold water.

Hypocalcemia or *alkalosis* from any cause may produce tetany and cramping pain. The disorder is thought to be due to an abnormality of the terminal motor nerve fibers rather than of intramuscular calcium metabolism.

Origin in Muscle

Cramps may be due to *sodium depletion*, for example, with heavy sweating (Stokers), dialysis, or other causes of unusual loss, renal or gastrointestinal; in adrenocortical deficiency: or with excessive ADH secretion. Reduced sodium intake, as in treatment of cardiac failure or hypertension, may also be responsible.

If the energy demand of muscles exceeds that available, as in *glycogen storage diseases* (Chap. 45), then some muscle fibers will be "caught" in contraction. The lack of available energy may prevent both calcium reuptake by the sarcoplasmic reticulum after contraction and the shortening of the crossbridges between actin and myosin. Such shortening, not associated with action potentials, is called a *contracture*. *Rigor mortis* is due to the same metabolic failure.

Origin in the Central Nervous System

Tetanus is cause of cramps and of stiffness at rest. Tetanus toxin is an inhibitor of inhibitory postsynaptic potentials, and the resulting excessive activity in the anterior horn cells is transmitted to the muscles.

The rare *stiff-person syndrome*** may have a similar pathogenesis, and a reduction of the inhibitory, with an increase in the excitatory, postsynaptic potentials affecting anterior horn cells also occurs in *parkinsonism, dystonias, phenothiazine* poisoning, and in occupational cramps. In many cases of upper motor neuron disease, such as multiple sclerosis and cord lesions, painful spasms of muscle groups occur as an excessive response to muscle stretch. When the cord is partially transected, extensor spasms are common. The severity of the spasm and of the pain can usually be lessened with baclofen.

---

*Really the "stiff-man syndrome," but it now has been described in a woman.

Occupational cramps, such as may be experienced by writers, telegraphists, and others, probably occur on the basis of some abnormal conditioned reflex induced by their repetitive activity and not as a result of any peripheral disease. In such cases the muscle may go into spasm, producing pain and tightness, but just as commonly there is no cramp at all; the patient can use the muscle satisfactorily for other tasks but not for the particular maneuvers that produced the symptom in the first place. In the short-term, the prognosis is excellent, and function quickly returns after a period of rest, but the patient may become seriously disabled by these symptoms if they continue; treatment using behavioral therapy or deconditioning has, at times, been effective.

MUSCLE STIFFNESS

Uncommonly, a patient's leading complaint is of undue firmness or failure of relaxation of muscles. *Tetany* (Chap. 42) usually produces this symptom locally (carpopedal spasm) and may be painless. *Pyramidal and extrapyramidal* lesions are next most often responsible for the symptom but may also cause pain. If no signs of these are evident, remember that *hypothyroidism* may present with slow muscle relaxation. Here, the failure of normal relaxation of muscles, best seen with the ankle jerk, is neither an electrical nor a biochemical abnormality but is due to mechanical difficulties which prevent the myofibrils from sliding past each other at a normal rate during relaxation.

In *myotonia* (Chap. 45) excessive irritability of the muscle membrane induces repetitive bursts of action potentials after a normal impulse has induced a contraction. Clinically, the muscle appears to relax very slowly after maximal activity or percussion. Stiffness is mild and cramp uncommon. The pathogenesis is uncertain, but it may be an alteration in membrane resistance, in sodium permeability, or of membrane cholesterol content.

In *pseudomyotonia,* repetitive electrical discharges of shorter duration occur. This is an EMG finding in muscles that are partly denervated and in cases of polymyositis or hypothyroidism.

Neuromyotonia is an exotically rare disorder of the terminal motor nerve fibers in which excessively abundant action potentials are transmitted to the muscles producing myotonia, myokymia, and stiffness. Cramps are not an important symptom. The excessive muscle activity leads to sweating and an increased metabolic rate, but symptoms respond dramatically to phenytoin or procainamide therapy.

MUSCLE PAIN

Pain and tenderness in muscles may occur in a large number of diseases, as listed in Table 27-1. Primary muscle diseases, muscle involvement in collagen-vascular disease, peripheral neuropathy, and various systemic conditions appear in that list, but the common factor that finally produces muscle discomfort or pain is not certain, in any case. The presence of some metabolic product within the muscle may be responsible.

In everyday language, *stiffness* within muscles means muscle tenderness on movement with discomfort on palpation. Cramp from any cause may leave residual muscle stiffness. The most typical form is that which occurs after unaccustomed heavy *exercise* or after an attack of *ordinary muscle cramps.* Painful stiffness may also be a presenting feature of certain collagen-vascular disorders such as *rheumatoid arthritis,* in which it occurs most characteristically in the morning,

Table 27-1   Causes of Tender Muscles

Muscle disorders

    Following cramps from any cause, flexor spasms, or direct trauma

Inflammatory myopathy	Polymyositis Polymyalgia rheumatica Infective (parasitic, bacterial)
Toxic myopathy	Alcohol Drugs (see Chap. 43)
Metabolic myopathy	$1°/2°$ hyperparathyroidism
Genetically determined	Glycogen storage diseases Other muscle enzyme deficiency states Idiopathic paroxysmal myoglobinuria

    Ischemia

    Deep vein thrombosis

Nerve disorders

Peripheral neuropathy	Alcoholism Guillain-Barré syndrome Vitamin B_{12} or vitamin C deficiency Diabetes Myelomatosis, amyloidosis

    Poliomyelitis

    Nerve root lesions (?)

Systemic causes

Infections	Mononucleosis, brucellosis, leptospirosis, mumps, influenza and coxsackievirus infections

    Hemophilia

    Leukemia

    Porphyria

    Uremia

Idiopathic

Depressive illness

decreasing as the patient continues with daily activities. In *polymyalgia rheumatica* there is stiffness in the proximal muscles without pain. Muscle discomfort will be felt following direct muscle *trauma* where, again, the cause is thought to be a local metabolic substance producing pain.

    The other myopathic causes are described in Chapter 45. Pain may also occur in muscles working in the presence of *arterial* or *venous insufficiency*.

Many *peripheral neuropathies* are painful because of hyperpathia, but those listed are also accompanied by muscle pain. In ischemic mononeuropathies, such as diabetic femoral neuropathy, the muscle pain is more symptomatic than the weakness. In certain *infectious diseases,* muscle pain is striking; why these and the other system diseases cause pain is poorly understood. A syndrome of leg muscle pain and fasciculations with an abnormal EMG is recognized and called, very reasonably, "painful legs and moving toes." Lumbar root disease is a possible cause, but its origin and nature are unclear.

A chronic syndrome of muscle pain at rest, made worse by exertion and unassociated with physical signs or abnormal enzyme, EMG, or biopsy studies, is a real clinical entity that awaits solution. Some of these patients lose their pain with small doses of baclofen, amitriptyline, or quinine. In most, no treatment works.

Finally, remember that *depressed* patients often complain of generalized muscle pain and tenderness.

BIBLIOGRAPHY

Layzer, R.B. *Neuromuscular Complications of Systemic Disease. Contemporary Neurology Series.* No. 25. Philadelphia, F.A. Davis Co., 1985.

28
Clumsiness

If you stand up, walk into another room, wind up your watch and set it correctly, and then turn out the light and leave without experiencing any difficulty in your motor actions, you then will have used successfully all the mechanisms upon which smooth coordination and powerful activity depend. The term *clumsiness* denotes any inaccuracy or difficulty in performing a motor act, compared with a hypothetical norm, and it indicates that some sensory, integrative, motor, or mechanical problem has interfered with the normal performance of motor acts. Because the symptom is nonspecific, all questioning must initially be directed toward finding out which system disorder has produced it.

CLINICAL APPROACH

One's approach must be to determine whether cortical, ocular, vestibular, cerebellar, upper or lower motor neuron, proprioceptive, or mechanical abnormalities are present.

Cortex

One of the most common reasons for being clumsy is lack of care, caused by preoccupation or distraction, often related to *emotional* factors such as depression or anxiety. Children with *minimal cerebral dysfunction* commonly have overactivity, gaucheness, and irritability; schizophrenics are said to be awkward in their movements. *Anticonvulsants, sedatives, and alcohol* may induce or worsen clumsiness in anybody.

In all such cases, the individual will seem to exhibit a lack of care, forgetfulness, or gaucheness in movement, rather than to show any specific motor or sensory

signs. Any tremor may produce clumsiness. People with lapses of attention because of petit mal or focal *epilepsy* may occasionally seem to be awkward in their
movements and may have accidents when their alertness is reduced because of a
(subclinical) seizure.

Eyes

The patient's visual acuity must be assessed. Most people will be aware of a refractive error themselves but those with a *visual field defect* may be unaware of
it and as a result have driving accidents, bump into things on one side, or knock
things over repeatedly. Double vision, oscillopsia, blurring, monocular blindness
with loss of stereoscopic vision, and tearing, all may produce difficulty with fine
movements such as threading a needle, putting objects on a surface, or writing;
or may lead to complaints similar to those resulting from a visual field defect.
Decreased visual acuity may also cause people to feel less secure in walking or
turning, thus they seem awkward. It will also produce a feeling of swaying if
peripheral sensation and eighth nerve function are diminished (the multisensory
syndrome).

Vestibular Apparatus

Disorders of the central or peripheral vestibular apparatus may produce vertigo,
a subjective sensation of movement of the self or of the environment. This is
likely to be the leading symptom, rather than clumsiness. Instability may however
result, with great difficulty in orienting the self in space, perhaps so great that
the patient has to remain lying down because he is afraid of falling off the bed or
chair. Vertigo was discussed in Chapter 24.

   Impaired balance will also be a feature of central cerebellar and of proprioceptive lesions (see later discussion).

Upper Motor Neuron

Corticospinal tract lesions may cause spasticity, weakness, clonus, and inability
to carry out fine movements. Visual and other sensory abnormalities often coexist. The weakness mainly affects the arm extensors and the leg flexors. The
loss of finely graded muscle control often reduces dexterity because power returns
more to proximal than to distal muscle groups.

   If the extrapyramidal system is involved, then abnormal movements, changes
in tone, or bradykinesia may distort normal movements (Chap. 29).

Cerebellum

Clumsiness caused by an isolated cerebellar lesion is uncommon. When it does occur, the patient's major problems will be ataxia of gait and incoordination of all
voluntary movements, especially fine ones (Chap. 2). Nystagmus will commonly
be present, adding to the patient's difficulty if it causes oscillopsia (in which objects appear to wobble, so fixation is hard to maintain). Corticospinal, propricep-
tive, or visual problems also frequently accompany cerebellar disorders.

   Some patients are referred because their family complain that their speech
is disjointed and hard to understand, or because the police or neighbors level unjustified accusations of insobriety. When walking, they veer to one side, and their
loss of manual dexterity may also be asymmetric.

With a central cerebellar lesion involving the flocculonodular lobe or the vermis, truncal ataxia is likely. In such cases, the usual tests of coordination may be performed normally while the patient is lying down, but he is hard put to maintain an upright posture, and walking may be impossible. The differing functions of the cerebellar lateral lobes and the older, central areas are well demonstrated in this circumstance. Tests of voluntary limb movements alone are never sufficient in evaluating cerebellar function and must always be supplemented by examination of upright stance and gait.

Lower Motor Neuron

Lower motor neuron disorders give rise to distal, more often than to proximal, weakness. If the symptom is due to a lesion of a nerve root, plexus, or peripheral nerve, the patient may be aware of atrophy, fasciculations, trophic changes, Raynaud's phenomenon, and sensory symptoms, all usually asymmetric. Distal weakness is manifest not in the more gross but rather in finer tasks, such as sewing, doing up buttons, and manipulating objects in the hand, e.g., picking up pins, paper, or coins.

Local Limb Lesions

Distal lesions, if caused by joint disease, may be accompanied by pain, swelling, stiffness, and deformity. Other local lesions should be obvious on inspection.

Proprioceptive System

Patients who are clumsy because of diminished or inaccurate proprioceptive feedback will have their greatest problems when visual cues are removed; thus at nighttime, in theaters, or in dimly lit corridors, walking may be impossible. Because discriminative touch sensation is mediated by the same pathways, except to hear complaints of heaviness, deadness, numbness, or paresthesia as well. Such patients have great difficulty in performing voluntary motor acts outside the range of their vision, such as finding objects in their handbags, taking a specific coin out of their pocket, brushing their hair at the back, and dressing. Other modalities of sensory loss may also be altered. The increased unsteadiness when visual cues are removed is demonstrated by Romberg's test. If there is a proprioceptive defect, the patient can stand with the eyes open but falls when he closes them. Medical students misinterpret this test as one for cerebellar disease, but it was described to demonstrate proprioceptive loss specifically.

BIBLIOGRAPHY

Gubbay, S. *The Clumsy Child. Major Problems in Neurology*, No. 5: Toronto, Saunders, 1975.

29
Disorders of Movement

There are many forms of involuntary movement, ranging from those caused by lesions of the muscle (myotonia, cramps) or spinal cord (fasciculations, cramps) to those caused by disorders of the brainstem (nystagmus, myoclonus) or of the brain itself (chorea, dystonias, epilepsy, etc.).

The following is a description of the different abnormalities with brief comments on what is known of their genesis.

IRREGULAR MOVEMENTS CAUSED
BY DISEASE OF THE BASAL GANGLIA

The extrapyramidal system is involved in motor control through a complex organization involving the cerebellum, basal ganglia, cortex, pyramidal tracts, vestibular nuclei, and the reticular activating system of the brainstem. Understanding the brain has been made harder by our habit of trying to define the function of a specific structure when it really operates as part of a complex mechanism. Such is the case with the basal ganglia, which function only within this complex motor system. However some specific lesions within the basal ganglia do give rise to typical signs in the area of motor control.

Rigidity

Rigidity is characteristically seen in Parkinson's disease and is manifest by a relatively constant resistance to muscle stretching in both flexors and extensors (plastic rigidity) or by a ratchetlike feeling when, for example, the wrist or arm is quickly flexed and extended (cogwheel rigidity). Rigidity differs thus from spasticity, which initially increases as more and more motor units are recruited until

inhibition of resistance is fired by the Golgi tendon organs. In rigidity, the stretching force induces some motor units to fire, but as the stretch continues, some drop
out as others are recruited, producing a smooth, constant resistance.

Bradykinesia

Although tremor and rigidity are the most dramatic aspects of Parkinson's disease,
the most disabling symptom is bradykinesia, an overall poverty of movement. Im-
plied in this term is a loss of automatic movements, accompanying both postural
and volitional activities. The patient begins to sit without making the normal small
alterations of posture, the shuffling and slight restlessness that one normally exhibits. The face becomes expressionless and tends to stare unblinking like a statue.
When the patient walks, he lacks the normal automatic postural corrections if he
gets off balance, does not swing his arms, and makes movements such as turning
as if his body were a single block. The loss of those automatic postural movements
that we take for granted makes it very difficult to reach for objects, to turn over
a bed, or to walk on uneven ground. Rigidity, tremor, and bradykinesia result from
lesions in the substantia nigra and globus pallidus; and perhaps in the RAS.

Athetosis

Athetosis is a writhing, sinuous, alternating contraction of agonistic and antagonistic muscles, more in the arms than the legs, which result from alternating contractions of flexors and extensors. As with many movement disorders, it is difficult
to define this one specifically enough to differentiate it clearly from others; different physicians seeing the same patient may describe the abnormality as myoclonus,
athetosis, chorea, or choreoathetosis. The lesion probably involves the putamen.

Chorea

Chorea is a sudden involuntary jerking movement involving a muscle or muscle
group, which can involve the arms and hands, tongue, legs, trunk, and even the
respiratory muscles but is best seen distally. Initially the patient is often able to
convert these into purposeful movements, thus masking them. An early sign is
often an inability to keep the tongue protruded and still because choreic movements
cause it to retract into the mouth. If the patient holds his arms over his head, they
will tend to take up a position of pronation with the palms facing forward and outward, the *pronator sign*. If very marked, the movements may interfere with posture
and walking and may give rise to a tragicomic gait. The lesion probably involves
the caudate nucleus most severely.

Hemiballismus

In this dramatic disorder there are flinging movements of one or both limbs on one
side of the body. The term *ballismus* would be used if the disorder was bilateral.
Because the movements may be continuous they can cause excessive fatigue or, indeed, exhaustion. Treatment with haloperidol or fluphenazine is effective. The
lesion involves the contralateral subthalamic nucleus.

Dystonia

Dystonia refers to a strong, sustained, and slow contraction of muscle groups that
cause twisting or writhing of a limb or of the whole body. This may occur in the

tongue, neck, trunk, or limbs: dystonias may be generalized or focal. The contractions are often painful and may result in gross disfigurement. Their strength may actually fracture bones or tear muscles. Dystonic movements last a minute or so, dystonic postures may be sustained for hours or even permanently and may persist in sleep. Sometimes dystonias are sparked off or stopped by certain movements; postural change and hypnosis may also inhibit them, leading to a wrong diagnosis of hysteria. Athetosis may blend into chorea if the movements are short and quick, it also blends into dystonia if it is slower and involves a more widespread contraction of muscle groups. Dystonia results from lesions in sites unknown. When there is no detectable CNS hereditary or acquired disease (of which a host are sometimes associated with dystonias), genetic causes are likely. Chemical and drug causes are listed in Chapter 43.

OTHER LOCALIZED IRREGULAR MOVEMENTS

At the level of the lower motor neuron, a number of abnormalities may occur. *Fasciculations* are brief, rippling contractions of the muscle fibers of a single motor unit (consisting of an anterior horn cell, its axon and divisions, the end-plates, and the muscle fibers that it supplies). Damage to the anterior horn cell may cause spontaneous, involuntary impulses to pass down the axon and produce contraction of all the muscle fibers in that unit. This is not enough to move a joint but may certainly be seen and is frequently felt by the patient. Exercise and tapping the muscle both make fasciculations more obvious. Although it is suggested that damage to the nerve and motor end-plate may produce fasciculations, it may be taken as a clinical rule of thumb that they imply damage to the anterior horn cell or the first few millimeters of its axon, close to the spinal cord (Table 29-1).

Fibrillations cannot be seen by the naked eye in the tongue or anywhere else. They are contractions of single myofibrils that become hyperresponsive to circulating cholinergic substances as a result of denervation.

Myokymia is a rippling contraction of muscles, with many causes (Table 29-2). It occurs most frequently around the periorbital muscles and also in the thighs of people who are tired. It is occasionally a sign of brainstem disease, as in multiple sclerosis. It may have the same mechanism as regularly occurring fasciculations in a group of cranial nerve nuclei or anterior horn cells.

Myotonia is a failure of immediate relaxation of a muscle. On the EMG it is manifest as a high-frequency but slowing discharge, which occurs following movement or after stimulation by moving the needle inside the muscle. It is a valuable sign of muscle disease, occurring in a number of dominantly inherited disorders and is probably caused by irritability of the myofibrillar membrane. Clinically, patients complain of inability to relax after making a movement, and it may also be shown in the reflexes by a "hung-up" response.

Neuromyotonia is a delayed relaxation of muscle following a voluntary contraction occasionally seen with chronic neuropathies or as part of a syndrome when combined with fasciculations, myokymia, and continuous discharges in motor neurons. The basis of the symptom is hyperexcitability of the nerves, and the treatment is carbamazepine.

In this section, we should also mention the effects of *abnormal reinnervation* of muscles after nerve injury. After severe damage to a peripheral nerve, fibers may sprout into incorrect channels. Thus an attempted movement may actually produce an entirely different one or lead to contraction of abnormally innervated muscles. This is not a common problem, but when it occurs one can usually obtain

Table 29-1   Causes of Fasciculations

Benign

Anterior horn cell/axonal lesions

    Motor neuron disease
    Hereditary motor neuropathies (spinal
      muscular atrophies) and other
      motor neuropathies
    Poliomyelitis and other myelitides
    Cord compression or other trauma
    Syringomyelia

Metabolic-endocrine diseases

    Uremia
    Hyperthyroidism
    Hyperparathyroidism, Na^+ deficiency
    Anticholinesterase toxicity

Jakob-Creutzfeldt disease

Polymyositis (uncommon)

Collagen-vascular disease

Table 29-2   Causes of Myokymia

Benign

Poisoning
    MAO inhibitors, lead

Brainstem disease

    Multiple sclerosis
    Encephalitis
    Vascular disease
    Tumor

Hyperthyroidism

Neuromyotonia

a history of previous paralysis in that area. The most distressing of these abnormal reinnervation syndromes is a group of peculiar facial movements that can follow facial palsy. These include jaw-winking, crocodile tears, and a type of *hemifacial spasm.*

Nystagmus is a recurring tendency of the eyes to deviate away from their point of focus and then to correct back again. It is described in Chapter 21.

Opsoclonus signifies brief, chaotic eye movements, most often seen in children with brainstem disease. *Ocular bobbing* refers to conjugate vertical movements of the eyes occurring in patients with pontine lesions, usually encephalitis, hemorrhage, or tumor.

Cramps (see Chap. 27) must be differentiated from muscle *contractures*. With contractures there is no electrical activity within the muscle, which is shortened, firm, and painful because of abnormal sudden biochemical changes such as lack of muscle phosphorylase or chemical poisoning. Contractures also may be due to chronic fibrotic changes within the muscle that prevent its relaxation.

Myoclonus caused by synchronous discharge of many motor neurons may be of cortical, brainstem, or spinal cord origin. It is described in Chapter 15.

Tetany is excessive, continuous muscle fiber activity caused by disease of the neuron, whether a result of alkalosis, hypocalcemia, or failure of those inhibitory mechanisms that would normally dampen neural transmission of impulses to the muscle. As in tetanus, "ordinary muscle cramps" may follow exercise or occur in deep sleep, especially in patients with thyroid disorders, in salt or water deficiency, in pregnancy, or with partial muscle denervation. The cause is uncertain. "Writers' cramp" and other *occupational cramps* are dystonias, and were described earlier.

Decerebrate rigidity is due to a lesion thought to lie between the superior and inferior colliculi. The unconscious patient develops (on one or both sides) a posture in which there are internal rotation of the shoulders, extension of the elbows, marked pronation of the wrist, and metacarpophalangeal flexion. In the legs, there are hip and knee extension with plantar flexion at the ankles. There may be accompanying hyperextension of the spine which, if marked, is called *opisthotonos* and which can also occur in tetanus, grand mal seizures, and hysteria.

Decorticate rigidity is due to a lesion just below the thalamus and produces a similar picture but with flexion at the elbows and strong adduction of the shoulders.

The classic movement disorders in *epilepsy* are the tonic and clonic phases of a grand mal seizure. Focal (partial) seizures, particularly involving the motor strip on one side, may cause localized tonic and clonic movements. Other abnormal movements seen in epilepsy are the fluttering eyelids in petit mal epilepsy and the generalized *automatisms* of temporal lobe seizures, in which the patient makes purposeful or semipurposeful movements without complete, or possibly any, awareness.

REGULAR MOVEMENTS
(TREMORS)

Tremors are more or less regular involuntary repetitive movements seen better distally in the fingers or wrists, but occasionally also in the eyelids, tongue, face, neck, or legs. They are characteristic of diseases affecting various sites in the nervous system, but they can be thought of as occurring in any combination of three situations. The first is *at complete rest,* as seen in Parkinson's disease. The second is while *maintaining a posture* of the hand or wrist, as in anxiety or benign essential tremor. The third is during *voluntary activity,* as in cerebellar disease.

Table 29-3   Common or Important Causes of Tremor

At rest

    Physiological

        High adrenergic tone,
          e.g., anxiety
        Drugs (see Chap. 43)
        Hyperthyroidism
        Parkinson's disease
        Delirium tremens
        General paresis
        Wilson's disease
        Mercury poisoning[*]

    Postural

        All of the above and
        Benign "essential" tremor
        Asterixis
        Red nucleus damage (rubral tremor)

    Action

        Cerebellar diseases
        Parkinson's disease (action component)

---

[*]Hardly common, but as relevant today as 100 years ago when hatters raised the nap on felt hats by brushing them with organic mercury. "Hatter's shakes" referred to the resulting tremor. The Mad Hatter probably would have had mercurial encephalopathy.

    The causes of tremor are many and varied (Table 29-3). If a normal subject extends his arms, they will probably show some fine irregular movements in the fingers, regarded as physiological. In some families such a tremor is coarser, markedly increased in amplitude, and made worse if a subject maintains a posture, e.g., arms extended. This is referred to as an *essential,* benign, or heredofamilial tremor; it should not be confused with parkinsonism. Patients who are markedly *anxious* also increase their physiological tremor, and the tremor of anxiety must be differentiated from that in hyperthyroidism (the only one that is likely to persist during sleep) and from essential tremor. *Hysterical* tremors are compound, asymmetric, frequently asynchronous, and completely atypical. However some bizarre tremors are due to organic causes (red nucleus tremor, for example), hence the diagnosis cannot be made just because the tremor looks odd. The diagnosis of hysteria must be made on positive grounds, and other aspects of the history and examination should confirm the diagnosis. In *hypothyroidism,* a tremor similar to that caused by cerebellar disease may be seen, while *hyperthyroidism* causes a markedly accentuated physiological tremor. Patients withdrawing from sedatives and those with certain disease such as *GPI, delirium tremens,* and *heavy-metal poisoning* may show a bilaterally symmetric, coarse tremor at rest, worse distally, and more severe in the arms than in the legs.

With *cerebellar disease* or disease of the *red nucleus,* tremor is observed that is a coarse, usually side-to-side movement of the arms or legs interrupting a voluntary action and absent at rest. This is the well-known *intention* or *action* tremor.

An irregular, flapping, coarse tremor of the hands, best seen at the wrists with the palms extended forward and upward occurs in chronic hepatic, renal, and respiratory disease (*asterixis* or flapping tremor). It is asymmetric, asynchronous, and bilateral.

A common sign of *basal ganglia* disease is a resting tremor at about 4 to 6 Hz (cycles per second). In the hands, especially in the thumb and index finger, it gives rise to the "pill-rolling" tremor, a term that harkens back to an age in which pharmacists rolled medicaments into small balls between their fingers. This tremor is prominent in the wrist, arm, and legs. Its development may be a random process, starting in any limb and later spreading to other areas. There has been some controversy over its origin; it probably arises from a lesion in the cerebellum or in the connections with the corpus striatum through the globus pallidus to the thalamus. The fact that stereotactic surgery may eliminate the tremor by placing a lesion in the thalamus does not solve the problem of where along this pathway it originates.

SEMIPURPOSIVE MOVEMENTS

Other cerebral cortical abnormalities produce a variety of movement disorders. In children, with or without diffuse brain disease, one may see tics, rhythmias, head-banging, and hyperkinesis. *Tics* are stereotyped simple movements, usually of nervous origin, that are repetitive, often unilateral, and more commonly occurring around the face or in the proximal parts of the limbs. An organic cause is seldom found, although some tics may result from a combination of organic and functional disturbances. In some children they begin as voluntary motor acts that relieve tension, but later they may become repetitive when they occur without any thought and are to a great extent involuntary, although they may be voluntarily suppressed. *Rhythmias* are repetitive, compound movements, usually side-to-side or to-and-fro, made with the trunk, head, and neck. They are usually seen in children with generalized brain disease. In adults a tremor of the head or neck of fairly large amplitude and at rates of 2 to 3 Hz may occur with brainstem disease as in multiple sclerosis; this is known as *titubation.* Children with generalized overactivity, frequently associated with spitefulness, head-banging, bad temper, brief attention span, and destructiveness are said to be suffering from hyperkinetic states, usually in association with localized or more generalized but minimal cerebral dysfunction (Chap. 39).

BIBLIOGRAPHY

Barbeau, A. (ed.). Movement disorders. In *Current Status of Modern Therapy,* Vol. 8. Lancaster, MTP Press, 1981.

Marsden, C.D., Fahn, S. (eds.). *Movement disorders.* London, Butterworth Scientific, 1982.

30
Pain in the Back

In the evaluation of back pain, the history is usually enough to enable distinction between the four major types of pain that occur. These are those due to root irritation; arising from muscles or ligaments; arising from vertebral structures; or referred to the back from elsewhere.

VARIETIES OF PAIN

Root Pain

Pain felt in root distribution may arise from traction, irritation, or compression of a dorsal root or its ganglion. In character sharp, knifelike, or continuously burning, it may be of any degree of severity. One can often localize the involved root as the pain is referred to a defined dermatomal area — L3 to the anterior thigh, calf, and dorsum of the foot; L4 to the shin; L5 to the dorsum of the foot; S1 to the posterior thigh, calf, and sole of the foot; and S2 to the back and buttocks. Coughing, local percussion of the spine, or spinal movement (particularly flexion) will aggravate root pain, while rest may relieve it to some extent.

Examination may show decreased or altered subjective sensation in the affected dermatomal area. Lower motor neuron signs and reflex changes may be present because of anterior or posterior root compression or irritation.

After some time, the pain acquires a more constant, dull aching quality, possibly because of spasm in the muscles innervated by that root.

Muscle and Ligamentous Pain

Another type of pain is recognized occurring in association with spondylosis or following slight or moderate trauma to the back. This type varies from a dull ache up to a sharp pain with a background of continual burning discomfort. It is often hard to localize exactly. This pain is reduced when the patient walks and is worse with standing in one position, lying in bed, sitting (especially in a car), with spinal flexion, and with coughing. The patient may have difficulty in localizing it. If it radiates, it does not exactly follow any dermatomal distribution but may be felt diffusely in the back or in the lateral spine but usually more laterally over the sacrospinalis or the pelvic girdle muscles, such as gluteus maximus or medius. Sensory features are usually entirely subjective, reflexes are normal, and there is no muscle wasting or weakness except that induced by the pain.

Bone Pain

This dull, deep pain has a boring or aching nature. It is again ill-localized, does not radiate unless vertebral collapse or root pressure produces a radicular element, and is usually of slow onset and continuous. If caused by bone trauma or neoplasm, especially if there is a pathological fracture, pain is frequently worse at night and is made worse still by any local percussion or jarring of the spine, such as occurs with walking down stairs.

Referred pain to the Back

Diseased abdominal and thoracic viscera may cause pain felt in the back if the lesion involves the posterior peritoneal or retroperitoneal structures. Cholecystitis, aortic aneurysm, retrocecal appendicitis, renal colic, pancreatitis, large-bowel disease, and gynecological diseases are examples, although the latter usually refer to sacral areas. The dull, aching, or burning pain is ill-localized, usually bilateral, and constant. Its severity varies with the cause, but it is not worsened by spinal percussion or movement. Skin hyperesthesia is often found in the relevant dermatomal areas.

EVALUATION

The cause may be obvious from the history in cases of trauma and referred pain from the abdomen, but in all cases a full history must document all the characteristics of the pain, as described previously, and in particular its mode of onset. Clinical evidence of neurological involvement (such as fasciculations, wasting, reflex or sensory change, or bladder involvement) and of intraabdominal disease is sought by a careful examination. Spinal evaluation then proceeds in four major steps.

Inspection

First examine the patient's *gait* and *standing posture* for pelvic tilt, kyphosis, lordosis, or scoliosis, and for the presence of muscle spasm on either side of the spine at any level. Examine the *shoes* for evidence of unusual localized wear or scuffing. Congenital spinal disorders may be accompanied by a lipoma, a midline cleft in the skin, horizontal silver striae, or an abnormal tuft of hair over the midline. *Trophic changes* and *muscle atrophy,* particularly in the quadriceps, anterior tibial muscles, or gastrocnemius should be noted.

The *range of movement* of the spine in flexion, extension, lateral flexion to both sides, and rotation in each direction must be assessed and the patient may be asked to cough or perform a Valsalva maneuver, which will worsen pain caused by root irritation. If the patient bends one knee on flexing his spine, this is another indication of root disease.

Palpation

Palpation may reveal areas of local tenderness within muscles (in which case a small knot of unusually firm muscles may be felt causing exquisite pain on pressure, *a trigger zone*) or on percussion of the spine, when the patient may feel pain in root distribution. Pressure on the iliac crests downward and sideways may elicit pain, suggesting sacroiliac joint disease. One must *measure* the circumference of the thighs and calves and also the distance on each side between the anterior superior iliac spine and the medial malleolus to detect leg length discrepancies. *Straight-leg raising* must be performed and later, when the patient is in the prone position, passive hip extension (femoral stretch) may increase pain with L2, 3, and 4 root disease.

Examination of the Nervous System

The usual examination of the nervous system may now proceed with exact testing of power within each muscle group, elicitation of knee and ankle reflexes, and examination of sensation with particular attention to altered sensation within any dermatomal distribution (see Chap. 2). Although there is often a good deal of overlap, it is true in general that hip flexion is supplied by L1, adduction by L2, knee extension by L3, ankle eversion by L4, dorsiflexion of the hallux by L5, and plantar flexion by S1.

Examination of the Abdomen
and Genitourinary Systems

Finally, examination of these systems, including a rectal examination, is required in all patients with back pain. It is also wise to check the femoral and distal pulses and to listen for femoral bruits. If pain is at a higher level, intrathoracic disease may be responsible through the mechanism of referred pain.

Investigations

Useful investigations include x-ray of the spine in almost all cases, although the yield is low in the absence of frank clinical signs. Views of the sacroiliac joints, hips, or pelvis may be required as well. Hematological screening, ESR, protein electrophoresis, screening for collagen diseases, urinalysis, and examination of the bone marrow are frequently necessary. Biochemical investigations of greatest yield include estimations of calcium and phosphate and of acid and alkaline phosphatase levels.

Computerized tomographic (CT) scanning is replacing myelography as the procedure of choice in the evaluation of low-back pain with physical signs. These, EMG, and the clinical examination, each produce abnormal findings in about three-quarters of patients with proved pathology.

DISEASES ASSOCIATED
WITH PAIN IN THE BACK

Pain may arise because of diseases of the spine itself, of its supporting ligaments and muscles, of the cord, and (through the mechanisms of referred pain) from intraabdominal structures. Psychogenic back pain is also described. Table 30-1 lists some of the more common causes.

Table 30-1   Common Causes of Back Pain

Age	Diagnosis
2-15 years	Postural (? secondary to leg-length discrepancy), osteochondritis, spondylolisthesis
15-30 years	Prolapsed disk, ankylosing spondylitis, ligamentous and muscle strain, arachnoiditis
30-50 years	Prolapsed disk, ligamentous and muscle strain, spinal stenosis, arachnoiditis
Over 50 years	Spondylosis, osteoporosis with collapse, osteomalacia, secondary neoplasm, myeloma, Paget's disease

Disease of the Spine

Certain *congenital* disorders of the lumbar spine may cause pain mainly by distortion and strain upon a supporting ligament. These include the presence of *hemivertebrae* and *spondylolisthesis.* The former may be suggested if scoliosis is seen, but it must be confirmed by x-ray. The latter condition is a forward slipping of one vertebral body upon the one below, usually L4 on L5. This may give rise to a palpable ledge and a restricted range of spinal movement. Again, radiography is necessary for certain diagnosis. Symptoms may include chronic low-back pain, bladder disturbances, and symptoms resembling intermittent claudication. Most patients show no physical signs but in some, weakness, a diminished ankle jerk, or slight sensory changes are found.

Spinal *inflammatory disease* may be pyogenic, occurring as a result of septicemia (osteomyelitis of a vertebral body) or tuberculous, but this latter is more usually seen in the thoracic or cervical regions. Vertebral osteomyelitis will produce a severe, deep-boring, or throbbing pain: marked local muscle spasm and the usual signs of infections are also present. Scheuermann's disease (osteochondritis) is a common cause of pain in the thoracic region in young people, but it is diagnosed radiologically, not clinically.

A compression *fracture* of the lumbar spine is common following trauma, especially road traffic accidents; it causes mild or moderate pain mainly resulting from protective muscle spasm. *Fracture-dislocation* may lead to pain in radicular distribution and signs of cauda equina compression may be detectable. These include symptoms of bladder involvement, impotence, and motor or sensory lesions at any levels between L1 and S4.

Primary tumors of bone are uncommon; hemangiomas and osteomas do occur but clinical diagnosis is difficult. Multiple myeloma and *secondary carcinoma* from the prostate or breast (osteoblastic secondaries with dense calcification) are the more common spinal secondaries. They cause dull, deep, and boring pain often with a radicular element because of root compression.

The usual *metabolic* bone disease affecting the lumbar spine is osteoporosis, seen particularly in elderly females and in patients taking steroid drugs. It may be accompanied by osteomalacia. A similar reduction in bone density occurs after prolonged immobilization. Diffuse low-back pain probably results from muscle spasm, caused in turn by vertebral collapse.

Diseases of the Spinal Cord

Because the lowest part of the spinal cord extends only as far as the level of L1 vertebra, pain caused by cord lesions must arise above that level. The cord itself is largely insensitive to pain, and myelitis, trauma, ischemia, or tumors cause pain by dorsal root irritation. Combined with this, the usual neurological signs of cord disease may be expected (see Chap. 9).

Joint, Ligamentous, and Muscle Disease

Cervical and lumbar spondylosis are discussed more fully in later sections of this chapter.

Degenerative arthritis of the spine with osteophytes, intervertebral disk space reduction, and subchondral sclerosis of the vertebral bodies is so common that it must be regarded as a normal wear-and-tear phenomenon; whether or not it causes many patients to complain of back pain is doubtful. Even prolapsed disks are not always symptomatic. In young males, back pain and stiffness may be due to *ankylosing spondylitis,* in which disorder tenderness of the sacroiliac joints, generalized flexion of the spine, and reduction in spinal mobility with reduced chest expansion, raised ESR, and specific x-ray changes, are the leading clinical features. The inflammatory changes may compress local nerve roots to produce cauda equina compression.

The sacroiliac joints may also be involved in *rheumatoid arthritis, psoriatic arthropathy,* and chronic brucella and salmonella infections. These are however probably the strongest joints in the body and so-called "sacroiliac strain" is not a respectable diagnosis.

Rheumatoid spinal disease is seen mainly in women and children and probably always involves other joints as well.

Most of the conditions discussed so far induce pain through ligamentous strain or muscle spasm. When muscle involvement is primary, the affected muscles contain small knots of fibers, acutely tender on deep pressure (trigger zones). From these, pain of a burning, steady nature may radiate diffusely down the leg, *not* observing dermatomal areas. Since weakness because of pain and reduced hip mobility are usually present, the differential diagnosis from spinal or disk disease can be difficult. But there are no hard neurological signs of a lower motor neuron lesion in these *myofascial pain syndromes,* nor are there any reflex nor objective sensory findings. Infiltration of the trigger point with local anesthetic may produce temporary relief, but this may have to be repeated a number of times for a permanent effect.

Minor *trauma, obesity, osteoarthritis* of the hip or knee, poor *posture* and some diseases causing proximal *muscle weakness* may all produce diffuse, chronic, low-back pain without neurological signs. The pain's origin is probably in protective muscle spasm or ligamentous strain secondary to the abnormal posture.

Referred Pain

Referred pain may arise from diseases of the kidneys, such as acute glomerulonephritis, hydronephrosis, or calculi; from a duodenal *ulcer* perforating back into the pancreas or from other causes of *pancreatitis;* from aortic *aneurysm* or *ischemia*

associated with aortic atheroma; and from *colonic disease*. *Gynecological* conditions, such as endometriosis or pelvic inflammation, may cause pain to be referred
to the sacrum. Pain from an inflamed retrocecal *appendix* may also be referred to
the back.

Psychogenic Pain

Psychogenic pain is a snare if not a delusion. It almost always arises out of a structural cause of back pain which has not settled or improved with time and treatment.
Depressed, anxious, and introspective patients fear somatic disease and may complain of low backache, although seldom as a leading symptom. Following surgery,
a few people will feign continuing back pain for economic gain (see Chap. 6 for the
examination of functional disorders). More commonly, muscle spasm or tension associated with abnormal affective states is the basis of the complaint; the diagnosis
of hysteria or frank malingering is best made only after exhaustive neurological,
orthopedic, and psychiatric assessment.

SPONDYLOSIS AND DISK DISEASE

In most people, the normal stresses upon the vertebral column cause its bony and
joint structures to degenerate somewhat by late middle age. If these stresses are
unusually severe, such degeneration may occur earlier. In association with dystonias or prior injury, and perhaps as an hereditary tendency, such lesions may occur
even in young adults.

In *spondylosis,* the vertebral bodies show outgrowths of bone (osteophytes) beside the disk, both anteriorly, projecting forward and posteriorly, projecting back
into the spinal canal. There is subchondral sclerosis of the vertebral bodies (Fig.
30-1). Osteophytes, infoldings of the ligamentum flavum and of the posterior
longitudinal ligament, and intervertebral disks may all project inward, narrowing
both the intervertebral foramina and the canal itself. Pressure upon the radicular
arteries may produce ischemia, and any subluxation of the vertebrae one upon
another may further diminish the diameter of the canal or cause more ischemia.
Patients who develop cord compression usually have a congenitally narrow canal.
Measurements of the canal width on the lateral cervical radiographs will thus help
in determining if a patient with cord signs has compression from cervical
spondylosis.

In *rheumatoid arthritis,* dislocation of the atlantoaxial joint or subluxation of
vertebrae because of softened and weakened ligaments may cause cord compression. Cervical canal narrowing is seen in a high proportion of patients with this
condition. *Osteoporosis,* particularly when caused by steroids, and *Paget's disease*
are other disorders affecting the spine with similar results. In all of these conditions, pressure upon the spinal cord and nerve roots may produce ischemia, leading
to pain and variable combinations of long-tract signs.

The soft nucleus pulposus is the central part of the interverbebral disk and is
enclosed within a strong circular condensation of cartilage. If this fibrocartilage
should rupture, some of the nucleus pulposus may herniate backward on one or
another side of the posterior longitudinal ligament (which tends to bind down the
central part of the herniated disk, preventing it from prolapsing in the midline).
If however this ligament is itself damaged or degenerated, then a *central* protrusion of the disk may occur. In the cervical region, disk prolapse most often occurs at C5-6 levels. While cervical disk prolapse is mainly seen among patients
with marked cervical spondylosis, prolapse of a lumbar disk occurs in younger

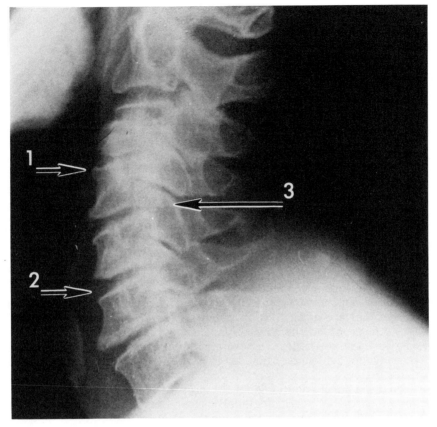

Figure 30-1   Cervical spondylosis; lateral rádiographs of cervical spine showing (1) Anterior osteophytes; (2) Narrowed C5-6 disk space (also C3-4 and C4-5 spaces are narrowed); and (3) Posterior osteophyte projecting into the cervical canal.

patients whose spines are usually otherwise healthy. This is most common at the L4-5-L5S1 levels. Pressure at both sites is usually upon the emerging nerve root on one side or the other, seldom both. With a central disk prolapse, the pressure may be on the anterior aspect of the cord at higher levels or upon nerve roots bilaterally.

Cervical Spondylosis

Cervical spondylosis is common in males over the ages of 50 or 60 years, with or without a history of previous neck injury. Symptomatic patients often complain of grating or crunching sensations with neck movement, the range of which is limited. Induced neck pain is often associated with muscle spasm, and sometimes the neck locks into one position for a short time. Pain and paresthesias may be felt in dermatomal distribution. Other complaints include weakness or clumsiness of the hands or arms, sometimes with loss of muscle bulk.

Examination reveals some straightening out of the normal cervical lordosis, perhaps with muscle spasm; evidence of a lower motor neuron lesion in the appropriate distribution, uni- or bilaterally; and subjective, if not often objective sensory changes. If disk prolapse occurs, the severity of the symptoms will be markedly increased, and if there is narrowing of the cervical spinal canal or ischemia because of compression of a radicular artery by osteophytes or by the ligamentum flavum, then the usual features of a progressive myelopathy will be apparent. However the abdominal reflexes are often retained, bladder symptoms are uncommon, and the plantar responses may remain downgoing until a late stage.

Lumbar Spondylosis

Lumbar spondylosis is extremely common in adult life; changes similar to those in the cervical vertebrae may give rise to root pain and sensory and motor symptoms. However the spinal cord ends at the lower border of L1, so the lesions will be entirely of the sensory or motor fibers of the cauda equina. If the lumbar disks are intact, patients complain of ill-localized pain and sensory disturbances without objective sensory change on examination, accompanied only by minor weakness. A reduction in the range of movement of the spine in all directions (flexion, extension, lateral flexion and rotation) will be seen as well here as in the neck.

Symptoms of disk protrusion in lumbar regions usually point to disease of the lowest lumbar levels, the patient complaining of diffuse and ill-localized back pain and then of pain felt in sciatic distrubution in the shin (L4 and 5), the lateral border of the foot (S1), or the back of the calf and thigh (S2). Thoracic and lumbar spinal roots are named from the vertebrae *below* which they leave the canal, so it is the L5 and S1 roots that are most often involved. If the disk presses further backward and damages other roots in the cauda equina, objective motor, sensory, and reflex changes may be found in the legs, asymmetrically. The situation becomes an emergency if there is any evidence of bladder involvement, which is an indication for immediate operation.

Apart from the purely neurological features, straight-leg raising will be markedly diminished on the affected side in all cases of disk prolapse. In addition, the normal lumbar lordosis will be lost, paravertebral muscle spasm will be marked with resultant postural deformity, the sciatic nerve may be tender when palpated in the buttock or thigh, and gentle compression of the two jugular veins of the neck by the examiner may produce markedly increased pain in the back and leg, much in the same way as will coughing or a Valsalva maneuver. The mechanism here is a rise in intracranial pressure transmitted to the lumbar theca causing further distortion of the entrapped nerve roots (Naffziger's sign).

Lumbar Spinal Stenosis

Lumbar spinal stenosis occurs mainly in males, in whom there is a marked diminution in the AP (sagittal) diameter of the canal. This may be a congenital anomaly or may be found in association with lumbar spondylosis, Paget's disease, or following lumbar surgery. The chronic low-back pain (which may be in bilateral root distribution), bilaterally reduced straight-leg raising, and variable motor, reflex, and sensory changes resemble those caused by spondylosis alone. Often they coexist. Sometimes there are symptoms suggesting intermittent claudication or signs of bilateral cauda equina damage such as bladder involvement.

In the syndrome of *neurogenic claudication,* the patient with spinal stenosis (or occasionally median disk protrusion) will complain of pain in the legs on walking, relieved by rest or by bending forward. This disorder is differentiated from vascular intermittent claudication by the presence here of sensory symptoms, increasing weakness, dropfoot, and reflex changes produced by walking but absent after rest. In vascular claudication, only pain develops. All too often the patient with lumbar stenosis is subjected to arteriography because the vascular syndrome is so much better known. The diagnosis is best made by CT scanning; decompressive surgery is invariably required and is frequently successful.

Investigations

At both cervical and lumbar levels, x-rays should show the changes of spondylosis and also a reduction in intervertebral disk spaces at the appropriate level. However the demonstration of degenerative changes is not the same thing as proving that they are responsible for the patient's symptoms. Myelography is indicated when there is any doubt about the causative pathology (a spinal tumor or intrinsic cord diseases could give rise to similar features), when the exact level or number of levels affected is not known, and when surgery is contemplated (Figs. 30-2A, B; 30-3A, B). The CSF protein level may be raised even to 1 g/L, but this is of no diagnostic value.

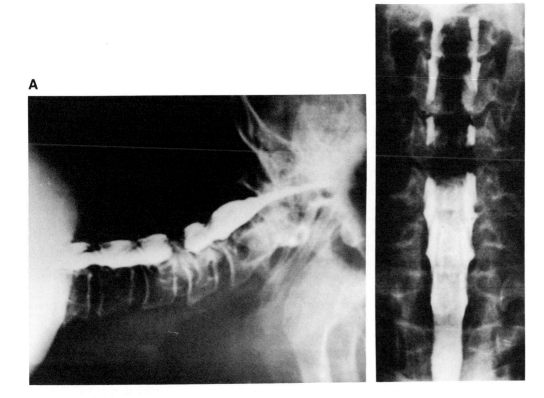

Figure 30-2 Iophendylate (Myodil) myelogram in a patient with cervical spondylosis. (A) With the patient lying prone, the dye column is indented posteriorly by the hypertrophic ligamentum flavum and a large osteophyte fragments the dye column at C3-4. (B) A transverse bar (probably a disk) cuts off the dye at C5-6 and C6-7.

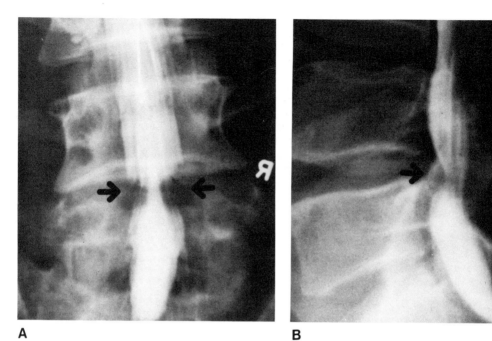

A   **B**

Figure 30-3   (A) AP and (B) lateral views of myelogram showing a large prolapse of the L-4 disk.

Management

Cervical

The natural history of cervical spondylosis is unusual in that there is evidence that the condition seldom gets very much worse after the patient first attends complaining of neck symptoms. Nevertheless, investigation is called for if there is any suggestion of myelopathy since surgery in such cases may be beneficial. Otherwise, immobilization of the neck with a soft or rigid cervical collar, or traction may be useful.

Because of pressure by osteophytes upon the vertebral arteries within the cervical spine, symptoms of vertebrobasilar insufficiency may occur particularly with neck rotation or extension, which compress the arteries yet further, even in normal subjects. In such patients and in those with obvious symptoms of root compression, a cervical collar may be of great benefit, probably because it stops the patient from moving the neck and thus exacerbating pressure on the roots. At operation, it is possible to stabilize the neck, to open up the foramina, and to remove bony, cartilaginous or ligamentous projections into the canal, thus relieving pressure on the cord or radicular arteries.

Lumbar

Acute back pain without neurological signs may be due to disk prolapse, muscle spasm, or both. Spasm in muscles with marked local and referred pain may be found in the paravertebral muscles or the glutei and is not always associated with underlying vertebral disease. Muscle and ligamentous pain is also common in patients who are anxious, depressed, or "neurotic" and again provides great problems in differential diagnosis and in management.

With any cause of acute back pain, rest is obviously essential (indeed anything else may be impossible). The patient should be kept in bed and given adequate analgesics to diminish his marked discomfort. The bed itself should be firm; this is most simply and cheaply achieved by sliding a piece of plywood under the mattress or by putting the mattress directly onto the floor.

In all cases, repeated careful neurological examinations of motor, sensory, and bladder functions are required to demonstrate any evidence of damage to the cauda equina. If any is found, the decision must be made about what type of mass is present — a disk, osteophytes, or a tumor — for which purpose myelography, often with CT scanning, will be necessary (see Fig. 30-3A, B). Patients without hard signs whose symptoms are still present after 2 weeks of bed rest, should also be considered for myelography or CT.

Surgical removal of protruded disks or decompression of spinal roots of the cord or of the cauda equina is best regarded as a last resort in patients who have persistent signs despite adequate conservative therapy; the natural history of the disease is toward spontaneous improvement. Extrusions of single disks may be relieved by chymopapain injections as an alternative to surgery. Frequent, if temporary, worsening of local pain and the risk of anaphylaxis temper our enthusiasm for this form of treatment, although it undoubtedly works well in 75 percent of the cases.

When chronic, recurrent, but not incapacitating low-back pain continues, the therapeutic options include exercises designed to strengthen the abdominal muscles and thus to prevent excessive postural lumbar lordosis; intermittent traction, (which probably works because it keeps the patient at rest in his bed); the use of a spinal corset or brace, to reduce all spinal movements (but at the expense of weakening the abdominal muscles by disuse); analgesics and muscle relaxants such as the benzodiazepines; and manipulation. Thought of the latter horrifies most doctors because they know little about it and consider it the province of the chiropractors. Yet manipulation can be strikingly effective in cases of minor disk prolapse at lumbar levels. We abhor manipulation of the neck however because of the risk of vertebral artery damage.

BIBLIOGRAPHY

Keim, H.A. Low back pain. *Clin. Symposia* (CIBA) *26*:2, 1981.

MacNab, I. *Backache.* Baltimore, Williams & Wilkins, 1977.

Wilkinson, M. *Cervical Spondylosis: Its Early Diagnosis and Treatment.* Toronto, W.B. Saunders Co., 1971.

31
Scoliosis

The spine is a flexible structure, straight when viewed from the front, but with a lordosis (convex forward) in the neck and lumbar regions, and a kyphosis (concave forward) at the thoracic level. The paravertebral muscles, by acting as stays, maintain the vertebrae in the normal resting position, support them in different postures, and move them. If the pull of these muscles is asymmetrically directed, then lateral and rotational curvature of the spine will occur — scoliosis. Scoliosis may be nonstructural or structural (Table 31-1). The former may represent a change of the spine's position to compensate, for example, chest wall deformity or a short leg. In such cases the patient may be able to correct the deformity himself, by raising the heel on the side of the shortened leg.

Structural scoliosis is a fixed deficit. No cause is found in 70 percent of cases, while the remainder have skeletal causes such as an extra half-vertebra or are secondary to neural or muscular disease.

Assessment

The following is a convenient scheme for the assessment of a patient with scoliosis.

First, determine if there has been trauma or surgery to the spine, or if there has been a history of pain in the back, pelvis, hips, or legs, or past poliomyelitis. In the acute stage of pain caused by a prolapsed intravertebral disk or other structural spinal diseases, scoliosis is common. In other cases, if you find abnormal movements, weakness, or clumsiness, consider cerebral palsy, spinocerebellar degeneration, spinal tumor, muscular dystrophy, or peripheral neuropathy: the history should already have alerted you to such possibilities.

Table 31-1   Causes of Scoliosis

Nonstructural	Postural
	Compensatory
Structural	Idiopathic
	Congenital
	Neuromuscular
	Neurofibromatosis
	Mesenchymal disorders
	Traumatic

With the patient standing, define the site, direction, and severity of the scoliosis, which is conventionally taken to be *toward* the *convex* side. Associated abnormalities will also be seen when the patient is standing, such as asymmetry of the pelvis, scapula, shoulders, and thorax.

Now determine whether or not the scoliosis is structural. On forward bending the angulation will remain in structural scoliosis but will disappear in nonstructural types. A single, short, angular curve may be associated with a skeletal abnormality at the site or with local neurofibromatosis.

Determine also if the legs are of equal length, and if they are not, whether or not correction by raising the heel of the short leg also corrects the scoliosis. Neurological disease (see Table 31-1) may be associated with leg shortening.

Note if there is any evidence of failed fusion of the neural arches such as spina bifida or meningocele. Spina bifida may be indicated by the presence of a local lipoma, a deep central cleft over the lumbar spine, or a tuft of hair in that region.

Look for complications. If the deformity is severe, root and musculoskeletal pains are common. Restricted ventilation secondary to thoracic deformity may ultimately lead to cardiac failure. The poor respiratory excursion in kyphoscoliosis is the reason for avoiding narcotics or other respiratory depressants in these patients. Severe scoliosis itself may lead to paraplegia.

Last, on general examination look for evidence of rheumatoid arthritis and other arthritic changes because these may be associated with vertebral involvement and resulting scoliosis.

BIBLIOGRAPHY

Goldstein, L.A., Waugh, T.R. Classification and terminology of scoliosis. *Clin. Orthop. Relat. Res.* 93:10, 1973.

Keim, H.A. Scoliosis. *Clin. Symposia* (CIBA) 31:1-30, 1979.

32
Abnormalities of Gait

A busman's holiday for a neurologist, physiatrist, or orthopedic surgeon would involve sitting in a sidewalk cafe observing the gait patterns of passersby, but observation of gait is more than an interesting diversion; it is an extremely important part of the neurological examination. It is unfortunate that examining rooms and offices are ill-designed to assess this essential function, and you must overcome this by using hallways and corridors.

The act of walking is a complex process involving brainstem and spinal cord postural reflexes that maintain tone in the antigravity muscles; tonic neck, labyrinthine and righting reflexes to maintain position in space; motor cortical control; automatic postural reflexes from the basal ganglia; proprioceptive mechanisms; muscle power; and bone and joint structures.

In walking, one leg supports weight while the other moves forward. When the supporting limb is extended, the heel lifts and the center of gravity is moved forward by slight trunk flexion. The progressing foot accepts the body weight first on the heel and then on the ball of the foot as the center of gravity moves forward. The pelvis rotates slightly forward on the side of progression and is elevated above the horizontal on that side by the trunk muscles.

In evaluating gait, the patient's normal resting position, his position when standing with eyes both open and closed, and his posture when walking and turning are inspected. He should be asked to initiate walking from a sitting position, to walk with heel-to-toe as on a tightrope, to stand on one foot, to walk on his heels and then on his toes.

Some of the more characteristic neurological gaits will now be discussed.

STEPPAGE GAIT

Weakness of dorsiflexion of the foot produces footdrop and a steppage gait, in which the leg is raised high and slapped down while walking. A lesion in the corticospinal tract, L5-S1 roots, or peripheral nerve may cause weakness of the dorsiflexors (tibialis anterior and extensors digitorum and hallucis longus) or these muscles may be primarily diseased. Common causes of footdrop include lesions of the common or deep peroneal nerves; a disk or other mass lesion compressing the L5 root of the cauda equina; or a cord lesion above the L5 level. Bilateral footdrop is seen in bilateral pyramidal lesions and peripheral neuropathies. The steppage gait is characterized by a down-pointing foot which is raised high in walking to prevent scraping the toe. The patient cannot dorsiflex the foot to stand on his heels. The steppage gait can be diagnosed by its characteristic sound before the patient actually enters the room.

One of the most common causes of dropfoot is a peroneal nerve palsy, often caused by pressure on the nerve in bedridden patients or those who have had their legs crossed for a long period.

THE DYSTROPHIC GAIT

Various myopathies can produce a characteristic waddling gait caused by weakness of the hip girdle muscles. It is most dramatic in muscular dystrophy, but it may be seen in any severe disease of proximal muscles. With the broad-based gait is seen as exaggerated rotation of the pelvis, the patient rolling or throwing the hips up and forward with each step to get the foot off the ground. There is accentuation of the lumbar lordosis and difficulty lifting the feet from the floor. Because of the proximal weakness, the patient has particular difficulty going upstairs, getting out of a chair, or getting up from the floor. This gait pattern has to be differentiated from the waddling gait seen with dislocation of the hips.

SPASTIC GAIT

A patient with spasticity on one side will show a tendency to extension of the lower limb and flexion of the upper limb. To keep the extended leg from scraping the floor when walking, the patient swings it out in a half circle (circumduction), to accomplish which the pelvis is elevated on that side. The phase of support on the affected side is shortened. Later, an equinus deformity may develop with shortening of the Achilles tendon producing functional lengthening of the leg; the patient may need to lean far over the strong side to raise the pelvis and leg on the weak side enough to allow progression. In cases of spastic paraplegia, the bilateral equinus position of the feet makes walking much more awkward. As a result of the spasticity in both legs therre may be accentuated adduction causing a "scissor" gait. The steps are short, the knees seem pressed together or the legs may actually cross, and the feet appear to stick to the floor, being scraped along with a characteristic sound.

ATAXIC GAIT

An ataxic gait may result either from a cerebellar abnormality or from a peripheral sensory proprioceptive problem.

The gait resulting from *cerebellar ataxia* has three characteristics (1) incoordination of the legs, (2) dysequilibrium with pitching and reeling, and (3) a disturbance of postural and walking reflexes. The incoordination, coupled with deviation of the path toward one side, indicates a unilateral cerebellar lesion on that side. Lesions of the vestibular portions of the cerebellum (flocculonodular lobe) produce dysequilibrium, preventing the patient from maintaining an upright posture in space. Posture and walking reflexes are under the control of the anterior cerebellum, and lesions of this area, e.g., alcoholic intoxication, may produce a stiff-legged, wide-based gait. Vision cannot compensate for a cerebellar lesion.

Sensory ataxia results from a lesion involving the proprioceptive system either in the peripheral nerves or the posterior columns. Ataxic gait may thus be seen in peripheral neuropathies, tabes dorsalis, subacute combined degeneration of the cord, multiple sclerosis, and Friedreich's ataxia. Position in space is maintained by the vestibular system, vision, and peripheral proprioception. Vision alone *may* be able to compensate when only the proprioceptive sense is lost, but if the subject closes his eyes, he is unable to maintain his position in space and falls. The gait disturbance is due to unawareness of the position and motion of the legs and sometimes of the body as a whole. The patient's walk may be broad-based, stamping, and jerky, particularly in the dark or on uneven ground. The steps are slowed and the patient watches the floor to know where his feet are. In early sensory ataxia there may not be any abnormality noted during the day, but he will comment that he is very unsteady if he gets up at night and attempts to walk without a light.

PARKINSONIAN GAIT

The patient with Parkinson's disease often shows rigidity, bradykinesis, and tremor when walking. A characteristic feature of parkinsonism is the loss of associated and automatic movements. The gait is slow and shuffling, and the patient's body appears to move *en bloc*. Arm swing is lost early, and there is an accentuation of dorsal kyphosis so the head is flexed and the whole body stooped. The patient may walk as if his center of gravity were ahead of him and he were chasing it. A tendency to fall forward when standing or walking is known as *propulsion*. A more dangerous situation is *retropulsion* in which he may suddenly begin to fall backward, and when starting to fall takes a series of rapid short steps in reverse. When walking down an incline, the patient may not be able to stop, and his short little steps get faster and faster until he falls or runs into something. The loss of automatic movements and postural reflexes makes it difficult for him to get out of chairs, to go up and down stairs, to roll over in bed, and to turn around. When starting to walk, or for example, in a doorway, there may be marked hesitation in initiating foot movements. This hesitation in initiating movement becomes characteristic of other motor acts as the disease progresses.

THE GAIT OF CEREBRAL ATROPHY

Patients with diffuse cerebral disease may manifest a number of unusual gaits. One of the best known is the *marche à petits pas* in which the patient walks with very short shuffling steps. There may be the same loss of associated movements as in parkinsonism. Other patients will show difficulty in initiating walking so that their feet seem stuck to the floor *(magnetic gait)* or they may take a series of tiny step movements and then stride out in a virtually normal gait. Some patients will walk quite well until they attempt to turn, which causes them great difficulty.

A *pathological fear of walking* may develop in these patients, despite a lack of objective abnormalities on examination. They seem to become fearful of falling and will resist attempts to make them walk, perhaps falling to their knees to protect themselves. Other patients may walk quite normally until they meet an obstruction or a narrow passageway when they will freeze, again sometimes falling to their knees. This tendency to freeze during movement is also seen in parkinsonism.

APRAXIC GAIT

An apraxic gait indicates an inability to use the motor function of the limbs despite a lack of objective weakness or sensory loss. It may be seen in patients with extensive uni- or bilateral cerebral disease, particularly of the frontal lobes. Such patients have difficulty in using their legs and feet for things people do automatically such as kicking a ball, dancing, or walking, although such movements are full and strong when they are lying down.

THE GAIT OF DYSKINESIAS

Gait may be markedly affected by involuntary movements. The gait of Huntington's chorea may take on a bizarre, dancelike quality as the jerking movements interrupt the normal pattern of muscle contraction. Athetosis may induce twisting movements of the body or limbs when walking, and dystonia musculorum deformans may become so marked as to preclude gait. Hemiballismus will interfere with walking because of the sudden, violent, flinging motion of the involved limb or limbs. Most tremors do not interfere significantly with gait, although they may be accentuated by walking.

HYSTERICAL GAIT

A number of psychiatric diseases have characteristic gaits (depression, catatonic schizophrenia), but the most dramatic are "hysterical" gait disturbances. Because the abnormality conforms to the patient's idea of how gait *should* look in his or her particular disorder, there is no characteristic or uniform pattern. What is characteristic is the absence of the other physical findings and symptoms that accompany organic gait disturbances. Also typical is the alteration of the picture with circumstance and by suggestion. The gait is often extremely bizarre and wild. The patient may bounce off the walls in a reeling fashion, but usually does so without falling and may continually head for the examiner. There is also a tendency to fall toward the bed or the wall. When turned around he tends still to fall toward the bed which is now, of course, on the other side. The patient may reel about with marked swaying and arm swinging, maintaining balance in a manner that actually demonstrates excellent equilibrium. Falling is often very theatrical but usually without significant injury.

BIBLIOGRAPHY

DeJong, R.N. *The Neurological Examination.* 4th Ed. New York, Harper & Row, 1979.

33
Abnormalities of Micturition

ANATOMY AND PHYSIOLOGY OF MICTURITION

Micturition is a coordinated contraction of the detrusor muscle of the bladder following release of cortical inhibition. In association with the detrusor contraction there is relaxation of the neuromuscular components of the proximal urethra. Control of the micturition reflex is not vested in a spinal center but rather in a neural circuit that extends from the pons to the sacral cord. Facilitatory and inhibitory influences from cortical and subcortical centers are exerted on this neural circuit, but the overall effect is inhibitory. Afferent and efferent nerve fibers connect the bladder to the sacral segments.

Disturbances of micturition are common with lesions in the frontal lobes, corticospinal tracts, spinal cord, or sacral nerves. The range of bladder symptoms caused by neurological lesions is wide and determined by whether the lesion primarily affects supraspinal control, the pontine-sacral neural circuit, or the sacral nerves; and whether these lesions are predominantly motor or sensory, or both.

The role of this innervation in bladder physiology is the key to understanding bladder dysfunction in neurological disorders. Sensory fibers subserving proprioception and muscle stretch sensation travel from the bladder wall in the pelvic nerves to the sacral cord (S2, 3, and 4) and motor fibers pass distally along the same paths (Fig. 33-1). Sensory impulses from the mucosa, particularly from the trigone, take the same afferent course or pass centrally in sympathetic nerves and are relayed to the cortex for conscious awareness through the dorsal columns and spinothalamic tracts. This conscious awareness produces the feeling of bladder fullness, the desire to void, and perhaps pain. Although the pontine-sacral neural circuit for micturition can function autonomously, it is controlled after infancy by higher inhibitory influences from the brain, which are under conscious, or at least preconscious, control.

378

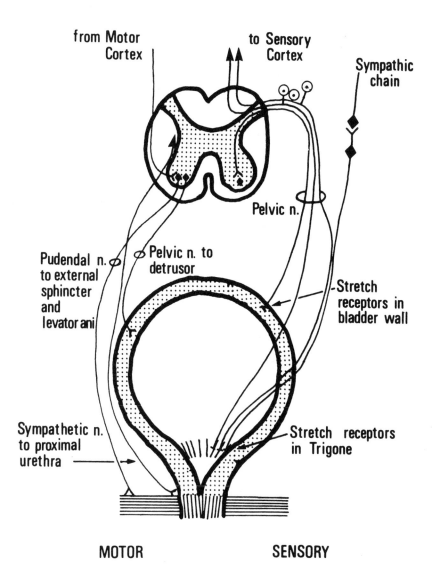

Figure 33-1   The innervation of the bladder.

The cortical areas influencing bladder control include the frontal lobes and paracentral lobules from which fibers pass to the pons and downward in the corticospinal tracts to the anterior and lateral horn cells at S2-4. Here the sacral outflow controlling the contraction of the detrusor is facilitated or inhibited. In addition, motor fibers run in the pudendal nerve to the external sphincter and to the muscles of the pelvic floor. Tone in the smooth muscle of the proximal urethra is maintained via the hypogastric (sympathetic) nerves.

Normally, the bladder will fill with urine slowly, stretching the detrusor muscle. The bladder has the ability to accommodate urine largely because of its viscoelastic property, a nonneural phenomenon. However beyond a certain volume (or degree of stretch), afferent stimuli running to the cortex increase central inhibition of the reflex, allowing the detrusor muscle to relax, the bladder to continue filling, and the sphincter to remain contracted. But when the bladder contains 400-500 ml of urine, there is cortical awareness of a desire to void. To initiate micturition, this inhibition of the bladder's reflex arc activity is voluntarily cut off, and voluntary relaxation of the pelvic floor muscles and external sphincter occurs. Reciprocal inhibition and relaxation of these muscles and of the sympathetically innervated smooth muscle of the proximal urethra also occur. The detrusor thus contracts against little resistance and the bladder empties completely.

DISORDERS OF MICTURITION

Hypertonic Bladder

If the amount of cortical inhibition running in descending motor pathways is reduced by a supraspinal lesion, such as a parasagittal meningioma, bilateral cerebrovascular disease, or multiple sclerosis, or by partial cord damage, there will be awareness of bladder fullness with diminished ability to inhibit the micturition reflex. This results in a hyperactive reflex arc and a "spastic" or hypertonic bladder.

When the bladder contains a comparatively small volume, inhibition of the reflex arc will fail and the detrusor muscle will contract. There may be some resistance from the external sphincter which cannot be adequately inhibited either, but this is usually not enough to prevent reflex emptying of the bladder. Patients with a spastic bladder will complain of frequency, urgency, and incontinence. They may have residual urine and thus become prone to bladder infections. Recurrent infections and inflammation of the bladder will actually increase the activity of the reflex arc and thus may worsen the patient's symptoms.

The investigation of patients with such problems is commonly undertaken by an urologist, using sphincter EMG and urodynamic pressure studies. These may demonstrate detrusor hypertonicity (the bladder contracts when containing only a small volume) or detrusor-sphincter dysynergia (the timing of the detrusor contraction is out of phase with relaxation of the sphincter, and as a result, the detrusor tries to expel urine against a closed sphincter).

The Bladder in "Spinal Shock"

Following acute spinal cord injury at a level above the sacral segments, the central synapses between the afferent and efferent arms of the micturition reflex will be rendered inactive. The detrusor will be paralyzed, and there will be no conscious awareness of bladder fullness. However the proximal urethra remains closed. The bladder will continue to distend because the reflex arc does not function and the detrusor will become hypotonic. The resulting retention of urine is followed by dribbling incontinence as a consequence of overflow. Infection resulting from the large amount of residual urine may become a serious recurrent problem. When infection occurs, the patient may in time feel poorly localized abdominal pain and may show signs of sympathetic stimulation (hypertension, sweating, "goose flesh," pallor of skin).

Automatic Bladder

An automatic bladder follows the stage of spinal shock resulting from a cord lesion above the S1 level. Consciousness of bladder sensation may not be totally absent but voluntary inhibition of the reflex arc and of the external sphincter are lost.

The initial retention of urine with overflow incontinence during the stage of spinal shock gives way to the effects of an augmented reflex arc and results in a small, spastic, and automatic bladder. The bladder empties incompletely because of the continuing uninhibited contraction of the external sphincter, so infection is likely. In time, reflex bladder contraction in response to skin stimulation may be learned, allowing the patient some voluntary control.

The Motor Paralytic Bladder

With a paralytic bladder there is a lesion of the lower motor paths at S2-4. Conscious awareness of bladder fullness and of pain will be retained, but the detrusor reflex and the ability to contract the external sphincter voluntarily are both lost. Because the detrusor cannot contract, the bladder dilates, with overflow incontinence and dribbling. Urine can be expressed by suprapubic pressure (Crede's maneuver) but complete emptying is seldom achieved.

The Deafferented Bladder

The deafferented bladder complicates tabes, diabetes, amyloidosis, and other autonomic sensory neuropathies. Awareness of bladder fullness is diminished or lost while voluntary contraction of the external sphincter is still possible. The reflex arc is broken on the afferent side, hence reflex contraction of the detrusor is not possible and the bladder dilates, with dribbling incontinence and infection as a result, although some external sphincter control is theoretically possible.

Some sensory perception may be maintained through the sympathetic nerves that conduct pain impulses from the mucosa. Because of the common anatomical path, structural lesions that produce a deafferented bladder will often produce motor paralysis.

MANAGEMENT

Urinary Retention or Obstruction

The concept of *intermittent catheterization* has revolutionized the management of the neurogenic bladder. In the stage of spinal shock or in patients with a permanent sacral cord lesion, intermittent catheterization (by sterile technique) is begun as soon as possible. This technique is far superior to an indwelling catheter; it must continue until recovery begins, which is often a month or so after injury.

The return of parasympathetic function is manifested by the ability to void or by return of function on the cystometrogram. Patients with sacral lesions may find straining useful; those with high lesions may learn to trigger the bladder reflex by rubbing or stroking the upper part of the thigh. This is done regularly every 3 or 4 hr during the day and preferably once at night. Postvoid residual urines should be checked frequently.

A detailed description of the management is as follows:

1. Record fluid intake and output.
2. Adjust the fluid input so that the urine output is 450 ml or less every 6 hr.
3. Encourage the patient to try and void every 3 to 4 hr (while sitting or standing, if possible). Every 6 hr, the patient is catheterized, whether or not he has voided. If the residual urine is large, i.e., >120 ml, catheterization should be repeated every 6 hr.

4. If the residual urine falls consistently below 120 ml, the catheterization inter-
    val is increased to 8 hr, gradually to 12 hr and later 24 hr, after which cathe-
    terization is discontinued provided the residuals remain low.
5. During this period, ascorbic acid (500 mg q.i.d.) is given to acidify the urine
    and methenamine mandelate 1 g q.i.d. is also prescribed. If a clinically ap-
    parent infection develops, trimethoprim/sulfamethoxazole, or another chemo-
    therapeutic agent is given after cultures are taken.

If residuals remain large, urodynamic evaluation such as a cystometrogram
with electromyographic study of the external sphincter should be done. Therapy
such as bethanechol chloride (5 mg SC or 25-50 mg p.o. q6h) may be useful to
stimulate the motor paralytic bladder. In the presence of a spastic external
sphincter, pudendal block or transurethral sphincterotomy may be necessary. In
general, these principles apply to the management of obstruction in any type of
neurogenic bladder.

Urinary Incontinence

In milder degrees of upper motor neuron lesion, incontinence because of detrusor
hyperreflexia may be the main problem. Anticholinergic drugs such as propantheline bromide or belladonna are effective in "sedating" the reflex activity, but it is
rare to control bladder reflex overactivity in complete upper motor neuron lesions.
Male patients with incontinence can wear a urinary appliance (a condom around
the penis connected to a leg bag). Female patients may require an indwelling catheter or urinary diversion (ileal or sigmoid conduit). Bladder denervation procedures
have not been very successful.

Treatment of Complications

Urinary infection, calculi (vesical or renal), vesicoureteric reflux, urethral trauma
and inflammation, balanitis, and epididymitis should be diagnosed promptly and ap-
propriately treated because neglect to do so could lead to ascending urinary infection and ultimately renal failure.

RECTAL CONTROL

The innervation of the rectum is very much the same as that of the bladder. Here
again, the parasympathetic system controls contraction of the sigmoid and rectal
musculature and relaxation of the internal sphincter. The role of the sympathetic
nervous system is not clear. Voluntary control is primarily through augmented contraction of the external sphincter to prevent defecation, rather than inhibition of
the parasympathetic reflex arc. To assist in defecation there is also contraction
of the muscles of the anterior abdominal wall with relaxation of the pelvic floor
musculature. With spinal lesions above the sacral level, both voluntary control of
the sphincter ani and the sensation of rectal fullness are abolished, leading to fecal
retention because the internal sphincter will probably be hypertonic except during
the period of spinal shock. With lesions in the sacral regions S3-5, fecal incontinence will occur because of paralysis both of the sphincters and of the levator ani.

BIBLIOGRAPHY

Krane, R.J., Siroky, M.B. *Clinical Neuro-Urology.* Boston, Little, Brown, 1979.

34
Impotence

Impotence refers to that distressing condition of connubial life in which the spirit is willing but the flesh is weak.[*] It is the inability to obtain or maintain penile erection. It does not encompass premature or failed ejaculation of semen.

When seeing a patient suspected of having a neurogenic cause of impotence, it is important to look carefully for other evidence of neurological disease because it will often be present. The autonomic (parasympathetic) outflow to the male genitalia may be directly damaged by neuropathies, most commonly those caused by diabetes. In any case you must examine motor and sensory functions in the legs and the reflexes, including anal and bulbocavernosus reflexes and must inquire into bladder and rectal function.

Causes of Impotence

Medication Effect

First, one should determine if the patient is taking any *medication* that may cause impotence: most of these are hypotensive agents, diuretics, vasodilators, or anticonvulsants (Chap. 43). Together they are responsible for about a quarter of the cases seen.

---

[*]Neurologists used to be regarded as therapeutically impotent but those days are long gone; people who make the statement nowadays usually need help upstairs.

Psychological Causes

Psychosexual difficulties are other common causes. Almost all overt emotions, apart from actual lust, tend to inhibit erection. The childhood years, parental identification, premorbid personality, sexual orientation and preexisting marital difficulties are important areas of inquiry and may require consultation with, and management by, a psychiatrist. If one is fairly sure that there is no underlying psychiatric disease as a cause, then spinal cord, cauda equina, or peripheral nerve disease must be excluded (Table 34-1).

Alcoholism leads to atrophy of the desire for almost everything but alcohol itself; sexual performance is much impaired as well. Alcoholism is responsible for about 10 percent of cases of impotence.

Neuropathy

Peripheral neuropathies with an autonomic component should be excluded by clinical examination, supplemented by electrodiagnostic studies if any abnormality is found. Diabetes is the leading cause in this category; one report suggests that about half of all male diabetics have weak or lost erections. The presence of diabetic retinopathy correlates with the incidence of impotence.

CNS Disease

A *spinal cord lesion* at the level of the parasympathetic outflow at S2-4 (such as tumors of the sacral cord, local congenital disorders, and syphilis (usually tabes dorsalis) is another possibility. This will always be accompanied by other signs or symptoms: it would be extremely unusual for impotence to present in isolation. Lesions of the low spinal cord, affecting the sacral segments, produce saddle anesthesia without somatic motor signs, while cauda equina damage produces bladder, motor, and sensory symptoms including pain in the legs. Above the sacral cord level, multiple sclerosis, strokes, or any other cause of bilateral corticospinal disease may cause impotence, among their usual neurological signs. Undiagnosed temporal lobe epilepsy ("complex partial seizures") has been shown to produce impotence. The patient's history may enable you to make the diagnosis, because other evidence of the seizure tendency (see Chap. 15) will be heard. In these patients, treatment of the seizure will correct the problem.

Endocrinopathy

Endocrine diseases are the cause in about one-fifth of the cases. Primary hypogonadism, both hyper- and hypothyroidism, and hyperprolactinemia, usually caused by a chromophobe adenoma, are all possibilities. Headache, visual loss, and the usual symptoms of the underlying disease may be expected in such cases.

Investigation

The first laboratory investigation to be performed is a nocturnal tumescence study; this is almost always required. If penile erections occur during sleep, psychological causes for impotence can be presumed. If they do not, then the other diseases discussed previously will have to be excluded. A glucose tolerance test, nerve conduction studies, radiographs of the dorsal, lumbar, and sacral areas, and spinal CT or myelography may be required as determined by the clinical findings. A cystometrogram and urinary flow studies may be used to evaluate bladder function and to give

Table 34-1   Causes of Impotence

Psychological disorders
Drugs (see Chap. 43)
Cauda equina lesions
Bilateral corticospinal disease
Tabes dorsalis
Autonomic neuropathy (diabetes, alcoholism)
Pituitary-hypothalamic disease
Hepatic or thyroid dysfunction

---

an indication of parasympathetic control. Other tests may be necessary to demonstrate lesions higher in the central nervous system, but these should have been suggested already by the results of neurological examination.

Treatment

This is almost always of the underlying cause, such as the discontinuation of drug therapy; but for patients with diabetic autonomic neuropathy, and other is whom specific treatment cannot be given, implantation of an inflatable penile prosthesis is of huge psychological benefit and is remarkably free from unwanted effects.

In summary, the clinical approach should be to identify the symptom of impotence, to explore the patient's drug history, psychiatric status, and past medical and psychosocial background; and only then to consider the possible neurological causes.

BIBLIOGRAPHY

McKendra, J.B. et al. Erectile impotence: a clinical finding. *Can. Med. Assoc. J. 128:*653-663, 1983.

35
Patterns of Sensory Deficit

Whether awareness of the various sensory modalities is altered, increased, reduced, or completely lost has much the same clinical significance. The degree of loss commonly reflects the severity of the pathologic process rather than its nature. The pattern of sensory loss that you detect depends upon the site in the sensory system involved (Fig. 35-1). Some of the possibilities, such as dissociated anesthesia, were discussed in Chapter 9.

Sensory impulses pass from the receptors through the peripheral nerves and enter the spinal cord by the dorsal roots. In the cord, the impulses pass upward via various tracts to the brainstem and thalamus, before finally reaching the parietal cortex. A lesion of any of these structures will result in sensory loss, its pattern suggesting the area of the nervous system involved. The following describes the major patterns of deficit that we expect to find.

PERIPHERAL LESIONS

Distal and Symmetric Sensory Loss

Distal and symmetric sensory loss is the common picture in a peripheral neuropathy. The deficit lessens as one tests more and more proximally and a level can be found where the abnormal becomes normal, although this cutoff is often indistinct. This pattern does not correspond with a root or an anatomical nerve territory and is usually symmetric, often in the distribution of a stocking (legs) or glove (hands and arms) pattern.

Although in most cases, all modalities of sensation are involved, sometimes only selected modalities of sensation are decreased in this distal and symmetric pattern. Thus *thick-fiber* function may be more obviously involved, as in early

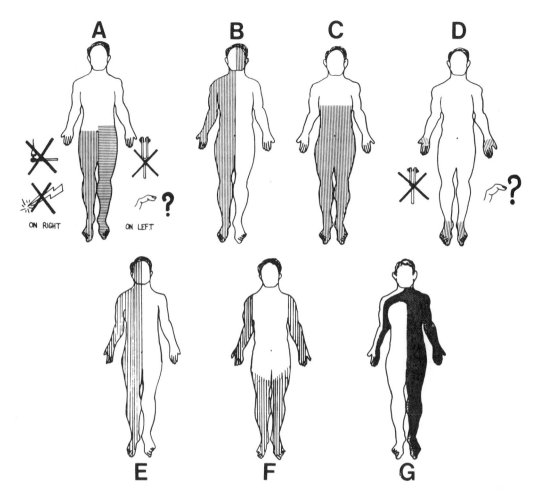

Figure 35-1 Common patterns of sensory disorder. (A) Unilateral cord lesion (Brown-Séquard). Loss of pain and temperature on opposite side and of vibration and joint position sense on the same side; (B) Alternating thermoanalgesia; brainstem lesion affecting face (same side) and body (other side) sensations of pain and temperature; (C) Anterior cord lesion; thermoanalgesia bilaterally below the lesion; (D) Early distal symmetric sensory neuropathy; (E) This pattern of sensory loss may be hysterical or may occur with a contralateral lesion of the thalamus or sensory radiation; (F) The exact cutoff at groin and shoulder with total or near total sensory loss in the limbs suggests a conversion reaction; (G) Typical areas in which pain and temperature sensations are lost in syringomyelia.

diabetic sensory neuropathy that affects vibration more than position sense, while pinprick pain and temperature are relatively spared. Demyelinating neuropathies, some dorsal root ganglion cell diseases (carcinoma, tabes dorsalis, herpes zoster), and dorsal column disease (subacute combined degeneration, multiple sclerosis) produce this type of picture. Selective *thin-fiber* dysfunction is a rarity but does occur in congenital insensitivity to pain, caused by a failure of the small dorsal root ganglion cells to develop.

Mononeuropathies

In single-nerve lesions (Fig. 35-2), all modalities of sensation are affected to a
similar extent in a distribution depending upon the nerve involved and the site of
its damage. Ischemic lesions, including compression palsies, are the most common
causes.

Root Lesions

Alterations of sensory function may be precisely confined to the dermatomal areas
in the limbs (Fig. 35-3), but on the trunk the overlapping areas of sensation from
neighboring roots makes any sensory deficit unlikely with a single-root lesion.
Root lesions cause pain that radiates in a more or less segmental fashion, and hyper-
or hypoesthesia. Although all modalities of sensation should be involved, pinprick
and light touch are most conveniently tested because it is almost impossible to test
proprioceptive sensation in one dermatomal area without involving the neighboring
root territory. The dermatomal areas are shown on the sensory charts in Chapter
2.

Plexus Lesions

All modalities of sensation are involved in a pattern corresponding to the fibers
damaged in a plexus lesion (Fig. 35-4). Figure 35-5 shows sensory loss in C8 and T1
dermatomes because of a lesion of the medial cord of the brachial plexus, which
distributes C8 and T1 fibers to the median, ulnar, and medial cutaneous nerves of
the arm and of the forearm. More complicated patterns may easily be imagined
in view of the complex anatomy of the brachial and lumbar plexuses.

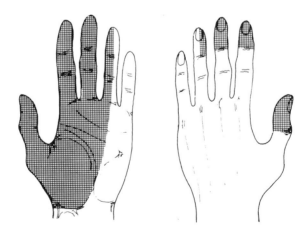

Figure 35-2   Mononeuropathy. In this case reduction in all modes of sensation
would be expected. The area involved demonstrates that the lesion is of the median nerve.

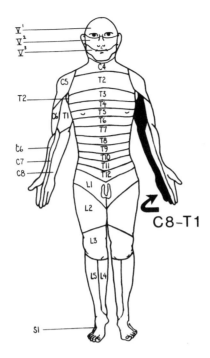

Figure 35-3   Area involved with a lesion involving C8 and T1 roots.

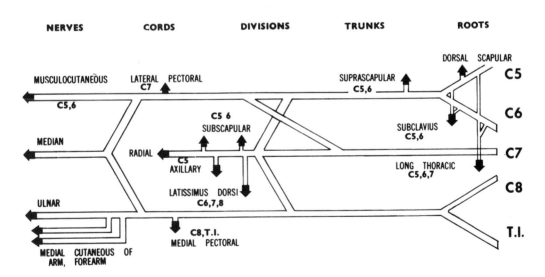

Figure 35-4   Diagram of the components of the brachial plexus.

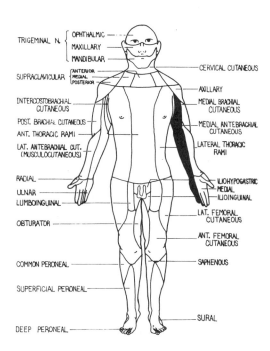

TRIGEMINAL N. {
OPHTHALMIC
MAXILLARY
MANDIBULAR
}

SUPRACLAVICULAR {
ANTERIOR
MEDIAL
POSTERIOR
}

INTERCOSTOBRACHIAL CUTANEOUS
POST. BRACHIAL CUTANEOUS
ANT. THORACIC RAMI
LAT. ANTEBRACHIAL CUT. (MUSCULOCUTANEOUS)

RADIAL
ULNAR
LUMBOINGUINAL

OBTURATOR

COMMON PERONEAL

SUPERFICIAL PERONEAL

DEEP PERONEAL

CERVICAL CUTANEOUS
AXILLARY
MEDIAL BRACHIAL CUTANEOUS
MEDIAL ANTEBRACHIAL CUTANEOUS
LATERAL THORACIC RAMI
ILIOHYPOGASTRIC
MEDIAL
ILIOINGUINAL
LAT. FEMORAL CUTANEOUS
ANT. FEMORAL CUTANEOUS
SAPHENOUS
SURAL

Figure 35-5   Area of sensory loss with damage to medial cord of the brachial plexus. Compare with Figure 35-3. The difference is in the fourth finger, where only the side supplied by the ulnar nerve is affected with a medial cord lesion.

SPINAL CORD LESIONS

Central Lesions

By interrupting the fibers crossing in the anterior commissure, a central lesion of the cord produces a loss of pain, temperature, and tickle sensation over a defined area, with regions of normality above and below. The analgesic areas involved are usually bilateral but asymmetric. In some cases, a "suspended" area of sensory loss to pain and temperature is found. Because of similar interruption of the afferent fibers running to the anterior horn cells inside the cord from the dorsal roots, and subserving the monosynaptic stretch reflex, tendon reflexes at that cord level are frequently lost. Because the sensory fibers derived from the sacral regions lie most superficially in the spinothalamic tracts, they may escape damage when there is a central cord lesion at or above thoracic levels.

Classic *sacral sparing* is produced however by an extrinsic lesion, such as a prolapsed disk that damages the cauda equina roots (e.g., L4, L5, or S1) but does not compress the centrally placed fibers coming from S3, S4, or S5. Contrast this with *saddle anesthesia* in which a lesion of the conus medullaris affects these low sacral levels only. Dorsal column sensation is usually unimpaired with central cord disease. Central lesions may result from acute cord trauma, ischemia, syringomyelia, and occasionally tumors.

Posterior Cord Lesions

Infolding of the ligamentum flavum, a neoplasm, or any other cause of mechanical compression of the posterior part of the cord may lead to patchy loss of joint position sense and perhaps vibration below that level. In such cases, Lhermitte's sign may be present. Most masses will impinge upon at least one entering dorsal root and cause pain in its dermatome. Expect to find irregular compensating ("pseudo-athetoid") movements of the outstretched hands in patients with proprioceptive losses.

Anterior Cord Lesions

Damage here is mainly to the ascending spinothalamic tracts, leading to deficits in pinprick pain, light touch, and temperature sensations, starting one or two segments below the level of the lesion. Dorsal column function is spared. Depending upon the size of the lesion (and thus on the area of the cord involved), there may be evidence of damage to the anterior horn cells at that level and perhaps signs of involvement of the lateral corticospinal tracts. Vascular insufficiency in the distribution of the anterior spinal artery is a typical cause.

Unilateral Cord Lesions

Damage to the right side of the spinal cord leads to loss of dorsal column function with impaired joint position sense, vibration, and discriminatory tactile sensation on the same side as the lesion. Damage to the right ascending spinothalamic tract will cause diminution of pain and temperature sensation on the *left* side of the body, starting a couple of segments below the lesion, because the fibers subserving these sensations have crossed from the left to the right side at a lower level and are now ascending in the right spinothalamic tract. Thus one set of modalities is affected on one side and another set on the opposite side. This is known as *dissociated* sensory loss (see Chap. 9).

Radicular pain often occurs in the distribution of the nerve roots at the level of the lesion, and evidence of corticospinal tract damage may also be found on the same side. If the cord lesion is compressive, the sacral fibers nearer the surface of the cord may be involved, causing saddle anesthesia on the opposite side.

With brainstem lesions, pain and temperature are most often involved, vibration, position, and localizing tactile sensations frequently being spared. One characteristic pattern of brainstem sensory involvement is an *alternating* sensory loss, i.e., one affecting one side of the face and the opposite side of the body. The localization of brainstem disease is discussed in Chapter 9.

THALAMUS

A lesion of the thalamus usually produces a marked or total hemisensory loss on the opposite side of the body, usually associated with hemiparesis and sometimes with a severe, agonizing, poorly localized, burning pain in the anesthetic areas. This *thalamic pain syndrome* may also result from a lesion in the thalamocortical radiation.

CORTEX AND SUBCORTICAL RADIATIONS

The deeper the lesion in the hemisphere, the more extensive the sensory deficit on the opposite side of the body. In the internal capsule, the picture may be very similar to the total hemisensory loss seen with a thalamic lesion. Higher up toward the cortex, the face, arm, and leg may be involved to a different extend depending upon which cortical area has been damaged. Although some awareness of pain and temperature may be possible at a thalamic level, sensory discrimination requires an intact cortex, and therefore cortical lesions cause decreased graphesthesia and two-point discrimination, astereognosis, and decreased sensory awareness of the opposite side of the body. Cortical lesions may leave vibration sense intact.

PSYCHOGENIC (HYSTERICAL) SENSORY LOSS

This pattern of sensory loss is often of the glove-and-stocking variety, but there is a precise cutoff from normal to abnormal sensation which may be altered by suggestion. The sensory loss is often symmetric, involves all modalities equally, is complete, and is usually not accompanied by other changes such as trophic disturbances or reduced reflexes. Hysterical hemianesthesia is similarly unphysiological in its distribution, ending at the exact midline and affecting all modalities from head to toe. For instance, the patient may state that he cannot feel the vibrating tuning fork on one side of the sternum or forehead but can do so on the other. This type of sensory disturbance may resemble a thalamic lesion, but there will not be any associated reflex changes or disorder of proprioception. Since the patient can walk and use his limbs in a manner that suggests awareness of limb position, one can tell that joint position sense is retained. The diagnosis of psychogenic sensory loss is made only with the greatest of care however, because some bizarre patterns do occur with organic lesions.

BIBLIOGRAPHY

DeJong, R.N. *The Neurologic Examination.* 4th Ed. Hagerstown, Harper & Row, 1979.

Shepherd, D.I. Sensory disturbances. *Br. Med. J. 288:*1147-1149, 1984.

36
Pain Syndromes

Pain is hard to characterize and its mechanisms are even harder to define. Although understandable as an endogenous warning signal, it far exceeds the boundaries of that role and is at times spontaneous, crippling, excessive, debilitating, and perhaps even pleasurable. Its anatomy and physiology are under careful research study and what follows is an attempt to summarize and synthesize current information without any dogmatic assertion about the complete truth of the interpretations made.

PHYSIOLOGY OF PAIN

Free nerve endings carry pain impulses but may subserve other forms of skin sensation as well. The stimulus initiating the afferent discharge may be physical distortion (compression or traction) or chemical irritation (e.g., release in the tissue of amines, such as bradykinin, serotonin, and histamine, or of prostaglandins). Physical causes may in fact act only through such a chemical link.

Both fast-conducting (myelinated A delta) and slow-conducting small (unmyelinated gamma) fibers run centrally, entering the cord or brainstem by the dorsal root, and the latter synapse with second-order neurons in the substantia gelatinosa. Those neurons rise for a few segments in Lissauer's tract before crossing to the lateral spinothalamic tract in the anterior commissure. Some A delta afferents may pass upward in the dorsal column and are responsible for both "deep pain" sensation and also for the fast cortical perception of any pain-producing stimulus. The gamma afferents are probably concerned with less exactly localized perceptions of pinprick or visceral pain; the two qualities of pain on banging a finger may rely upon the speeds of conduction of the two sizes of fiber. Thus the immediate hurt, with withdrawal occurring at once, is followed a second or so later by a much more intensely unpleasant and less localized, longer-lasting sensation. Central mechanisms *could* be responsible for this however.

From the lateral spinothalamic tract (or the bulbothalamic tract in the case of the fifth, seventh (intermedius), ninth, and tenth nerve fibers), impulses pass to the posteroventrobasal thalamus and thence bilaterally to the somatosensory, frontal, and temporal cortices to subserve, respectively, the perceptual, emotional, and memory aspects of the painful sensation. Finally, some fibers leave the ventrobasal thalamus and pass downward to the reticular activating system (RAS) and hypothalamus, presumably subserving autonomic and other reflexes associated with pain.

Some spinal second-order neurons however do not take this well-defined path but ascend diffusely and probably bilaterally in the cord as the spinoreticulothalamic pathway, passing with numerous synapses in the brainstem RAS to the midline intralaminar and reticular nuclei of the thalamus and thence diffusely to perhaps all cortical areas.

The anatomy of painful sensation is thus diffuse and even the scheme just presented is still under critical study. The physiology of pain is even less understood, but opinions are becoming more unified with the elaboration of the gate theory of pain propounded initially by Melzack and Wall (1965). This does not rely upon the suppositions that specific pain receptor pathways and brain centers exist (the older "specificity" theory), nor that patterning of afferent impulses control the circumstances and forms of pain feeling, but rather proposes that specialized inhibitory and facilitatory mechanisms at cord level modulate input into the CNS pain pathways.

Thus the large (A delta) and small (gamma) fibers both carry impulses centrally to the second-order neuron or transmission (T) cell in the cord. When they are excited peripherally by a pain-producing stimulus, the large fibers can activate a mechanism in the substantia gelatinosa (SG) that *inhibits* transmission of impulses onward to the T cell in both small and large fibers (closing the gate), while the small fibers inhibit this inhibitory mechanism, thus "opening the gate." Descending impulses from the RAS and cortex may also inhibit T cell activation. If the stimulation of T cells reaches a certain point, the central pain-experiencing mechanisms are activated.

As a corollary, it might be expected that the more thick-fiber activity, the less pain would be experienced; and the less the relative amount of thick-to-thin fiber input, the more open the gate will be, so more pain will be felt. Neuropathies that affect primarily the largest fibers may open the gate to minimal stimuli, and more pain or even spontaneous pain may be felt (hyperpathia or dysesthesia). It will be seen that this does in fact explain some clinical observations, e.g., vibration or rubbing a painful part diminishes the amount of pain felt. Mothers of small children have known this for thousands of years, but the fact has only recently been appreciated by medicine. Again, it is noted that prolonged pain may occur despite normal proportions of thick and thin fibers; this is explicable if excessive or long-continued painful stimuli produce a prolonged "bias" in the gate. This bias is also affected by emotion and by stimulation at distant sites. It may be returned to normal by increasing or decreasing the total sensory input.

In the nervous system, a number of chemical substances affect the interaction between nerves. These include neurotransmitters, neuromodulators, and neurohormones, all are generally classed as neuroregulators. Some naturally occurring morphinelike substances called endorphins act in all three of these categories in different circumstances. They are found in high concentration particularly in the dorsal horns of the spinal cord, the periaqueductal gray matter, the basal ganglia, the limbic system, and the hypothalamus. In at least some of these sites they are able to block the behavioral responses to pain, a property that is reversed by the administration of the morphine antagonist, naloxone. Because these substances are endogenous morphinelike agents, the term *endorphin* has been used for them. The physiology of the endorphins is now under intensive study; although not yet proved, it seems at least possible that many of the ways we have of relieving pain depend upon the liberation of endorphins centrally; hypnosis, acupuncture, counterstimulation, and perhaps even some drug effects might be explicable in this way.

Pain produces long-lasting changes in CNS activity and is itself produced by diffuse and interdependent patterns of stimulation of central pathways. The examples of painful syndromes that follow are still not founded upon a secure physiological basis of knowledge but will be more easily remembered if a widely applicable theory of pain, such as the gate theory, is used to interpret them.

CLINICAL SYNDROMES

The pain history was outlined in Chapter 1, but remember to ask about the impact it has on sleep, mood, and physical activity, and about the drugs used to control it. The pain's character, severity, and spatial and temporal characteristics, and associated symptoms must be learned: they present diagnosis.

Pain with Peripheral Nerve Lesions

Neuralgia means nerve pain, which is obvious and thus tells us nothing at all. Ischemia (often caused by compression) and stretching of nerves both lead to pain in the general area supplied by the nerve but not exactly, however, while paresthesias are well localized to the appropriate dermatome or area of nerve distribution, pain is felt in sclerotomes which, although similar, do not quite correspond with dermatomes in extent.

Such nerve-derived pains may be intermittent or continuous. *Cranial neuralgias* (Chap. 22) exemplify the former type, but other nerves may be involved, including the *femoral* (usually caused by diabetic ischemic neuropathy and occasionally by trauma or compression from mass lesions) and *pudendal* nerves ("proctalgia fugax"). *Root lesions* also may produce sudden stabs of pain such as the lightning pains felt approximately in root distribution in diabetes, early herpes zoster, and tabes dorsalis. The cause of the symptom is possibly the particular susceptibility of thick fibers to pressure ischemia or to the tendency of these infective processes to involve the *large* rather than the *small* dorsal root ganglion cells. The resulting relative thin-fiber predominance and the ability of stimuli from elsewhere converging upon the appropriate segmental dorsal root entry zone to trigger the T cells are likely to be responsible for the pain.

More continuous neuralgic pains may again involve the nerves or roots mentioned before, *postherpetic* neuralgia being an example, but almost any nerve that is partially damaged may produce continuous burning or aching pains. The same mechanism, with an added effect from bias of the gate, is presumably responsible. Pain felt up the arm and into the hand from median nerve compression in the carpal tunnel, in the shoulder or wrist from the cubital tunnel syndrome of ulnar nerve compression, and down the leg with lumbar root compression are other examples.

Such *partial nerve damage* (mainly involving the largest fibers) is commonly accompanied by hyperalgesia on clinical testing with a pin, although thick-fiber function (e.g., two-point discrimination) is actually reduced. Pinprick stimulation of the skin produces a peculiar and unpleasantly increased sensation of pain with delay in its application, overreaction to it, and a continued after-sensation when the stimulus is ended. The whole sensory effect is known as *hyperalgesia* or *hyperpathia.* The same unusually unpleasant, long-lasting pain sensation may also occur with thalamic lesions. Relief is sometimes attained by artifically increasing the thick-fiber function at nerve or at cord level, e.g., by vibrators placed on the skin, or by rubbing the affected area. Implanted extradural electrodes, which can stimulate the dorsal columns electronically, are available and by increasing thick-fiber function centrally, also seem to be capable of reducing pain of this type. Regional guanethidine infusion may be of value.

The intermittent neuralgias may be more responsive to drug therapy. Because the psychological and attentive components of pain are in part mediated by poly-synaptic paths, including the RAS, so agents raising synaptic thresholds along these paths such as carbamazepine and phenytoin may be of the greatest value in reduc-ing neuralgic pains of all types.

Causalgia is a different condition and is due to partial damage to a large senso-rimotor nerve. It is most commonly found in the arm associated with partial median nerve lesions. Severe spontaneous burning pains occur with swelling, sweating, and pallor of the limb. Osteoporosis of the underlying bones is usual. The condition is markedly worsened by emotion, and the mechanism probably involves activation of sympathetic afferents. Treatment is possible with oral phenoxybenzamine 10-40 mg q8h. If that fails, intraarterial guanethidine may succeed. If it does not, the best therapy is surgical, removing the T2-4 sympathetic ganglia. All analgesics lead to habituation and are not advised except on a short-term basis.

Phantom-Limb Pain

All amputees feel the amputated limb to be present and, in a third of the cases, it is painful. The stump may be hypoesthetic but any stimulation that is perceived is unpleasant — a dull, boring, or stabbing pain, made worse by any form of stress. Repeated percussion of the stump, tricyclic drugs, local anesthesia, sympathetic block, or transcutaneous stimulation may be effective therapies.

Root and Cord Pain Syndromes

Intermittent pains caused by *dorsal root lesions,* such as lightning pains and continu-ous ones also felt in girdle distribution have been mentioned previously. The lesion is usually of the larger cells in the dorsal root ganglion, which are most susceptible to pressure and to ischemic, inflammatory, or other metabolic involvement (herpes zoster, B_{12} deficiency). They all produce sensory neuropathy and mainly affect thick-fiber function so that vibration, joint position sense, and deep tendon reflex-es are all reduced, and thin-fiber function is relatively preserved; thus pinprick and cotton-wool sensation may be tested and found to be normal.

Lesions that avulse roots of the *brachial plexus* from the cord are caused by traction on the abducted arm or distraction of the neck and the shoulder (as when a motorcyclist comes off his machine and lands on his shoulder). In the latter case the C5, 6 roots of the upper brachial plexus will be involved. Traction on the ab-ducted arm might occur when someone grabs onto a window ledge when falling. In these cases the C8 and T1 root fibers of the lower brachial plexus will be damaged. Such injuries may lead to severe distal pain between 2 and 4 weeks after the injury. The injury has probably damaged the dorsal root entry zone *within* the cord and sympathectomy is of no value. The lower cord is a more common site of damage than the upper.

Neuralgic amyotrophy is a severely painful condition, which is usually unilater-al but occasionally is bilateral and follows viral infections, surgery, or immunologi-cal challenges such as injections of serum or vaccination, but often there is no recognized preceding event. Pain is felt continuously in C5 and C6 areas and the local sclerotomes. The causes are unknown but the disorder is likely to have an immunological basis. In association with the pain but following its onset, weakness and wasting in C5 and C6 may occur and may persist for months, although the pain usually clears within a few weeks at most. Sensory testing may reveal some diminution of sensation in the C5 and C6 dermatomes, but this is inconstant. If the disease is autoallergic, it is odd that it is so consistently found at this level and that it does not involve other segments as well.

The phenomenon of *referred pain* probably operates at spinal cord level. The presently favored postulate is that afferent impulses from the viscera and from the skin converge upon the same afferent pathways in the CNS, and the cortical perception is thus of pain arising from the area "known by" and thus localizable by the cortex. Examples are: upper surface of diaphragm to C4,5 over the shoulder; lower surface of diaphragm to T7-10 abdominal wall; maxillary antrum to upper molars and premolars; ethmoidal sinus to upper molars; heart, pericardium, and upper esophagus to C8, T1, and T2 inside the arm.

Similar *radicular pain syndromes* often accompany myelopathies and occur also in diabetic patients. These result from central stimulation, for example along the spinothalamic paths resulting from ischemic irritation of the dorsal root entry zone, of the crossing fibers, or of the ascending tract. The pain is felt as a sharp stabbing or a more continuous burning sensation in segmental or girdle distribution.

Brainstem Pain Syndromes

The cranial neuralgias are described in Chapter 22.

Thalamic Pain

Despite its name, this severe pain may be the result of RAS rather than of actual thalamic lesions, because it is uncommon in association with localized thalamic tumors. The pain is burning, long-lasting, and provoked by normally nonpainful stimuli at a higher threshold than usual. It long outlasts the duration of the stimulus. Vascular disease is the usual pathology. The pain is indistinguishable from hyperpathia secondary to a peripheral nerve lesion except that it involves one-half of the body.

Abnormal electrical excitation of the bulbar RAS may stimulate the associated thalamic nuclei and projection areas of cortex upon which somatosensory afferents from the other side of the body converge. Pain is then referred to the face, uni- or bilaterally. The syndrome is mainly seen in females over the age of 40 years who complain of up to 15 min of throbbing or burning pain on one or both sides of the face with or without other focal epileptic phenomenon. The pains are prevented by phenytoin, phenothiazines, apomorphine, and stereotactic thalamotomy and are accompanied by slow-wave discharges on the EEG.

Cortical Pain Syndromes

Pain is probably not initiated at cortical levels, although the cortex is certainly concerned with its perception, localization, memory, and emotive appreciation. All of these factors are enhanced with greater arousal and, conversely, diminished by RAS depressants such as hypnosis, yoga, or opiates. High arousal occurs with anxiety states and in many depressive syndromes. When the cortical appreciation of pain is enhanced, corticofugal (descending) impulses "open the gate" and allow further impulses subserving pain to arrive. Patients with such psychological states as anxiety and depression therefore may not only feel pains more acutely, but probably also become aware of pains that have no current pathological basis but reflect only old, but reconstituted, bias settings of the gate.

Autonomic Pain Syndromes

The role of the sympathetic afferent system in causalgia has been discussed previously. The autonomic system is also involved in the *shoulder-hand syndrome,* seen after myocardial infarction, strokes, or thalamic damage, and with cervical osteoarthritis. The syndrome includes pain in the shoulder with stiffness, swelling, and pain in the hand; symptoms of capsulitis (frozen shoulder) may also occur. The symptoms last for some months and are accompanied by marked osteoporosis of the affected hand, often with flexion contractures of the wrist and fingers. Although presumably based upon some autonomic afferent pain pathway, its precise pathogenesis is uncertain. Stellate ganglion block has been reported as of some benefit and steroids may also hasten recovery.

THE MANAGEMENT OF CHRONIC PAIN

First, always assume that the pain is indeed as bad as the patient claims, and take the history prepared to believe what you hear. Logical management of any pain syndrome is not possible until a diagnosis of the cause has been made and some idea of the mechanism whereby pain has been produced has been obtained. In treatable diseases, it is only correct to prescribe analgesics if the pain is temporary, e.g., traumatic, or caused by myocardial infarction and so on. Analgesics may also be used in the waiting period before specific treatment can be given, e.g., before removal of stones in a case of renal colic. Wherever possible, the specific therapy for the disease should be given rather than relying upon analgesia to mask the main complaint. Patients with chronic pain who do not have significant physical symptoms and signs have a high prevalence of depression and respond well as a group to high-dose tricyclic drug therapy.

Cancer Pain

When the pain is derived from disease of the CNS, specific treatment is unlikely to be available in most cases. In such patients, if the prognosis for life is short, as with carcinomatous infiltration of the spinal cord (or brachial plexus), narcotics are the correct treatment. In the late stages of malignancy, pain may be the single most grievous problem to the patient, capturing almost all of his awareness, its duration and severity both apparently unlimited. Depression, anxiety, misinformation, or ignorance and isolation compound the misery; all are treatable and so is the pain.* In the terminal patient we are concerned with relief of pain, not the inconsequential possibility of addiction.

When pain is mild, use aspirin or paracetamol on a strict 4-hourly basis, adding or changing to codeine 30-180 mg p.o., oxycodone 5-10 mg q4h p.o., pentazocine 50-200 mg p.o., or meperidine (Demerol) 50-300 mg p.o. as pain worsens.

Severe pain demands morphia. This may be given as an elixir, 5-100 mg q4h p.o. Prochlorperazine 5 mg p.o. may be added as necessary, titrating both the dose

---

*But never with placebos, although it is a hallmark of genuine pain that there will be some initial placebo response.

and the frequencies until the patient is free of it. *The next dose must always be given before the last one has completely worn off* (usually q4h). If the patient is vomiting, intramuscular injection of a smaller dose will have to replace oral treatment.

Even though the pain may be due to incurable malignancy, a number of other therapies may be tried to reduce drug dependency. Local nerve or regional blocks, deep x-ray therapy (DXT), and steroid therapy, all may help to reduce the pain perceived and are valuable complementary treatments.

Other Chronic Pain Syndromes

In patients who do not respond adequately to these measures, other forms of therapy may be employed. With the gate theory of pain before us, we may predict that to increase thick-fiber function will be to close the gait, diminishing the number of centrally directed impulses arising from the first transmission cell (T cell). Therefore some therapies directed toward relieving pain of neurological origin seek to increase the activity of thick fibers for this purpose. Other forms of therapy recognize that sympathetic afferents may carry impulses appreciated as painful; try to diminish the polysynaptic pathways at RAS or at substantia gelatinosa level, with resulting effects mainly upon thin fibers; or try to alter the cortical appreciation of pain at an emotional level, e.g., by anterior thalamotomy, cingulectomy, or orbitofrontal leukotomy. Thus the hyperpathic state caused by partial nerve damage (as with nerve trauma or in postherpetic neuralgia), may be treated by local rubbing, pressure, or vibration in the affected area. Initially, this seems to cause an increased amount of pain, but after it has been continued for a few seconds or minutes, pain is markedly diminished, and (perhaps because of altered setting of the bias of the gate) this pain relief may be extremely prolonged through hours initially and, later, days. Postherpetic neuralgia may respond to oral chlorprothixene (Taractan) 50 mg three or four times daily, and amantadine also has been found helpful. When there is partial nerve damage, as with the carpal or cubital tunnel syndromes, decompression of the nerve is probably all that will be required. In causalgia, sympathectomy is frequently curative.

With pain syndromes resulting from *damage to the root or cord,* little can be done and in such conditions, as with some patients with infiltration of nerves by tumor, no local therapy is possible. In these cases, anterolateral cordotomy will interrupt the ascending pathway carrying pain impulses in the lateral spinothalamic tract, and in a proportion of cases has good effect, although this is by no means always so, and operations at successively higher levels, involving the ventrobasal thalamus, the thalamic radiations, or the cortex may be required. Since it is probable that pain impulses travel upward *bilaterally,* it is not altogether surprising that some of these patients get no relief from operative intervention.

In other cases however, both surgical and nonsurgical attacks upon the entering dorsal roots may be of value. Surgical rhizotomy interrupts all entering afferents, but alcohol or phenol injections into the subarachnoid space (with the patient properly positioned so that only certain roots are bathed in the chemical) will selectively damage the entering thin fibers, leaving the thick fibers relatively unaffected. If the phenol is allowed to descend to sacral levels, for example, bladder and sexual functions will be lost, so the method is not without risk and demands a good deal of experience in its use.

Dorsal column stimulation has been previously mentioned. Percutaneous stimulation should be tried first; if successful, dorsal column stimulation, at a rate and strength chosen by the patient by means of an induction coil strapped to the overlying skin, may be used on a more permanent basis. The firm indications for such therapy are not clear and the apparatus is expensive.

In the case of *acute lumbar disk protrusion,* ice-cold saline injections extra-durally and local steroid injections have been found useful in diminishing pain, presumably by reducing local nerve edema and thus nerve pressure (which may be supposed preferentially to damage the heavily myelinated fibers more than the unmyelinated thin fibers).

Direct nerve blocks are seldom of lasting benefit, but in *causalgias,* sympathetic blockade may well forecast the success of more permanent surgical treatment. Fortunately, the cranial neuralgias usually respond to carbamazepine, baclofen and/or phenytoin, but if they do not, then sectioning the appropriate root or alcohol injection of the gasserian ganglion may provide specific relief of pain with minimal loss of common sensation. These techniques however are chosen by the operating surgeon and are outside the scope of this book.

Finally, it has already been mentioned that anxiety and the ubiquitous condition of the human frame that we call depression, are both potential causes of the appearance of pain without any demonstrable pathological basis and of the intensification of pain from whatever cause. Every patient who is in pain is likely to be unhappy, and many of them may be suffering a true clinical depressive state. The use of a tricyclic drug, or at least of tranquilizers (e.g., phenothiazines which augment the analgesic properties of most other drugs) should always be considered when a chronic pain problem is encountered, whether or not a primary pathology has been identified. Tricyclics have a specific value in the treatment of chronic pain, aside from their antidepressant value.

BIBLIOGRAPHY

Bond, M.R. *Pain: Its Nature, Analysis and Treatment.* Edinburgh, Churchill-Livingstone, 1979.

Edmeads, J. The physiology of pain: A review. *Prog. Neuropharmacol. Biol. Psychiatry 7:*413-419, 1983.

Fields, H.L. Pain II: New approaches to management. *Ann. Neurol. 9:*101-106, 1981.

Lipton, S. (ed.). *Persistent Pain. Modern Methods of Treatment.* New York, Grune & Stratton, 1977.

Livingston, W.K. *Pain Mechanisms. Physiological Interpretation.* New York, Plenum Press, 1976.

Melzack, R., Wall, P.D. Pain mechanisms: A new theory. *Science 150:*971, 1965.

IV
IMPORTANT NEUROLOGICAL DISORDERS

INTRODUCTION TO PART IV

When a patient brings a complaint to you, you must first try to determine *whether or not his lesion is in the nervous system.* This may be the most difficult decision of all. The data upon which that decision will be based were given in Parts I and III. If you conclude that it is the nervous system, you must then determine *what level* it appears to involve and how extensively. Information allowing that decision is discussed in Part II.

Only when these points are solved are you in a position to try to determine what the underlying *pathology* is and finally, at the highest level of problem solving, to decide the *etiology* of the process.

Sometimes you will be able to go through all of these steps and to institute correct management, but if you cannot, and get stuck at one of the four steps listed, you must make another decision; this time, about the urgency with which you must deal with the situation. Whatever the symptom, the need for speedy referral is in direct proportion to the rate of progress of the condition.

You need never apologize for calling a neurological center with the simple statement, "I am not sure exactly what is going on but I feel that this patient has a progressive neurological problem that requires further evaluation." You have done enough by taking the solution of the problem as far as you can and by recognizing that unless special facilities are available, further progression will occur. You are now in a position to demand that the patient has the benefit of assessment in a neurological center.

In the remaining chapters of this book, we offer a brief outline of clinical neurology. In no case do we suggest that we have covered the subject in adequate depth to take you further than your first contact with the patient with the disease in question, and for this reason, we have included suggestions for further reading in each chapter in case you want to go further than the larger textbooks of medicine. Mainly, these references are to texts chosen because they present recent, readable, relevant, and fairly comprehensive coverage of the disease in question .

We have however tried to emphasize and describe in slightly greater detail those diseases that we ourselves saw most commonly in general practice and that we still have referred to us in our outpatient clinics most often. In addition to those that are common, we have also included others because they demand emergency management, because there is treatment available even though the disease may not be seen by a general practitioner more than once every 2 or 3 years, or because they illuminate recent advances in the neurosciences and may be expected to grow yet further in importance in coming years.

When we mention diseases that are rare, culled from the garden of neurological exotica, it is solely so that you need not feel insecure when somebody else mentions these recherché diagnoses. Common things occur commonly, and we have tried to make sure that it is those that you will meet most commonly in the succeeding chapters.

37
Strokes

A stroke is a focal neurological disorder developing suddenly because of a pathological process of blood vessels. Strokes are the third most common cause of death in our population (10.6 percent of deaths) with an incidence of about 200 cases per 100,000 population per year. But death resulting from stroke is only one aspect of the problem, because a depressing number of the patients who survive are disabled by their cerebrovascular disease. These are people who are usually quite well until the moment of their sudden stroke. Perhaps 70 percent of them have had their first stroke in the age range of 45 to 65 years.

CEREBROVASCULAR FLOW DYNAMICS

There are a few basic concepts important in understanding the dynamics of cerebrovascular disease. We stress the term *dynamics* because the older idea that the brain is supplied by a number of end arteries is incorrect. Three factors that must be considered in understanding cerebral blood supply are the anatomy of the cerebral circulation, cerebral blood flow, and collateral blood supply.

Anatomy

There are two systems supplying the brain: the carotid and the vertebrobasilar systems (Fig. 37-1). These are connected by the circle of Willis. The textbook picture of the circle of Willis is unusual, as congenital variations are seen in perhaps 85 percent of people. The circle may not be complete, and even major vessels may be absent or extremely small. The normal anatomy will not be considered here, and you should refer to your anatomy textbook for this information.

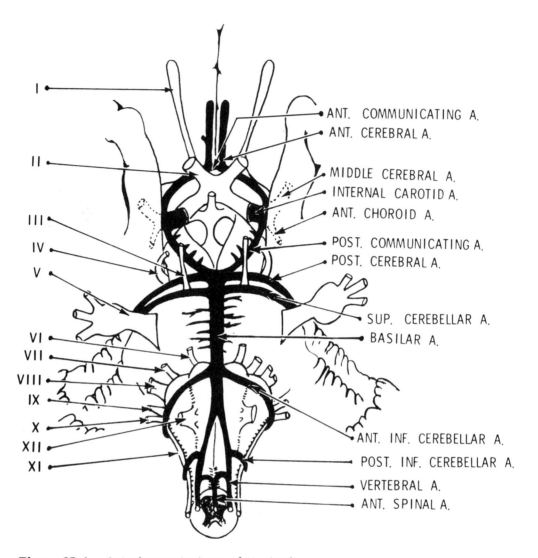

I

ANT. COMMUNICATING A.
ANT. CEREBRAL A.

II

MIDDLE CEREBRAL A.
INTERNAL CAROTID A.
ANT. CHOROID A.

III

POST. COMMUNICATING A.
POST. CEREBRAL A.

IV

V

SUP. CEREBELLAR A.
BASILAR A.

VI
VII
VIII
IX

X
XII
XI

ANT. INF. CEREBELLAR A.
POST. INF. CEREBELLAR A.
VERTEBRAL A.
ANT. SPINAL A.

Figure 37-1   Arteries at the base of the brain.

Collateral Supply

Many collateral vessels connect the major vessels supplying the brain (anterior
cerebral, middle cerebral, and posterior cerebral arteries) and the brain stem
(various branches of the vertebrobasilar system) (Fig. 37-2A-C). The circle of
Willis acts as a collateral connection between many of these major divisions and
particularly between the carotid and vertebrobasilar systems. There are also
collaterals connecting the extracranial to the intracranial vessels.

The branches of the major intracerebral vessels form an extensive collateral
bed. Thus with an occlusion of a middle cerebral artery (MCA), the posterior
cerebral (PCA) artery can supply much of this area through its collateral connection. As a result, most infarctions do not exactly demarcate the anatomical distribution of a vessel involved. Occasionally, this anastomotic area between two

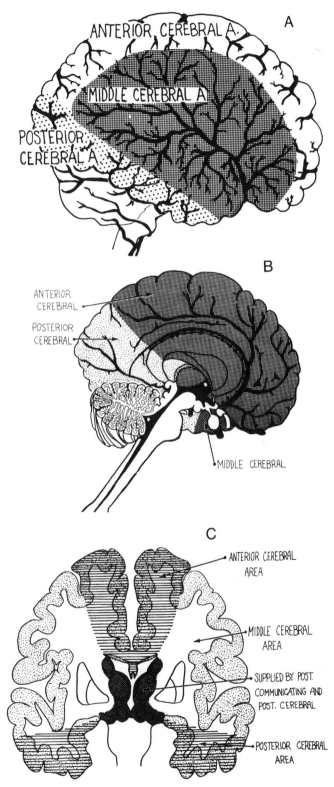

Figure 37-2 Anatomy of the cerebral vascular territories. (A) Lateral; (B) Medial; (C) Coronal views.

cerebral arteries ("watershed") is the site of infarction when both vessels are partially occluded and this border zone becomes ischemic.

An occlusion of a major intracerebral artery may be compensated for by redirection of the flow of blood within the circle of Willis. For example, one anterior cerebral artery can be supplied from the othre side through the anterior communicating artery.

Extracranial anastomoses can also supply intracranial structures. Carotid occlusion seldom causes blindness of the eye on that side because of the collateral connections between the external carotid artery and the ophthalmic artery. Meningeal, occipital, thyrocervical, costocervical, and caroticotympanic arteries can reverse their flow and dilate, thus supplying the brain if an appropriate vessel obstruction has occurred.

This potentially extensive collateral system can almost immediately come into play and this explains many peculiarities about strokes, particularly why they do not occur in some situations. The efficiency of the collaterals depends upon

Their anatomy: Some congenital anomalies remove potential collateral patterns. Thus agenesis of the posterior communicating artery will make infarction of the occipital lobe on that side more likely if there is an occlusion of the vertebrobasilar system. If the posterior communicating artery is not functioning, the carotid system cannot deliver blood back to that side.

The cross-sectional area of the lumina of the collateral supply: If the total area is equal to that of the occluded vessel then the anastomoses will probably be adequate.

The location of the collateral vessels: If the site of anastomosis is nearer the heart and is proximal to the occlusion, it tends to be more efficient. This of course depends upon the number of anastomotic channels.

The state of the vascular system: Atherosclerotic lesions, for example, will impair the potential for the opening of collaterals.

Timing: A *sudden* occlusion will allow little time for the collateral circulation to adapt to the altered flow patterns, while *gradual* occlusions can be compensated for by an efficient collateral circulation with perhaps little or no neurological deficit developing.

Cerebral Blood Flow

The cerebral vessels are different from peripheral vessels. The sympathetic fibers anatomically present appear to have little functional significance except perhaps to regulate blood pressure effects in the larger vessels around the circle of Willis. The regulation of cerebral blood flow is essentially by *autoregulation.* If blood pressure is reduced in the cerebral circulation, dilatation of the vessels occurs to maintain blood flow at a constant rate. In hypertension, cerebrovascular constriction will again keep the flow constant. Cerebral blood flow is dramatically changed by altering arterial CO_2 content because carbon dioxide is the most powerful cerebral vasodilator known. An increase in arterial oxygen tension will cause vasoconstriction, as will alkalosis, but both of these factors and blood pressure are weak in comparison with the effect of carbon dioxide. Drugs appear to have little effect on cerebral blood flow and this includes the many medications advertised for their effect of "dilating the cerebral vessels of your patient with cerebrovascular disease." Intracranial pressure, sleep, CSF pH, and body temperature all have relatively little effect on cerebral blood flow.

Cerebral blood flow is kept strikingly constant in spite of a variety of anatomical and metabolic variations. Autoregulation is an intrinsic mechanism regulating vessel diameter. Only in extreme situations do the vessels fail to compensate, allowing a fall in cerebral blood flow. A stroke represents such an extreme situation, involving a decrease in blood supply to a localized area, for which cerebral autoregulation and the presence of collaterals cannot compensate. The power of autoregulation may be lost if there is a severe fall in diastolic blood pressure below 50 mmHg or a rise above 150 mmHg. Autoregulation may also fail in the area of a cerebral infarction or when there is severe vascular disease, such as widespread atherosclerosis or intracranial arteritis. When autoregulation fails, the cerebral blood flow has a linear relationship to the blood pressure. Elderly patients tend to lose some of this autoregulatory compensation and are prone to the symptomatic effects of hypotension and hypertension.

CLASSIFICATION OF STROKES

There is an essential differentiation to be made between ischemic infarction and hemorrhage when considering the pathological basis for strokes. Sometimes however these occur together, as when spasm of cerebral vessels occurs distal to the site of a ruptured aneurysm that has produced a hemorrhage; the spasm itself may produce ischemia and perhaps infarction.

Four classes of ischemic stroke are defined, as follows:

1. *Transient ischemic attacks* (TIAs): Brief ischemia, most often caused by an embolus, produces focal symptoms and signs lasting (quite arbitrarily) less than 24 hr.
2. *Reversible ischemic neurological deficit* (RIND): The same as TIA, but signs persist for longer than 24 hr before full clinical recovery.
3. *Evolving stroke:* Ischemic or hemorrhagic stroke worsening under your clinical scrutiny, usually in a step-wise fashion.
4. *Completed stroke:* Ischemic or hemorrhagic stroke that has caused maximal deficit and that may now start to show improvement.

The lesion causing cerebral ischemia may be within the vessel (embolus), in the wall (spasm, arteritis, or atherosclerosis), or entirely extracranial (hypoxemia or reduced cardiac output). Anoxia may produce relatively minor transient symptoms and signs, or it may lead to infarction, an irreversible state of ischemic damage from which the brain cells cannot completely recover.

Intracranial hemorrhage may occur because of rupture either of the smallest vessels deep in the substance of the brain or of an aneurysm, situated usually at the base of the brain or close to the circle of Willis. Less common causes of hemorrhage are bleeding from an arteriovenous malformation or hemorrhagic infarction resulting from an embolus.

The relative frequency of the three types of strokes (ischemic, embolic, hemorrhagic) is in some dispute. For many years, thrombosis was considered by far the most common cause; for instance, the middle cerebral artery syndrome was thought to be due to occlusion of the middle cerebral artery until it was shown that almost 50 percent of these cases had a significant thrombotic lesion in the large vessels in the neck, usually in the internal carotid artery. We are now recognizing that emboli from these sites are a common cause of transient attacks and strokes, rather than decreased blood flow because of the arterial narrowing or occlusion itself. The heart is a much more important cause of ischemic symptoms, either because of an arrhythmia or to cardiac emboli, than was previously thought. This has been made plain by long-term cardiac monitoring and telemetry. It has also been noted that in many cases of cerebral infarction with no significant arterial disease at postmortem, there is evidence of a cardiac origin of an embolism. This probably accounts for the strokes that had previously been ascribed to arterial spasm or hypotension. It is beginning to appear that "atherosclerotic occlusive thrombosis," a time-honored diagnosis in clinical neurology, might be quite unusual.

Although middle cerebral artery infarction is the most common clinical stroke, only 4 percent can be shown at autopsy to have an actual occlusion of that vessel. About 75 percent of these patients have internal carotid artery lesions and 75 percent have evidence of embolism. Therefore interest in the pathogenesis of stroke has shifted outside the head to the large vessels in the neck and to the cardiovascular system.

In assessing any acute cerebral catastrophe we must consider the differential diagnosis of ischemic, embolic, and hemorrhagic stroke from other common non-vascular pathologies that may also cause the sudden appearance of neurological signs. Epileptic seizures with Todd's paralysis are sometimes indistinguishable from strokes when first seen, particularly because emboli and hemorrhages may sometimes present with seizures. Multiple sclerosis, tumors, cerebral abscesses, and extra- or subdural hematomas can all mimic stroke patterns, and one should never assume that an elderly patient with a sudden onset of a grave neurological disorder is necessarily suffering from a stroke. In younger patients, diseases of the arterial wall that are not atherosclerotic (associated with infection, syphilis, diabetes, and collagen-vascular disease) have to be considered.[*]

PATHOGENESIS

Thrombosis and Embolism

Atheromatous occlusion of the great vessels in the neck is particularly common at sites of bifurcation or change in course of the vessels (Fig. 37-3). Thus the origins of the innominate, carotid, subclavian, and vertebral arteries, the bifurcations of the carotid arteries, and the more tortuous portions of the cerebral and carotid arteries are the major sites of atherosclerotic plaques, ulcers, and stenosis (Fig. 37-4).[†] Exposed collagen at these sites causes the platelets in the blood flowing past to adhere to the wall because of a difference in electrical charge. The platelets that adhere to the collagen release ADP which results in platelet aggregation producing a platelet thrombus. The platelet aggregates are friable, hence they break up easily and may embolize. They may become more organized and form thrombi when fibrin is laid down. The thrombus then becomes organized and may be dislodged as a more solid embolus. The friable platelet emboli typically lead to only transient, if any, symptoms, but a firm, organized embolus tends to produce a more solid vascular obstruction and is more likely to produce an infarction.

---

[*]Largely because of the control now obtained over hypertension, the prevalence of stroke (and of myocardial infarction) is showing a decline in the Western world. Drugs are partly responsible but refrigeration (leading to a decline in the use of salt as a preservative) is probably just as important.

[†]Examination of the neck vessels is a vital part of the workup of the stroke patient, but although an editorial in *Stroke* once advised that patients with TIAs should be "carefully osculated for cervical bruits. . . , we would not go that far and advise you not to either.

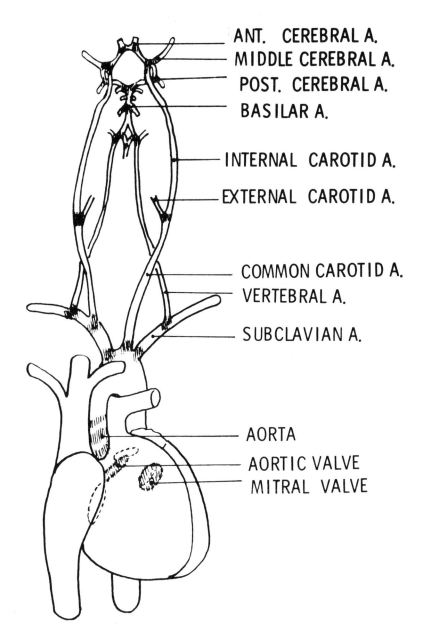

Figure 37-3   Common sites of atheromatous stenosis or ulceration in the neck vessels.

Atherosclerosis is a disorder of the larger arteries and it is unusual to find typical changes of the condition more distal than the larger branches arising from the circle of Willis. This is in contrast with the vascular change typical of hypertension, which is primarily found in arterioles. Thrombosis of the extracranial vessels and embolism from these lesions or from the heart should be considered in any case of stroke.

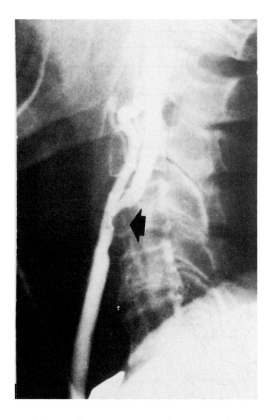

Figure 37-4   Left carotid arteriogram. Irregular stenosis and ulceration at the carotid bifurcation.

Cerebral emboli are usually composed of platelets and fibrin if they arise from extracranial vessels, although cholesterol and atheromatous material from ulcerated plaques may also embolize (Fig. 37-5). In comparison, emboli arising from the other sites listed in Table 37-1 are rare. Except for infective emboli that may produce a *mycotic aneurysm,* the clinical features of all emboli are more or less similar. These will be discussed in the next section.

Emboli may cause either transient ischemia of an area of brain or infarction. If the ischemia is transient, the blood supply may be reinstituted by the opening of collateral vessels, or the emboli may break up allowing blood to flow again. Undoubtedly in many instances, emboli do not produce either transient ischemic attacks or infarction and are completely asymptomatic.

There are a number of risk factors that predispose to the development of atherosclerosis of the cerebrovascular system, and these are essentially the same as those for coronary and peripheral vascular disease (see Tables 37-2 and 37-3). The most important include hypertension, both systolic and diastolic, hyperlipidemia, and diabetes. Obesity and the presence of ischemic heart disease are others. Smoking, hyperlipidemia, and increased triglycerides rather seem to predispose to ischemic heart disease. In cerebral emboli, atrial fibrillation (from any cause), cardiomyopathy, valve prostheses, recent myocardial infarcts, and prolapsed mitral valve are the major risk factors.

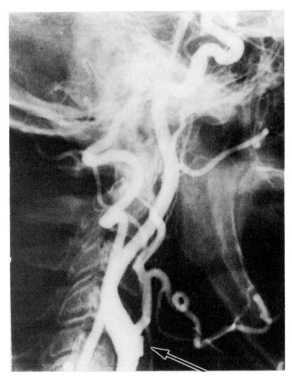

Figure 37-5   Right brachial angiogram, lateral view. The arrow shows a well-defined punched-out rulcer below the bifurcation. The patient was experiencing TIAs.

It is important to remember that virtually all can be treated, even with the family history of disease in many cases, because this may be of hypertension, hyperlipidemia, diabetes, or other manageable problems.

Transient ischemic attacks are usually embolic, as was mentioned. There are other mechanisms however that can also produce brief ischemia, including vascular spasm from migraine and severe hypertension and severe generalized reduction in cerebral blood flow caused by cardiac arrhythmias or hypotension. Ischemia is particularly likely to occur if there is any preexisting obstruction in the cerebral vessels. Ischemia may also occur when an obstruction causes blood flow to be "stolen" from another area. A classic example of this is the *subclavian steal syndrome* (Fig. 37-6). To compensate for stenosis or occlusion of the first part of a subclavian artery, blood is diverted from one vertebral artery *down* the other one so that it supplies the occluded subclavian at a point distal to the obstruction and prevents the normal flow of blood from the healthy vertebral into the basilar artery. Ischemia can also result from polycythemia, due to slowed circulation or occlusion because of the sludging effect of high-viscosity blood, or from marked anemia.

Intracranial Hemorrhage

Although hypertension has been mentioned as a risk factor in the development of atherosclerosis and of thrombotic or embolic cerebral vascular disease, it also

Table 37-1   Origins of Cerebral Emboli

Cardiac

    Atrial fibrillation
    Mural thrombi after myocardial infarction
    Acute and subacute bacterial endocarditis
    Aortic and mitral valve disease, including prolapsing mitral valve
    Nonbacterial thrombotic endocarditis
    Paradoxical embolism
    Complications of cardiac surgery and prosthetic valves
    Atrial myxoma

Noncardiac

    Atheroma of aorta, carotids, and vertebrals
    Atheroma of largest intracranial vessels
    Pulmonary vein thrombi
    Fat emboli
    Tumor emboli
    Air emboli
    Complications of pulmonary and neck surgery

Uncertain

Table 37-2   Risk Factors for Stroke

    Advanced age
    Cardiac disease
    Hypertension (diastolic and systolic)
    Hyperlipidemia
    Diabetes mellitus
    A family history of vascular disease
    Smoking
    Physical inactivity
    Oral contraceptive pills
    Abnormal ECG
    Polycythemia
    Severe anemia

Table 37-3   Causes of Hemorrhagic Strokes

Intracerebral hemorrhage

> Hypertensive intracerebral hemorrhage*
> Trauma
> Hematological disorders
> Anticoagulant therapy
> Hemorrhage into tumors
> Septic embolism or mycotic aneurysms
> Amyloid angiopathy
> Vasculitis
> Vasopressor drugs
> Encephalitis and postinfectious encephalopathy

Subarachnoid hemorrhage

> Ruptured saccular aneurysm
> Ruptured angioma
> Trauma
> Anticoagulant therapy

*About 10 percent of all strokes.

predisposes to the development of sudden intracranial hemorrhage. In most cases one of two pathological lesions is present. In the first, fibrinoid necrosis of arterioles deep in the white matter causes weakening of the arteriolar wall with the production of tiny aneurysms bound by glial tissue (Charcot-Bouchard aneurysms). With continuing arteriolar damage and disruption of its muscular coat, further weakening of the wall may lead to hemorrhage that cannot be prevented by arteriolar constriction. The severity of a hemorrhage is widely variable. On the one hand, there may be no more than a few milliliters of blood released, splitting local white matter fibers and producing a smaller area of local damage. Later a small cavity results, called a *lacune*. If the hemorrhage is more severe it will act as a quickly expanding mass lesion, producing compressive brain destruction (Fig. 37-7). The blood will track further afield and often enters the CSF or the ventricles. The sudden hemorrhagic mass lesion produces widespread pressure changes that may compress the brainstem structures, causing hemorrhages in the pons (Duret hemorrhages). Most intracranial hemorrhages occur in the deep central area of the brain and the small lacunes are found particularly in the putamen, the internal capsule, corona radiate, and in the pons and deep white matter of the cerebellum.

The second lesion causing intracerebral hemorrhage is a ruptured aneurysm. The aneurysm is a dilatation of an artery and varies from a few millimeters to 2 or 3 cm in diameter, occurring at the bifurcation of a vessel where the media is weakest (Fig. 37-8). In the presence of hypertension, raised pressure in the weaker areas may produce dilatation and, in time, rupture with sudden bleeding into the subarachnoid space and often into the brain itself. The local vascular spasm caused by both the vessel rupture and the presence of blood in the subarachnoid space results in further widespread vasospasm increasing the risk of severe brain damage. Thus although the bleeding may remain in the subarachnoid space, there may be a pale infarct in the distribution of the vessel intracerebrally.

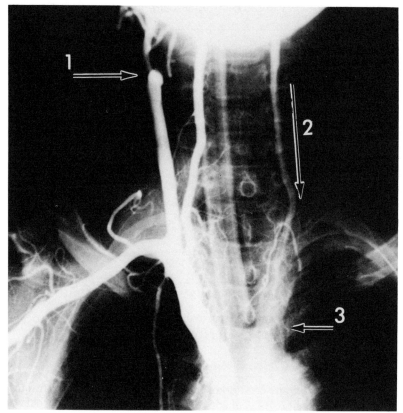

Figure 37-6   Arch angiogram in subclavian steal syndrome. (1) Occlusion of the right ICA at its origin; (2) Downward flow of (dye) blood in left vertebral artery; (3) Failure of left subclavian artery filling at its take-off from the aorta.

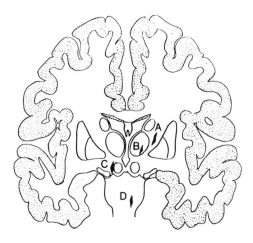

Figure 37-7   Usual sites of lacunar hemorrhages in the deep white matter. (A) Internal capsule/putamen; (B) Thalamus; (C) Mesencephalon; (D) Pons.

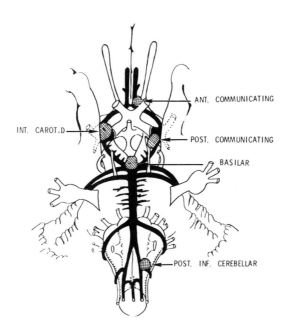

ANT. COMMUNICATING

INT. CAROT.D

POST. COMMUNICATING

BASILAR

POST. INF. CEREBELLAR

Figure 37-8   Common sites of aneurysm formation at the base of the brain. All but mycotic aneurysms tend to occur on the vessels of the circle of Willis, or before the second bifurcation of vessels arising from it.

The other causes of intracranial hemorrhage in Table 37-3 are comparatively rare. About 90 percent of subarachnoid hemorrhages are due to ruptured berry aneurysms.

We have now discussed the three common variaties of stroke; thrombosis, embolism, and hemorrhage. For more complete lists of causes see Tables 37-1, 37-2, and 37-4, but many of these are uncommon and will not be described.

CLINICAL FEATURES OF STROKES

Transient Ischemic Attacks

Transient ischemic attacks (TIAs) are brief, transient and focal disturbances of neurological function that clear with little or no residual deficit within 24 hr. We have not been as strict in this definition as some authors, who regard any mild residual deficit after 24 hr as representing a cerebral infarction rather than a TIA, because our management of these patients who rapidly recover is the same as for TIAs. Transient ischemic attacks were formerly referred to as little strokes, but they are harbingers of more serious ones. A careful history in stroke patients will elicit evidence of previous transient disturbances of function in about half the subjects.

If a group of TIA patients are followed over the long-term, 5 to 10 percent will have a major infarction each year, but the greatest risk is in the first 3 months

Table 37-4   Causes of Transient Cerebral Ischemia

Emboli (see Table 37-1): Cardiac origin
                          Noncardiac origin
                          Uncertain origin

Carotid artery stenosis or occlusion

Subclavian steal syndrome

Polycythemia, anemia

Carotid sinus sensitivity

Hypertensive crises

Other causes of syncope (see Table 10-3)

Migraine

following the first TIA episode. A patient has about a 40 percent chance of a major cerebral infarction within 5 years of a TIA.*

Clinical Features

Symptoms may involve either the carotid or the vertebrobasilar system. Transient dysphasia, hemiparesis, or hemianesthesia involving the face, arm, and leg, or monocular visual disturbance are typical symptoms with TIAs in the carotid territory. In such cases, abrupt, painless loss of function occurs, reaching its maximum within minutes or less, and clearing progressively over minutes or hours. A patient may describe monocular visual loss "like a curtain being drawn" over part of his visual field, during which period a pale embolus may be visible in a retinal arteriole (see Fig. 20-2)†

Vertebrobasilar symptoms include brief unconsciousness, vertigo, visual hallucinations, hemianopic visual loss, drop attacks, bilateral weakness, diplopia, and ataxia. Alternating hemiplegia (involvement of the face on one side and the arm and leg on the other) also indicates a lesion of the vertebrobasilar territory in the brainstem. Because such TIAs cause no lasting deficit, it is very important that the patient be correctly diagnosed and treated to prevent the occurrence of further attacks and strokes in the future. Although in perhaps 40 percent of the cases the attacks may stop spontaneously, the chances of stroke are still high and an aggressive attitude toward therapy is warranted. The various causes are shown in Table 37-4.

All of the pathologies that may lead to TIAs should be considered, as also the conditions that may masquerade as them, before a diagnosis of TIA resulting from platelet embolism is made (see Chapter 9 and Table 37-5).

An atherosclerotic basis is suspected if there is evidence of vascular disease elsewhere such as intermittent claudication, angina, or a history of myocardial infarction. There may also be atherosclerotic changes in the fundi, an absence of peripheral pulses, or hypertension. A carotid bruit may be found localized to the

---

*Actually, the major cause of death is not a stroke but a myocardial infarction, which affects 20 percent of patients with TIA within 5 years. In fact a TIA is a better predictor of MI than is angina.

†But remember that under the age of 40, this symptom (amaurosis fugax is its older name) is probably caused by migraine.

Table 37-5   Leading Causes of Transient Episodes of Neurological Dysfunction

Migraine
Transient ischemic attacks (see Tables 10-3 and 37-4)
Seizures
Acute hyperventilation syndromes
Cerebral tumor or subdural hematoma
Multiple sclerosis
Hypoglycemia
Labyrinthine vertigo including Ménières syndrome
Cataplexy
Leaking intracranial aneurysm or AV malformation
Ingested drugs or toxic agents

bifurcation in the neck. However this is an overrated sign of carotid vascular disease because many patient with carotid stenosis do not have a bruit, and occluded carotid vessels are silent. Also many normal people have bruits of no significance.

Embolic and Thrombotic Infarction

Embolic and thrombotic infarctions (also known as atherothrombotic brain infarcts, ABIs) are classed together here, first because a clinical differentiation is often impossible; second, because both are often operational in the patient; and finally because the authors feel that thrombotic strokes *per se* are uncommon compared with embolic strokes (Table 37-6).

In ABI the onset may be acute and sudden; progressive over a short period of hours; or step-wise over a 24 hr period or longer. There may be a history of similar brief transient episodes in the days, weeks, or months preceding the stroke in half the cases. The patients are often elderly, but strokes do occur in younger-aged groups. There is frequently evidence of atherosclerotic disease in the peripheral or cardiac vessels by history or examination; and hypertension, diabetes, or xanthomatosis may also be found. Many of these patients do not lose consciousness but drowsiness, confusion, and stupor are common if strokes involve large areas. Unconsciousness often results if the brainstem RAS is involved (Chapter 10).

The focal abnormalities that result from a stroke depend entirely upon which area of the brain has suffered ischemic damage. Some of the common syndromes are described in the following section. There are many variations on these patterns and partial syndromes are very common. It is important to remember that an infarction in the distribution of a vessel does not necessarily mean that there is any pathological process in that vessel itself. The problem is often in the neck vessels or heart, or the ischemia may be due to hemodynamic change from hypotension, cardiac arrhythmia, anemia, or polycythemia.

Carotid Syndromes (see Table 37-7)

Middle Cerebral Territory Infarction: This is the most common pattern of stroke. Typically, the eyes are deviated toward the infarcted hemisphere and there is a spastic hemiparesis on the opposite side, with the arm involved more than the leg, and with a lower-quadrant facial weakness. Tone may initially be decreased, but spasticity will develop over days or weeks. Sometimes the leg has no significant

Table 37-6   Causes of Cerebral Infarction

Atherosclerosis

Arteritis
    Infections (syphilis, meningitis)
    Collagen-vascular diseases (temporal arteritis, lupus)

Hematological disorders
    Polycythemia
    Sickle-cell disease
    Thrombotic thrombocytopenia
    Macroglobulinemias

Trauma to the carotid artery

Complications of angiography

Dissecting aortic aneurysm

Hypotension

Migraine (vasoconstrictive phase)

Hypoxia

Radiation

Closed head injury

Table 37-7   Common Stroke Syndromes

Carotid

    Middle cerebral artery infarction 86%
    Anterior cerebral infarction 1%
    Posterior cerebral artery infarction 3%

Vertebral basilar 10%

---

sensory or motor involvement, and the arm may appear to be primarily involved. Hemisensory loss in the face, arm, and leg is common on the side opposite the infarction, but the trunk tends to be much less involved. Homonymous hemianopia indicates involvement of the optic radiation. If the dominant hemisphere is involved, an expressive and/or a receptive dysphasia may occur, while in the non-dominant hemisphere a parietal lobe syndrome may result. Right hemisphere lesions often cause a confusional state; those on the left commonly lead to depressive syndromes in the later stages.

Brain swelling may cause coning (see Chapter 10) and occlusion of one or both PCAs, producing a hemianopia or cortical blindness. Figure 37-9A,B illustrates MCA infarcts.

With occlusion of the internal carotid artery in the neck by the thrombosis, the anterior cerebral artery usually gets enough blood through the anterior communicating artery from the opposite side to prevent infarction in the frontal and medial portions of the hemisphere. The posterior cerebral should get an adequate

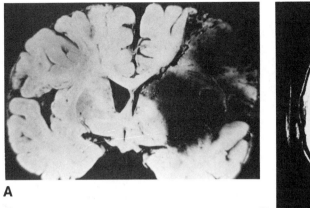
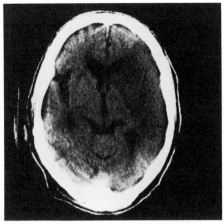

Figure 37-9 (A) Coronal section of brain. Hemorrhagic infarction in the territory of the right MCA. The adjacent territories of the ACA and PCA are seen to be spared; (B) Unenhanced CT scan. A large wedge-shaped, low-density area is seen in the territory of the right MCA, with some mass effect.

supply from the vertebrobasilar system. Thus carotid occlusion often manifests as an infarction in the territory of the middle cerebral artery but not in the entire carotid distribution.

Although the presence of a localized bruit over the bifurcation of the carotid may be of some help in determining the presence of a stenotic lesion, palpation of the vessel is of dubious value because the presence of the external carotid may enable one to feel a normal pulse in that area. However a marked difference in the carotid pulse on the two sides may indicate common carotid artery occlusion on the side of the reduced pain. Occlusion of the ICA may be suggested by relatively increased pulses in the facial or superficial temporal vessels on that side, because these are branches of the ECA, which is now receiving all the carotid blood supply. This is a difficult judgment to make however. Orbital bruits may be due to ICA stenosis.

Anterior Cerebral Territory Infarction: This is a much less common type of stroke and is characterized by more marked weakness of the leg than of the arm. The face is usually spared. The patient's head and eyes are deviated toward the infarcted side. Sensory changes in the leg are minimal or absent. Urinary incontinence and personality changes may be seen. If the dominant hemisphere is involved, an expressive dysphasia is common, while if the nondominant hemisphere is involved, apraxia of the opposite limbs or of all limbs may be found. Occasionally a cerebellar-like syndrome can result from disruption of fibers connecting the frontal lobes to the cerebellum (Bruns's ataxia). This manifests primarily by incoordination and ataxia on the side opposite the infarction. Nystagmus and speech abnormalities are less common than with cerebellar lesions, and another clue to the frontal localization is the finding of unilateral cerebellar signs on the same side as pyramidal changes.

Watershed infarcts comprise 10 percent of all. They are usually due to an abrupt fall in blood pressure or to ICA occlusion and lead to syndromes of dysphasia, hemianopia, and sensory or motor deficit because of ischemia of the areas of brain situated between the territories of supply of the middle and anterior, or middle and posterior cerebral arteries.

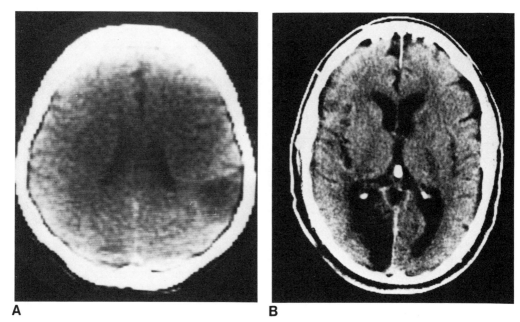

A   **B**

Figure 37-10   (A) Unenhanced CT scan. Small infarct in right parietal lobe; (B) Enhanced CT scan, showing an infarct in the left occipital lobe and ventricular dilatation.

Cerebral hypoperfusion syndromes occur in patients with severe extracranial arterial disease affecting more than one vessel. They complain of light-headedness, imbalance, and weakness of the limbs. Examination reveals such nonspecific findings as poverty of speech, mild dementia, and impaired memory. There is no orthostatic hypotension, but the symptoms improve with recumbency. Endarterectory is usually advised.

Vertebrobasilar Syndromes

Posterior Cerebral Territory Infarction: The clinical picture is variable in this type of stroke, depending upon whether the infarction occurs in the distal or more proximal distribution of the artery (Fig. 37-10A,B). With a distal infarct, a homonymous hemianopia and receptive dysphasia (if the infarction is on the dominant side) with transient confusion and memory loss result. If the artery is occluded near its origin, then branches to the thalamus and brainstem may be involved, produring a mild hemiparesis, a thalamic syndrome, or cerebellar ataxia. If ischemia occurs in the territory of *both* posterior cerebral arteries, as from hypotension or basilar artery occlusion, the patients often develop cortical blindness, sometimes with denial of the blindness (Anton's syndrome), and agitated delirium. Variable visual field defects can be documented as the patient progressively improves.

The vertebral arteries give rise to the posterior-inferior cerebellar arteries which in turn supply the lateral medulla and inferior cerebellum. Occlusion or ischemia in this area will give rise to a classic *lateral medullary syndrome.* Damage to the inferior cerebellar peduncle produces a homolateral cerebellar ataxia; damage to the nucleus ambiguus causes dysarthria and dysphonia; and involvement of the descending sympathetic fibers causes a Horner's syndrome on the same side. The descending nucleus and tract of the fifth nerve will be involved producing loss of pinprick and temperature sensation on the same side of the face, while the adjacent ascending lateral spinothalamic tract involvement produces similar findings in the arm, trunk, and leg on the opposite side of the body. Vertigo, because of ischemia of the vestibular nuclei, and hiccups are also frequent symptoms. Because the pyramidal tracts and the medial lemiscus are are centrally placed and are supplied by paramedian branches of the vertebral and basilar arteries, they are not affected by this condition.

In a stroke patient, if the eyes deviate conjugately toward the hemiparetic side, the lesion is probably in the brainstem. Other brainstem ischemic syndromes probably will cause alternating hemiplegia, as well as signs indicating damage to, for example, the RAS, cerebellum, and sensory tracts, with marked changes in blood pressure, pulse, and respiratory rate and possibly homonymous hemianopia because of PCA occlusion.

Occlusion of the *basilar artery* is often fatal. Because so many ascending and descending tracts and cranial nerve nuclei are closely applied in a small volume of the brainstem, symptoms and signs will be severe, extensive, and bilateral, although not necessarily symmetric. Involvement of any of the cranial nerves from III to XI, of the cerebellum, of the corticospinal and corticobulbar tracts, and of the reticular system are seen. These patients are usually admitted to the hospital in coma and seldom survive.

Vertebrobasilar insufficiency (VBI) is the term used for brainstem ischemia resulting from hypertension, hypotension, atherosclerosis, or steal syndromes. Cardiac emboli usually land in the carotid territory. Cervical spondylosis predisposes to VBI by compressing the vertebral arteries as they run through the bony canals of the cervical vertebrae. Symptoms sometimes can be produced by extending or rotating the head and neck to one side or the other. Turning the head will occlude one vertebral artery even in normal people. Symptoms of VBI (i.e., brainstem symptoms) include vertigo, tinnitus, diplopia, blurring of vision, hemianopia or even total blindness, ataxia, limb weakness, and occipital headache. Occasionally a brainstem infarction is accompanied by vomiting, transient paresthesias in the face or limbs, transient reduction in consciousness, deafness, and unilateral or bilateral limb paralysis. On examination these patients may show nystagmus, patchy pyramidal tract signs, cerebellar incoordination, and variable signs of cranial nerve involvement. There may be a subclavian bruit or differences between systolic blood pressures in the arms of 20 mmHg or more.

In the event of cerebellar infarction, the same symptoms are accompanied by signs of a mass lesion compressing the brainstem and raising intracranial pressure. The prognosis with small infarctions in the vertebrobasilar territory is better than with those in the carotid territory, and recovery from a mild vertebrobasilar infarction is often excellent. Angiography is seldom warranted in patients with VBI, because surgery in this area is less well developed than in the carotid system, and a specific lesion is found less often in this territory. The management of the patient is thus seldom altered by the angiographic findings. However if a cerebellar infarct is diagnosed, surgery can be lifesaving and recovery of useful function is sometimes gratifying.

Spinal Cord Infarction

Thrombosis of the anterior spinal artery is rare and is usually secondary to trauma or cervical spondylosis. Infarctions of the spinal cord are usually caused by occlusion of a radicular artery by an atherosclerotic plaque, by a ruptured intervertebral

disk, by direct trauma, or (more commonly) by atheroma or aortic aneurysm blocking the supplying arteries as they leave the aorta. Infarction can also occur during
aortic surgery. Whether or not embolism is involved in spinal cord infarction is not
really certain.

The clinical features are those of involvement of the anterior two-thirds of the
spinal cord in the distribution of the anterior spinal artery (the posterior third of
the cord is supplied by the two posterior spinal arteries, which have more extensive
anastomoses). Damage to the corticospinal tracts produces paraplegia with a spastic bladder. Spinothalamic involvement gives rise to loss of pain and temperature
sensation up to the level of the infarction, and damage to the anterior horn cells
produces a lower motor neuron lesion with fasciculations at the level of the lesion.
Pain is usually not a feature because the posterior sensory roots are supplied by
the posterior spinal arteries.

Venous infarcts of the cord occur in patients already predisposed to venous
embolism (pregnancy, thrombophlebitis, polycythemia, etc.); spinal pain with
sensory and motor long-tract signs are characteristic features.

Hemorrhagic Strokes

Intracerebral hemorrhages may be small (producing a small lacune) or large (producing a sudden increase in intracranial pressure because of the enlarging clot). Both
types are associated with hypertension, which can also produce strokes in other ways.
In malignant hypertension intracranial arteriospasm and cerebral edema sometimes
produce reversible focal and general ischemic damage characterized by decreasing
consciousness, seizures, fundal hemorrhages, and papilledema. This is called *hypertensive encephalopathy.* Congenital berry aneurysms bleed when the blood pressure
is elevated. Hypertension also accelerates the development of atheroma.

Lacunar Strokes

Lacunar strokes may be the most common vascular lesions occurring in the brain.
These small, healed hemorrhages or ischemic infarcts can be found in many routine
autopsies, particularly on patients who have a history of hypertension, most commonly in the thalamus, striatum, internal capsule and pons, and occasionally in the
cerebellum and the corona radiata. Most patients are asymptomatic, but in about
20 percent a stroke syndrome occurs. Representative syndromes (from about 20
defined) are

1. A *pure motor hemiplegia:* Here the lesion is in the internal capsule or in the
   base of the pons.
2. A *pure hemisensory syndrome:* The lesion is in the ventrolateral nucleus of
   the thalamus.
3. *Cerebellar and pyramidal signs* occurring together in the same leg and less
   obviously in the arm: The lesion involves the superior cerebellar peduncle
   fibers after they have crossed, and the corticospinal fibers at the level of
   the midbrain.
4. A syndrome of *slurred speech, facial weakness, and clumsy hand:* This is due
   to a lacune in the base of the pons. Involvement of the face and tongue may
   account for the dysarthria. The clumsy hand is probably a manifestation of an
   upper motor neuron lesion or of a mild cerebellar syndrome.

5. Unilateral third nerve palsy with contralateral hemiplegia (Weber's syndrome).
6. Cerebellar ataxia and crossed third nerve palsy (Claude's syndrome).
7. Hemiballismus from a lesion in the subthalamic nucleus.
8. Locked-in syndrome caused by bilateral lesions of the ventral pons.
9. "Top of the basilar artery" syndrome with unilateral or bilateral third nerve palsies, paralysis of downward gaze, and drowsiness resulting from infarction in the territory of a penetrating arteriole arising from the posterior cerebral artery.

These syndromes are relatively mild and often are transient. They have a very good prognosis, particularly if the patient's blood pressure is carefully controlled. If they are recognized, they usually do not require extensive investigation because the angiogram, brain scan, EEG, and other investigations are usually normal. The CT scan shows a small area of infarction in 25 percent of cases.

Parenchymal Hemorrhage

In contrast to the relatively benign lacunar syndromes, primary hypertensive intracerebral hemorrhage is frequently fatal. In this situation a Charcot-Bouchard aneurysm or a small artery ruptures, causing a fiber-splitting hemorrhage, which can be small, but is more commonly moderate or massive. The intracerebral bleeding stops only when the blood pressure falls, or when either pressure within the clot rises or vasospasm in the artery prevents further bleeding.

Parenchymal hemorrhage occurs in hypertensive patients in the same sites that lacunar strokes develop (Figs. 37-11A-C and 37-12A,B) (putamen 55 percent, thalamus 25 percent, cerebellum 10 percent, subcortical 10 percent, pons 7 percent).

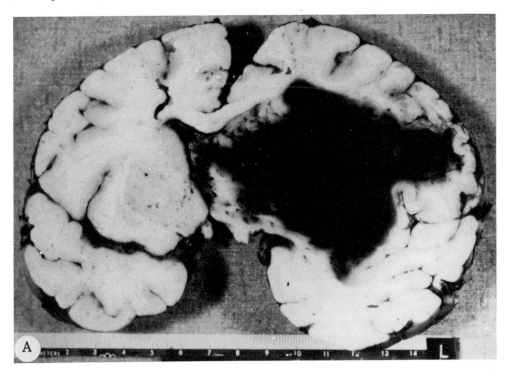

Figure 37-11A   Typical primary intracerebral hemorrhage. Large parenchymal hemorrhage into the putamen with rupture into the ventricle and through the brain tissue.

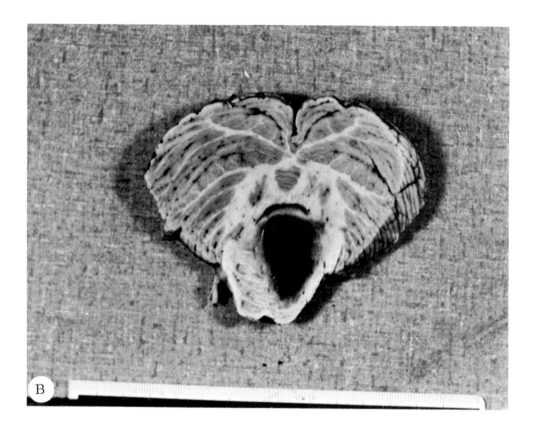

Figure 37-11B   Typical primary intracerebral hemorrhage. Pontine hemorrhage.

The most common area is that supplied by the deep penetrating vessels branching from the middle cerebral artery around the internal capsule. Symptoms are usually sudden and severe and most often occur during the day, unlike ischemic strokes, which often occur at night. The deficit is maximal within minutes of the onset of hemorrhage and the patient often loses consciousness after complaining of a severe headache with nausea and vomiting. It is one of the most common causes of sudden death.

A grand mal seizure may occur, with or without a focal onset. The severe headache and early vomiting are highly suggestive of an intracerebral hemorrhage but may also occur with a subarachnoid hemorrhage. In those patients who do not immediately lose consciousness, confusion and complaints of headache and hemiparesis are usual. Signs of raised intracranial pressure often develop.

The focal signs that might enable one to localize the lesion arre usually clouded by the presence of coma, meningism, or raised intracranial pressure. With hemorrhage into the *putamen,* both eyes are often deviated conjugately to the side of the cerebral lesion and away from the hemiparesis. With *thalamic* hemorrage, the eyes are deviated downward, the pupils are small and sluggish to reaction, and there may be aphasia and sensorimotor deficit. If the patient is conscious, marked sensory changes can be found. With *pontine* hemorrhage the patient is usually comatose, with Cheyne-Stokes or neurogenic hyperventilation, pinpoint

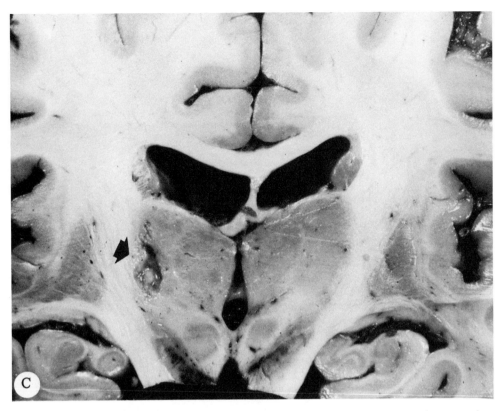

Figure 37-11C   Typical ischemic or hemorrhagic lacune in thalamus (arrowed).

pupils, hyperpyrexia, facial weakness, and flaccid quadriplegia. Decerebrate rigidity is typical. With *cerebellar* hemorrhage there may be conjugate deviation of eyes or a sixth nerve palsy without pupillary signs and often without any hemiparesis. These patients may have only a transient period of unconsciousness, awakening with vomiting and severe occipital headache. When they can cooperate, facial weakness, cerebellar signs, and meningism will usually be found. There is a particular danger of tonsillar herniation because of raised intracranial pressure, but if the syndrome is recognized, immediate neurosurgical intervention may allow excellent recovery. Although angiography can demonstrate the mass effect of a hemorrhage in the cerebellum, it is best seen by the noninvasive and more rapid CT scan, angled to see the cerebellum and brainstem.

It has been suggested that because the hemorrhage splits fibers apart rather than destroying them, patients recover better than from an ischemic infarction if they survive the initial event.

The differentiation of bleeding at other sites is probably less important, but the recognition and removal of a large intracerebral clot by the neurosurgeon can result in excellent improvement in some patients.

Hemorrhages sometimes occur from arteriovenous malformations, in bleeding diatheses, after trauma, or from disease of the vessel wall such as cerebral amyloid angiopathy. In many of these conditions, the CT scan (you will not make the diagnosis any other way) shows that the bleed is in or just under the cortex — very atypical sites in primary intracerebral hemorrhage.

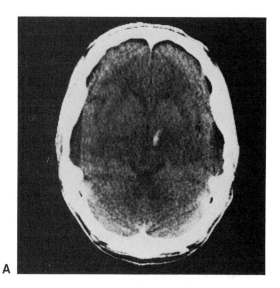

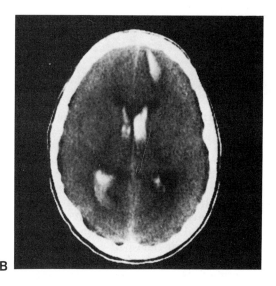

Figure 37-12   (A) Unenhanced CT scan showing a small hemorrhage in the basal ganglia; (B) Unenhanced CT scan; hemorrhages in the frontal lobe and left basal ganglia, extending into the ventricles.

Subarachnoid Hemorrhage

Most patients with subarachnoid hemorrhage (SAH) have bled from a ruptured berry aneurysm. Such intracranial aneurysms are usually found on the vessels around the circle of Willis or on the arteries directly leading from it (Fig. 37-13A,B).*
    They occur at bifurcations where the muscular medial coat is deficient and the elastica and intima may be damaged by hypertension. Under these circumstances the intima is unable to withstand the increased intraluminal pressure and bulges out. Because the intracranial vessels are not covered by any adventitia, the aneurysm so formed expands and those over 10 mm in diameter often rupture. Before doing so, it may compress local structures, usually the second or third nerves.
    The risk of SAH is much increased in smokers and in women taking oral contraceptives.

Clinical Features

A rupturing aneurysm bleeds into the subarachnoid space producing sudden, severe, explosive headache with transient or prolonged loss of consciousness in about half the patients (Fig. 37-14). Occasionally a grand mal seizure may occur. If the patient is awake, severe headache and meningism are the major complaints. Examination may show confusion, Babinski's signs, and other focal neurological deficits. Preretinal (subhyaloid) hemorrhages may be seen on fundoscopy.

---

*The sites of bleeding aneurysms are quite easy to remember; about one-third occur on the MCA, a quarter on the ACA/A Comm A, a fifth on the ICA/P Comm A and a sixth on the basilar A or its branches. One in five patients will have multiple aneurysms.

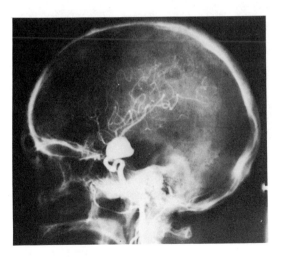

Figure 37-13A   Left carotid angiogram, lateral, showing a huge ICA aneurysm in the cavernous sinus.

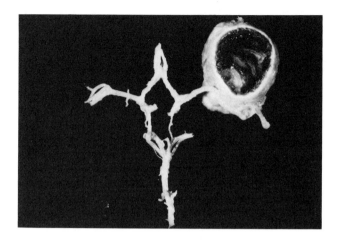

Figure 37-13B   Giant middle cerebral aneurysm.

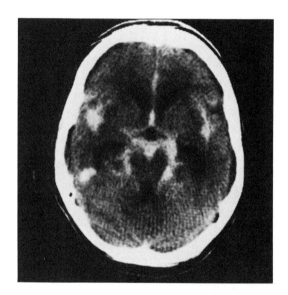

Figure 37-14   Unenhanced CT scan, showing blood in the basal cisterns, inter-hemispheric fissure, and insulas of temporal lobes. Subarachnoid hemorrhage.

Monocular blindness and a severe confusional state may attend the rupture of an aneurysm on the anterior communicating artery while a third nerve palsy is commonly found with an aneurysm on the posterior communicating artery. Apart from these, few signs exist to help one clinically to locate the site of the aneurysm, although motor asymmetries may assist in lateralization. Minor bleeding may have occurred in the past, producing only headache, nuchal rigidity, or transient mild CNS dysfunction which were ignored.

Metabolic changes associated with SAH frequently include diencephalic stimulation with alteration of sympathetic function. Both blood sugar levels and blood
pressure tend to be elevated, and ECG abnormalities are common. The latter may
be due to alteration in sympathetic tone and include bradycardia with a prolonged
QT interval and large upright or deeply inverted T waves. The ECG changes often
suggest a myocardial infarction and appropriate treatment may therefore be with-
held if it is not recognized that such changes are extremely common in SAH.

In patients who have had an acute onset with coma, the diagnosis from primary
intracerebral hemorrhage can be difficult. In these cases the CSF can be examined,
but this is potentially dangerous, particularly in the patient with an intracerebral
clot. If the diagnosis of SAH can be made clinically with confidence, there seems
little point in performing a lumbar puncture, especially since the CT scan can determine the presence of blood in the subarachnoid space and in the basal cisterms,
as well as showing any intracerebral bleeding. The absence of blood in the cisterns
in SAH is a good prognostic sign.

Differential Diagnosis

Other conditions may be confused with SAH or sentinel headache. Meningitis or
encephalitis of sudden onset may mimic it, and if there is any doubt about the
diagnosis and the question of meningitis has been raised, lumbar puncture is justi-
fiable. Some red cells may be found in the CSF in cases of herpes simplex encephalitis and also with embolic infarction, as a result of migration of red cells from
the damaged brain into the subarachnoid space. These conditions do not give rise
to frank blood in the CSF however. Patients taking monoamine oxidase inhibitors
who eat foods containing tyramine may have symptoms and signs similar to SAH
with increased blood pressure and severe headache without any actual bleeding,
although SAH has also complicated this situation. Severe migraine headaches
(particularly in patients who have not had migraine before), coital cephalgia, and
severe cluster migraine may suggest a diagnosis of SAH, but these patients will
have a clear CSF. Acute neck strain, pituitary infarction, hypertensive encephalopathy, and severe systemic infections may also cause difficulty in diagnosis.

About one in ten cases of SAH are due to bleeding from an arteriovenous
malformation (Fig. 37-15). Such patients may have a history of previous subarachnoid bleeding, and there is a history of recurrent seizures in 30 percent,
recurrent vascular headaches in 10 percent, and focal neurological findings in 50
percent. Patients with angiomas are usually in a much younger age group than
those with SAH caused by a ruptured aneurysm. Any premonitory features preceding the typical signs of a subarachnoid hemorrhage in a young person should
suggest the diagnosis of arteriovenous malformation. Patients with bleeding disorders and those taking anticoagulants may rarely bleed into the CSF, but in
these cases bleeding is seldom severe and the correct diagnosis is often suggested
by the history, physical examination, and initial laboratory values. The risk of a
subarachnoid hemorrhage from a ruptured aneurysm is four times higher in smokers, but the reasons are unclear.

Spinal subarachnoid hemorrhage is distinctly uncommon. The clinical features
include sudden severe root pain with incapacitating backache and meningism. This
triad is virtually diagnostic and early transfer to a neurological unit is mandatory.

Prognosis

The prognosis in SAH is not good. About half of the patients who have a bleed die
within the first month; by the end of the first year over half have died. Death

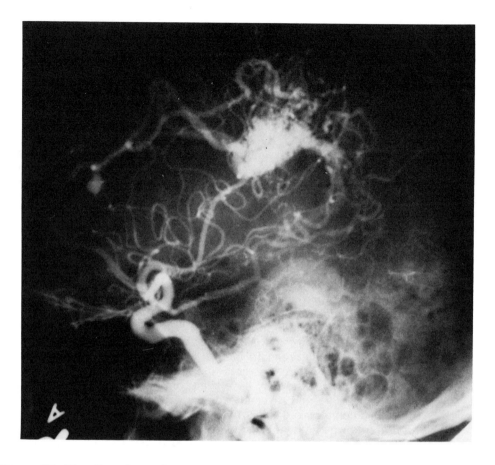

Figure 37-15   Carotid angiogram; arteriovenous malformation.

may be due to brain destruction or distortion, rebleeding, raised intracranial pressure, or compression of the brainstem. Vasospasm is one cause of secondary deterioration of consciousness with increasing physical signs. It is usually treated with blood volume repletion but calcium-channel blockers are currently under intensive study. Hyponatremia, hydrocephalus, infarcts, cardiac dysrhythmias, seizures, and rebleeding are the other leading causes. Epsilon-aminocaproic acid reduces rebleeding but may increase the risk of ischemic complications.

The prognosis in an arteriovenous malformation is much better, although they also tend to bleed again. The greatest mortality is within the first 10 days after an SAH with a further chance of rebleeding when the clot around the ruptured aneurysm lyses at 14 days. If the patient survives the first 3 months, the mortality rate for the next 5 years is only about 10 percent.

The management of SAH is considered in the following section.

Given successful surgical intervention after a SAH and good control of the blood pressure in future, a further subarachnoid hemorrhage is not likely, although the patient always has a slightly increased risk particularly if there is another aneurysm present. The dangers of blood in the CSF include both acute and normal pressure hydrocephalus, and of course, the patient may be left with some deficit after the initial episode. However these complications are not common. In about

25 percent of cases, no cause for the bleeding is ever diagnosed; these patients may have an even better prognosis than those operated upon. It is possible that in many of them, the aneurysm was destroyed by the bleed or else arteriospasm prevented further loss of blood and spontaneous healing occurred. Sometimes, a repeat angiogram after 2 weeks will show an aneurysm that was not seen during the first study, probably because of vasospasm.

MANAGEMENT OF STROKES

Some details of management have already been given but the following is a general outline for the acute, postacute, and long-term or chronic stages.

Acute Management

The initial history and findings are particularly important in determining those specific measures that must be taken for each individual patient. An assessment of the patient's general status including pulse rate, blood pressure, respiratory rate and pattern, and hydration, and of neurological signs (level of consciousness, speech, pupils, and limb movements) are essential. Observation for changing signs is far more useful than any single evaluation, however precise.

In all patients who are comatose, the support measures outlined in Chapter 10 must be provided, including the establishment of an airway and, if necessary, assisted ventilation. An IV line should be introduced to maintain fluid and electrolyte balance and all patients need intermittent catheterization.

Few investigations are required in the acute stage. You are trying to prove the diagnosis of stroke rather than, for example, tumor; to assess its extent; and to note any complications at this stage. An ECG, x-rays of chest, and routine hematological and biochemical tests will be required, and an early CT or isotope scan will be of value, particularly when contrasted with a second one a week later. Angiography may be useful in certain circumstances but this decision will be taken by a neurologist.

At this stage the awake patient may be supported by reassurance and explanation of the nature of his disease, while the family should be told of the diagnostic possibilities and the likely prognosis, although prognoses given at an early stage are often embarrassingly wrong. The uncertainty of the situation however should be recognized by the family.

Postacute Stage

Transient Ischemic Attacks

Because the symptoms and signs are transient, the patient requires an explanation and reassurance about the nature of the problem to convince him of the need for further investigations. They are indeed necessary both to assess the various risk factors and to determine the nature of the TIA that has occurred. Selective arteriography is the most useful test but one may also need to look for evidence of the conditions listed in Tables 37-4 and 37-5. We use as routine tests a complete blood count, including platelet estimation and ESR, BUN, syphilitic serology, uric acid, AC and 2-hr PC sugar, serum lipid profile and electrophoresis, a glucose tolerance test in some cases, ECG, and chest x-ray. The CT scan is negative in TIAs but positive within a day of a completed stroke.

The treatment for TIAs is currently undergoing careful study. If localized atherosclerotic stenosis of the carotid or subclavian artery can be identified, then surgical *endarterectomy* may be the appropriate treatment. The value of this procedure over other "medical" forms of therapy in preventing a future stroke is not yet proven.[*] "Operable" lesions are commoner in patients with prior TIAs, hypertension, claudication and a carotid bruit. However, only half of the patients with TIAs actually have a demonstrable ipsilateral lesion at all.

Anticoagulant therapy diminishes or completely stops the TIAs in 80 percent of the patients, but again there is, as yet, no firm evidence that anticoagulants significantly reduce the ultimate mortality. There is some evidence however that anticoagulants may prevent strokes in the most dangerous period, namely the 3 months after the first TIA, but there is little evidence that they are effective thereafter. In assessing surgery and anticoagulants, we must recall that many patients with TIAs are not candidates for either because other serious medical disease is present.

Because most transient ischemic attacks appear to be due to platelet emboli, therapy with platelet-inhibiting agents, such as aspirin and dipyridamole, is used. Aspirin alone has been successful in treating patients with typical TIAs and has been shown to reduce strokes and deaths, at least in elderly, normotensive male patients.

Therefore patients who present with transient episodes of neurological dysfunction of sudden onset and brief duration should be referred for further investigation, and if a localized area of arterial disease can be demonstrated on arteriography, then either some form of drug or surgical therapy may be considered. If no lesion is found and the diagnosis remains TIA, probably due to platelet emboli, then anticoagulants or platelet suppression should be employed.

Infarction

Most of these patients should be admitted to the hospital. Many will have an altered state of consciousness, and continued attention to the airway, ventilatory function, blood pressure, skin, bladder and bowel care, fluid and electrolyte balance, and calorie and vitamin intake will be necessary. Investigation of value are the same as for TIAs.

The place of anticoagulants is ill defined. If you are sure that the stroke is due to a cardiac lesion, and if the infarct is neither large nor the blood pressure grossly raised, then heparin may be given after 24 hr. In patients whose stroke deficit is evolving under observation and whose CT scan shows no hemorrhage, we recommend anticoagulants. In all other cases we advise against them in the acute or postacute stages, but we will use them for a flurry of TIAs not prevented by antiplatelet agents.

---

[*]The trouble is that while endarterectomy may reduce stroke morbidity, it has obviously no effect on mortality, which is more often due to myocardial infarction; and one has to consider the morbidity of angiography and of the surgical procedure itself (variously 2 to 20 percent) when determining the relative risks of operating and of not doing so. In the words of one expert: "Patients leaving hospital by the front door and with patent carotids do better than others . . . (but) . . . fewer patients leave hospital by the front door without a stroke after surgical than after medical therapy."

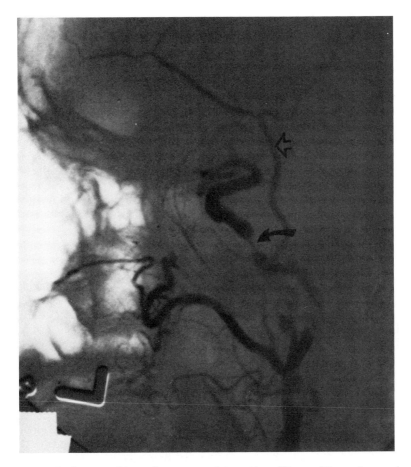

Figure 37-16   Left carotid angiogram, subtraction films. There is marked stenosis of the intracranial ICA. This lesion cannot be directly attacked.
might be a candidate for an extracranial-intracranial bypass operation.

If it is thought that some form of surgical treatment might be possible, or if
the diagnosis is in doubt, an angiogram may be required, but it is otherwise not indicated in a completed infarct. A lumbar puncture would only be indicated if
meningeal infection were suspected. An isotope scan during the first 3 or 4 days
should be negative, but it becomes positive at about 6 days. If it is positive on the
first day, suspect a cerebral tumor or arteriovenous malformation. The history,
examination, and investigation for risk factors required are again the same as the
TIAs.

Bad prognostic factors are increased age, reduced conscious level, and severe
hemiplegia, hemianopia, or higher cerebral dysfunction. Female patients and those
with hypertension or past myocardial infarcts also do less well.

When the type and site of the lesion have been diagnosed, and as soon as the
patient's condition is stable and he is conscious and rational, he should be allowed
up in bed and later in a chair and physiotherapy begun. As early as possible, active
physiotherapy should replace passive, and ambulation encouraged with gait training
and use of the limbs. Hemiparesis also causes some diminution in ventilation, so

that chest physiotherapy may be required. As soon as it is practical, catheterization should be stopped, if it has been necessary at all. Antiepileptic drugs are not routinely given because seizures follow strokes in only about 10 percent of cases, usually as a late complication.

Parenchymal Hemorrhage

The management of such patients is almost exactly the same as those with infarct. Greater attention however must be paid to reduction of blood pressure to normal levels, always attempting to keep the diastolic pressure below 100 mmHg, and preferably lower than 90 mmHg. A CT scan will be positive immediately. If there is any suggestion of cerebellar hemorrhage, lumbar puncture must be avoided and a urgent call placed for a neurosurgeon. Patients with lacunar strokes diagnosed by CT scan can be managed as those with TIAs except that angiography is usually negative.

Subarachnoid Hemorrhage

While still in the emergency room, order urinalysis, ECG, routine hematology, biochemistry tests, and a coagulation profile, and arrange for an urgent CT scan. Sedate the awake patient in pain with phenothiazines or meperidine (Demerol), treat hypertension above 100 mmHg diastolic, and restrict fluids, but catheterize the patient anyway. The earlier you can get an angiogram done and the aneurysm surgically attacked, the better.

The patient should be transferred to a neurosurgical unit when his condition is stable (signs are static or improving and the blood pressure is normal). In a neurosurgical unit, CT scanning and four-vessel angiography will be performed. Twenty percent of cases have multiple aneurysms, and it is important to note the angiographic changes that may indicate which aneurysm has bled. Aneurysms in most sites are susceptible to either direct or indirect surgical treatment, the approaches varying from tying the carotid artery in the neck to a direct attack, clipping the aneurysm itself, wrapping it with muscle or plastic resins, or thrombosing it with foreign material. The chance of rebleeding may be lessened by a number of regimens, including the use of epsilon-aminocaproic acid and therapy for arteriospasm, and raised intracranial pressure will also be required in some patients.

Cerebral Venous Infarction

This subject is treated in Chapter 40 because it is most often a complication of infection.

Long-Term Management

There are three important aspects of late management that are often overlooked. The first is the availability of many rehabilitation services. *Speech therapists* may assist the patient's recovery of some degree of useful language communication and may also provide a great psychological boost to the patient who is continually frustrated by his difficulties in communicating. *Physiotherapists* may aid in gait and arm retraining, and *occupational therapists* aid in developing competency in the activities of daily living. *Social services* can greatly help the patient to realize those benefits to which he is entitled by his sickness, and they may arrange suitable placement. *Home care* and *social* and *nursing services* may also be called in to assist the patient in returning home earlier, and they may provide follow-up assessments of his ability to function in the home as well as his reliability in taking prescribed medication.

The second factor, often overlooked, is the importance of *continuing therapy to prevent further strokes.* The proper treatment for hyperlipidemia, use of antiplatelet agents, weight reduction, diets, and specific treatment for hypertension, diabetes, and other risk factors have a very large part to play in the prophylaxis against further attacks. In cases where they may be familial risk factors, such as hyperlipidemia, hypertension, or diabetes, other family members should be assessed to prevent vascular disease occurring in them as well. It has been well shown that the prognosis in patients following a stroke can be dramatically improved if all risk factors are continually monitored. In one study the 5-year mortality in those who were followed carefully, managing all risk factors, was about 15 percent, compared with 65 percent in the patients who were not so treated.

The third factor that always warrants careful attention is the presence of *depression.* A stroke is well named, for it often strikes men and women down in their years of greatest achievement and happiness, devastating their ambition, and chilling them with the fear of impending renewed disaster. Depression is not just a neurotic tilt at the windmill of an unkind world, nor is it purely an expression of chemical dysfunction in the limbic system. It is, in part, both of these, but in addition, a near-universal response of the mind to damage of its own substrate, the brain. When the stroke patient seems to perform well on formal examination but does not go to work, can climb the stairs to his bedroom but will not visit across the road, and writes his will but will not read a book, then you must search for other somatic and mental symptoms of depressive illness. When you have found them, do not regard them as the inevitable and immutable consequences of brain damage, but rather a further challenge to your diagnostic and therapeutic skills that you can, and must, meet.

BIBLIOGRAPHY

Buonanno, F., O'Toole, J.F. Management of patients with established ("completed") cerebral infarction. *Stroke 12:*7-16, 1981.

Easton, J.D. et al. Diagnosis and management of ischemic stroke (Parts 1 and 2). *Curr. Probl. Cardiol. 8:*Nos. 5, 7, 1983.

Harrison, M.J.G., Dyken, M.L. *Cerebral Vascular Disease.* London, Butterworths, 1983.

Hines, R.C., Kirsten, J.P. Intracranial arterial aneurysm: An update. *Curr. Concepts Cerebrovasc. Dis. Stroke 18:*No. 1, 1983.

Illis, L.S., Sedgwick, E.M., Glanville, H.J. *Rehabilitation of the Neurology Patient.* Oxford, Blackwell Scientific, 1982.

Kirsten, J.P. et al. Therapy of cerebral vascular disease due to atherothrombosis. *N. Engl. J. Med. 311:*27-34, 100-105, 1984.

Ojemann, R.G., Heros, R.C. Spontaneous brain hemorrhage. *Stroke 14:*468-475, 1983.

Warrow, C. Carotid endarterectomy; does it work? *Stroke 15:*1068-1076, 1984.

Weir, B. Medical aspects of the preoperative management of aneurysm: A review. *Can. J. Neurol. Sci. 6:*41-50, 1979.

38
Head Injuries and Spinal Trauma

As you read this, 1 percent of the working population is disabled because of head injuries, road traffic accidents accounting for most of these. Brain injury may occur with or without a fracture of the skull. The injury may be a simple *concussion,* a brief and entirely reversible reduction in consciousness caused by traumatic disruption of physiological activity of the brain; a direct *contusion* of the brain; *compression,* which usually results from a subdural or extradural bleed; or *laceration,* caused by direct shart injury, including that caused by depressed skull fragments. All of these are accompanied by at least some degree of cerebral *edema,* magnifying the direct effects of the original trauma to a greater or lesser extent.

Skull fractures may involve the vault, the base of the skull, or both. The fracture line may extend into one of the sinuses or the middle ear, where it ranks as a compound fracture with the danger of infection. The same will be true of any depressed skull fracture, which not only may be compound (communicating with the outside through a scalp laceration), but may directly injure the underlying brain. The fracture line also may cross the middle meningeal groove, and the shear stresses produced may rupture that vessel, causing an extradural hematoma.

The patient with a head injury runs an added risk from extracranial complications, such as respiratory inadequacy and hypoxia, blood and fluid loss, and metabolic disorders related to the brain injury.

Simple *concussion* occurs when a closed head injury results in a brief period of unconsciousness without brain damage or residual deficit. Unconsciousness occurs because of the effect upon the brain of the sudden acceleration or deceleration of the head, generating a tremendous rise in intracranial pressure and perhaps shearing synapses. The period of unconsciousness is seldom more than a few minutes, although longer periods may be ascribed to the presence of diffuse cerebral edema in more serious injuries.

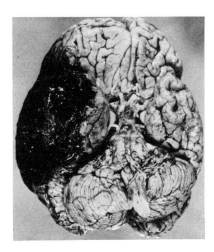

Figure 38-1 Base of brain, showing necrosis and hemorrhage in the right hemisphere following violent injury.

In very severe injuries (Fig. 38-1), brain damage is caused by trauma either at the site of the blow or on the opposite side. This "contrecoup" injury occurs when the head is struck, causing the skull to accelerate before the brain, which is thus pushed up against the struck area. When the skull decelerates suddenly, the brain continues its momentum and smashes against the inner wall of the skull. Damage is particularly likely to involve the anterior temporal lobe in the middle fossa, the tips of the frontal lobes, and the occipital lobes. With both frontal injuries and those to the back of the skull, direct or contrecoup damage to the frontal and temporal lobes are most frequently found. The sudden movement from a head injury may also tear meninges and blood vessels resulting in subdural or extradural hematomas. If a fracture occurs, it may tear a meningeal artery while a fracture through the petrous bone may damage the seventh and eighth nerves.

GENERAL MANAGEMENT
OF HEAD INJURIES

Whatever the degree of severity of the injury, one's first tasks are to ensure the patency of the airway, and the adequacy of ventilation and to control hemorrhage anywhere. Only when these have been attended to should one turn to the patient's neurological status. A summary of the immediate steps in management is given in the following checklist.

Checklist

1. Airway/ventilation
2. Signs of hemorrhage
3. Level of consciousness

4. Pupillary size and light response
5. Evidence of cranial/spinal injury
6. Examination of the patient in coma (Chap. 7)
7. Examination of other systems

Initial management is simple if the patient was not unconscious or has re-covered and has no neurological deficit. It consists of a period of observation (usually 24 hr) during which time narcotics and sedatives may not be used. Skull x-rays are indicated if the scalp is bruised or swollen, if there has been any loss of consciousness or amnesia, with a penetrating injury, and if there is a CSF leak or any neurological signs on examination. Admission of mild head-injured patients is advised if there is no responsible person to watch them at home, if there is per-sistent confusion or any CNS signs, if there is a skull fracture, or if assessment is made difficult because the patient has epilepsy or has taken alcohol.

If the patient is unconscious when first seen, then a rapid examination of respiration, pupils, and response to pain will provide a great deal of information on the urgency of the situation. If there is no evidence of a depressed or compound fracture, respirations are normal, the patient's pupils are equal and reactive, and there is no evidence of any motor deficit on painful stimulation, then the patient can be safely observed until he recovers consciousness and for at least 24 hr there-after, preferably in a neurosurgical unit.

If a pupil dilates, or with any other evidence of an expanding intracranial le-sion, then 200 ml of 20% mannitol should be infused intravenously in 20 min and intramuscular dexamethasone (10 mg) given. There is no evidence that routine steroids have any beneficial effect in head-injured patients. A catheter should be inserted into the bladder and the patient then transferred immediately to the care of a neurosurgeon. Deteriorating consciousness, seizures, confusion, slowing of respiration, rise in blood pressure, evidence of hemiparesis or other focal signs, or the presence of a depressed, basal or compound fracture are other indications for the transfer.

The head injury itself is not a contraindication to moving the patient as long as

• Any emergency surgery that could be performed in the referral center is undertaken before the patient is moved. This includes control of any hemor-rhage, laparotomy, chest drainage, and possibly the placing of burr holes.
• Unstable fractures are reduced or at least splinted.
• Clinical examination and x-rays of the entire spine have excluded a spinal spinal injury. Cervical and lumbar sites are the most common. Adequate fixation is necessary before the patient is transported. You must never for-get that spinal injuries often occur in association with head injuries, particu-larly after road traffic accidents.
• The airway is clear and the patient is either breathing spontaneously or has been ventilated. Transportation must therefore be in a vehicle equipped with oxygen and suction apparatus, and with competent attendants. If possible, the patient should be transported in the semiprone position.
• Full clinical data detailing the initial level of consciousness and physical signs, accompany the patient.
• No narcotics, sedative agents, nor drugs that have any effect upon the pupils are given.

To maintain a good airway is of prime concern. Probably more patients die because of an obstructed airway than from any other cause after head injury.

Check the mouth for foreign bodies and suction the pharynx if needed. The ears and mastoid regions should be checked for evidence of blood or of CSF leak, and the patient should be examined carefully for trauma elsewhere. Do not miss a ruptured liver or spleen in a comatose patient.

If the patient remains unconscious for over 24 hr, then a nasogastric tube can be inserted for hydration and feeding. Strict attention to the care of the bladder, bowels, skin, and eyes is imperative. Watch for pressure points over peripheral nerves and keep the limbs in a physiological position to minimize later contractures. Cerebral oxygenation during this critical period might be reduced by hypoventilation, hypotension, raised intracranial pressure, or vascular damage. All must be looked for and corrected if further needless damage to the brain is to be prevented.

Because water and sodium are retained by head-injured patients through increased aldosterone and ADH secretion, restrict salt in the first few days while urinary output is still low.

COMPLICATIONS OF HEAD INJURIES

Avoidable causes of morbidity and mortality mainly concern the complications of head injuries, some of which are presented in Fig. 38-2. The biggest problems are delays in the diagnosis of intracranial bleeding, of extracranial injuries, and of open-skull injuries, leading to delay in referral.

Extradural Hematoma

A tear in the middle meningeal artery, usually from a fracture of the squamous temporal bone, may result in a hemorrhage into the extradural space, stripping the dura off the skull and compressing the brain. This complication of head injury fortunately is rare, because it is often fatal. Typically, the patient loses

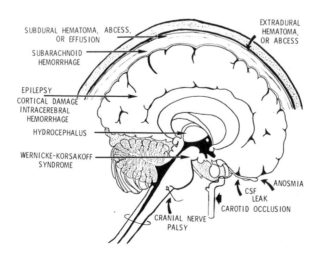

Figure 38-2   Some complications of head injuries.

consciousness at the time of the injury because of concussion, then awakens for a few hours (the "lucid interval") before lapsing into a coma with hemiplegia caused by brainstem compression secondary to the expanding hematoma. The hemiplegia is usually on the opposite side but is sometimes homolateral to the hematoma owing to a shift of the brainstem across the midline, which presses the opposite cerebral peduncle against the edge of the tentorium (Kernohan's notch). Patients usually deteriorate within hours after the accident; rarely the complication develops slowly over days or weeks. The first sign of serious compression is a dilated pupil from third nerve compression as the medial temporal lobe herniates over the edge of the tentorium.

While a CT scan can be diagnostic (Fig. 38-3), when it is unavailable plain skull x-rays should show a fracture line on the side of the hematoma and an arteriogram will demonstrate the characteristic avascular area over the surface of the brain with displacement of the midline structures to the opposite side. In cases showing rapid deterioration, there is no time for any tests, and burr-holes should be drilled for diagnosis and therapy.

An extradural hemorrhage is probably the complication of head injury most likely to be fatal if untreated. Even with an experienced neurosurgical team in a head injury unit, up to 50 percent of patients die despite control of bleeding and drainage of the clot.

Subdural Hematoma

Accumulation of blood within the subdural space occurs most frequently after severe head injuries but may follow relatively minor trauma in the elderly and in alcoholics (Fig. 38-4). Occasionally it occurs in patients with bleeding disorders or in those taking anticoagulants, or complicates a traumatic delivery in the newborn. In such patients, the cortex is relatively thin and the width of the subarachnoid space relatively great, so that the bridging veins have further to go and are more likely to rupture with shearing stresses, leading to oozing of blood.

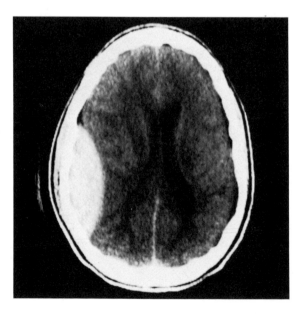

Figure 38-3   Unenhanced CT scan. Large lens-shaped extradural hematoma following trauma.

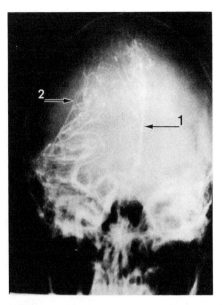

Figure 38-4 Right carotid arteriogram. Marked right-to-left shift of the anterior cerebral vessels (1) due to a large acute right subdural hematoma (2).

However because half of all patients with subdural hematoma give no history of trauma, this diagnosis must be suspected not only in anybody who develops even minor disorientation and certainly focal signs after trauma, but in anyone within the population most at risk who shows a subacute evolution of dementia, confusion, or focal signs at any time.

The symptoms of an acute subdural hematoma (see Fig. 38-4) may develop within a few hours and comprises headache, pupillary changes, altered consciousness, and hemiparesis because of compression of the underlying brain and eventually of the brainstem.

In more chronic cases (Fig. 38-5A,B) the same changes occur, but over a longer period, and the symptoms and signs may wax and wane. Seventy percent of such patients are male, usually over the age of 50. Their initial complains are of headache, and their family may have noticed mild but progressive personality change. Hemiplegia or a contralateral upper motor neuron facial palsy occur in half the patients and seizures in about 5 percent. Aphasia, papilledema, and hemianopia are unusual. In about 10 percent of the patients, a chronic subdural is present bilaterally (see Fig. 38-5B). The CT scan may grant you a diagnostic triumph in such cases, but an isodense hematoma or a "hypernormal" brain appearance (the sulci are small) may make interpretation tricky.

Lumbar puncture is contraindicated, but if performed, the CSF is found to be xanthochromic owing to raised protein levels, and under increased pressure. Skull films seldom show a fracture, the EEG may show reduction in electrical activity over the affected hemisphere. The best diagnostic test is the CT scan, which should be performed with enhancement since many subdurals are isodense with brain, and therefore they cannot be seen on the unenhanced scan. Bilateral cerebral arteriography is an alternative if no CT scanner is available.

Evacuation of the clot is the best therapy. Some patients get along well when treated with steroids and without surgery, but we prefer to advise surgery if the patient's state permits, which it usually does. Anticonvulsants will be needed thereafter.

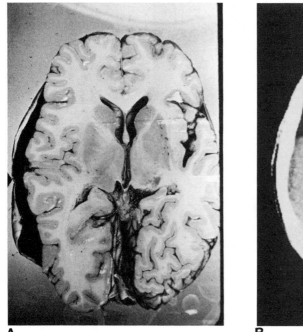 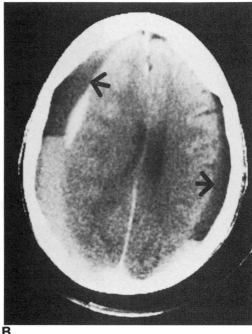

A   B

Figure 38-5   (A) Chronic subdural hematoma; (B) CT scan of bilateral chronic subdural hematomas with fluid levels and a left-to-right midline shift.

Subdural Hygroma

A head injury may tear the arachnoid, allowing the CSF to enter the subdural space. The clinical features resemble those of a subdural hematoma and the treatment is surgical.

Intracerebral Hemorrhage

Hemorrhage can occur in the brain from contusion or laceration or from tearing of large or medium-sized blood vessels. Many of these hematomas are small, but a large one may require surgical removal. Severe contusion with resulting edema, itself causes a high mortality, even without hemorrhage (Fig. 38-7).

Carotid Thrombosis

Neck injury may result in carotid stenosis, or thrombosis may be due to the shearing force of sudden head movements, although it is more commonly due to localized vessel trauma in the neck or inside the mouth. Thus children who fall on pencils held in their mouths may injure the carotid artery near the lateral pharyngeal wall.

Arteriovenous Fistulas

A tear in the internal carotid artery as it passes through the cavernous sinus may result in a fistula between these two vascular channels, but this occurs more often as a spontaneous event in middle-aged women. The patient suddenly feels and hears a pulsating bruit behind one eye and may develop sudden exophthalmos with venous distension, paralysis of the oculomotor nerves, and numbness in the first division of the fifth nerve. The common carotid artery may be ligated in the neck, but a more direct attack upon the fistula (e.g., balloon occlusion) is preferable.

Intracranial Infection

Infection may occur in the extradural, subdural, subarachnoid, or intracerebral areas. The organisms may enter through the wound or through a fracture of the frontal or petrous bones, producing an extra- or subdural abscess or meningitis. Intracerebral abscess however is uncommon and usually occurs with a penetrating injury or in association with an infected scalp wound.

Cerebrospinal Fluid Leaks

Fracture of the cribriform plate may produce a connection between the CSF space and the nose (Fig. 38-6). Although this leak usually stops spontaneously, it does provide a portal for infection. Occasionally, patients note CSF drainage into the postnasal area when they lie down, which is stopped by sitting up. The site of the CSF leak can sometimes be disclosed by a RISA scan.

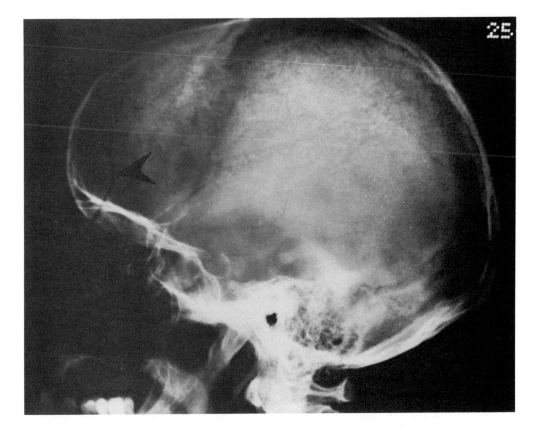

Figure 38-6   Lateral skull radiograph showing a frontal linear fracture.

A fracture of the petrous temporal bone may cause CSF to leak out of the ear. This usually seals spontaneously, seldom requiring surgical closure.

Cranial Nerve Palsies

The most common cranial nerve problem after a head injury is *anosmia* caused by disruption of the olfactory nerve fibers passing through the cribriform plate. If unilateral, the patient often remains unaware of it, but if bilateral, he will notice a change in flavor discrimination or its total loss. Occasionally, parosmia (perversion of smell sensations) results. Optic nerve lesions also may follow trauma, resulting in optic atrophy.

While trauma may damage the oculomotor nerves, dysfunction is often transient. The sixth nerve is more commonly damaged than the other two, but trauma is the single most common cause of a fourth nerve palsy. Lesions of the fifth nerve intracranially are unusual with trauma, but seventh nerve palsy is common (and eighth nerve damage can occur) with fractures through the petrous temporal bone. Because the facial nerve is superficial, it may also be damaged by a direct blow, and by stab or gunshot wounds behind the angle of the jaw. Occasionally it is damaged by obstetric forceps. The bulbar nerves are seldom involved except by direct trauma.

Other Complications of Head Injuries

Some patients may remain in a prolonged state of unconsciousness following the injury, presumably because of diffuse brain damage. A *pneumocele* is an unusual complication in which air enters the intracranial cavity following an injury that tore the meninges behind the frontal sinuses. *Leptomeningeal cysts* are fluid-filled spaces formed between the pia mater and the arachnoid membrane. *Osteomyelitis* may develop in the skull when a scalp laceration becomes infected. Transient *diabetes insipidus* is seen in a few patients with severe head injury and *pituitary infarction* has been reported. *Narcolepsy* has a relationship with head injury in half the cases, presumably because of hypothalamic damage. *Posttraumatic parkinsonism* may be due to anoxia at the time of injury. *Venous sinus thrombosis* (Chap. 40) is recorded as another complication.

SEQUELAE OF HEAD INJURIES

Posttraumatic Syndrome

About 40 percent of patients who sustain a head injury of any severity develop a stereotyped syndrome consisting of headaches, dizziness, insomnia, irritability, nervousness, personality change, memory disturbance, depression, paroxysmal sweating, vertigo, diplopia, decreased libido, effort fatigue, and intolerance of alcohol. There has been a medicolegal controversy for years as to whether this is primarily organic or psychogenic, but evidence is accumulating that it has an organic basis in damage to fiber tracts in the upper brainstem.

There are a few myths attached to the syndrome, including the widespread belief that it does not occur with severe injuries, that the prognosis is usually good, and that the patients are merely seeking compensation (as the symptoms may disappear when the claim is settled and it is less commonly seen after amateur sporting injuries). Although long-standing, such opinions cannot be substantiated and these patients have been harshly treated by the courts and by our profession for many years. The development of the syndrome does not relate to possible compensation or insurance payments.

The relationship between this syndrome and the previous personality of the patient is uncertain, but the personality change now incurred, with irritability and depression, does influence the other complaints. The prognosis is not necessarily good, and although many of the milder cases clear within 6 months, other patients may never completely lose their symptoms.

The best method of management appears to be strong encouragement, explanation, and reassurance, helping the patients to return by stages to their normal home and working lives. Tranquilizers and antidepressants are often helpful. Severely injured patients will need prolonged rehabilitation efforts.

Posttraumatic Epilepsy

Perhaps 15 percent of epilepsy relates to previous trauma but the true figure may be higher. Wounds penetrating the dura cause seizures in over 50 percent of the cases. The likelihood of seizures is related to whether or not the injury occurred to a brain area with a high or a relatively low threshold. Seizures are more common with parietal and temporal than with frontal polar or occipital lesions (Fig. 38-7).

If the seizures occur *at the time* of the trauma, it does not necessarily mean that severe brain damage has occurred, and they may never recur. It is difficult to prevent these seizures with anticonvulsants. Seizures occur more commonly in the acute phase if there has been focal damage or hemorrhage. If focal signs persist following a head injury, the likelihood of seizures is between 30 and 50 percent, but in cases without posttraumatic deficit the risk is less than 5 percent. *Delayed* seizures tend to recur, but are usually easily controlled. The delay *may* be up to many years but usually the first seizure occurs within 6 to 24 months of the accident. If no seizure has occurred within 2 years, then future epilepsy is unlikely. The presence of early seizures, a hematoma, or a depressed fracture all predispose to the development of epilepsy later resulting from adhesions, vascular change, or

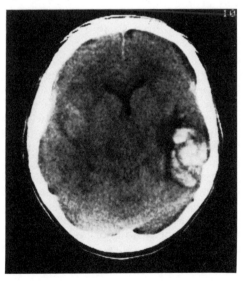

Figure 38-7   Unenhanced CT scan. Traumatic right temporal lobe hematoma with a little contrecoup bleeding on the left.

gliosis in damaged areas. Around a scar, the number of capillaries are reduced and the neurons are damaged by mild chronic ischemia. As the scar contracts, there is further traction on vessels and more neurons are damaged in a wider area. This development was called "focus ripening" by Penfield.

The EEG often reveals suppression of cerebral activity immediately after a seizure but later will show abnormal focal discharges and/or evidence of focal damage in many cases. It is useless as a predictor of future seizures.

Mental Changes

The punch-drunk syndrome* of dementia and parkinsonism is well known to occur after repeated head injuries and occasionally after a single head injury. Some patients develop a transient acute psychotic episode following a head injury and some develop a Korsakoff-type memory loss indicating bilateral temporal lobe, fornix, mammillary body, or thalamic damage. The amount of retrograde and anterograde amnesia at the time of injury reflects the severity of brain damage. The picture of traumatic amnesia which is indelibly engraved in the mind of every moviegoer — that of a person wandering about trying to find his past life — is not due to brain injury and is usually a conversion reaction.

Minor changes in personality, increased nervousness, and anxiety related to the traumatic event are common after moderate or severe head injuries. Seventy-five percent of patients recover well from these symptoms, even before compensation claims are settled. Normal pressure hydrocephalus is yet another uncommon long-term effect (Chap. 16); dementia is one of its features.

Recurrence

Certain occupations predispose to recurrent head injuries, but two other situations should be called to mind. Alcoholics are particularly susceptible to head injury because of falling as well as from social altercations; and in children less than 3 years old, the presence of retinal hemorrhages should make you very suspicious that you are seeing a "battered child."

PROGNOSIS

Prolonged coma, abnormal motor movements such as hypotonia and decerebrate posturing, older age, and major surgical complications all are associated with a worse prognosis. The best prognostic factors are the clinical state on initial examination as determined by e.g., the Glasgow Coma Scale (see Chap. 10) and the length of posttraumatic amnesia (PTA), the period between the original injury and the end of that stage in which the patient is not able to lay down permanent new memory traces. This amnesic period ceases when the patient's continuous memory reappears. The simplest way to test this is to ask the patient when he woke up.

If the PTA is less than 1 hr, then the head injury is only mild and full functional recovery may be expected if complications do not ensue. If it is longer than 24 hr, then the head injury is classed as severe (with a rate of over 2000 each year in Canada). Perhaps 25 percent of these will never regain their former working ability. With a PTA of over 7 days, the head injury is classed as very severe; a significant proportion of such patients will require extended care for the remainder of their lives.

---

*No extra marks for calling it "pugilistic encephalopathy."

TRAUMA TO THE SPINE

The spinal cord can be damaged through direct trauma or, more commonly, indirectly by flexion-extension injuries as sustained in motor vehicle accidents or falls, or during a difficult delivery in the case of the newborn.

Concussion of the spinal cord results in transient dysfunction probably caused by an electrical or biochemical disturbance in the damaged area, although swelling, edema, and vascular congestion may play a part.

Compression, contusion, and *laceration* may also damage the cord. Bleeding from venules occurs in the center of the cord in many cases, secondary ischemic changes occurring locally with edema and producing a central core of necrosis that extends both above and below the level of trauma. Penetration by a bony spicule produces a laceration, the extent of which cannot be determining at the time of acute injury because of secondary vascular and inflammatory changes. Such direct trauma to the cord also occurs with stab wounds and may produce a Brown-Séquard syndrome or any other combination of motor and sensory signs below the level of the lesion (see Chap. 9).

Hemorrhage into the cord is usually central and produces a cavity in communication with the central canal — *hematomyelia.* Because of the arcade of anastomoses between the anterior and posterior spinal arteries and the radicular arteries, the outer circumstance of the cord is little involved, the most severe bleeding (or in other cases, ischemic infarction) being in the territory of the sulcal artery which arises from the anterior spinal artery and passes backward in the anterior median sulcus.

Immediately after a severe spinal injury there is often a period of *spinal shock* with total absence of deep reflexes, an atonic, paralyzed bladder and rectum, complete flaccid paralysis, and loss of sensation. The patient may still be fully conscious. If the injury is below C4, breathing should be normal, but if it is above that level, phrenic paralysis may lead to early death. Incomplete lesions of the cervical cord may cause Horner's syndrome and any degree of corticospinal and long sensory tract involvement. Examination may also show angulation or deformity of the spine, and protective muscle spasm may be visible, at least in the muscles on the cranial side of the injury. Spinal shock may last weeks and may be prolonged by the presence of bedsores or urinary tract infection. As the period of shock clears, there is a return of reflexes and the patient enters a spastic stage.

With complete transection, the eventual picture is of paraplegia-in-flexion (i.e., with the greatest reflex contraction in the flexor muscles, and perhaps flexor spasms). With incomplete lesions, paraplegia-in-extension may be seen, in which the antigravity muscles dominate their antagonists.

Unless the cord is completely transected, some degree of recovery is usual, but many patients are left with marked spasticity and weakness, some loss of bladder and bowel control, and impotence. Poor vasomotor control in the paralyzed extremities results in orthostatic hypotension, adrenergic crises with bladder distension, and disturbances of sweating and of heat regulation.

Stable injuries to the *vertebrae* include compression and wedge fractures of the vertebral bodies and fracture-dislocation of the thoracic vertebrae, the spine here being splinted by the ribs. Fracture-dislocations of the cervical or lumbar spine however are not stable, and any further flexion will magnify or add to the original injury (Figs. 38-8, 38-9).

Impairment of *the blood supply* to the cord is usually due to radicular artery compression (e.g., by a prolapsed disk). If compression from a hematoma extends over a number of segments, then the collateral supply will fail, causing infarction.

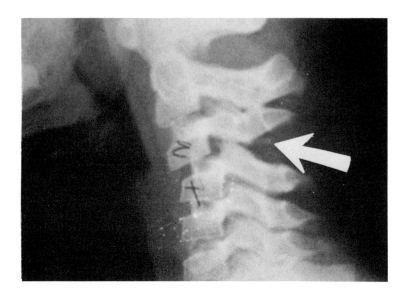

Figure 38-8   Lateral radiograph of cervical spine, showing a fracture-dislocation at C3-4.

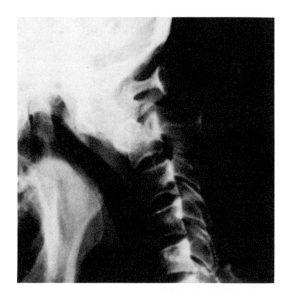

Figure 38-9   Lateral radiograph of cervical spine, showing a fracture-dislocation following a fall to the knees while blueberry picking. The patient walked into the emergency department a week later complaining of headache.

Damage to the *lower motor neurons* in the lumbar region (the cauda equina) results in flaccid paralysis of the legs, sensory loss, and paralysis of the bladder and rectum.

Management

Emergency treatment of patients with spinal injury aims to ensure adequate ventilation and to prevent further movement of the spine. This may be done immediately with a cervical collar, which must be put on the subject before he is moved. If it is available, a spinal board can be used instead to maintain spinal immobility.

The patient must not leave your presence until you have

1. Ruled out injuries to other body areas
2. Examined the entire length of the spine and the CNS
3. Inserted a catheter if a severe cord lesion is likely

Only then may you permit the patient to be transferred to a neurosurgical or spinal injury center, although you should have arranged for this earlier. In the treatment of spinal cord trauma, minutes count.

In a treatment center, cardiorespiratory function and spinal fixation will be checked first, after which the entire spine will be x-rayed, and myelography, spinal tomography, CT scanning, and/or evoked potential recordings will be used to localize and quantify the injury. Any continuing compression or fracture-dislocation will always merit surgery. Myelotomy, steroid therapy, local cord cooling, mannitol, and diuretics to slow ischemic cord damage; treatment of hypotension; and initiation of rehabilitation procedures are the main treatment options.

Skin care should begin immediately to prevent bedsores. Apart from direct attention to the condition of the skin, in particular keeping it dry and supple, frequent turning and the use of air mattresses are the first steps in preventative nursing because ulcers are likely to develop in the skin wherever there are bony prominences pressing on the sheets or mattress (sacrum, trochanters, heels, ischium, knees, and anterior-superior iliac spines).

If ulcers occur, numerous local treatments including the use of sugar, oxygen, hydrogen peroxide, and antibiotics can be employed. Occasionally plastic surgery is required.

The physiotherapy program will include massage, muscle training, movement of all joints and eventually the application of braces and the beginning of gait therapy.

Bladder care is of particular importance because urinary infection shortens the patient's life expectancy. The simplest and best method is intermittent catheterization under sterile conditions, while encouraging the patient to drink large amounts of fluid. Frequent urine cultures are mandatory, and appropriate antibiotics must be used for any significant infection. Patients can be trained to control the emptying of their bladder by various maneuvers involving skin stimulation (Chap. 33).

Adequate *nutrition* with a high vitamin intake is an important component in the management of these patients, and a high-protein diet is advisable, particularly in the presence of bedsores. If spasticity is prominent, painful muscle spasms may occur frequently. Diazepam, dantrolene sodium, and baclofen reduce spasticity and flexor spasms. If they fail, surgical procedures such as myelotomy or root section may be considered.

Pain occurs in about 25 percent of paraplegic patients either within the area of the lesion or referred to dermatomes. Carbamazepine may be effective in reducing it.

The *rehabilitation* program for spinal cord injuries is vital, and certain centers specializing in spinal cord injuries have produced magnificent results as regards freedom from bedsores and from urinary infection. Utilization of returning reflexes may allow appropriate bladder function, and sometimes even some form of motility can be restored.

BIBLIOGRAPHY

Jennett, B., Teasedale, G. *The Management of Head Injuries.* Contemporary Neurology Series. Philadelphia, F.A. Davis Co., 1981.

Jennett, B. et al. Guidelines for the initial management of head injuries in adults. *Br. Med. J. 288:*983-985, 1984.

Leffert, R.D. Brachial plexus injuries. *N. Engl. J. Med. 291:*1059, 1974.

Tator, C.H., Rowed, D.W. Current concepts in the immediate management of acute spinal cord injury. *Can. Med. Assoc. J. 121:*1453, 1979.

39

Cerebral Palsy and Mental Retardation

CEREBRAL PALSY

The term *cerebral palsy* encompasses all of the many disorders affecting the nervous system around or before birth. Such damage may declare itself in numerous ways. If the motor pathways of the brain are involved, cerebral palsy results. If a widespread abnormality affects intellectual functions but largely spares the motor pathways, then mental retardation results. Should an irritative brain lesion be present, seizures may occur. If the brain disorder is only slight, it may produce the syndrome known as *minimal brain dysfunction.*

The term indicates a lesion of the brain that is permanent but nonprogressive and involves mainly the motor pathways of the CNS. Primary manifestations include impaired motor control, tone, coordination, and posture, but other neurological symptoms and signs may be present too. Intellectual deficits do not necessarily accompany these abnormalities.

Causes of Cerebral Palsy

Cerebral palsy may originate in the prenatal, perinatal, or postnatal period, and it has been estimated that from two to six cases occur among every 1000 live births.

The stage of pregnancy at which the cause exerts its effect determines to a large extent the type of pathological abnormality. Problems in the first 4 months are more likely to produce major brain malformations (and by implication bilateral involvement of the brain, probably leading to mental retardation), such as microcephaly, hydranencephaly, and malformations of the gyri of the cerebral cortex. By contrast, lesions that occur in the last 5 months damage an already-established brain and mainly affect white matter, particularly that surrounding the lateral ventricles. In premature infants or in full-term deliveries, cysts and areas of localized atrophy of the cortex are more common.

453

In addition, brainstem lesions from hypoxia and asphyxia during labor, intracranial hemorrhage, and damage to the temporal lobes from effects of brain edema and asphyxia may complicate a difficult delivery. Newborn monkeys subjected to prolonged partial asphyxia lasting 7 to 12 min frequently develop cerebral palsy; there are obvious parallels with intrapartum obstetrical hazards.

Although the timing of the damage largely determines the nature of the lesion, the etiology is also important.

Prenatal Causes

The TORCH (toxoplasmosis, rubella, cytomegalic inclusion disease, herpes simplex) group of congenital infections, and syphilis and influenza may all cause either cerebral palsy or mental retardation and are most damaging when they affect the fetus during the first trimester. Newborn infants may show features of the infection or may be asymptomatic. Subsequent mental retardation, or less often cerebral palsy, may only become evident in later childhood.

Irradiation and teratogenic drugs such as aminopterin, may cause fetal damage; less severe effects may result from an extensive range of drugs or other chemicals ingested by the mother, particularly in the first trimester.

Familial cerebral palsy is rare and should make one reconsider the diagnosis and search for an underlying genetically determined degenerative disease. However, *ataxic diplegia* may be inherited as a sex-linked trait. Conditions that adversely affect the intrauterine environment of the fetus often result in cerebral palsy. These include preeclamptic toxemia, maternal diabetes, renal disease, hypertension, viral hepatitis, and placental insufficiency with associated intrauterine growth retardation; and prematurity.

Babies who are small-for-dates, but not necessarily premature (for example, because of chronic maternal disease or placental insufficiency), represent with the premature babies a significant proportion of the children whose later diagnosis is cerebral palsy, hyperkinetic states, or minimal brain dysfunction.

Perinatal Causes

By far the most common cause of cerebral palsy is hypoxia and asphyxia that are manifested during labor by the clinical features of fetal distress and are associated with prolonged labor, complicated delivery, or premature birth.

In complicated or difficult deliveries, intracranial bleeding is common, particularly in premature infants; it may cause brain damage directly or may affect the brainstem circulatory and respiratory centers, resulting in further anoxia. Subarachnoid bleeding or intracerebral petechiae are common after a traumatic birth, and intraventricular hemorrhage may complicate or follow a difficult delivery. Subarachnoid bleeding may lead to communicating hydrocephalus.

Although it is becoming much less common, hemolytic disease of the newborn may result in yellow staining of the basal ganglia *(kernicterus)* with disturbances of function in the jaundiced areas of the brain. Although bilirubin is mainly concentrated in the basal ganglia, the olives, eighth nerve, corticospinal tracts, and the cortex may also be affected.

Postnatal Causes

The newborn are susceptible to infections in the nursery; thus a gram-negative meningitis may cause brain damage manifested later as cerebral palsy, but any severe infection may interfere with the infant's development or cause hypoxia.

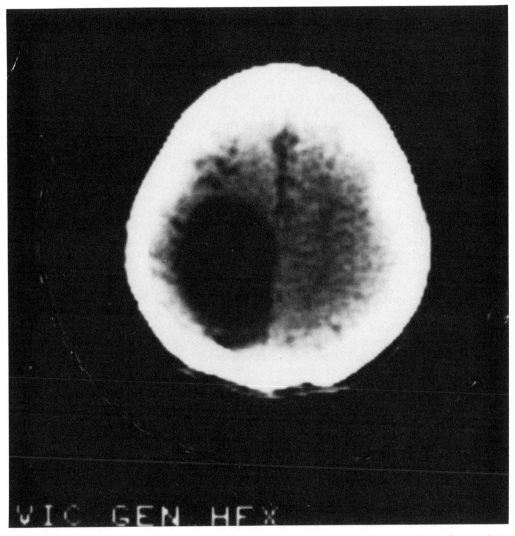

Figure 39-1 Unenhanced CT scan. Large porencephalic cyst resulting from birth trauma.

Types of Cerebral Palsy

Spastic Cerebral Palsy

Hemiplegic Form: This is the most common single type of cerebral palsy, accounting for over a third of all cases. It may have multiple causes, two-thirds of which are of prenatal origin with an increased prevalence of complicated pregnancies (toxemia, antepartum hemorrhage, or prolonged or precipitate labor). The remaining third are postnatal in origin. Occlusion of the middle cerebral artery may be suspected in some from the presence of atrophy or porencephalic cysts within its territory, while infections, trauma, high fever, or prolonged convulsions may be causal in others (Fig. 39-1).

The later development of unilateral neurological defects in an infant may be suggested by unilateral fisting, persistence of infantile reflexes, increased tone, or a decided preference for using one hand, but the hemiplegia is seldom recognized until 6 to 12 months of age. Subsequently, the classic picture emerges with increased tone, hyperreflexia, decreased use of the limbs, and extensor plantar responses. Flexion contractures, e.g., at the ankle, elbow, or shoulder, may develop subsequently. However, the superficial reflexes such as the abdominals and cremasterics are preserved.

Cortical sensory loss may lead to loss of fine discrimination, largely responsible for the limited use of the hand. Homonymous hemianopia may reflect involvement of the optic radiation or occipital cortex. Lack of growth of the affected side may be present, probably caused by parietal lobe involvement. Seizures occur in up to half the patients. Hemiplegic cerebral palsy has the best prognosis for intellectual development, normal IQ levels being found in over 50 percent of the cases.

Spastic Diplegia: Spastic diplegia refers to a form of cerebral palsy in which the legs are affected either alone or more severely than the arms. Typically there is a history of prematurity or breech delivery. The most common pathological abnormality is periventricular leukomalacia — damage to the white matter around the lateral angles of the lateral ventricles affecting the pyramidal tract fibers destined for the lumbosacral cord.

The usual presentation is of an infant with delayed crawling, sitting, or standing. Only when the problem is mild will the child achieve a gait pattern close to normal. Scissoring (excessive adduction with crossing of the legs) is characteristic. Slight involvement of the hands accentuates the child's disability. Strabismus is often found. The overall outlook regarding intelligence is less favorable than in the hemiplegic form and tends to be worse in proportion to the severity of the motor defect overall.

Complex Diplegia: Complex diplegia refers to a form of cerebral palsy in which the involvement of all four limbs is of approximately equal extent (quadriplegia, tetraplegia). This may be combined with other motor deficits such as ataxia or athetosis. Because the diffuse and severe CNS involvement indicates both cortical and subcortical damage, the prognosis is poor for walking, for independent living, and for the development of normal intelligence. This form of cerebral palsy usually follows a complicated pregnancy or delivery. As infants, such patients are likely to have seizures, and primitive reflexes (tonic neck, Moro, sucking, grasp) persist well beyond the normal age (see Chap. 4). The limbs may not become spastic until the end of the first year. In the first few months the children may appear flaccid at rest, but when stimulated they may change from the flaccid frog-leg position to the extensor, spastic position. Reflexes may not be strikingly increased in the first few months, but later all the feared evidence of widespread brain damage is remorselessly displayed.

Extrapyramidal Cerebral Palsy

Involvement of the extrapyramidal pathways typically results in athetoid or dystonic movements of the limbs, often accompanied by severe difficulties in articulation, drooling despite normal intelligence, and emotional lability. Delayed motor milestones and particular difficulty in reaching out and grasping and transferring objects in the latter part of the first year are often the first indications of the problem. Speech may be delayed further by accompanying sensorineural deafness. The eyes and sensory functions are spared.

Formerly, hemolytic disease of the newborn was the major cause, but with the development of Rh immunization this has been significantly lessened and anoxia has become a relatively more common cause. The clinical features of abnormal movements are described at length in Chapter 29.

Ataxic Cerebral Palsy

After about 6 months, when babies normally begin to sit up and reach out purposefully, about 10 percent of children with cerebral palsy demonstrate poor coordination and balance. Muscle tone is typically decreased and they remain clumsy throughout their development. How well they compensate depends in part upon whether or not there is associated spasticity or choreoathetosis.

Associated Neurologic Abnormalities

More than half the children with significant cerebral palsy have associated mental retardation, but the remainder have normal intelligence even if their disabilities make them appear dull. It requires a long period of training and rehabilitation in the face of their motor deficits to enable them to realize their true intellectual potential. There is also an increased frequency of minimal brain dysfunction (described later). Unfortunately, social isolation of these children often accentuates any mental impairment because of their limited stimulation and experiences and the decreased expectations of parents and teachers. Further impairment may result from sedation, tranquilizers, or anticonvulsants.

Epilepsy is a common accompaniment of cerebral palsy, particularly of the spastic forms, but it can usually be well controlled by anticonvulsant drugs.

Associated physical defects often found among these children include developmental abnormalities, contractures, and dislocation of the hips: this last requires early recognition to avoid the added complication of painful arthritis. Optic atrophy, choroiditis, refractive errors, and cataracts may be present. About 10 percent of children with cerebral palsy have impaired hearing, usually of the sensorineural type. This makes it hard for them to understand the spoken word, which further impairs their social and language development and gives the impression of mental retardation. The child's ability to communicate may also be impaired by interference with speech mechanisms resulting from the spastic, extrapyramidal, or cerebellar lesions.

Differential Diagnosis

Because the conclusion that the child has cerebral palsy implies a nonprogressive defect, it is important to rule out progressive or treatable diseases. Metabolic disorders such as phenylketonuria and other aminoacidopathies should be considered. Hearing and vision must be assessed carefully, perhaps repeatedly, especially in the face of inappropriate delay in speech development. The family history should be examined to see if the problem could be genetically determined, particularly in ataxic forms. If there is no history to explain cerebral palsy, one should recall the possibility of a subdural hematoma, brain tumor, or infection. Hemiparesis should be particularly suspect, since the cause may be a treatable mass lesion; in one series of patients with cerebral palsy, 5 percent of those who died had an unsuspected brain tumor, which was usually benign and slow growing.

Investigation

The investigations to be carried out depend upon the age at which the condition is suspected and the type of handicap. When the defect is confined to the legs, an origin in the spinal cord should be excluded. The spine should be x-rayed and my-lography may be appropriate. In hemiplegic forms, skull x-rays, CT scan, and EEG may suggest unilateral cerebral atrophy. Developmental retardation requires a search for aminoacidurias. In extrapyramidal forms, minor degrees of sensorineu-ral deafness must be excluded by audiometry. If there is any suggestion of a progressive lesion, the child should be investigated for a tumor, subdural hematoma, or one of the rare degenerative diseases. Psychological testing should be done shortly before school entry, when it will help in planning the child's education and appropriate streaming within the school system.

Therapy

Prevention is the best treatment. Very high standards of obstetrical and perinatal care have led to a great reduction in the incidence of cerebral palsy in the United Kingdom and Sweden in the past 15 years, mainly because of a fall in the number of cases of spastic diplegia and athetoid cerebral palsy.

While much has been written on the child with cerebral palsy, there are few controlled studies of the different forms of treatment. Using a team approach the work of many disciplines must be coordinated, most efficiently from a rehab-ilitation center.

Physiotherapy should begin as soon as the problem is recognized, with programs to prevent those contractures that may lead to subsequent deformity, to correct any established deformity, and to provide sensory stimulation of paretic limbs. These may be hospital-based or the mother may be taught how to apply them at home. The *occupational therapist* will teach skills related to the activities of daily living. *Orthopedic surgery* may be required, e.g., the release of tight tendons such as the hamstrings, adductors, or the tendo-Achilles or the treatment of dislo-cated hips. In severely handicapped spastic patients, these procedures may reduce pain and deformity and enable easier management of incontinence. Nonsurgical orthopedic treatment with braces and splinting may also be considered.

Medical treatment of *seizures* follows principles similar to those in epilepsy from other causes (Chap. 15). *Drug therapy* in the management of either spastic or extrapyramidal forms is, genetically speaking, disappointing, although drugs may help to maximize gains from physiotherapy. They include dantrolene sodium, baclofen, and benzodiazepines such as diazepam, for spasticity, while L-dopa, carbamazepine, and benztropine have been used with occasional success in extra-pyramidal disorders. The role of surgery in these situations is still unresolved.

In later years the physician's task is to ensure that these children achieve their full potential. This requires not only medical and physical therapy but also support of the whole family unit of which the child is a member. Ideally, the child will live at home and attend a normal school, thus establishing relationships with his peers. More is asked of the parents of a cerebral-palsied child than of one who is physically adept, and they will need help in understanding the child's and their own problems as they face the difficult task of rearing someone who may be mentally as well as physically handicapped.

Course and Prognosis

The course, by definition, should be nonprogressive, but in fact some children's defects either appear for the first time or become accentuated as they grow older, while others manage to compensate better as they grow up. The physical handi-caps of cerebral palsy have their maximum effect in preschool years. The ultimate place of these children in society is mainly determined by the extent of their mental and physical handicaps. The hemiplegic person usually has the best outlook, with a 30 percent chance of being able to earn his living. The prognosis of those with extrapyramidal forms is less than would be predicted by their intelligence alone; only one-quarter manage to work. The overall figures for cerebral palsy indicate however that about 60 percent lead "twilight lives," depending upon their parents or others, or functioning only in sheltered workshops. Only a small proportion of patients with cerebral palsy every marry.

MINIMAL BRAIN DYSFUNCTION

At one time it was thought that the nervous system was either normal or had an evident structural abnormality. In the past 25 years the concept of *minimal brain dysfunction* has emerged, which (by contrast with the obvious brain dysfunction of cerebral palsy and mental retardation) is characterized only by minor symptoms. These include an attention deficit; disorders of motor function and of the central processing of information; perceptual disturbances; and delay in the development of language and auditory comprehension. These exist either alone or in combination and may be combined with minor neurological signs.

The clinical characteristics of minimal brain dysfunction include average or above average intelligence; specific learning disabilities; visual and/or auditory perceptual difficulties; visuomotor incoordination; confused or crossed laterality; hyperkinesis, distractability, and short attention span; emotional lability and a number of so-called soft neurological signs. Many of these children also have abnormal EEGs. As an example of this class of disorder, the hyperkinetic syndrome will be described.

The Hyperkinetic Syndrome

The hyperkinetic syndrome in children has achieved wide publicity in recent years, but there are still many gaps in our understanding of the disorder. It is an example of the "borderland" between psychiatry and neurology in which there is an overlap of behavioral and organic phenomena and the relative importance of genetic, environmental, psychological, and structural factors is never clear.

The syndrome is more common in boys, usually becoming manifest in the preschool years. The chief characteristics are

1. Excessive motor activity
2. Distractability and impulsive behavior
3. Emotional lability and exaggerated responses to external stimuli
4. Low frustration tolerance and impatience
5. Uneven academic performance with underachievement in relation to intelligence
6. Specific learning disorders

The most obvious characteristic of these children is their overactive, impulsive behavior with decreased sleep requirements, often exhausting their parents whose total life-style is compromised.

From 5 to 15 percent of the childhood population is estimated to suffer from this problem in North America; in England the prevalence is considerably lower, probably because of differences in diagnostic criteria. Its genesis is uncertain; some deny that it is due to brain damage and suggest either that it has a biochemical origin or that it reflects maturational delay. Others regard it as a mild form of cerebral palsy.

It is hard to define suitable diagnostic criteria because most normal children will show some of the features listed earlier, and hyperkinetic children do not show all of the features all the time. Hence it is important to get information from the teacher, or day-care center staff, as well as from both parents, to determine if overactivity, distractibility, disorders of attention, and frustrated behavior do truly interfere with the child's daily life. All pediatricians have experienced the "office wrecker," who is constantly on the move flitting from object to object, picking them up in rapid succession only to pass on to another when the first has briefly held his attention; however some hyperkinetic children can control their symptoms for a time, so behavior in front of the physician may not be diagnostic and the history of their daylong behavior is all-important.

During the *examination,* note should be made of poor following movements of the eyes, clumsiness or awkwardness particularly with hand movements, inability to maintain a steady posture of the outstretched arms, and the presence of any lateralizing neurological signs. Diagnosis is difficult because one has to decide whether one is dealing with a behavior problem in an essentially normal child or with true though minimal cerebral dysfunction. If any soft neurological signs, such as those mentioned previously, are found in a hyperactive child, referral to a developmental clinic or pediatric neurologist is advisable.

Other causes of a high level of activity in children include emotional disturbance, disrupted family life, cultural factors, and (rarely) organic medical disease such as hyperthyroidism or rheumatic chorea.

Management begins with an explanation of the problem to the parents. This relieves any guilt they may feel and also allows one to outline a management plan. These children need a structured environment, and the parents must decide exactly how much overactive or bad behavior they are prepared to tolerate, then apply sanctions quickly and consistently. The child's teacher must be made aware of the problem and must work with the parents to achieve the same goals in the same way.

Drug therapy with methylphenidate (Ritalin), caffeine, or occasionally dextroamphetamine (Dexedrine) may be valuable. These medications should be adjusted one or two times a week until an optimal dose is achieved without such side effects as insomnia, anorexia, or depression. These stimulants have the paradoxical effect of quietening children. They should be used at a dosage level which normalizes activity without producing sedation. It is wise to order a "drug holiday" one or two times a year to check whether or not the agent is still needed because the requirement may be outgrown after a few years.

The *prognosis* for hyperactive children is for a diminution of the overactivity in time, but there are long-term concerns about their future social integration. Distractibility persists, and there is an increased prevalence of adjustment and behavioral problems in the teens. The value of drugs in preventing this aspect of the problem is uncertain.

Learning Disorders

Ten to fifteen percent of children have a level of academic attainment that is inappropriate for their intelligence. This school failure often is due to learning disorders. Most children who fail to learn effectively do so because of various sociocultural factors such as lack of opportunity, ghetto environments, overcrowding, inadequate education, and disruptive family life. The importance of adequate nutrition in facilitating normal neurological development is becoming more generally recognized because the part that undernutrition plays in hindering such development is now apparent in the countries of the Third World.

Of more relevance to the Western neurologist is the problem of the child with a learning disability caused by his inability to process information from outside because of altered brain functioning. This may be due to disorders of visual or of auditory perception, causing the child to experience difficulty with the central processing of visual or auditory stimuli. Particular difficulty with reading results; the child may fail to recognize the differences among letters and may reverse them; making similar mistakes when attempting to write. Other children have their greatest problem with arithmetic, with space-form perception, or in more than one area. Defects of attention, recall, abstract reasoning, comprehension, and motor coordination also occur, the last caused by movement disorders or by the effects of minimal brain dysfunction.

In a small group of children who are severely affected, the analysis of this problem requires careful neurological assessment to recognize the specific learning handicaps, which are often multiple. Following this, a suitable plan to help solve the child's problems must be devised, taking into account his most effective pathway of learning, his need to be taught how to make the best use of his handicapped channels where possible or practical, and the value of a multidisciplinary approach.

If an early diagnosis is made, the children can often be taught to compensate for their handicap and maybe to achieve this potential. Early identification also prevents the common psychological traumas that they may otherwise experience, for if allowed to fail repeatedly because of a learning disability, they may develop a self-image of inadequacy, stupidity, and worthlessness.

The parents and the classroom teacher can all supply valuable information, and all will need the results of the physician's and psychologist's assessments. The physician should ensure that the parents understand the nature of the problem, what may reasonably be anticipated in the future, and what their contribution to management should be. Given suitable support, most children can be significantly helped, although it is difficult to single out one particular item as the most important therapeutic aid, unless it is the dedicated teacher who has the time and the skill to give to that particular child's problem.

Etiology has not been discussed because once a progressive lesion has been excluded, it is unimportant whether the cerebral dysfunction results from an *organic* cause, such as prematurity or neonatal asphyxia, is *maturational* because of unevenness or delay in the acquisition of specific skills, or is *biochemical* such as might be due to inadequacy of central neurotransmitters. We have as yet no specific treatments.

MENTAL RETARDATION

Mental retardation is defined by the World Health Organization as an incomplete or insufficient general development of mental capacity encompassing a global delay in the normal development of motor, language, and social adaptive skills. As there is a continuum of mental ability from negligible function up to genius, the division into levels of mental retardation is necessarily arbitrary. Borderline (IQ 75 to 85), mild (50 to 75), moderate (25 to 50), and severe (below 25) degrees are recognized. Mentally retarded individuals however are more practically designated in terms of their function rather than by category. For instance, a person with an IQ between 50 and 70 may be a slow learner but educable, and one with an IQ below that level may still be trained in certain simple skills.

Two to three percent of the population can be defined as mentally retarded (IQ below 75) but almost all are educable or trainable. Only a tenth of them require permanent institutional care.

Table 39-1   Treatable or Preventable Causes of Mental Retardation

Cause	Treatment
Prematurity	Proper antenatal care with early admission in high-risk cases
Obstetrical hazards	Early admission, anticipatory care
Subdural hematoma	Evacuation of the clot
Hydrocephalus	Shunt procedure
Craniostenosis	Surgical suture separation
Syphilis	Penicillin
Phenylketonuria	Intrauterine diagnosis, genetic counseling; diet
Galactosemia	Intrauterine diagnosis, genetic counseling; diet
Erythroblastosis	Intrauterine diagnosis; exchange transfusion anti-D immunization
Pyridoxine deficiency	Pyridoxine
Hypoglycemia	Glucose; treat underlying cause
Hypothyroidism	Thyroxine
Wilson's disease	Penicillamine, K_2S
Lead poisoning	Chelating agents
Cultural deprivation	Family therapy, social rehabilitation
Battered child	Placement away from home; treat parents

Causes of Mental Retardation

Of the many causes of mental retardation, we list in Table 39-1 only those that can be treated and therefore demand early diagnosis. One should be alerted to the possibility of mental retardation if there is a history of maternal illness during the pregnancy or a positive family history of similar disease, if the pregnancy or labor was complicated, if the child appears abnormal at birth, or if there is a failure in the normal course of development (see Chap. 4).

In considering the etiology of mental retardation, it is convenient to group the causes under the following headings.

Prenatal

1. Genetic
2. Inborn errors of metabolism including many degenerative and storage diseases of the nervous system
3. Chromosomal anomalies
4. Neurocutaneous syndromes
5. Intrauterine infections
6. Fetal irradiation and toxic causes
7. Other causes that adversely affect the intrauterine environment including maternal and placental disorders

Perinatal

1. Trauma: birth injuries with associated anoxia and asphyxia
2. Hemolytic disease producing kernicterus

Postnatal

1. Infections of the central nervous system
2. Nutritional
3. Deprivation and trauma
4. Toxins; and the sequelae of immunization

Prenatal Causes

Genetic: Obviously a family history of any of the chromosomal or genetic disorders must alert one to the possibility that a new member of the family has the same disease. Consanguinity, low parental intelligence and a history of previous fetal or neonatal death or of prematurity are risk factors. Some two-thirds of the mentally retarded have no identifiable cause. Most of them are only mildly retarded, and they may not be identified as such until beyond infancy, during the preschool or early school years.

These children show no distinguishing clinical features. It is generally accepted that multiple factors account for this group, including unfavorable combinations from the total gene pool, and that it largely represents the lower end of the normal distribution curve of intelligence. There is however an increased prevalence of adverse obstetrical circumstances, poor prenatal care, and low-birth-weight infants, and an increased probability of the child being reared in poor socioeconomic circumstances. There is thus a greater likelihood of poor nutrition, sociocultural deprivation, lack of community support, inadequate education, and lack of opportunity in older childhood or adult life, all contributing to the problem. Less often, conditions such as hydrocephalus and microencephaly may be inherited on a mendelian basis, and therefore a careful family history must be taken to allow risk estimation.

Spinal dyraphism, hydrocephalus, and craniosynostosis may have genetic bases in some instances or may be associated with environmental factors; because of the resulting brain damage they may be associated with mental retardation; the diagnosis is seldom difficult in such cases.

Inborn Errors of Metabolism: The importance of inborn errors of metabolism, which are relatively rare and form only a small proportion of the total number of cases of retardation, is that they do include treatable conditions such as phenylketonuria and maple syrup urine disease.

Most of them present with mental retardation and many include seizures. Generally speaking, the *aminoacidopathies* are not characterized by any distinctive phenotypic appearances, but children with *mucopolysaccharide* disorders (e.g., Hurler's syndrome or gargoylism) have notably coarse facial features and visceromegaly. Some diseases of *lipid storage* such as Niemann-Pick disease also have enlarged viscera, while the *cerebroretinal degenerations* such as Tay-Sachs disease do not. A few inborn errors cause progressive mental retardation, which must always make one exclude such disorders. Inborn errors of *thyroid* metabolism may also present in this manner.

Many of these diseases permit prenatal diagnosis by amniocentesis and examination of cultured fibroblasts from the amniotic fluid for specific enzymatic defects. If the parents have had a previously affected child, this enables a rational approach to the question of therapeutic abortion to be taken, should this be consistent with the parents' views. Where an affected child is a sibling or close relative of a potential patient, the question of carrier status may often be resolved by means of a specific loading test, e.g., phenylketonuria.

Chromosomal Anomalies: The best known of the chromosomal anomalies is mongolism or *Down's syndrome* in which the characteristic features, present at birth, include a reduced head size, obliquely slanted palpebral fissures, epicanthic folds, a flattened facial appearance, and a small mouth cavity giving the appearance of a large tongue. These infants are floppy at birth. They have a single transverse palmar crease and short digits. There may be a large cleft between the first and second toes. One must recognize the condition at birth; mental retardation is a constant feature and counseling and support of the family, who often recognize the unusual appearance of the infant themselves, must start at once. Most children with Down's syndrome are of gentle and affectionate disposition, and many have only moderate mental retardation.

The prevalence is highest (1 percent) in the children born to mothers aged over 40 years. Confirmation of the diagnosis can be made by a chromosome count and is mandatory when the infant is born to a younger mother, because instead of trisomy of the 21st chromosome, a translocation of chromosomes is more likely among young mothers and may well happen again.

Chromosomal abnormalities should also be suspected in infants and children with the characteristic features of certain identified syndromes and those with multiple congenital anomalies. Many of these syndromes can be identified in utero by culture of the shed epithelial cells and subsequent karyotyping. Some geneticists recommend this as a routine procedure in pregnant women over the age of 40 or 45, provided the information gained would be used therapeutically.

Neurocutaneous Syndromes: Also known as *phakomatoses,* neurocutaneous syndromes are congenital disorders of ectoderm, involving both the skin and the central and peripheral nervous systems. Mental retardation is frequently associated. Six of the most distinctive will be described briefly.

Tuberous sclerosis: Tuberous sclerosis is inherited as an autosomal-dominant trait, although about a third of cases are due to spontaneous mutations. Masses of glial tissue (hamartomas) occur in the brain, eye, bones, heart, lung, thyroid, and other glands (Fig. 39-2). In the cortex, they may give rise to grand mal or other seizures and are frequently associated with mental retardation. If large hamartomas project into the ventricles they may cause obstruction to CSF flow. Patients with tuberous sclerosis may die young, often in status epilepticus.

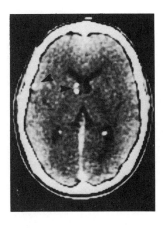

Figure 39-2 Unenhanced CT scan. Tuberous sclerosis, with multiple masses especially in subependymal areas.

In the skin, adenoma sebaceum (which looks like severe acne) is typically seen over the butterfly area of the face, and lipomas, depigmented nevi, and fibromas underneath the nails may be seen. Renal cysts or tumors occur in 80 percent of these patients.

Neurofibromatosis: Neurofibromatosis is inherited as an autosomal-dominant trait; only about 10 percent of the patients are retarded. There are four major groups of abnormality.

Skeletal lesions include kyphoscoliosis, macrocephaly, spina bifida, pes cavus, and syndactyly.

In the *skin* café au lait spots are seen; these are brown macules which must number five or more (at least one having a long axis greater than 1 cm) to be significant (Fig. 39-3A, B)

In the *peripheral nervous system,* neurofibromas may be single or multiple and may be seen or felt in the skin.

In the *central nervous system,* there is an association with mental retardation and with seizures of any type. Neurofibromas occur mainly on cranial nerves VIII, V, and II, and there is a markedly increased prevalence of benign and malignant cerebral tumors, particularly meningiomas and gliomas. Hypertension may occur because of renal artery stenosis or pheochromocytoma. As in tuberous sclerosis, renal phakomas may be seen.

Sturge-Weber syndrome: In the Sturge-Weber syndrome, a large port-wine stain is seen over one or more divisions of the fifth nerve. If the first division is affected, glaucoma and enlargement of that eye may occur. Small pial angiomas may coexist, leading to upper motor neuron or cortical sensory deficits, seizures, and/or hemianopia (Fig. 39-4). Skull x-rays show "tramline" calcification caused by calcium deposits in the cortex; this may be seen at a young age on a CT scan (Fig. 39-5A, B). Mental retardation is an almost invariable feature but may be minimized by removal of the affected hemisphere, so early diagnosis is important.

Ataxia telangiectasia (Louis-Bar syndrome): The Louis-Bar syndrome is an autosomal-recessive condition manifested by a mild cerebellar syndrome or choreoathetotic movements in early childhood. After the age of 4 or 5, telangiectasas appear progressively on the face, bulbar conjunctiva, and limbs. Frequent infections, usually of the upper or lower respiratory tracts are associated with a diminution of gamma globulins, particularly IgA and IgE.

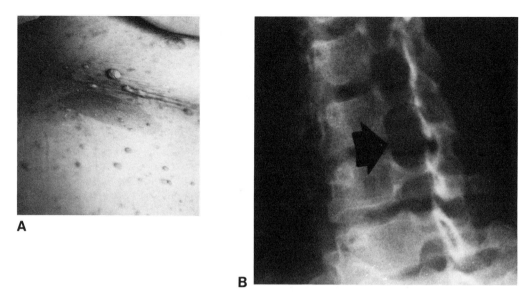

Figure 39-3   (A) Skin lesions in neurofibromatosis; (B) Lateral radiograph of cervical spine. Expansion of many intervertebral foramina by "dumbbell" neurofibromas.

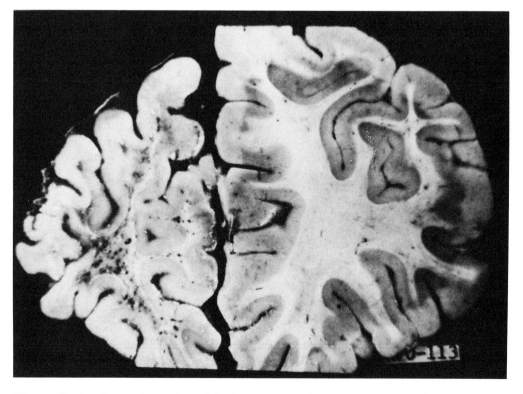

Figure 39-4   Coronal section of brain, with hemiatrophy because of Sturge-Weber syndrome.

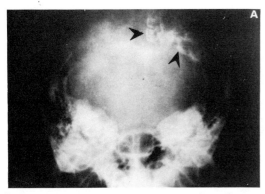 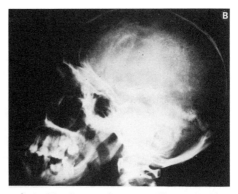

Figure 39-5A, B   AP and lateral radiographs of skull. Posterior tramline calcification in Sturge-Weber disease.

Incontinentia pigmenti: In this rare condition, female infants develop vesicles and darkly pigmented macules arranged longitudinally on the limbs and transversely on the trunk. They fade as the child grows older and may be forgotten. Cerebral palsy and mental retardation are often associated. The cause is not known.

Von Hippel-Lindau disease: Von Hippel-Lindau disease is an autosomal-dominant or sporadic disease characterized by the development of hemangioblastomas of the neuraxis and cysts of the kidneys, liver, and pancreas. The former usually produces a typical cerebellar syndrome. Because of excessive production of erythropoietin, primary erythrocytosis may coexist. This syndrome is rarely associated with mental retardation and is only included here for completeness among the other neurocutaneous syndromes. Pheochromocytomas and renal carcinomas are sometimes described.

Intrauterine Infection: Maternal infections (such as rubella, toxoplasmosis, cytomegalic inclusion disease, syphilis, infectious hepatitis, mumps, influenza, or malaria) may lead to eventual mental retardation with or without neurological and skeletal abnormalities in the infant.

Fetal Irradiation and Toxins: Lead, mercury, lysergic acid diethylamide (LSD), ethanol, nicotine, and many other drugs may produce mental retardation in the infant when they have been ingested by the mother, particularly during the first 3 months of pregnancy. X-rays are well known to produce damage to the fetus and stringent precautions are taken with pregnant women to prevent unnecessary irradiation.

Other Causes: There is a statistical association between mental retardation and maternal age under 16 or over 40 years, in the latter case mainly because of the increased likelihood of Down's syndrome. It is widely considered that obstetrical complications during pregnancy may cause or contribute to mental retardation. Poor health in the mother caused by toxemia of pregnancy, thyroid disease, hypertension, diabetes, and so forth, may adversely affect the fetus. Placental abnormalities including infarcts and retroplacental hemorrhage may lead to small-for-dates infants, who are vulnerable to hypoxia. Threatened miscarriages may indicate the presence of a fetus with developmental abnormalities, and it is relevant here that two-thirds of the fetuses with Down's syndrome fail to survive to term. The obstetrical histories of mothers with myotonic dystrophy are often appalling and the risk of severe hypotonia to the live-born child, as well as later mental retardation as part of the whole syndrome, are high.

Perinatal Damage

Birth Injury: Probably the most common causes of damage to the fetus and the newborn are anoxia, intracerebral hemorrhage, and other birth traumas. These are particularly dangerous to premature babies, and often occur in cases where other risk factors, such as previous premature births, maternal diabetes, and so on, have been identified.

Hemolytic Disease of the Newborn: Hemolytic disease is an important cause of later deafness, choreoathetosis or other forms of cerebral palsy, and mental retardation. This disorder may be diagnosed prenatally and will be minimized by energetic treatment measures even before birth. Its prevalence has been greatly reduced by prevention of Rh sensitization using human anti-D globulin after delivery in Rh-negative mothers.

Postnatal Causes

Infections of the Nervous System: Viral infections of the nervous system, particularly the common childhood illnesses, may also result in mental deficiency, in addition to specific neurological sequelae. Meningitis may result in significant brain damage in the infant or child, and hyperpyrexia from any cause, even from trivial infections, may do the same either alone or if complicated by recurrent seizures. Postinfective encephalopathy (ADEM) may complicate smallpox, measles and, rarely, other viral infections and may lead to brain damage and other specific residua (see Chap. 40).

The term *infantile spasms* describes a serious disease of children usually less than 1-year-old who present with listlessness, failure to thrive, and sudden, brief, generalized myoclonic jerks with the arms flung out, forward and upward, the legs flexing or extending, and the trunk flexing. In older children these seizures have been described as *salaam attacks.* They are evidence of diffuse cerebral pathology and the prognosis is poor; almost all these children develop severe mental retardation and many die.

Nutritional and Metabolic Causes: Malnutrition during the growth period, when cell proliferation is taking place, leads to a permanent reduction in the number of cells in the body, including the brain. In numerical terms, 300 million children are currently undernourished in the world. This must be viewed as one of the most important causes of developmental retardation. Iodine deficiency may lead to severe mental retardation resulting from hypothyroidism in those parts of the world where iodine is deficient in the food, water, or salt. Damage to the nervous system occurs in the children of malnourished mothers, and in infants marked deficiency of protein results in kwashiorkor, signs of which include decreased intellectual development. Hypoglycemia and severe dehydration (as with gastroenteritis) may both lead to later brain damage and retardation.

Deprivation and Trauma: Many factors in the child's environment may contribute to his failing to develop his potential. These include inadequate mothering, frank neglect, and the consequences of ghetto upbringing with poor schooling and few opportunities for advancement.

Trauma accounts for only about 15 percent of cases of mental retardation but operates mainly at the time of birth. Postnatal or infantile trauma also causes brain damage, and there is increasing concern today about the residual CNS effects of repeated physical trauma at home — "the battered baby."

Among other traumatic causes, subdural hematomas from direct injury or the "whiplash-shaken" infant may be important, as may the injuries to which accident-prone children are subject.

Toxicity and Immunizations: Acute disseminated encephalomyelopathy is a rare sequel to immunizations, particularly against smallpox and measles. The relationship between pertussis immunization and the development of infantile spasms is not clear but has been postulated.

Status epilepticus may occasionally cause mental retardation because of acquired brain damage, but excessive anticonvulsant medication is probably a more common cause. Phenobarbitone is the agent usually responsible.

Hexachlorophene, used to wash the skin, is a potential cause of brain damage in premature infants.

Diagnosis

Any child with any degree of mental retardation or any neurological deficit should be referred for specialist assessment. This will not only increase the chance of successful treatment but also will allow some idea of prognosis to be given to the parents; the institution of those measures that may enable the child to utilize what abilities he has, and the provision of advice on diagnosis, which may lead to successful genetic counseling.

Mental retardation cannot be diagnosed clinically in the neonatal period, but it may be predicted in some instances by the presence of abnormal physical findings (see Chap. 4), as in Down's syndrome, hydranencephaly (in which transillumination of the skull demonstrates replacement of the cerebral hemispheres by fluid), or microcephaly.

The neonate should be carefully examined for unusual physical characteristics that will enable any of the above syndromes to be recognized. Because of the proliferation of syndromes it is impossible to remember more than a few common ones, but reference atlases are available so that clinical observations can be compared with known conditions. This may enable a diagnosis to be reached, may initiate a search for important associated malformations, and may permit genetic counseling to be undertaken and recurrent risks to be quoted.

In familial retardation with no particular distinguishing features, particularly if severe, the possibility of inborn errors of metabolism must always be considered, and a ferric chloride test and an amino acid chromatogram are valuable and generally available screening tests. Where appropriate they may be supplemented by other tests such as examination of the urine for mucopolysaccharides.

Differential Diagnosis

Recognition of the normal variations in child development are important to avoid a wrong diagnosis and unnecessary anxiety to the parents.

Isolated motor delay may be just a benign familial condition, but *cerebral palsy* may also present thus. Failure to talk, unaccompanied by other features of generalized developmental retardation, can be due to *deafness* or to an *isolated speech delay,* and particularly in the very young child, *poor vision* may not always be obvious as a cause of delayed milestones. Childhood psychosis or *autism* is a rare condition in which the child treats humans impersonally, is distressed by interruption of his set routines, indulges in repetitive, meaningless movements, and is often speechless. *Progressive retardation,* with or without features of raised intracranial pressure, must raise the suspicion of one of the *degenerative* diseases of childhood, of subacute *encephalitis,* or of cerebral *tumor.* Finally, a child whose parents show features of lack of appropriate concern and are themselves vulnerable or inadequate, or a child brought in who is bruised without explanation or who is unusually passive or terrified, should raise the question of child *abuse.*

Management

Management begins with recognizing that there is a problem. The most important task of the family physician will be to introduce the parents gently but firmly to a realization that their child is mentally retarded and requires from them a whole new set of expectations. The time at which the situation is accepted may vary between the two parents, although the very act of one parent having sought medical advice in the first instance suggests that realistic concerns were present. It is best that the mother not be informed of the news in the early postpartum period, at which time women are frequently emotionally unstable, and that the bad news be introduced calmly and gently to both parents. Their reactions are frequently rejection of the diagnosis and of the doctor, dismay, guilt, and final acceptance, with then the understanding that allows constructive planning for the future. Sometimes however, acceptance of the diagnosis leads to rejection of the child. Any guilt that parents feel must be quickly and firmly dispelled. Advice about subsequent pregnancies is not usually welcomed at this time. If it is requested however, the answer depends upon the diagnosis.

The impact on the parents of this tragedy is hard to describe. It has been said that it constitutes a dual burden; the death of their hopes for the normal child they had expected and the burden of the handicapped child whom they had not expected.

Counseling, as a continuing service, must dispel guilt and provide genetic information. The physician must point out the realistic accomplishments that may be achieved and supervise the provision of ancillary services from day care to appropriate schooling. He must also function as an advocate where necessary. He should remember that while he is a valued advisor, his role is to act as a member of a team of specialists, medical and nonmedical, to provide the family with information on which they make decisions about present and future care.

After the diagnosis of neurological abnormality has been made, the child should be referred to a specialized assessment center for final steps in diagnosis and for pediatric, neurological, orthopedic, and physiatric evaluation. Treatment will be given by the pediatrician for those disorders listed in Table 39-1. The family physician should work closely with the assessment center and their social service department to ensure that the parents are aware of all of the benefits available to them.

Finally, any child is heir to intercurrent physical ailments, and the retarded may develop intercurrent illnesses in the same way as other children. These may be harder to recognize, but they need the same treatment.

BIBLIOGRAPHY

Baird, H.W., Gordon, E.C. Neurological evaluation of infants and children. *Clin. Develop. Med.* No. 84/85, Oxford, Blackwell, 1983.

Dycken, P., Krawiecki, N. Neurodegenerative diseases of infancy and childhood. *Ann. Neurol. 13*:331-364, 1983.

Ingram, T.T.S. The neurology of cerebral palsy. *Arch. Dis. Child. 41*:337, 1966.

Levine, M., Brooks, R., Shonkoff, J.P. *A Pediatric Approach to Learning Disorders.* New York, John Wiley & Sons, 1980.

Pellock, J.M., Myer, E.C. *Neurologic Emergencies in Infancy and Childhood.* London, Harper & Row, 1984.

Pincus, J.H., Glaser, G.H. The syndrome of minimal brain damage in childhood. *N. Engl. J. Med. 275:*27, 1966.

Scott, C.L., Thomas, G.H. Genetic disorders associated with mental retardation. *Pediatr. Clin. N. Am. 20:*121, 1973.

40
Infectious Diseases of the Nervous System

The central nervous system has no lymphatic system as such, and although usually well protected from direct infection, its resistance to any infection that does occur is low. The patterns of infective illness are relatively few, but the organisms that can produce disease are many. This chapter will outline the kinds of infection, paying particular attention to those that are most common (Table 40-1).

MENINGITIS

Meningitis is always a neurological emergency. It is most common in the earliest years of life, particularly in premature infants, of whom half may die as a result. The peak incidence is in the first 2 years, and about three-quarters of all cases occur before the age of 10. The death rate in older patients has decreased to 10 percent but continuous developments in therapy do not seem to have lowered it further.

When handling a case of possible mengingeal inflammation, the first step is to confirm the diagnosis, and the second is to identify the organisms responsible. Third, one must immediately start appropriate therapy, and fourth, assess why *this* patient developed *this* infection at *this* time. The most common organisms responsible for septic meningitis in people over the age of 2 months are *Neisseria meningitidis, Haemophilus influenzae,* and *Streptococcus pneumoniae.* However other organisms must be considered in neonates, in patients with CNS defects or local infections, and in those with immunological suppression.

Most cases of meningitis are associated with infection in the upper respiratory tract, but one should always consider whether the patient may have a lowered resistance to infections or an abnormal portal of entry for organisms to reach the nervous system; and whether an unusual organism may be present.

Table 40-1   Overview of CNS Infections

Meningitis

   Acute*
   Subacute*
   Chronic*
   Recurrent*

Encephalitis

   Viral: general, herpes simplex, rabies, polio
   Fungal
   Parasitic

Abscess

   Extradural, subdural, intracerebral, spinal epidural abscess

Other

Herpes zoster	Tetanus
Cytomegalovirus	Botulism
Coxsackievirus	Toxoplasmosis
Infectious mononucleosis	Reye's syndrome (?)
Influenza	Syphilis
Tick paralysis	Behcet's syndrome

Slow virus infections

   Jakob-Creutzfeldt
   Subacute sclerosing panencephalitis
   Progressive multifocal leukoencephalopathy

Neurological complications of other infections

   Acute toxic encephalopathy
   Acute allergic encephalomyelitis
   Bacterial endocarditis
   Cerebral thrombophlebitis

*These may be bacterial, viral, fungal or parasitic.

Although the word *meningitis* suggests an inflammation of the meninges only, there is always some involvement of the most superficial parts of the brain and often alterations in the flow of CSF. An occlusive arteritis is common in the subpial cortex, so meningitis may usefully be considered as a meningoencephalitis in all cases. Causative organisms include bacteria and spirochetes, viruses, fungi, rickettsiae, and protozoa; sometimes carcinomatous invasion of the meninges produces meningeal inflammation that is hard to differentiate clinically from infective meningitis.

Meningitis may present as an acute, subacute, chronic, or recurrent inflammation of the meninges. It is classed as *septic* or purulent when organisms are isolated by routine culture methods. With bacterial infection, polymorphonuclear (PMN)

leukocytes predominate in the CSF. Viruses usually cause an *aseptic* meningitis in which mononuclear cells predominate and routine cultures do not grow the organism. The same CSF picture can be seen with tuberculous and fungal infection.

Certain pathologic conditions consistently predispose to CNS infections and in any patient seen they must be considered, if not in the acute stage, at least immediately after it. Thus patients with leukemia or lymphoma, receiving immunosuppressive drugs including steroids, and after splenectomy, are at risk of infection by measles, herpes zoster, and cytomegaloviruses, fungi, streptococci, listeria and gram-negative bacilli. Skull defects and cranial trauma, including CNS surgery, may make pneumococcal, staphylococcal and gram-negative infections more likely. Progressive multifocal leukoencephalopathy is always associated with impaired immune responsiveness. Toxoplasmosis has been found in patients with the acquired immunodeficiency syndrome (AIDS).

Clinical Presentations

Acute Meningitis

Acute septic meningitis evolves over hours or, at the most, days. Patients who have been quite healthy or have only had an upper respiratory infection now begin to complain of the symptoms of meningeal irritation and of raised intracranial pressure. Malaise, fever, headaches of traction type, nausea, vomiting, anorexia, stiff painful neck, and photophobia are the usual initial symptoms. Then there may follow depression in the level of consciousness, delirium, seizures, and various focal neurological signs. The association of fever and any form of mental deterioration must make one consider meningoencephalitis as a possible diagnosis. The inflammatory cells in the CSF and accompanying cerebral edema may cause a rapid rise in intracranial pressure and produce false localizing signs (see Chap. 16).

Examination shows the signs of meningism with stiff neck and resistance to flexion of the spine or to straight-leg raising. Such signs may be absent in neonates, who may just show features listed in Table 40-2. A bulging fontanel, neck stiffness, and drowsiness are late signs of meningitis in neonates. Hepatosplenomegaly and skin rashes are common in neonates and young children. Prematurity, perinatal complications, and neural tube defects are predisposing factors for the meningitis that is usually caused by gram-negative organisms.

Children may also show head retraction which can be so marked as to warrant the term *opisthotonos*. General examination may show a rash (particularly if the meningococcus or ECHO or Coxsackie viruses are involved); signs of infective disease in the eyes, joints, bones, chest, or heart; and sometimes purpura and hypotension. Shock is common if a gram-negative organism is the cause of septicemia with secondary meningitis and in meningococcal septicemia causing adrenal infarction (Waterhouse-Friedrichsen syndrome). Infections with *Escherichia coli, Pseudomonas, Proteus, Listeria monocytogenes, Streptococcus,* and *Staphylococcus aureus* can also produce this picture.

Examination of CSF in Meningitis: A lumbar puncture is indicated whenever there is evidence of meningeal inflammation. Before it is performed, intracerebral abscess or expanding mass lesions, particularly in the posterior fossa, must be considered and ruled out. In the presence of any focal signs an EEG and isotope or CT scan are necessary. In infants, lumbar puncture is indicated in the investigation of pyrexia of unknown origin and may be indicated in any ill child with fever or septicemia, with or without neurological signs, and in the investigation of failure to thrive and of seizures. If the result of the first LP is not conclusive, i.e., no organisms are seen and the cells present are not polymorphonuclear leukocytes (PMNs),

Table 40-2   Signs of Meningitis in Infants and Children

Neonates	Older Infants	Over Age 2
Fever	Fever	Fever
Lethargy	Vomiting	Drowsiness
Anorexia	Irritability	Headache
Vomiting	Drowsiness	Stiff neck
Respiratory distress	Convulsions	Vomiting
Convulsions	Bulging fontanel	Convulsions
Irritability		
Jaundice		
Bulging fontanel		

then the patient can be carefully observed for a period without antibiotics and the test repeated in 12 to 18 hr with a greater chance of finding organisms or diagnostic cell patterns.

The CSF pressure need not be taken if the initial fluid is cloudy or bloodstained since raised pressures do not help diagnosis in these circumstances. The fluid may be turbid or clear; microscopy may show any number of mononuclear or polymorphonuclear cells. The PMNs almost always predominate in acute bacterial meningitis, but lymphocytes may predominate in the very earliest stages and in the later stages during recovery from such infections. Mononuclear cells usually predominate in the other forms (caused by *Mycobacterium tuberculosis,* viruses, or fungi). CSF protein is raised in all forms of meningitis, particularly those of longer duration or with very high cell counts. Apart from gram and Ziehl-Neelsen stains, auramine stains for *M. tuberculosis,* india ink preparations for fungi, special stains for other organisms and specific antigen or antibody studies may be needed. The sample should be examined immediately; to leave it for hours or until the next day allows disintegration of most of the cells, and the results are then dangerously misleading. If laboratory analysis isn't immediately available, do a simple gram stain yourself.*

A simultaneous blood sugar estimation is mandatory when the lumbar puncture is done. With most viral meningitides and parameningeal foci of infection, CSF sugar values are often normal. Values will be low (i.e., less than two-thirds of the

---

*A rapid Gram stain can be performed by drying and fixing the centrifuged deposit of CSF and staining it with gentian violet for 2 sec and Gram's iodine for 2 sec. The sample is then rinsed in water, 95% ethyl alcohol is dripped onto the slide until the gentian violet is completely eluted (up to 3 sec), and the slide rinsed in water, counterstained with 2% safranin or carbolfuchsin for 3 sec, and then again rinsed in water.

blood level) in bacterial meningitis. High polymorphonuclear cell counts are to be expected in all cases — over $50,000/mm^3$ if the meningitis is due to rupture of an abscess. If the cell count is surprisingly low, consider agranulocytosis or immuno-suppression.

If CSF cultures are negative despite suspected bacterial meningitis, the pa-tient may have been given antibiotics prior to the collection of CSF, in which case counter-immunoelectrophoresis to detect bacterial antigen in the CSF may be helpful in diagnosing infection with S. pneumoniae, *N. meningitidis* or *H. influenzae*. However, blood cultures will probably be positive anyhow.

Haemophilus influenzae is common in children up to the age of 2 years but is rarely seen after the age of 5 years. Patients have often had recent otitis or upper respiratory infection. *Meningococcus* meningitis has a peak appearance between the ages of 2 and 25, and *pneumococcal* meningitis occurs in childhood and through-out adult life but has a peak incidence in old age. In the first 3 months of life, other commonly responsible organisms include *Escherichia coli, Streptococcus* (group B), *S. aureus, L. monocytogenes* and Enterobacteriaceae.

Specific organisms causing meningitis may be suggested by specific clinical signs. Disseminated intravascular coagulation and a purpuric skin rash suggest meningococcemia. Shock may also result from adrenal hemorrhage. *Neisseria meningitidis* tends to occur in epidemics (Table 40-3).

Pneumococcal meningitis is mainly a disease of adult life, particularly com-mon in subjects with an obvious focus of infection elsewhere (ears, chest, recent skull fracture with CSF leak, or ENT operation); in patients with immunological deficiency, and in alcoholics. Adults infected with *H. influenzae* may have a CSF leak or immunological deficiency.

Staphylococcal and *gram-negative meningitis* are usually complications of en-docarditis or prior head trauma. In such cases the CSF may not show many leuko-cytes and may be sterile; however a blood culture is mandatory in all cases of meningitis so that the correct diagnosis should not be missed.

Listeria monocytogenes infections occur in neonates, the elderly, and in pa-tients with compromised immunological defenses. The abrupt onset of signs sug-gesting meningitis, encephalitis, or abscess in such patients with upper or lower respiratory infections, otitis, or conjunctivitis, may make one consider this diagnosis.

Aseptic meningitis may be due to many agents, including viruses. The syn-drome is characterized by fever, headache, and meningeal signs. Change in con-sciousness and frank localizing neurological signs are rare, and the patients look

Table 40-3   Organisms in Bacterial Meningitis (Adults)*

N. meningitidis	30%-40%
H. influenzae	5%
S. pneumoniae	40%-50%
Other organisms	10%

*In about 10 percent of the patients, usually because of prior antibiotic treatment, no organisms can be cultured.

wretched but not severely ill. The CSF examination will usually show an increase in mononuclear cells to fewer than $500/mm^3$ (although polymorphonuclear cells may be increased in the early stages); the protein level is normal or only slightly elevated and the CSF sugar level is usually normal except with mumps infection.

Unless there is a good history of recent infection, it may be hard to differentiate bacterial meningitis from the autoallergic acute disseminated encephalomyelitis (described later). Cerebral abscesses usually have a less acute onset, but thrombophlebitis in association with chronic mastoid or sinus infection and the toxic encephalopathy associated with bacterial endocarditis may present similarly, except that focal signs and evidence of increased intracranial pressure are usual in all of these latter conditions.

If there is clinical uncertainty about the presence of bacterial or aseptic meningitis, as long as the patient is not seriously ill, you may properly maintain careful observation, withhold antibiotics and repeat the lumbar puncture in 12 to 18 hr. With aseptic meningitis the second CSF sample will almost always show a shift toward mononuclear cell predominance while later examinations show the eventual disappearance of all the polymorphonuclear cells. In bacterial meningitis, these cells increase quickly, the CSF sugar level falls and the protein level rises.

As can be seen from Table 40-4, 70 percent of the known causes are common viral infections (Coxsackie, ECHO, mumps, and LCM). In about 25 percent of the cases the virus is not defined. The remaining long list of viruses identified includes measles, chickenpox, infectious mononucleosis, and influenza. Rarely, the clinical picture of aseptic meningitis may be seen in the preicteric stage of infectious hepatitis or in uremia. A similar picture occurs with inadequately treated bacterial meningitis.

The term *meningismus* refers to the condition of meningism without any actual infection of the meninges. Tonsillitis, cervical adenitis, pyelonephritis, and lobar pneumonia are common causes; other sources of meningeal irritation include blood in the CSF from any cause, otitis, sinusitis, spinal osteomyelitis, and epidural abscess (all *parameningeal foci*).

Treatment of Meningitis

Aseptic meningitis requires only analgesics and reduction in fever, but urgent management of *septic forms* is vital because severe cortical damage or death can result from delay. An immediate lumbar puncture must be performed whenever the diagnosis is suspected, and the CSF sent to the laboratory for smear and culture. Antibiotic therapy is started immediately if the CSF is cloudy, indicating that the cell count is high. Whenever the diagnosis of meningitis is suspected, the lumbar puncture must be done even though there is clinical evidence of raised intracranial pressure. Some patients with meningitis show early papilledema. In this situation an expert opinion should be requested if available, but the lumbar puncture will still have to be done because identification of the organism and determination of its sensitivities are essential. If any focal signs are detected, an EEG and isotope or CT scan are indicated to demonstrate a lesion such as cerebral abscess, because lumbar puncture would have been dangerous in this circumstance.

Having obtained the CSF in a case of suspected meningitis, it should be held up to the light to see if it is clear or cloudy (over 500 cells/ml) and then taken to the laboratory, preferably by you. A Gram stain, culture, cell count, and differential should be carried out and the protein and sugar levels estimated. Virus cultures and cytology might be indicated if septic meningitis is excluded by these tests.

Table 40-4   Aseptic Meningitis

(Routine cultures negative)

Common viral causes (70% of cases)

Mumps	ECHO
Coxsackie	Polio
Lymphocytic choriomeningitis (LCM)	

Less common viral causes

Measles	Infectious mononucleosis
Rubella	Arbovirus
Chickenpox	Encephalomyocarditis (?)
Herpes simplex	Behçet's disease (?)
Influenza	

Nonviral causes

Tuberculosis	Chemical meningitis
Brucellosis	Cerebral abscess
Syphilis	Collagen-vascular disease
Leptospirosis	Preicteric phase of infectious hepatitis
Malignancy	
Fungi	Inadequately treated bacterial meningitis

No cause determined (25% of cases)

Start antibiotic therapy at once if infection is confirmed. The smear will indicate the type of organism responsible and thus the correct therapy. For the dosages of antibiotics commonly used in meningitis see Table 40-5. The antibiotics usually used against each organism are listed in Table 40-6.

It is fine to know which antibiotics to use in which infection, but in most instances you will not know the exact organism until the cultures return. You cannot wait that long before starting treatment so unless clinical clues suggest one particular organism, start the patient on one of two antibiotic regimens — either triple therapy with penicillin, sulfadiazine, and chloramphenicol, or ampicillin and chloramphenicol in high dosages (see Table 40-7).

Many antibiotics will not normally enter the brain or CSF because of the blood-brain barrier, but when there is inflammation of the meninges, many of them will cross the barrier and thus will reach therapeutic levels in the CSF. Chloramphenicol and the sulfonamides always cross the blood-brain barrier, whereas ampicillin, carbenicillin, and cephalothin cross well only when there is inflammation of the meninges. Even with inflammation however, penetration into the CSF is poor with tetracyclines, streptomycin, kanamycin, gentamicin, polymyxin, and colistin, all drugs more likely to be needed for meningitis in children. Thus the choice of agents is crucial and the dosage should be arrived at by consideration of the severity of the infection and the age of the patient. After lumbar puncture, an initial

Table 40-5   Dosages of Antibiotics Commonly Used in Meningitis

Drug	Child	Adult
Penicillin G*	1 MU IM or IV stat 50-75,000 U/kg q4h 0.5 MU IV q3h	1.2-2.4 MU bolus IV q4h
Ampicillin[a]	100-200 mg/kg/day in 4-6 doses IV or IM	1 g IV stat and q3h
Cloxacillin*	40 mg/kg IV q4h 4-6 doses IV or IM	2 g IV q4h
Chloramphenicol	25 mg/kg q6h	1-2 g IV q6h to max 6 g/day initially
Penicillin G[a]	(less for neonates)	(100 mg/kg/day)
Gentamicin	1.5 mg/kg IV q8h	
Tobramycin	5-10 mg intrathecally q24h	1 mg/kg t.i.d. IM or IV[b]
Sulfadiazine	100 mg/kg/day in 6 doses	2-4 g IV stat; 6-8 g daily IV in 4 doses
Moxalactam	100 mg/kg loading; 50 mg/kg q3h IV	
Nafcillin	40 mg/kg IV q4h	
Ticarcillin	40 mg/kg IV q4h	50 mg/kg q6h
Amikacin	(Intraventricular) 5 mg q24h 7.5 mg/kg IV q12h	same dosage

[a]If the patient is allergic to penicillin, use chloramphenicol.
[b]If renal function is normal.

dose of the appropriate drug can be given and the child transferred to a pediatric center for therapy, both of the meningitis and of its potential complications.

In adults, treatment should begin as soon as the lumbar puncture has been performed. Seventy-five percent of the cases will be due to *H. influenzae,* meningococcus, or pneumococcus. Ampicillin is probably the drug of choice given intravenously in high dosages. In children 150 mg/kg/day can be given in six divided doses and in the adult 1 g of ampicillin is given intravenously every 3 to 4 hr. If

Table 40-6   Treatment of Acute Meningitis

Organism	Antibiotic	Other
Meningococcus	Penicillin, ampicillin, or chloramphenicol	Hydrocortisone Heparin Fresh-frozen plasma
H. influenzae	Ampicillin[a] and chloramphenicol Moxalactam Cefotaxime	
Pneumococcus	Penicillin, cephaloridine, ampicillin, or chloramphenicol	Prednisolone orally
Group B streptococcus	Ampicillin	
Staphylococcus	Nafcillin Cloxacillin	
Coliform organisms	Chloramphenicol Gentamicin/tobramycin Co-trimoxazole	
Pseudomonas and gram-negative organisms	Gentamicin and ticarcillin	
L. monocytogenes	Ampicillin[b]	

[a] *Haemophilus influenzae* is now resistant to ampicillin in 20 percent of cases.
[b] Four weeks of 16 g/day (100–150 mg/kg/day) with drainage of any abscess. Aminoglycoside may also be needed.

the patient is severely ill, double this dosage, and if haemophilus infection is at all likely, give chloramphenicol as well. Take cultures of blood, throat, and nose swabs and smears of any skin lesions before the antibiotic therapy is started. Monitoring of electrolytes, blood gases, and fluid balance should be carried out. Steroids and anticonvulsants are seldom needed at this stage. Antibiotics must be given for at least 10 days, and for 2 weeks with pneumococcal infections. Isolation of patients

Table 40-7 Treatment of Meningitis of Uncertain Etiology

Antibiotic	Dosage
Ampicillin[a]	1 g IV q3h
and Chloramphenicol	1 g IV q6h
Penicillin	1-2 MU q2h IV
and Sulfadiazine	2-4 g IV stat and q6h IV
and Chloramphenicol	1 g IM or IV q6h

[a]The authors' preference

with meningococcal disease is wise for the first 24 hr after treatment is started. Prophylaxis should be used for all household contacts and others closely associated with patients suffering from meningococcal disease, e.g., children in the same nursery school. Rifampin 600 mg b.i.d. for 2 days is a recommended treatment for adult contacts.

Gram-negative meningitis in adults usually complicates trauma, surgery, spinal anesthesia, or chronic debilitating diseases, but it is uncommon. *Pseudomonas* is the organism most often cultured. Moxalactam (6-8 g/day) or ticarcillin (12-24 g/day) with tobramycin (5 mg/kg/day) are probably the best agents. If gentamicin has to be given, a 5-mg dose may be given intrathecally twice daily for the first 2 days because of the poor CSF penetration of this drug, but in such cases referral to a neurological center will have occurred.

Aseptic meningitis is usually associated with a viral illness and has a much more benign prognosis than bacterial meningitis. The patient is seldom as ill and usually recovers readily. Measures to relieve headache and reduce fever are the only available treatment. One may attempt to identify the virus using acute and convalescent serum antibody titers. Enteroviruses are most frequently implicated, but usually no agent is incriminated. Infectious mononucleosis is probably a common cause.

Subacute Meningitis

Inadequately treated bacterial meningitis, fungal infections, and particularly tuberculous meningitis (TBM) are the more common causes of subacute meningitis. Viral causes are much less common. Tuberculous meningitis is the prototype and will be discussed here.

Tuberculosis is most likely to occur in North America among the Inuit and Indian populations, among alcoholics, and in those patients with immunological deficiency or generalized illness. A third of the cases occur before the age of 10. About half the patients will be known cases of tuberculosis. The illness usually occurs in the active stage of primary infection but may only present years later. Old tuberculin tests are positive in 85 percent of cases. The organism can be recovered in the sputum and from gastric washings as well as from CSF.

Tuberculous meningitis produces moderate but increasing signs of meningeal inflammation over many days or weeks. Children present with lethargy, failure to thrive, anorexia, irritability, nausea, and vomiting. In adults, similar symptoms lead on to a mild and gradual reduction in conscious level with confusion and head-ache, occasionally seizures, but only moderate evidence of meningeal irritation. Symptoms may have been precipitated by an initial flu-like illness or measles. If untreated, there occurs the slow but relentless progression of extraocular palsies, deafness, cerebellar signs, convulsions, optic atrophy, pupillary abnormalities, de-lirium, and possibly dementia. In the latest stages decerebrate rigidity occurs. The CSF contains mainly mononuclear cells, up to $500/mm^3$; the protein level is high and the sugar level low.

The lesion is essentially a basal meningitis with secondary vasculitis. An ac-cumulation of purulent cellular infiltrate over the inferior surface of the brain and brainstem, blocking CSF flow through the fourth ventricle roof foramin, is respon-sible for the cranial nerve palsies and raised intracranial pressure. (In meningococ-cal and pneumococcal meningitis the purulent material is seen all over the brain surface.)

Unusual presentations include a single seizure in infants and children, isolated focal neurological signs, the picture of acute meningitis, transverse myelopathy, or a preponderance of psychiatric symptoms in adults.

Complications of TBM include blindness, deafness, hydrocephalus, spinal block, hypothalamic abnormalities, focal signs from persistent arachnoiditis, and cortical damage caused by subpial vasculitis and predisposing to seizures.

Cryptococcal meningitis also has an insidious onset with evidence of a confu-sional state with focal signs and raised intracranial pressure. Although a smoulder-ing meningitis is the usual presentation, abscesses may form. Again, this condition occurs particularly in those with immunological deficiencies, diabetes, or chronic alcoholism. It is more likely to occur in those in contact with bird droppings — pigeon fanciers for example. A clinical point of interest in cryptococcal meningitis is the prolonged and severe nature of the headache that precedes any signs of men-ingism or increased intracranial pressure. Diagnosis may be made with india ink CSF preparations, but cryptococcal antigen should be detected in the blood. The treatment is with amphotericin B, 0.3 mg/kg/day IV with oral 5-fluorocytosine, continued for 6 weeks.

Infiltration of the meninges by carcinoma, lymphoma, larval cysts, fungi, or sarcoidosis, and secondary syphilis and brucellosis are uncommon causes of a simi-lar subacute syndrome.

CSF Findings: The CSF findings in subacute meningitis include the presence of large numbers of lymphocytes and elevated protein levels. In TBM, polymorpho-nuclear cells may predominate in the early stages and the glucose level is almost always depressed, even to zero. The chance of finding the organism varies with the time taken looking for it on the Ziehl-Neelsen smears. Other causes of lympho-cytic meningitis are listed in Table 8-4.

Treatment: Tuberculous meningitis can be treated successfully in almost all cases if therapy is started before the patient becomes unconscious. The generally accepted antibacterial regimen consists of triple therapy, with any three chosen from isoniazid, streptomycin, rifampin, and ethambutol, all but streptomycin being given orally (see Table 40-8).

There is disagreement about the use of intrathecal therapy, particularly with antibacterial agents, but it is a good general rule not to inject anything into the intrathecal space if possible. Perhaps the use of steroids intrathecally in TBM is an exception, because this tends to reduce the fibrotic reaction that may block CSF pathways as healing takes place, but as better antituberculous agents are developed, the need for intrathecal steroids is decreasing. There is increasing experience with rifampin, along with isoniazid and ethambutol and an improved regimen using these drugs may be developed in the future. However

Table 40-8   Treatment of Tuberculous Meningitis (Adult)

Drug	Dosage
Isoniazid[a]	10-20 mg/kg/day orally up to 300 mg/day
Streptomycin[b]	15 mg/kg/day (1 g daily)
Rifampin	10 mg/kg/day orally (usual dosage 600 mg/day)
Ethambutol	15 mg/kg/day orally

[a] The usual regimen comprises isoniazid and two of the three other drugs listed. Pyridoxine 40 mg daily should be added to prevent neuropathy caused by isoniazid.

[b] Assuming normal renal function.

currently the experience in TBM is still not adequate to give comparisons. The dosage of rifampin is 600 mg/day in a single dose each morning. We still use oral or parenteral corticosteroids to relieve initial cerebral edema.

Chronic Meningitis

Chronic meningitis is uncommon. The characteristic symptoms include mild fever, headache, depression and malaise, and subtle personality changes leading to confusion. The signs include meningism and frequently cranial nerve palsies and evidence of raised intracranial pressure.

The CSF may show a persistent lymphocytosis with high protein and low glucose levels. In such cases viruses, fungi, or bacteria (including *Leptospira, Treponema,* and acid-fast bacilli), and malignant cells have variously been found. In sarcoidosis, a chronic basal meningitis may cause focal neurological signs and rarely hydrocephalus, cranial nerve palsies, paraplegia, optic atrophy, or seizures. Meningeal carcinoma or leukemia cause headaches and cranial nerve palsies but seldom long-tract signs.

The appropriate treatment of chronic meningitis depends, naturally enough, upon its cause and will not be detailed here.

Chronic spinal arachnoiditis is usually caused by intrathecal injection of x-ray contrast media, steroids, anesthetics, or antibiotics. Spinal injury or surgery, prolapsed intervertebral disk, and numerous infections (tuberculosis, syphilis, viral) have also been held responsible. The thickened meninges, usually in the lumbar region, entrap the nerve roots, causing bilateral, burning leg pain at many root levels and local backache. Signs of multiple root lesions are usually detectable, and there may be loss of bladder function. The symptoms may have their onset acutely after spinal surgery with fever and severe local pain.

Myelography (often suspected to be the cause) will confirm the diagnosis. The only treatment is surgical but it is not very effective.

Recurrent Meningitis

Recurrent meningitis should lead one to search for the reason *why* repeated infections have involved the CNS. While spontaneous repeated infection by different organisms is possible, some defect opening up a pathway allowing organisms to penetrate the nervous system is far more likely. In such cases a midline sinus running to the meninges from the upper respiratory tract or from the skin of the head, neck, or spine should be carefully sought, even with a magnifying glass. Chronic mastoiditis, sinusitis, agammaglobulinemia and immunodeficiency syndromes are other possibilities. The condition may occur after splenectomy, in infancy, and also in association with skull fractures, particularly if there has been CSF rhinorrhea. Pneumococcal infection is the most common. When meningitis is recurrent, it usually is of the acute or subacute variety.

Differential Diagnosis

Acute meningitis may be mimicked by a subarachnoid hemorrhage, by the encephalopathy of bacterial endocarditis, malignant hypertension, lead poisoning or porphyria, and by migraine, viral encephalitis, or a cerebral abscess. Subacute or chronic meningitis can be confused with cerebral tumors, subdural hematoma, and with a rapid progressive dementing illness such as Jakob-Creutzfeldt disease or the nonmetastatic encephalopathy of carcinoma.

Certain causes of endarteritis such as diabetes and collagen vascular disease may also give rise to a similar picture. Slow virus infections, neoplasms seeding throughout the CSF, and local infections such as spinal osteitis or cranial osteomyelitis (parameningeal foci), may also be mistaken for meningitis.

Complications

In patients who recover from meningitis there may be evidence of significant *brain damage* because of vasculitis, cortical infarction, or hydrocephalus. *Seizures* occur in 10 percent of those recovering. In infants, *subdural effusions* and *deafness* may be associated with *H. influenzae* and pneumococcal infections, whereas acute or chronic *obstructive* or *normal-pressure hydrocephalus* may occur following meningitis from any cause. Obstructive hydrocephalus is particularly common with TBM, as are *deafness* or other lower *cranial nerve* palsies which occur in 15 percent of patients. *Hypothalamic damage* and *optic atrophy* are much less common, except in chronic basal meningitis (Fig. 40-1). Small infants and children who recover from meningitis may show signs of *cerebral palsy,* and such upper motor neuron signs may occur temporarily in adults recovering from a severe

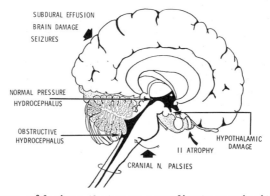

Figure 40-1 Diagram of lesions that may complicate meningitis.

meningitis. Because of the dangers of serious neurological impairment, early diagnosis and the appropriate specific therapy are essential to prevent such tragedies.

ENCEPHALITIS

Infection of the brain parenchyma is most commonly viral. This encephalitis may
be widespread or focal. Both DNA and RNA viruses may be responsible, certain
viruses in each group having a particular affinity for the nervous system. These
neurotropic viruses include polio, rabies, herpes simplex, and arboviruses. Those
that are usually *nonneurotropic* but that *may* involve the nervous system include
herpes simplex, mumps, measles, Coxsackie, ECHO, cytomegaloviruses, and the
Epstein-Barr virus responsible for mononucleosis. Finally, measles, the papova-
viruses and perhaps others may give rise to *slow virus* infections. Other organisms
causing encephalitis are listed in Table 40-9.

In the following discussion, the classic picture of encephalitis in general, and
that due to herpes simplex in particular will be discussed. Some other viral infective syndromes will be mentioned in brief. Most of the viruses causing encephalitis cannot be differentiated clinically however, and specific identification techniques are needed to determine which one is involved.

Typical Encephalitis

Arboviruses have their reservoir in ticks and mosquitos. They include the Eastern
and Western equine, St. Louis, and Japanese B varieties. Such enteroviruses as
polio, Coxsackie, ECHO, and those viruses responsible for rubella, measles, chickenpox, mononucleosis, mumps, viral hepatitis, and influenza, can all produce a more
or less similar clinical picture caused by direct parenchymal invasion of the nervous system and the subsequent antibody reaction. Major pathological features
include edema and petechiae within the brain, with mononuclear perivascular
cuffing and neuronal degeneration, mainly in the gray matter — the cortex and
the deep nuclei of the brainstem.

In North America, herpes simplex, enteroviruses (polio, ECHO, and Coxsackie),
and arboviruses are the most common, with lymphocytic choriomeningitis (LCM)
and mumps next most frequently identified. The prognosis in mumps and LCM is
excellent, while the arbovirus and herpes simplex infections are sometimes lethal
or leave severe sequelae. Enteroviral infection is most common in the summer
months; the arbovirus infection spread by ticks occurs mainly in the spring and
that by mosquitos in the late summer. Mumps is the most common cause of encephalitis in the earlier part of the year, whereas LCM is more common in the fall
and winter. During the great influenza pandemic of 1917, many patients developed
the syndrome of von Economo's encephalitis characterized by marked drowsiness
(sleeping sickness) which often developed years later into a form of Parkinson's
disease with oculogyric crises. It is not certain whether or not such an illness still
exists sporadically because the virus was never isolated.

In North America, arboviruses apart from the three listed in Table 40-9 are
rare indeed, as are *protozoal* and *metazoal* infections. Bacteria, meningovascular
syphilis, and fungi produce an encephalitis, usually only in association with frank
meningitic signs. While the herpes and other arbovirus infections are often exceedingly severe, most other viruses produce a milder illness. Tertiary neurosyphilis
smoulders on to produce the features of general paresis or tabes (see later discussion) or meningovascular syphilis. Obviously many of the causative agents listed are unlikely causes of encephalitis in, for example, eastern Canada, but one

Table 40-9   Causes of Encephalitis

Viruses

    Sporadic

        herpes simplex type 1[a]
        herpes zoster
        monkey B virus
        cytomegalovirus
        EB virus (mononucleosis)[a]
        mumps[a]
        lymphocytic choriomeningitis[a]
        rabies

    Epidemic

        arboviruses: E and W equine, St. Louis, etc.[a]
        enteroviruses: polio, Coxsackie, ECHO
        measles

    Slow viruses

Bacteria and spirochetes

    Cerebritis: early cerebral abscess
    Treponemas

Fungal

    Candida albicans[a]
    Cryptococcus neoformans
    Histoplasmosis
    Aspergillosis

Protozoal and metazoal

    Malaria
    Toxoplasmosis
    Amebiasis
    Echinococcus, cysticercosis, and trichiniasis
    Schistosomiasis, trypanosomiasis

Possible viral

    Encephalitis lethargica
    Behçet's syndrome
    Encephalomyocarditis
    Subacute myelo-optico neuropathy

[a]The more common conditions in North America.

always must ask about visits a patient may have made to another country in these days of frequent air travel.

Clinical features of typical encephalitides include fever, meningism, and signs of raised intracranial pressure. Reduction in conscious level from drowsiness to coma, seizures which are often focal, and various other focal signs as described in Chapter 9, also occur depending upon which areas of brain are particularly involved by the inflammatory process. As with cerebral abscesses, the combination of fever and meningism with evidence of cerebral dysfunction, either generalized (delirium, seizures, coma) or focal (hallucinations, hemiparesis, and so forth) must make one consider encephalitis.

The *differential diagnosis* is long. Any form of meningitis may be accompanied by evidence of cortical inflammation. Abscesses, septic emboli, cortical septic thrombophlebitis and postinfectious and toxic encephalopathies may be hard to distinguish from encephalitis. All are described later. Subdural and subarachnoid hemorrhage, bleeding into a tumor, porphyria, poisoning, and even multiple sclerosis can produce encephalopathy with meningism and sometimes fever.

Cerebrospinal fluid taken during the acute stage of encephalitis shows a moderate rise in protein level and contains lymphocytes up to about $250/mm^3$. The sugar level is usually normal, except in mumps encephalitis when it is less, as it is with bacterial, fungal, and carcinomatous meningitis. Specific laboratory diagnosis requires a fourfold increase in the level of viral antibody titers between acute and convalescent sera or virus isolation from the CSF or brain. Specimens must be frozen immediately after collection and shipped in dry ice to the laboratory for direct virus isolation, while acute and convalescent paired serum specimen can be sent unfrozen. If enterovirus infection is suspected, feces, CSF, or throat washings may be used for virus isolation. Throat washings and CSF are used for mumps idententification, blood and CSF for LCM, and CSF or occasionally brain biopsy material for herpes simplex. Other viruses may be isolated from blood or CSF and cytomegalovirus can be found in the urine, saliva, or liver biopsy specimens. Cryptococcal or other fungal antigens may need to be sought as well.

Encephalopathy without actual invasion of the brain substance occurs with bacterial endocarditis, rickettsial infections, pertussis, typhoid, and typhus. These cannot be differentiated by their neurological signs from viral encephalitis, but other systemic effects may allow diagnosis.

Treatment of encephalitis is improving. General measures maintain the patient's hydration and metabolic status, reduce fever, and prevent seizures. In mild cases, the headache may be reduced by repeated lumbar punctures. Antiviral agents are now available for treatment of herpes simplex (discussed later) and hold promise of effect with other agents. Steroids have been used on the premise that "encephalitis" is in part an allergic response and in part caused by edema as a direct effect of the virus. Opinions of their use are divided.

Herpes Simplex Encephalitis

Herpes Simplex is the most common cause of acute, sporadic, severe encephalitis. Both human and monkey types of herpes virus occur and both can cause neurological infection, although the latter is usually seen only in laboratory workers. Symptoms occur at any age, but particularly in the first three decades. Of the two serological types of human herpes simplex, type I gives rise to sporadic encephalitis and to oral ulcers, whereas type II produces aseptic meningitis and genital ulceration. In adults, nearly all herpes virus infections are of type I.

Herpes simplex encephalitis may have an acute or subacute onset. Typically, a few days of malaise, fever, headache, anorexia, nausea, and other nonspecific symptoms progress to a subtle change of personality with evolving depression, paranoia or abnormal behavior, and confusion. Photophobia, signs of raised intracranial pressure, meningeal irritation, and focal signs appear next; the latter include hemiparesis, facial weakness, dysphasia, dysarthria, decerebrate rigidity, ocular palsies or nystagmus, seizures, and in the late stages stupor or coma. Although the whole brain is involved, the temporal lobes are particularly affected.

The *CSF* shown an increase in pressure and in protein levels; lymphocytes and red cells are often present. A characteristic *EEG* appearance (diffuse, mainly temporal region slow activity with periodic discharges) is described, but it is not specific. The CT scan may demonstrate swelling and enlargement of the temporal lobes (usually asymmetrically). The only specific method of diagnosis is fluorescent antibody staining on either a *brain biopsy* specimen or on CSF cells. This test should be available in the laboratories of all major hospitals. However because of the mass effect of the lesion, lumbar puncture may be dangerous and CT scanning should be done first to rule out the presence of a pressure cone.

Drug treatment with acyclovir reduces mortality and morbidity if it is given early. In cases diagnosed by brain biopsy, acyclovir, 5 mg/kg given IV q8h for 10 days, reduces mortality to about 20 percent, and half the patients recover completely. Vidarabine, 15 mg/kg/day given IV for 10 days, is less effective. The role of steroids is disputed in this condition; if they do help, they do not help much. Acyclovir may become the treatment of choice against all herpes infections; it is also effective against the EB virus and varicella.

RABIES

The virus of rabies is introduced into the body through the bite of an infected bat or other wild animal. It travels centrally along peripheral nerves and produces a focal encephalitis, mainly involving the cervical cord, the brainstem and the temporal lobes. The latent period between the bite and the clinical features of the disease may be as long as a year.

Clinically, early irritability and agitated delirium lead to muscle hypertonia, especially affecting the pharyngeal muscles which go into spasm — hence the term *hydrophobia*. Convulsions and death usually occur within 10 days of the onset. Human diploid vaccine however has been found to be strongly immunogenic and its introduction may be an important breakthrough in the prevention of rabies. If unavailable, a duck embryo vaccine is used.

BEHÇET"S SYNDROME

The viral etiology of Behçet's syndrome is questionable. Oral and genital ulcers and uveitis are the main nonneurological features, but in up to a quarter of the cases, seizures, meningoencephalitis, cranial nerve palsies, and a residual organic brain syndrome also occur. Treatment involves oral chloroquine and for the neurological complications, high-dosage steroid therapy.

ACQUIRED IMMUNODEFICIENCY SYNDROME (AIDS)

The syndrome known as AIDS signifies a disturbance of cell-mediated immunity that predisposes to opportunistic infections and to Kaposi's sarcoma. The cause of the immunodeficiency is not clear. Multiple viral infections have been described, including herpes, cytomegalovirus, and hepatitis. Human T-cell leukemia virus III is thought to play a major role in T-helper cell suppression.

The syndrome has been diagnosed mainly in Haitan people, in the homosexual population, and in users of mainline heroin or other agents. In one-third of the cases, the presentation is neurological; toxoplasma encephalitis (abscesses) is the most common single syndrome, but tuberculous and cryptococcal meningitis and spirochetal or viral encephalomyelitis have been recorded, as have progressive multifocal leukoencephalopathy, CNS lymphomas, and peripheral neuropathy. The diffuse encephalopathy produces such features as memory loss, seizures, confusion, psychomotor retardation, dementia, and coma.

Human T-cell lymphotropic virus-lymphadenopathy-associated virus (HTLV-III/LAV) is thought to be the most likely viral causative agent in this condition, although herpes viruses have also been isolated from patients with the disease.

Acquired immunodeficiency syndrome remains a fatal disease, but prompt diagnosis and treatment of the opportunistic infections have prolonged survival. Toxoplasmosis can be treated with pyrimethamine, 75 mg, then 25 mg daily and sultadiazine 4 g/day.

ABSCESS

Abscesses may occur in the epidural or subdural spaces or within the substance of the brain, in which they are examples of suppurative bacterial encephalitis.

Intracranial epidural abscess is usually associated with a local skull fracture, osteomyelitis, or inflammation of the transverse or sagittal sinuses. The abscess is frequently situated over the convexity of the brain and the clinical features are those of a generalized infection of a local destructive lesion compressing the brain, and of raised intracranial pressure.

Spinal epidural abscesses are usually caused by staphylococcal infections in the lumbar region or by tuberculosis at thoracic levels. In tuberculosis, granulation tissue, pus, and vertebral body and disk collapse cause cord compression and local pain. Acute angulation (angular kyphosis) may result from the local infection and should be treated first by the usual antituberculous agents to render the contents of the abscess sterile; it can then be drained surgically with later reconstruction of the spine. Should it cause neurological signs, emergency surgical intervention will be required.

Problems may arise in the differential diagnosis of acute lumbar spinal epidural abscess from acute transverse myelopathy, which is usually of viral origin (and eight times as common). Both cause root pain in girdle distribution, stiff neck, marked muscle spasms, and local tenderness of the spine, the usual neurological deficit of paraparesis with a sensory level, fever, and increased cells and protein in the CSF. However the ESR is always high in epidural abscesses, not necessarily with transverse myelitis. Evidence of block of CSF passage, x-ray findings of osteomyelitis of the appropriate vertebrae, recent bacterial infection elsewhere, and perhaps slower clinical development (so that the maximal deficit is not reached until the third or fourth day) are all factors in favor of epidural abscess. Also, transverse myelitis is more common at thoracic, not lumbar levels. In children transverse myelitis sometimes presents without any pain in the back.

Subdural Abscess ("Empyma")

The cause in at least 80 percent of cases of subdural abscess is disease of the nasal sinuses or of the middle ear, when it occurs by direct extension or secondary to thrombophlebitis. Paranasal infection commonly gives rise to frontal, otitis to posterior cerebral and cerebellar abscesses.

A subdural infection occurs when a subdural hematoma or effusion (particularly if secondary to meningitis in infants) becomes infected; when a cerebral abscess ruptures into the subdural space; or following a penetrating wound.

The organisms are usually anaerobic streptococci, less commonly staphylococci, gram-negative bacteria, or clostridia. The disease occurs particularly between the ages of 10 and 20 years, with paranasal infection, and after the age of 40, with an otitic origin.

The usual *clinical features* include evidence of skull osteomyelitis (local tenderness, swelling, and cellulitis), systemic signs of infection, headache, fever, meningism, and focal neurological signs appropriate to the area of cerebral involvement. Seizures of any type are common.

The diagnosis is suggested by the findings of nasal sinus or middle ear infection in the presence of these signs. The EEG will show local slow-wave activity, whereas plain skull x-rays may show sinus opacity, osteomyelitis, and sometimes a shift of the pineal gland. The enhanced CT scan localizes the abscess, enabling the neurosurgeon to drain the infection when it has become encapsulated. A catheter may be inserted and antibiotics instilled into the abscess cavity after drainage. Cloxacillin and chloramphenicol are recommended, and treatment should be continued for a month. The mortality in subdural abscess is about 25 percent; residual seizures and focal neurological deficits are common, so anticonvulsants are prescribed routinely in these patients.

Intracerebral Abscess

Over half of all cases of intracerebral abscess complicate an ear or paranasal sinus infection. Skull fractures, facial or dental infections, and congenital heart disease also predispose, and hematogenous spread of infection from chronic lung disease (bronchiectasis, lung abscess) is responsible for another 20 percent. The intracerebral abscess is truly a local purulent encephalitis and while usually single and well localized to frontal or temporal regions when the infection extends from an adjacent source, multiple abscesses can occur with hematogenous spread (Fig. 40-2A, B). This usually occurs in elderly patients, particularly diabetics, among whom multiple staphylococcal microabscesses are becoming more common. Neonates, diabetics, the immunocompromised, heroin and alcohol addicts, patients with prosthetic or congenitally damaged heart valves, and those with lymphomas are especially at risk. The immunocompromised patients may develop candidial abscesses with intracerebral vasculitis; they present with fever but few focal signs. In many patients the infection can be traced to endocarditis or other septic foci.

An abscess may spread directly or by septic thrombophlebitis, in which the infected clot may extend backward along a large vein to infect other areas of the brain. The organism most frequently cultured from cerebral abscesses include streptococci, staphylococci, *Klebsiella, Proteus, Bacteroides,* pneumococcus, and anaerobic organisms.

The *symptoms* may for a time be vague and nonspecific and include fever, mild drowsiness and headache.[*] These may be followed by evidence of focal brain destruction, meningism, and raised intracranial pressure. Seizures are particularly common with cerebral abscesses in the frontal, temporal and parietal regions.

_____

[*]Legg's aphorism, "Infection somewhere plus something wrong in the head means abscess or some other form of encephalitis," is valid.

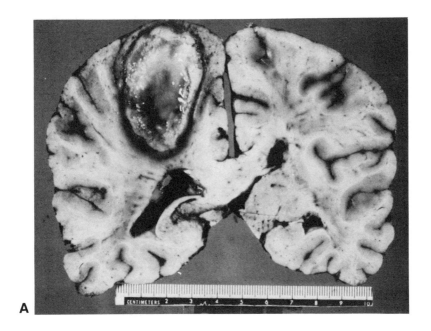

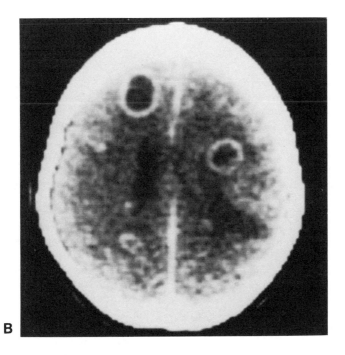

Figure 40-2   (A) Coronal section of brain; chronic right frontal lobe abscess; (B) Enhanced CT scan; multiple abscesses with enhancing rim margin.

Often there is little evidence of sepsis and lethargic delirium is the main clinical feature. Cerebellar abscesses however produce rapidly rising intracranial pressure and brainstem signs.

Diagnosis of an intracerebral abscess is suggested by the clinical picture of lung, ear, or sinus disease with signs of intracranial infection and seizures; "meningitis" with a focal deficit; "stroke" with fever; or raised intracranial pressure with no obvious cause. The EEG is invariably abnormal, with local slow-wave formation. The isotope scan shows a clearly localized area of increased uptake. A CT scan will localize the abscess even more accurately and will determine the degree of capsule formation. Lumbar puncture is potentially lethal.

Treatment employs massive antibiotic coverage such as methicillin or nafcillin, 12 g/day, plus chloramphenicol 4 g or ampicillin 12 g/day (plus moxolactam 8–12 g/ day, if renal function permits), followed by surgical intervention when the abscess has localized and formed a capsule, as shown by CT scanning. Since anaerobic organisms are frequently present, especially with otitic abscesses, the addition of metronidazole is favored by some clinicians.

If intracranial pressure is much raised, steroids may be prescribed as long as antibiotic treatment is under way, but steroids should not be used routinely. Patients who have recovered from an acute cerebral abscess frequently progress to seizures. If it is likely that the abscess developed by hematogenous spread, congenital heart disease with a right-to-left shunt, pulmonary disease, and sepsis elsewhere in the body must be excluded.*

Cerebral abscesses are serious emergencies and require rapid diagnosis so that antibiotic therapy can be begun and surgical intervention speeded. Sadly, they still carry the 40 percent mortality recorded in 1893.

OTHER NEUROLOGICAL INFECTIONS

Herpes Zoster

The varicella-zoster virus is neurotropic. After many years of latency, it may be activated (by unknown mechanisms) when it primarily affects the dorsal root ganglion cells of spinal nerves and the sensory ganglia of cranial nerves, certainly the gasserian (V) ganglion and perhaps the geniculate (VII). At the spinal level, the involvement is usually unilateral and 75 percent of cases occur in the abdominal or upper thoracic regions. The virus will occasionally attack anterior horn cells of the spinal cord. Edema, monocytic infiltration, and perivascular cuffing with neuronal degeneration are seen histologically, with later fibrosis and secondary degeneration of the distal part of the nerve fiber.

There may be a history of chickenpox in the family, as the virus of chickenpox and herpes zoster is the same. Among elderly patients, recurrent herpes should put one on guard for the presence of an underlying malignancy, lymphoma, or immunological deficiency syndrome. Chickenpox itself may be complicated by acute allergic encephalomyelitis (see later), polyradiculitis, and cerebellar ataxia.

Burning or shooting pain with local hyperalgesia within the affected dermatomes is followed in 3 or 4 days by a typical vesicular eruption. This fades in the next two days with scarring and depigmentation of the skin. Over the area, the skin may be anesthetic but at the same time painful or itchy. Motor involvement may affect the face, eye, diaphragm, or limb musculature.

_____

*And look for needle marks; many younger patients are using dirty syringes to mainline drugs.

Postherpetic neuralgia is exceedingly unpleasant and is discussed in the chapter on pain syndromes. During the acute phase, 35% idoxuridine may be applied to the skin over the whole of the affected dermatome for 3 or 4 days to speed recovery. Steroids are only recommended for elderly patients; vitamin B_{12}, which once enjoyed popularity, is ineffective.

Herpes zoster ophthalmicus may produce corneal damage and secondary infection which are feared complications; the eye should be treated immediately with topical idoxuridine. The region of the forehead and eye may be exceedingly painful at the time and postherpetic neuralgia may follow. In such cases, excision of affected skin or local injection with steroid and local anesthetic may markedly reduce pain. When zoster attacks the seventh nerve, the fifth nerve is often involved as well, which explains the vesicles in the auricle and inside the mouth.

Intracranial CNS involvement is uncommon, but meningoencephalitis is occasionally seen. Acyclovir and vidarabine are both effective for reducing the amount of pain during the acute illness, and the frequency of complications, if treatment is started early.

Cytomegalovirus

Cytomegaloviruses are members of the herpesvirus family which may cause eye and brain damage in utero. In adults (most of whom are immunocompromised), meningoencephalitis and polyneuropathies may be caused. Treatment with vidarabine is under study.

Poliomyelitis

There are three types of neurotropic poliovirus; type I is the most common. Spread from person to person is by fecal contamination. After entering the gastrointestinal tract, the virus passes into the blood stream to invade the nervous system. The incubation period is 7 to 14 days and in nonimmunized populations the disease may be either epidemic or sporadic. Subclinical infection frequently occurs and produces immunity, which is the basis of live virus immunization.

After the polio virus invades the nervous system, producing a focal encephalitis predominantly of the spinal cord or brainstem, a *minor illness* occurs with headache, drowsiness, fever, and mild gastrointestinal symptoms. The illness may stop at that stage, or after 1 or 2 days of apparent remission, severe muscle pains, meningism, and delirium lead to sudden appearance of asymmetric or generalized paralysis within 24 hr *(paralytic form of major illness)*. The muscles are tender and fasciculations may be seen (and felt) in the earliest stages. This stage is over in a week, when some degree of improvement usually begins. Truncal and bulbar involvement may give rise to severe respiratory and bulbar paralysis requiring artificial ventilation and skilled nursing attention in an intensive care unit. The lower motor neuron lesions produced may eventually lead on to contractures, trophic changes, failure of growth of limbs, and joint disorganization.

A *nonparalytic* form of the major illness also occurs, with signs of meningoencephalitis, as in the paralytic form, but without anterior horn cell involvement.

In the earliest stages, the disease can only be diagnosed early during an epidemic because the mild symptoms resemble many other nonspecific viral illnesses. A paretic illness can also be caused by other enteroviruses, in which case the prognosis is much better. Weakness may also occur in association with other inflammatory bone or joint diseases. The differential diagnosis of muscle pain is given in Chapter 27. Other fast-advancing peripheral motor neuropathies include those caused by porphyria, the Guillain-Barré syndrome, and polyarteritis nodosa. Lower motor neuron lesions seldom complicate other CNS infections, although mumps may rarely produce an encephalomyelitis. Other causes of myelitis are discussed in Chapter 50. Even in these days however, the presence of an acute infective illness associated with signs of anterior horn cell involvement must always make one suspect poliomyelitis.

Coxsackievirus

Although coxsackievirus infection may cause aseptic meningitis, *epidemic myalgia* is a more common manifestation. In this condition, the sudden onset of acute chest pain with severe tenderness of the intercostal muscles in one or more spaces and great difficulty in breathing because of pleuritic pain frequently raise suspicion of pulmonary embolism, pneumonia, or even myocardial infarction. The pain may occur so acutely that patients sometimes fear that they may have had a heart attack. Very few systemic signs are associated, and after a few days of useless symptomatic treatment, complete recovery occurs.

Infectious Mononucleosis

About 5 percent of patients with infectious mononucleosis develop neurological complications. The most common of these is aseptic meningitis, a benign and relatively transient disorder. Encephalitis and encephalomyelitis may present with seizures, reduction in conscious level, raised intracranial pressure, focal neurological signs and meningism. A generalized peripheral neuropathy indistinguishable from the Guillain-Barré syndrome is well recognized, but patients may also have mononeuropathies and virtually every cranial nerve has been affected in this condition.

Influenza

The neurological complications of influenza are usually indirect, taking the form of an acute postinfectious encephalomyelitis. Depression frequently occurs following influenza, and some patients with multiple sclerosis may have a relapse following even a mild attack. *Neuralgic amyotrophy* (Chap. 44) is another occasional complication.

Tick Paralysis

Particularly in western North America, wood ticks may attach themselves to people exploring the undergrowth, especially children. The tick is usually found attached to the head or to any other hairy parts. There may result a rapidly progressive, symmetric flaccid paralysis, caused by a neurotoxin elaborated by the tick. Weakness may be so severe that respiratory and bulbar paralysis occur, and the patient may die of respiratory insufficiency. The sudden onset of such profound weakness over the course of a day or less should make one think of tick paralysis. The neurotoxin affects the neuromuscular junction and produces signs resembling a severe myasthenic crisis.

Treatment consists of the removal of the tick, but this may be difficult to find and may require shaving the child or searching through the hair with a fine comb. With supportive measures, recovery should occur within a few days.

Tetanus

Although *Clostridium tetani* is not as common now as it was in the days of horse-drawn transport, tetanus still constitutes an important, if rare, disease despite a fairly high level of immunization in Western communities. The organism enters a wound (which may be very small) or follows surgical procedures, otitis media, or puerperal or umbilical sepsis. Its toxin then ascends the peripheral motor nerves to block inhibitory postsynaptic potentials playing on the anterior horn cells. After an incubation period of up to 3 weeks, symptoms of pain and stiffness of the muscles, especially in the neck, back, and abdominal wall develop. Trismus, dysphagia, and reflex spasm are common. These often begin in the back, neck, and jaw muscles and last 15 to 30 sec. Because of the strong muscular contractions, hyperpyrexia and respiratory arrest may occur, while laryngospasm, chest infections, and cardiac arrest are occasional lethal complications.

Diagnosis is achieved early only if you maintain a high index of suspicion. Treatment is along several lines. Human antitetanus immunoglobulin has replaced horse serum antitoxin and 2000–4000 U are given IM, after which a course of IM penicillin is necessary. Tetanus toxoid will also be required for active immunization. The wound must be excised and cleaned, all dead tissue being removed. Symptomatic treatment depends upon the severity of the case. Mild cases will need diazepam and sedatives only. Respiratory difficulty requires tracheostomy and possibly curarization as well as the other measures listed. The most severe cases must be anesthetized and paralyzed, so all patients must be transferred urgently to an intensive care unit; many metabolic and urinary problems complicate the acute illness and close nursing attention is essential. Even in the best facilities, about 10 percent of patients die, mainly because of the complications. The most seriously affected patients are those with cephalic tetanus and those in whom symptoms begin within a few days following wounding.

Botulism

The toxin of *Clostridium botulism* impairs ACh release at motor nerve endings. Most of it is ingested in improperly canned foods; wounds sometimes are the portal of entry. In infants, progressive weakness, hypotonia, poor gag and suck reflexes, and constipation arre the main signs. In adults, extraocular muscle, facial and bulbar palsies occur; the limbs are flaccid and paretic and the reflexes lost. The pupils are usually dilated and unresponsive. Treatment consists of urgent ventilatory support with neutralization of toxin using the specific trivalent antiserum.

Toxoplasmosis

Toxoplasmosis may occur as a congenital infection or may be acquired later in life, usually in immunosuppressed patients. The protozoan organism commonly affects the nervous system and produces an inflammatory reaction with formation of miliary granulomas. These may later calcify or undergo necrosis, resulting in hydrocephalus, or they may be completely asymptomatic.

Congenital toxoplasmosis may be evident shortly after birth. Failure to thrive, convulsions, spasticity, opisthotonos and eye defects such as chorioretinitis or microphthalmos, are possible presentations. Optic atrophy is a common later development, as is hydrocephalus. Some children do not develop symptoms until the age of 4 or 5, when hepatomegaly and splenomegaly are found. X-ray of the skull often shows scattered calcifications.

The *acquired* form of the infection is often traceable to infected animals. The toxoplasma may cause skin lesions, pulmonary and lymphatic involvement, acute meningitis, encephalitis, myositis, and chronic granulomatous meningitis.

The laboratory findings will depend upon the type and extent of involvement. The CSF may be under increased pressure, and the protein level will usually be increased with a slight or moderate increase in mononuclear cells. Skull x-rays and fundoscopy are often extremely helpful in making a diagnosis, but more definite support comes from complement-fixation and fluorescent antibody tests.

Children with symptomatic congenital toxoplasmosis often have significant mental and neurological defects, if they survive. In the adult form, which is much less common, the prognosis depends upon the severity of the involvement. Those with encephalitis do poorly. Treatment is with sulfonamides combined with pyrimethamine.

Syphilis

Although a request for specific serology is (or should be) routine on all patients admitted to neurological wards, the overall return on these tests is relatively small. The request is still important because the prevalence of syphilis is probably increasing and the number of patients who are coming for treatment is not, suggesting that we are going to be faced with an increasing amount of late and of congenital syphilis in the future.

Serodiagnostic tests for syphilis may be classified as reagin tests and specific antitreponemal antibody tests. In the former group, the most commonly used in North America is the rapid plasma reagin (RPR), a slide test that detects the presence of cardiolipin antigens. This gives a figure of between 75 and 95 percent positive in patients with primary, secondary, late, or latent syphilis. Unfortunately, false-positive tests are common with reagin tests, being seen in conditions accompanied by abnormal globulins or excessive normal globulins. These include almost all of the collagen-vascular diseases, pregnancy, vaccination for smallpox, Hansen's disease (leprosy), infectious mononucleosis, measles, and atypical pneumonia. Narcotic addicts and patients with chronic rubella, viral hepatitis or viral pneumonia, hemolytic anemia, and the tropical diseases yaws and pinta may show such biological false-positive reactions (Table 40-10).

The specific antitreponemal antibody test in common use is the microtreponema pallidum hemagglutination test (MTPHA). It is the first to become positive in syphilis, and is positive in about 95 percent of cases of primary, secondary, late, and latent syphilis. It can be performed on the CSF as well as on the blood and is seldom positive in the conditions causing false-positive RPR reactions, except for yaws and pinta, when it may give a weak positive reaction.

One single positive serological test for syphilis does not make the diagnosis however, and clinical evidence or repeated testing by different methods is always necessary. In the following discussion, the classic patterns of syphilis are described but nowadays the intercurrent use of penicillin has changed the clinical picture and seizures, strokes, confusional states, depression and visual field alterations may be the sole presenting signs (Table 40-11).

In *primary* syphilis, the chancre is the only lesion. It appears after an incubation period of 3 weeks to 3 months. There may be some increase in CSF lymphocytes at this time, but no clinical signs appear.

Secondary syphilis follows immediately upon primary, 2 or 4 months after the appearance of the chancre. Constitutional symptoms are those of fever in association with a symmetric, nonitchy skin rash over all of the body, but particularly on the palms and soles. Snail-track ulcers (mucous patches on the mucosa of the

Table 40-10   Causes of Biological False-Positive Serological Tests

Transient (negative after 3 months)

 Recent vaccination, TAB inoculation

 Infective hepatitis

 Infectious mononucleosis, measles, zoster-varicella

 Viral encephalitis

 Pregnancy

 Undetermined (30%)

Persistent (positive after 3 months)

 Collagen-vascular disease, Hashimoto's thyroiditis

 Rheumatic heart disease

 Hepatic cirrhosis

 Hemolytic anemia

 Chronic nephritis

 Peripheral vascular disease

 Undetermined (50%)

Table 40-11   Forms of Neurosyphilis

Primary	CSF lymphocytosis
Secondary	Acute syphilitic meningitis
Tertiary	*Meningovascular*; cerebral or spinal endarteritis; cerebral or spinal leptomeningitis; meningomyelitis
	Parenchymatous; general paresis; tabes dorsalis; isolated optic atrophy
Congenital	

mouth and genitalia), generalized lymphadenopathy, loss of hair, and iritis may occur. A meningoencephalitis with the usual features of fever, meningeal irritation,
raised intracranial pressure, and occasionally focal signs including seizures, is the
main neurological presentation. The CSF shows a small increase in protein concentration but a marked increase in lymphocytes, reduced glucose level and positive
serological reactions.

After the lesions of secondary syphilis clear, a latent stage occurs, even in untreated cases, when there are no signs of the underlying infection. Tertiary or late
syphilis may appear years later, involving the skin, mouth, eyes, bones and joints,
gut, or genitourinary system. In the cardiovascular system, there may be aortitis,
granulomas of the myocardium or arterial walls (called gummas), or a generalized
vasculitis. The nervous system may show a variety of abnormalities. The diversity
of involvement led to the old adage that syphilis is the great mimicker of virtually
every known medical disease.

In the *meningovascular* form of tertiary syphilis, a chronic basal meningitis
results in increased intracranial pressure, cranial nerve lesions, or cerebral infarction. The CSF will show positive serology, increased protein and lymphocytes and
occasionally decreased sugar.

Tabes dorsalis is characterized by degenerative changes in the posterior roots
and root entry zone of the spinal cord (Fig. 40-3). This results in numerous sensory
signs. Because of the atrophy of the large sensory fibers in the posterior roots and
dorsal columns, the patients show poor proprioception, loss of deep pain, absent
reflexes, hypotonia, a "stamping" gait, and a positive Romberg's test. Lancinating
pains may be felt in girdle distribution or in the smooth muscles of the bowel, bladder, or larynx. They can be much improved with carbamazepine. The loss of "thick-
fiber" or "dorsal column" sensation may result in ulcers of the feet and painless
destruction of joints (Charcot's joints). Impotence and bladder dilation due to de-
afferentation are also common; optic atrophy, ptosis, and Argyll Robertson pupils
complete the clinical picture.

General paresis is a subacute meningoencephalitis, characterized by progressive
dementia with major frontal lobe signs and evidence of involvement of the motor
cortex and of the parietal and temporal lobes (Fig. 40-4). Tremors and a parkinsonian picture may also result from basal ganglion involvement. Optic atrophy and
Argyll Robertson pupils are usually found. Seizures are frequent and may be the
presenting problem. The basal ganglion and corticospinal lesions combine to produce severe dysarthria with tremors of the tongue and lips and variable motor disturbances in the arms and legs (Fig. 40-5). These patients often show marked
emotional changes as well as mental deterioration, and stereotypically have delusions of grandeur. It is the patient with general paresis who has been typified as
the "insane" patient who believes that he is God, Napoleon, or Batman.

Syphilitic *gummas* may be single or multiple. If they occur intracerebrally,
they may mimic a brain tumor. If they are multiple and involve the meninges,
the patient may present with dementia and focal neurological signs.

Congenital syphilis affects the nervous system in about 10 percent of children
of mothers who have seropositive syphilis. Either meningovascular or parenchyma-
tous (general paresis, tabes, optic atrophy) syndromes may occur. Seizures and
mental defects are common, as are a number of other manifestations, including
gummata of the musculoskeletal system, bilateral painful joint effusions, osteochondritis, skin lesions and abnormalities of the brain.

Management

Given a positive RPR on a patient, a further history and examination is required
with the specific aim of finding evidence of any disease that may cause a biological

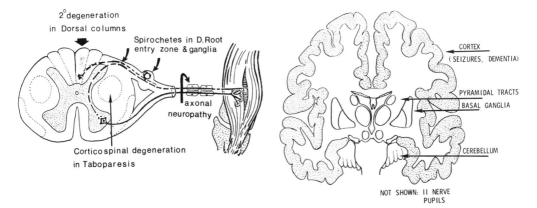

Figure 40-3 Sites of primary pathology in tabes dorsalis.

Figure 40-4 Sites of primary pathology in general paralysis of the insane (GPI).

false-positive reaction.* One should also seek evidence of a previous syphilitic infection. The RPR should be repeated and the MTPHA performed to have two separate positive serological tests at different times. The CSF should be examined for cells, serology, sugar, and protein.

If the CSF serology is positive, CSF must be rechecked every 6 months after treatment for 2 years to ascertain that the infection has cleared, the best indicators of which are the levels of cells and protein in the CSF.

For early syphilis (primary, secondary, or latent for less than 1 year) a single injection of benzathine penicillin 2.4 MU IM or procaine penicillin, 600,000 U IM daily for 8 days are adequate treatment. In tertiary stages however, benzathine penicillin 2.4 MU IM followed by 1.2 MU IM twice weekly to a total of 12 MU is required. Syphilis of the CNS requires IV benzylpenicillin therapy for 1 week.

In patients allergic to penicillin, tetracycline or erythromycin 500 mg q.i.d. for 20 to 30 days may be used. The latter is the drug of choice in allergic subjects, in women who are pregnant, and in young children.

SLOW VIRUS INFECTIONS OF THE NERVOUS SYSTEM

In 1957 an unusual disease was described in the Fore tribe of New Guinea. Its cause was traced to cannibalism and to the ceremonial rubbing of the blood and brains of the deceased over the bodies of those taking part in the ritual. Brain material from those who had died of kuru was injected into chimpanzees; some 19 months later they developed evidence of the disease.

Using a concept developed by Siggurdson, a Scandinavian veterinarian, the researchers postulated a slow virus infection — one caused by a transmissable agent presumed to be a virus particle, with a very long incubation period and slow course to death. Other conditions in this category have now been recognized.

In retrospect, it need not surprise us that an infection can occur but only produce disease months or years later. It has long been known that warts are due to a similarly prolonged latent phase and rabies is recognized as having a prolonged

---

*Always give people at least the benefit of the doubt.

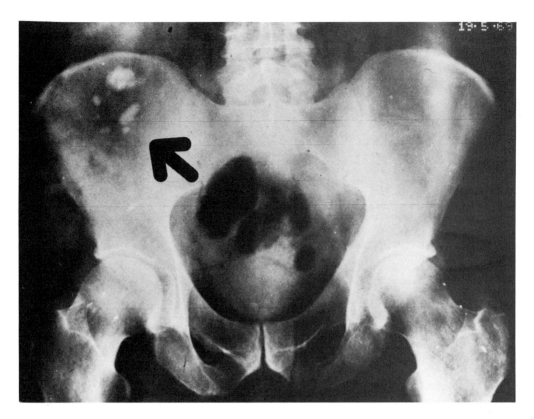

Figure 40-5   Radiograph of pelvis. Patient with GPI, formerly treated with bismuth injections.

incubation period. Herpes zoster has long been known to remain in dorsal root ganglia, often causing no clinical disease for many years. Other "slow viruses" include cytomegalovirus and the viruses of rubella and infectious hepatitis.

Jakob-Creutzfeldt Disease

Jakob-Creutzfeldt disease is an unusual condition, clinically and pathologically almost identical with kuru, and characterized by a spongiform degeneration of the cerebellar cortex, some subcortical structures, and the cerebellum. The clinical features include onset in later middle-age of personality change leading to dementia; slowly progressive spasticity; cerebellar and extrapyramidal signs; fasciculations and myoclonus. The patients usually die within 2 years. Gajdusek and other have been successful in transmitting the disease to chimpanzees through five consecutive passages, but the agent that is transmitted has not been isolated although it is presumed to be a virus.

Subacute Sclerosing Panencephalitis (SSPE)

Subacute sclerosing panencephalitis is a delayed measles encephalitis associated with a defective host immune response. It is becoming less common, perhaps because of widespread measles immunization. Typically, children or young adults

show mental and behavioral changes that lead to progressive dementia, myoclonic
jerking, seizures, and increasing motor disability. The patients deteriorate and die
in 1 to 3 years. The EEG characteristically shows periodic slow-wave and sharp-
wave discharges (Fig. 40-6), and the CSF contains excessive IgG; positive oligoclonal banding and a high titer of antimeasles antibody are also found. The para-
myxovirus has been isolated from the brains of many such patients.

The measles infection probably occurred up to 10 years before the onset of
SSPE, so this condition is a convincing argument for the existence of persistent
virus-induced autoimmune diseases of the nervous system.

Children born with the congenital rubella syndrome may develop a similar disease. Treatment in the past has been fruitless but early results using isoprinosine
give some hope for the future.

In immunosuppressed patients, e.g., those with lymphomas, a similar syndrome
may occur because of progressive measles encephalitis, but here the CSF is normal.

Progressive Multifocal Leukoencephalopathy (PML)

This is a fatal brain disease seen only in immunosuppressed patients. Progressive
demyelination occurs in the white matter of the cerebellar hemispheres and
sometimes that of the brainstem, cerebellum, and spinal cord. The patchy areas
of demyelination show preservation of axis cylinders, and the astrocytes are
large with abnormal nuclei and many mitoses. The supportive oligodendrocytes
are reduced in number and contain inclusion bodies. Crystalline arrays of papova
virions are seen at the periphery of the lesion.

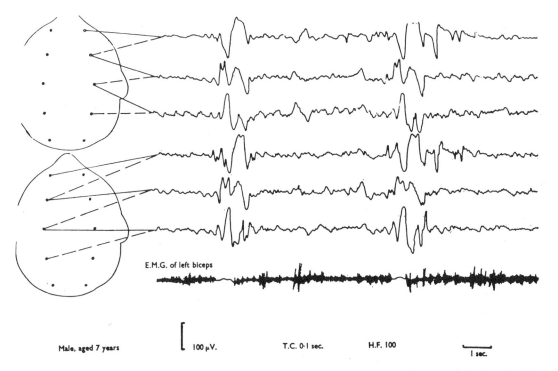

E.M.G. of left biceps

Male, aged 7 years   100 μV.   T.C. 0-1 sec.   H.F. 100   1 sec.

Figure 40-6   Subacute sclerosing panencephalitis. The EEG shows typical periodic
complexes.

This disorder is often a terminal event in Hodgkin's disease and lymphoma, occasionally in sarcoidosis, tuberculosis, and other conditions marked by immunological incompetence. It is due to a polyoma viral infection acting as a slow virus. Patients are within 3 years after a progressive downhill course characterized by behavioral change and developing ataxia, aphasia, blindness, paralysis, and ultimately coma.

These are just a few examples of disease that had been considered to be degenerative in nature but are now known to be due to viruses acting in an unusual way. It appears that the virus can stay in the nervous system for prolonged periods before causing a progressive disease. Interestingly, the brain lesions often look more degenerative than inflammatory or infective underthe microscope, and one naturally begins to wonder about other "degenerative" processes such as Alzheimer's disease, motor neuron disease, Parkinson's disease, and multiple sclerosis.

NEUROLOGICAL COMPLICATIONS OF OTHER INFECTIONS

The classification of the infectious encephalopathies has been clarified by Ropper, who suggests four categories of disorder. First there is encephalitis caused by direct viral invasion of the brain. Next, acute toxic encephalopathy with brain swelling rather than inflammation. Postinfectious or postvaccinial encephalopathy is also called acute allergic encephalomyelitis and is a multifocal demyelinating disease with an immunological basis. Finally, an inflammatory encephalitis occurs with EB virus, influenza, and mycoplasmal infections, which cannot be distinguished clinically from ordinary viral encephalitis, but the agent is not recoverable from the brain. The first of these has already been discussed; we will describe the next two under the older, popular headings.

Acute Toxic Encephalopathy

During or within 2 weeks of acute specific (e.g., measles) or nonspecific infections in children, during the acute illness in bacterial endocarditis in adults, or following vaccination in anybody, fever and acute neurological signs may suddenly appear. The latter include acute obtundation and delirium, seizures, myoclonus, signs of raised intracranial pressure, meningism, cerebellar signs, and chorea. The CSF is usually normal. A few patients recover completely but most are left with significant residual neurological deficits or epilepsy. No infective agent has ever been isolated from the brain in these cases, and the etiology is presumed to be an allergic vasculitis.

In children and young adults, possibly as a complication of a preceding influenza or varicella infection, *Reye's syndrome* of encephalopathy (delirium, seizures, coma, and inconstant focal signs) follows a period of malaise and fever with persistent vomiting. Fatty degeneration of the liver and cerebral edema with a marked rise in intracranial pressure are the pathologic basis of these signs. Because intensive metabolic therapy may be lifesaving, immediate referral is essential whenever even drowsiness follows prolonged vomiting in young people. It is possible that some environmental chemical agents predispose to the development of this reaction to viruses that are otherwise usually innocuous. This can be regarded as a special form of acute toxic encephalopathy.

Acute Allergic Encephalomyelitis

Alternative names for this condition are postinfectious or postvaccinal encephalomyelitis. These are a group of similar disorders characterized by a monophasic course following a febrile illness or vaccination. Multiple perivenular foci of demyelination and lymphocytic infiltration appear in the nervous system with secondary damage to axons. Thus unlike the acute encephalitides, the white rather than the gray matter is primarily affected.

The characteristic of this disorder is its occurrence 1 to 2 weeks after an acute infection or immunological challenge. The presumed pathogenesis is an autoimmune reaction to brain myelin, either following vaccination (e.g., against rabies or smallpox) or following infection with measles, rubella, chickenpox, smallpox, mumps, leptospirosis, etc. Injections of antitetanus serum may give rise to the same clinical picture. About a third of the cases diagnosed as encephalitis may in fact be of this type.

The incubation period is 8 to 15 days. Following this there is an abrupt onset of headache with signs of raised intracranial pressure and drowsiness which may progress to coma. Before coma develops, the patient may have nausea, vomiting, high fever, meningism, myoclonus or seizures, flaccid paralysis, and variable sensory loss. Cerebellar ataxia is sometimes the main feature. The brunt of the disease may be borne by the brain, the spinal cord, or occasionally by the spinal nerve roots (producing a radiculopathy). The CSF is under increased pressure and contains excess protein and sometimes increased mononuclear cells, but no virus is isolated.

Steroids in high dosage in the early stages are probably effective in reducing the immunological reaction, and concern about spreading a viral infection is probably unjustified. At the other end of the scale, the clinical picture may be identical with that of epidemic myalgic encephalomyelitis (see following section), while illnesses of any intermediate stage of severity are also possible. Despite therapy, most patients will either die or be left with serious neurological deficits. The others recover, often with some neurological sequelae.

The distinction from multiple sclerosis is made by the presence of fever, the monophasic character of the illness without any past history of neurological symptoms, a painful radiculopathy in many cases, and the *flaccid* paresis. The EEG shows bilateral delta activity in a high proportion of patients but is not diagnostic, although such records are not commonly seen in multiple sclerosis.

Epidemic Myalgic Encephalomyelitis

The organicity of this condition has been questioned but certain test results, such as raised serum lactic dehydrogenase (LDH), abnormal lymphocytes, and a raised CSF protein level, suggest that it is not psychogenic; it may be a mild form of acute allergic encephalomyelitis. In summer, young adults complain of headache, myelgia, fever, fatigue, and labile emotions. Lymphadenopathy and various mild brainstem and cord signs may be found. After some weeks and a long convalescence, all symptoms usually remit. The cause is, frankly, unknown.

Bacterial Endocarditis

Over a third of the patients with bacterial endocarditis present with neurological signs. Half of these appear to have cerebrovascular disease (usually an infarct, but occasionally a hemorrhage), and in the later stages, mycotic aneurysms may rupture, causing a subarachnoid hemorrhage. Acute toxic encephalopathy with delirium can be seen and some patients will show a clinical picture indistinguishable from acute meningitis or cerebral abscess. In these cases the CSF usually contains mononuclear cells but no organisms, although *S. aureus* is the most common infecting agent. Other complications of bacterial endocarditis include retinal hemorrhages, seizures, and recurring headaches (Table 40-12).

**Table 40-12   Neurological Presentations of Bacterial Endocarditis
(30% of All Cases)**

Cerebrovascular disease	Infarct	40%
	Hemorrhage	10%
Acute toxic encephalopathy		20%
Acute meningitis		5%
Headache, seizures, coma, retinal changes, etc.		25%

Children with bacterial endocarditis often show a rash in association with fever and delirium, and this picture must be differentiated from that caused by the acute specific fevers such as scarlet fever, measles, rubella, entero- and adenovirus infections, and by allergic and drug reactions. *Purpura with fever* may occur in mononucleosis, rickettsial disease, Henoch-Schönlein purpura, and with other causes of allergic vasculitis.

Cerebral Thrombophlebitis

Cerebral abscesses in association with sinus infection or otitis usually occur because of direct extension of the infection within or alongside the dural sinuses and the other large intracranial veins. Sometimes the brain itself is not directly involved, but the infection in the walls of the veins causes venous thrombosis, with venous infarction of the portions of the brain damaged by the occluded vessels. In children, sinus thrombosis can occur with no local infection at all, as when the child is markedly dehydrated or has a high fever. Sinus thrombosis may also complicate sickle-cell anemia. At any age, severe cachexia can cause sinus thrombosis, usually involving the superior sagittal sinus, and this may also occur in women in the postpartum period or in those who are taking the contraceptive pill. Underlying lymphomas, including polycythemia, are also associated.

The *clinical features* are those of local ear or sinus infection, seizures, raised intracranial pressure because of failure of venous drainage, meningism, and sometimes focal neurological findings resulting from venous infarction. Otitis usually produces thrombophlebitis in the transverse sinuses, and there may be little in the way of focal signs. General examination may show evidence of the systemic disorders such as reticulosis, cachexia, and so forth, listed in Table 40-13.

Sinus thrombosis complicating mastoiditis may also present subacutely with raised intracranial pressure without meningism, a condition described as "otitic hydrocephalus." With *superior sagittal* sinus occlusion, seizures and uni- or bilateral corticospinal signs in the legs are to be expected, because the territory infarcted is the motor strip region for the lower limbs.

Cavernous sinus thrombosis (Fig. 40-7) may complicate infections of the face or nasal sinuses; signs of raised intracranial pressure, exophthalmos with marked edema of the conjunctiva, chemosis and often ophthalmoplegia, and bilateral second nerve damage. There may also be evidence of meningitis. This condition has a grave prognosis.

Table 40-13   Causes of Intracranial Venous Thrombosis

Cachexia

Dehydration

Mastoiditis, sinusitis

Trauma

Polycythemia, sickle-cell anemia

Superior vena caval obstruction

Cardiac failure

Pregnancy, postpartum

Birth-control pill

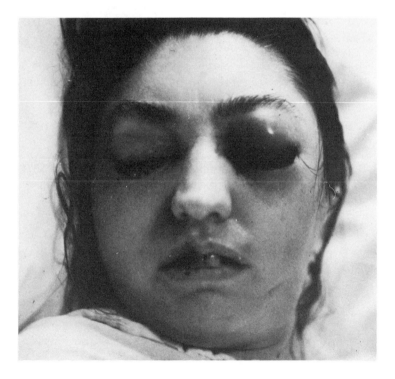

Figure 40-7   Cavernous sinus thrombosis; bacterial panophthalmitis was followed by septic thrombophlebitis.

The differential diagnosis of sinus thrombophlebitis from cerebral abscess or meningitis may be difficult. Brain scanning and EEG will probably not show the clear-cut localizing features to be expected with cerebral abscesses. The diagnosis is probably best made by CT scanning, orbital venography, and carotid arteriogram. The CSF pressure, lymphocyte count, and protein level are high. Red cells may be present with thrombophlebitis, but organisms are not detected and are cultured only from the blood.

If cerebral abscess seems clinically likely however, LP is best deferred until the patient is in a neurological center, as it is dangerous and unnecessary when a CT scan is available.

Treatment consists of attempts to lower the intracranial pressure with steroids or dehydrating solutions and the use of high dosages of broad-spectrum antibiotics. Ligation of the infected veins is of questionable value. Where specific underlying medical disease is found, this may be treatable. Anticoagulants are of uncertain value in sinus thrombosis.

BIBLIOGRAPHY

Advisory Committee on Venereal Disease Control. Recommended treatment of syphilis and gonorrhea. *Can. Med. Assoc. J. 117:*250, 1977.

Bell, W.E. Treatment of bacterial infections of the central nervous system. *Ann. Neurol. 9:*313-327, 1981.

Bell, W.E. Treatment of fungal infections of the central nervous system. *Ann. Neurol. 9:*417-422, 1981.

Edmondson, R.S., Flowers, M.W. Intensive care in tetanus. *Br. Med. J. 2:*1401-1403, 1979.

Ellner, J.J., Bennett, J.E. Chronic meningitis. *Medicine 55:*341, 1976. Johnson, R.T. *Viral Infections of the Nervous System.* New York, Raven Press, 1982.

Kennard, C., Swash, M. Acute viral encephalitis: Its diagnosis and outcome. *Brain 104:*129-148, 1981.

Lehrich, J.R. Case Records of the Massachusetts General Hospital. *N. Engl. J. Med. 306:*93, 1982.

Mandell, G.L. *Principles and Practices of Infectious Diseases.* New York, John Wiley & Sons, 1979.

Miller, A., Nathanson, N. Rabies: Recent advances in pathogenesis and control. *Ann. Neurol. 2:*511-519, 1977.

Ropper, A.H. Case Records of the Massachusetts General Hospital. *N. Engl. J. Med. 305:*507-514, 1981.

Snider, W.D. et al. Neurological complications of the acquired immune deficiency syndrome. *Ann. Neurol. 14:*403-418, 1983.

41
Neoplastic Disease

Most reports of the incidence of brain tumors come from neurosurgeons who only see a selected series of patients, as most people with multiple metastatic lesions involving the brain are treated by physicians and radiotherapists without the benefit of neurosurgical referral.

The true incidence of tumors is probably in the order of 5 per 100,000 population per year for primary tumors of all types, while secondary tumors must have at least an equal incidence whether or not they are actually detected. Table 41-1 lists the more common types. Tumors may arise from any intracranial component except the CSF, which however provides a pathway for seeding of some tumors from the intracranial to the intraspinal compartment.

Little is known about the specific factors causing brain tumors. Congenital anomalies of embryonic tissue may undergo malignant change. Neurofibromas and acoustic neuromas may have a genetic basis, as may some gliomas, especially when they arise in patients with tuberous sclerosis, but to state that a process is "genetic" does not explain its etiology. A number of viruses are oncogenic in laboratory animals, but there is no clear association with human brain tumors. Trauma is not a cause.

Brain tumors cause about 1 percent of deaths in our population and 2 percent of the deaths due to cancers. They represent the second most common tumor site in children. Ninety percent of them are malignant, but early diagnosis may improve the life expectancy and quality of that life even in these, whereas in patients with benign tumors, surgical removal is often possible, effecting a complete cure. The relative frequency of intracranial tumor types is given in Table 41-2.

A graph of the incidence of tumors by age would show three peaks: one between the ages of 5 and 9 years (because of an increased number of cerebellar gliomas, pinealomas, craniopharyngiomas, teratomas, and granulomas), a second

Table 41-1   Types of Intracranial Mass Lesions

Primary extracerebral

Skull	hyperostosis
	osteoma
	angioma
	metastasis
	granuloma, including xanthomatosis
Meninges	meningioma
	secondary carcinoma
	reticulosis
Cranial nerve	optic glioma
	neurofibroma (V or VII)
Ductless glands	pinealoma
Congenital tumors	cholesteatoma
	chordoma
	teratoma and dermoid cysts

Primary intracerebral

Supportive tissue	gliomas
Blood vessels	hemangioblastoma
	angiomas
Granulomas	tuberculoma
	gumma
Parasitic cysts	echinococcus
	cryptococcus

Metastases

Hemorrhage: epidural, subdural

in the 50s (because of a high proportion of gliomas, pituitary tumors, neurofibromas, and meningiomas), and a third in later life (when the frequency of metastases is high). The site of tumors is interesting because the pattern is an exact reversal when childhood and adult tumors are compared. In children, 80 percent of tumors are infratentorial, while in adults 80 percent are supratentorial.

The clinical features of almost all forms of cerebral tumor are essentially similar, with certain variations depending upon the site of origin. Signs of raised intracranial pressure will occur at some time in all but will be particularly early in tumors within or pressing upon the ventricular system, such as tumors in the posterior fossa, third ventricle cysts, pinealomas, and deep midline gliomas, e.g., of the thalamus. Secondary tumors, because of their rapid growth, also produce an early rise in intracranial pressure. Slow-growing tumors, such as meningiomas, on the other hand, may attain a very large size since their slow growth causes them to compress and cause atrophy of brain tissue rather than an increase in intracranial pressure.

Table 41-2 Relative Frequency of Glioma Types

Type of Glioma	Percentage
Glioblastoma	50
Other astrocytomas	30
Medulloblastomas	6
Ependymoma	7
Oligodendroglioma	5
Other	2

The CT scan has markedly improved the assessment of tumor size and location, accurately outlining the limits of the tumor edge, and can improve the focus of radiation therapy. This improved delineation of the tumor and of the edema around it makes it much easier to decide whether any new symptoms are due to tumor growth and invasion, to hemorrhage, or to local or general edema.

Seizures are common with all fast-growing tumors, such as gliomas and secondaries and also with meningiomas but unusual with other extracerebral tumors. Focal signs such as those of dementia, cranial nerve signs or personality change, visual deficits, dysphasia, hypothalamic dysfunction, corticospinal deficits, etc., may suggest the likely site of the lesion.

The onset of symptoms is seldom abrupt; even in the case of malignant tumors, progress is over the course of weeks or months. Sometimes a seizure may be the first sign of the lesion, a Todd's paralysis drawing attention to the focal origin of the attack and thus to the likely site of the tumor. Apart from some *true* localizing signs, *false* ones also occur, owing to raised intracranial pressure. In the following discussion, a detailed description of the clinical features of each particular tumor type will not be given because this would be repetitive and the information can be found elsewhere in this book, particularly in the appropriate sections on localization of lesions, seizures, and raised intracranial pressure in Parts II and III.

Tumor Types

Gliomas

Gliomas arise from the glial cells that are the supporting tissues of the brain, brainstem, and spinal cord. Astrocytomas arise from astrocytes and oligodendrogliomas from oligodendrocytes. The latter are rare, relatively slow-growing tumors, often containing calcium which may be seen on a skull x-ray. Much more common is the astrocytoma, which is graded into four histological types on the basis of the degree of malignant change within it histologically. Grade I is the most benign and grade IV, also known as *glioblastoma multiforme,* is the most malignant (Figs. 41-1; 41-2). This tumor is most common in adult males (incidence is 4/100,000 per year) and tends to arise in the temporal lobes, the thalamus, basal ganglia, deeper parts of the cortex, or corpus collosum. It spreads rapidly through the adjacent brain and produces even greater dysfunction owing to the presence of local edema and sometimes hemorrhage (Fig. 41-3).

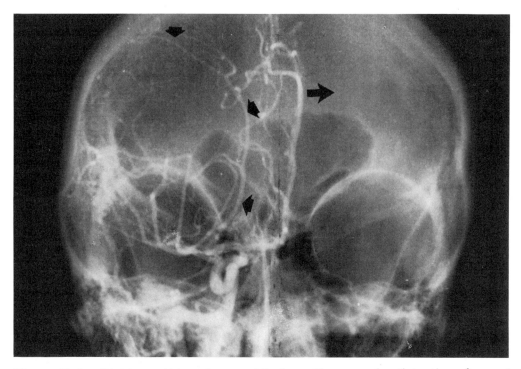

Figure 41-1   Right carotid angiogram AP view. New vessels, distortion of vessels and "square-shift" of the ACA resulting from a large right hemispheric glioma.

Other astrocytomas are less malignant than the glioblastoma but unfortunately are much less common. They arise in the cerebellum or brainstem (Figs. 41-4 to 41-6) or the optic nerve in children, but in adults are mainly in the cerebral hemispheres. They all infiltrate widely, explaining the surgeon's difficulty in achieving total removal in most cases, although within the cerebellum the tumors are often cystic and can be removed totally, giving an excellent prognosis.

Medulloblastomas are less common gliomas that arise from the roof of the fourth ventricle or the vermis of the cerebellum, mainly in children. These are highly malignant, may seed in the CSF to give rise to secondaries within the spinal cord, and carry a bad prognosis. As may be expected, their initial symptoms and signs are of cerebellar involvement and of obstruction to CSF flow. *Ependymomas* also occur in young people and are slow-growing, infiltrating tumors that arise from the ependymal lining of the ventricular system or filum terminale. Again, they cause a rise in intracranial pressure and bulbar and cerebellar signs. A choroid plexus *papilloma* may be an indolent form of ependymoma.

Despite their malignancy, it is always worth pursuing the diagnosis of astrocytomas because therapy occasionally is successful. If a tumor arises from the frontal lobe or from the anterior part of the temporal lobe, it sometimes can be removed completely without leaving any significant residual defect. If the patient has a progressive deficit from the effect of the tumor's expansion, removal of most of it may at least relieve the intracranial pressure rise and may make radiotherapy more likely to be effective. A shunt procedure may also be helpful in this situation. Nevertheless, the prognosis for the most malignant gliomas is death within 6 months of diagnosis in two-thirds of cases.

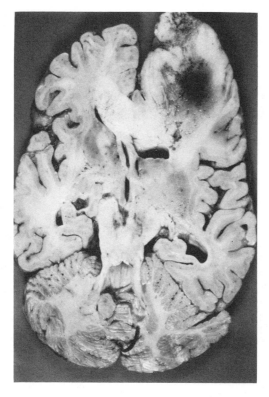

Figure 41-2   Horizontal section of brain. Glioblastoma multiforme in right frontal pole crossing the midline in the corpus callosum.

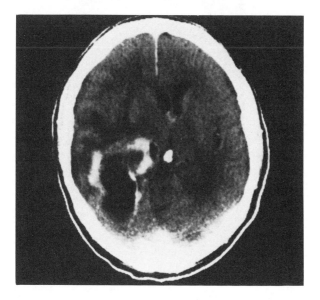

Figure 41-3   Enhanced CT scan. Irregular low-density area in the left parietal lobe with irregular enhancement of its wall, marked local edema, and midline shift. Glioma.

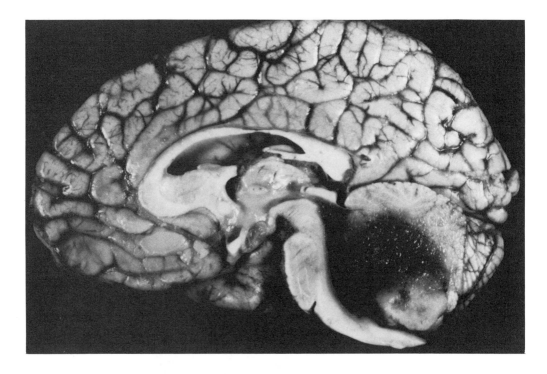

Figure 41-4   Saggital section of brain; large hemorrhagic ependymoma filling the fourth ventricle and invading the cerebellum.

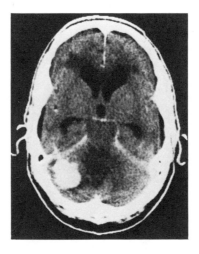

Figure 41-5   Enhanced CT scan. Large enhancing mass in the posterior fossa with local edema and obstructive hydrocephalus.

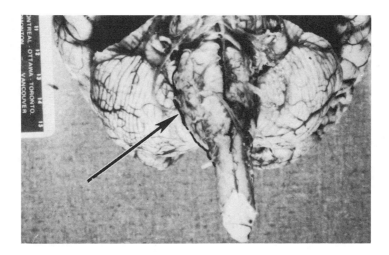

Figure 41-6   Pontine glioma.

Meningiomas

Meningiomas probably arise from arachnoid cell rests in the dura mater or the choroid plexuses. They are firm, round masses of connective tissue cells containing
collagen fibers and often deposits of calcium. Usually they occur singly and arise
from the meninges, causing neurological deficit because of pressure on the local
brain, but they do not infiltrate the brain, rather they remain within a capsule.
There may be localized reactive bone formation of the skull in the area of the tumor, particularly if it takes the form of sheets of cells rather than a circumscribed
mass — "meningiomas en plaque." When this occurs, the site of the tumor is usually on the floor of the anterior or middle cranial fossae.
    Meningiomas (incidence about 1/100,000 per year) are most common in women,
usually at or around middle age. Frequent sites of involvement are the parasagittal areas, the sphenoidal ridge, and the floor of the anterior or middle fossae. Within the skull, they tend to be located in anterior (frontal or temporal) rather than in
posterior (parietal or occipital) areas. Although the meningioma makes its presence
known by pressure on the nearby brain, there are a few specific presentations that
are worthy of comment.

    Parasaggital meningiomas may sit between the two hemispheres and by
    pressing on the leg areas of the motor strip, produce weakness and spasticity
    in the legs, a picture that at first sight may be thought to be due to a spinal
    lesion (Fig. 41-7).
    Meningiomas situated medially on the sphenoid ridge cause visual loss, ho-
    molateral optic atrophy, and contralateral papilledema because of raised
    intracranial pressure (the Foster-Kennedy syndrome); also proptosis and ocu-
    lomotor palsies. More laterally placed tumors cause only papilledema bilater-
    ally. Those situated far laterally produce riased intracranial pressure and
    homolateral proptosis, pain in the eye, and visual loss. Headache, seizures,
    and mental change are common to all of these sites.

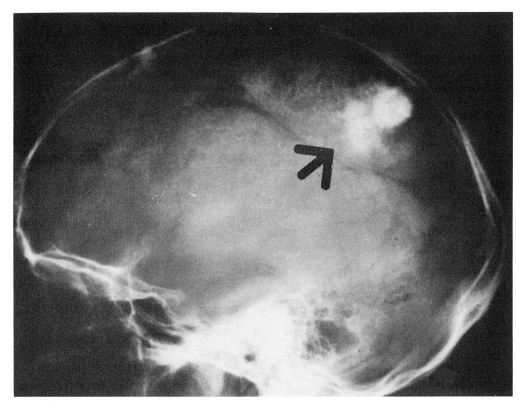

Figure 41-7   Lateral radiograph of skull. There is calcification in a recurrent parasaggital meningioma. The lucencies are burr-holes made at the previous craniotomy.

Olfactory groove meningiomas cause anosmia, visual loss, and sometimes the Foster-Kennedy syndrome.

Suprasellar meningiomas may produce either slowly progressing visual dimming with especially diminished color perception, or a bitemporal hemianopia with optic atrophy and progressive visual loss. If skull x-rays are normal in this circumstance, remember that aneurysms can also occur in this region.

The slowest-growing meningiomas are commonly in the frontal region, where they may grow to a large size over many years without significant symptoms. Often, the first sign is a change in intellectual function or in personality.* Seizures, visual deficits, and headache are also common, and clinical testing may detect unilateral anosmia because of pressure on the first nerve. Meningiomas are usually very vascular and show a blush on the arteriogram in the capillary phase (Fig. 41-8). Because they arise from the meninges, they will be supplied

---

*Never for the better. When the cabinet minister embezzles, the vicar is tactless with the choirboys, or the neurologist passes water in Grand Rounds, it is possible that the CT scan would be a better defense than the attorney could otherwise muster.

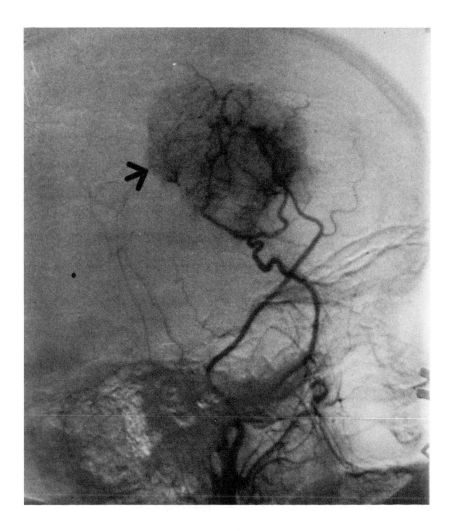

Figure 41-8   Right external carotid arteriogram showing the characteristic "blush" of a meningioma, here situated in the right midfrontal parasaggital region.

at least in part by the external carotid artery, usually through its middle meningeal branch, and therefore an x-ray of the base of the skull may show an enlarged foramen spinosum.

They are also well demonstrated on isotope and CT scans and even a plain x-ray film shows an increase in bone formation in about half the cases. Malignant transformation is very uncommon but recurrence is not.

Acoustic Neuroma (Schwannoma)

The schwannoma is a tumor of middle adult life that arises from the vestibular portion of the eighth nerve, disturbing both vestibular and cochlear functions. Initially, complaints of deafness, unsteadiness on turning the head, suboccipital discomfort, and tinnitus are more frequent than those of vertigo. As the tumor expands and widens the medial portion of the internal auditory meatus, it may also compress the fibers of the fifth nerve, the cerebellar peduncles, and the seventh nerve (Fig. 41-9). When it becomes very large it produces bulbar, corticospinal, and posterior column signs and raised intracranial pressure. Examination will almost invariably show an absent corneal reflex on that side and as with other tumors of the cerebellopontine angle (cholesteatoma, meningioma, metastasis, aneurysm), a combination of fifth, seventh, and eighth nerve symptoms and signs with a cerebellar deficit is extremely suggestive. Audiometry, caloric testing, brainstem evoked responses and x-rays of the internal auditory meatus should be requested (Fig. 41-10), but CT scanning demonstrates the tumor most accurately. The CSF protein level is often extremely high.

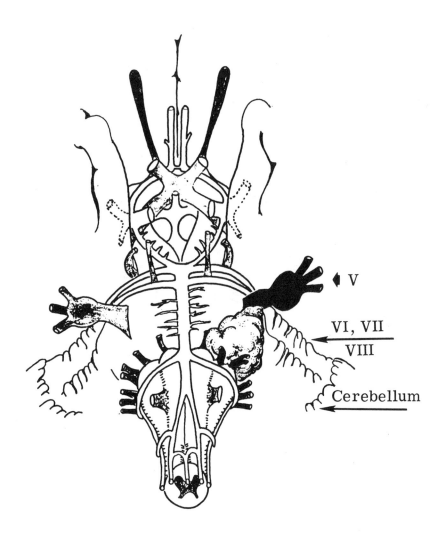

Figure 41-9   Diagram of a cerebellopontine angle mass. Pressure may be exerted on the fifth, seventh, and eighth cranial nerves and the inferior cerebellar peduncle by such lesions.

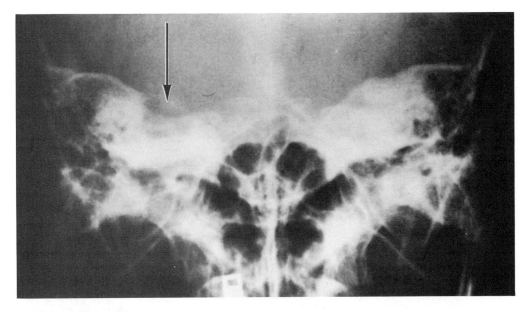

Figure 41-10 Skull radiograph; right acoustic schwannoma with expansion of the internal auditory neatus (arrowed).

If the tumor is bilateral, one should consider von Recklinghausen's disease (see Chap. 39), which is associated with almost every other intracranial tumor much more frequently than can be explained by chance.

Craniopharyngioma

Craniopharyngiomas arise mainly in childhood and youth, occasionally in patients over the age of 50 years. They originate from Rathke's pouch, an embryological remnant in the roof of the mouth, and form cystic, often calcified tumors involving the bone around the pituitary fossa and extending upward into the hypothalamic area, sometimes compressing the third ventricle (Fig. 41-11). As a result, sexual immaturity, growth failure, and other signs of pituitary dysfunction are common. Pressure upward and backward on the third ventricle may lead to obstructive hydrocephalus; the tumor may also compress the optic nerve, producing atrophy, and the ascending RAS, causing drowsiness or, in time, coma. By mechanisms not entirely understood, it may cause alterations in intellectual function from mild memory loss to profound dementia. Surgical removal is frequently possible.

Pituitary Tumors

Pituitary tumors are usually adenomas, 90 percent of which are *chromphobe adenomas*. These may cause growth failure or, alternatively, excessive production of growth hormone with giantism in children and acromegaly in adults. As with craniopharyngiomas, their enlargement puts pressure on the optic chiasm, producing bitemporal hemianopia. Raised intracranial pressure with headache; damage to the third, fourth, and sixth nerves because of lateral expansion in the region of the cavernous sinus; pressure on the fifth nerve; extension laterally into the temporal lobe, with features of temporal lobe seizures; and erosion of bone, with CSF

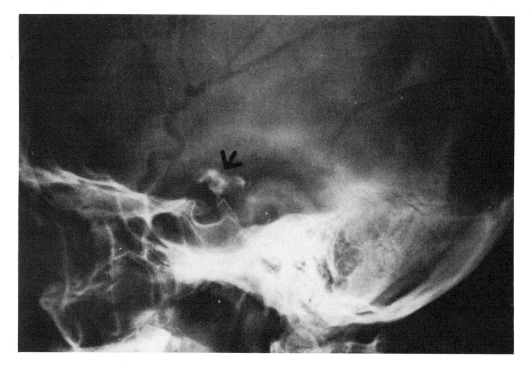

Figure 41-11   Lateral skull radiograph.   Calcification in a craniopharyngioma.

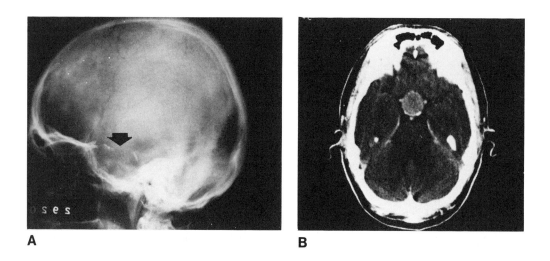

A   B

Figure 41-12   (A) Expansion and destruction of the pituitary fossa by a chromophobe adenoma;   (B) Enhanced CT scan.   Large pituitary adenoma extending up into the suprasellar cistern.

rhinorrhea and proptosis, are other possible manifestations because these tumors may become very large (Fig. 41-12A, B). Chromophobe adenomas may also contain cells producing melanin, corticotrophin, or prolactin. When such tumors are very small (microadenomas), the more common clinical manifestations include infertility, menstrual problems, and galactorrhea in women, and impotence in men. Preoperative diagnosis (first, think of the possibility; next, order serum prolactin levels) is essential because microsurgical trans-sphenoidal removal of the tumors is comparatively simple and safe. *Eosinophilic adenomas* comprise less than 10 percent of pituitary tumors. They produce growth hormone, but themselves seldom are large enough to produce more than visual symptoms. *Basophil* adenomas make up the remainder. These may secrete excessive follicle-stimulating hormone, corticotrophin, or thyrotrophin, causing Cushing's syndrome or hyperthyroidism. In many cases, the tumor is presumed rather than identified because it is small, and when removed the pituitary shows no more than an increased number of basophilic cells without any evidence of a true mitotic lesion.

Because pituitary tumors arise within the sella turcica, skull x-rays often demonstrate the signs of raised intracranial pressure and erosion of the floor of the pituitary fossa and of the posterior clinoids, sometimes with expansion of the size of the fossa. The tumor may be defined with a CT scan or angiogram. Hormonal disturbances should be defined by specific testing. Unlike craniopharyngiomas, pituitary adenomas do not calcify.

Metastatic Tumors

At least 40 percent of brain tumors arise outside the nervous system. The most common sites of the primaries that metastasize to the head are the lung, breast, stomach, kidney, and thyroid (see Table 41-3). Melanomas also often metastasize to the head. Breast and prostate neoplasms metastasize to the subarachnoid space and meninges as well as to the brain parenchyma, and malignant cells then spread throughout the CSF causing widespread scattered neurological deficits, often with involvement of cranial and spinal nerve roots. The CSF will have high protein and low sugar levels and malignant cells will be found. Obstruction to CSF flow will result in hydrocephalus.

Table 41-3   Relative Frequency of Intracerebral Tumors[a]

Secondary carcinoma	40%
Gliomas, all types	40%
Meningiomas	13%
Pituitary adenomas	3%
Neurofibromas	
Congenital tumors	
Tumors of blood vessels	4%
Other tumors	

[a]These figures apply to adult populations. In children, about three-quarters of cerebral tumors are gliomas.

Secondaries in the skull and brain are frequently multiple (Figs. 41-13 to 14-15). They give rise to headaches, mental clouding and depression, seizures, signs of raised intracranial pressure, and a variety of focal signs. The diagnosis is made by CT scanning, which is positive in 95 percent of cases. Up to 40 percent of carcinomas of the lung metastasize to the brain and although the prognosis in this type of tumor is awful (the median survival is only 6 months), there is some hope of therapeutic success if the metastatic lesion is single. Steroids in high dosage (dexamethasone 20-40 mg daily) are the mainstay of treatment, but the prognosis is improved by irradiation of the whole head, not just the metastatic lesion. Surgical removal may be warranted for a single metastasis as judged clinically and by CT scan, as long as others are not found elsewhere, and for cerebellar secondaries. Chemotherapy is of value only in treating leukemia and diffuse lymphomas.

Pinealoma

The pinealoma is a rare neoplasm of young males (Fig. 41-16). It has a close histological relationship to teratoma. Arising from the pineal gland, it is bounded in front by the third ventricle, behind the cerebellum, and below by the brainstem at the level of the superior colliculi.

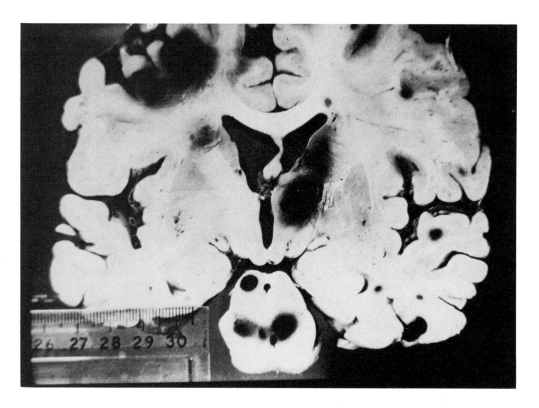

Figure 41-13 Coronal section of brain; multiple secondary renal cell carcinoma deposits.

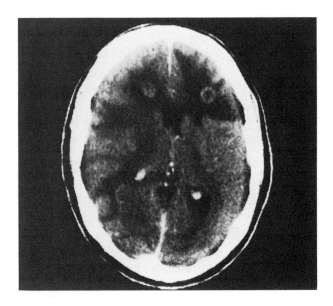

Figure 41-14A   Enhanced CT scan.   Multiple irregular enhancing metastatic tumors with surrounding edema.

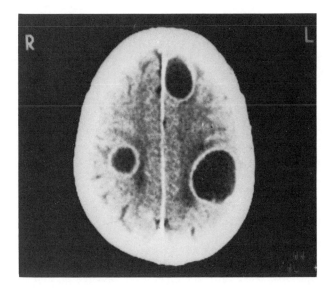

Figure 41-14B   Large ring lesions due to metastases.

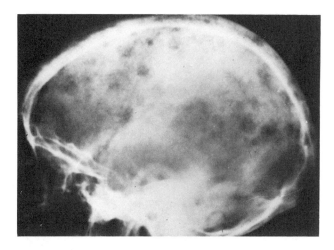

Figure 41-15   Lateral skull radiograph.   Multiple irregular and blurred lucencies caused by metastatic carcinoma.

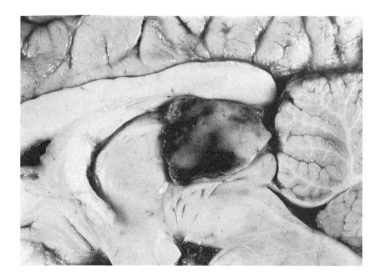

Figure 41-16   Sagittal section of brain; pinealoma. The downward compression of the tumor on the third ventricle and superior colliculi is shown.

Damage to the hypothalamus may lead to diabetes insipidus, precocious puberty, or hypogonadism. Pressure on the superior cerebellar peduncle gives rise to a typical cerebellar syndrome, and on the superior colliculi, to failure of upward gaze. Further pressure damages the third and fourth nerves and the associated autonomic nuclei controlling pupillary function; thus the pupils are often unequal with impaired responses to light or accommodation. Finally, pressure on the aqueduct leads to hydrocephalus. These tumors are usually benign, but their surgical removal is extremely hazardous and because radiation is of only limited value in treating them, the prognosis is grave.

Colloid Cysts

Although often detected only by chance at postmortem, these small tumors may cause acute obstructive hydrocephalus and transient loss of consciousness by compression of the periventricular RAS (Fig. 41-17A, B).

Angiomas

Most commonly in association with other evidence of congenital vascular disturbances, such as von Hippel-Lindau disease, these hamartomas may sometimes attain a large size, in which case focal seizures and vascular headaches are the usual features, although damage to the underlying brain may produce corticospinal or sensory signs. A bruit may be heard over the larger ones. They seldom bleed but should they do so, the results are not catastrophic, as they are with aneurysms. Symptoms usually occur before the age of 30, so this is not a likely lesion when a patient complains of vascular headaches with onset in adult life.

Hemangioblastomas are malignant vascular tumors presenting most frequently between the ages of 20 and 40 years and are sometimes associated with von Hippel-Lindau disease. Polycythemia, renal tumors, and pancreatic cysts may coexist. The most common site in the nervous system is the cerebellum where operative intervention may be successful. The family history is sometimes positive for similar tumors.

Tumors of the Nasopharynx

Carcinomas, and less commonly sarcomas, occur in the lateral nasopharyngeal wall, mainly in adult males. They usually compress the emerging cranial nerves III, IV, V, VI, and VIII. If the tumor spreads backward, the bulbar nerves may be involved as well. Other symptoms include proptosis, Horner's syndrome, and nasal obstruction, discharge, or bleeding. Skull involvement frequently produces headache or facial pain, and nodes are often palpable in the neck. Specific bulbar palsies and isolated trigeminal sensory loss should put one on guard for the presence of such tumors. Even with surgical removal and irradiation, the prognosis is poor because recurrence is likely.

Lymphomas

The *leukemias* may produce a picture of subacute basal meningitis with cranial nerve pain and CSF obstruction, leukoencephalopathy, or intracranial bleeding probably caused by a reduction in platelets. Opportunistic CNS infections by fungi or viruses are also common, and cerebral atrophy often complicates cranial irradiation and methotrexate therapy. *Polycythemia* affects the nervous system almost entirely through occlusive cerebral vascular diseaese, including sinus thrombosis.

In *Hodgkin's disease*, 25 percent of patients have some evidence of neurological disease. Hodgkin tissue may invade the meninges intracranially or intraspinally, frequently compressing the cauda equina. In such cases, CSF cytology may be positive. Chronic basal meningitis may produce raised intracranial pressure or any cranial nerve palsies. As with other tumors, cerebral and cerebellar cortical degenerations, peripheral neuropathies, a myasthenic syndrome, or proximal myopathy can occur. Amyloidosis, tuberculosis and opportunistic fungal infections are other complications. A search for this or similar tumors should be made in any adult with herpes zoster. Progressive multifocal leukoencephalopathy (discussed later) is yet another complication of Hodgkin's disease.

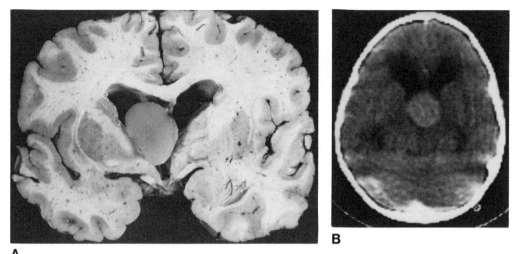

A

B

Figure 41-17 (A) Coronal section of brain. Colloid cyst of the third ventricle; (B) CT scan of a colloid cyst.

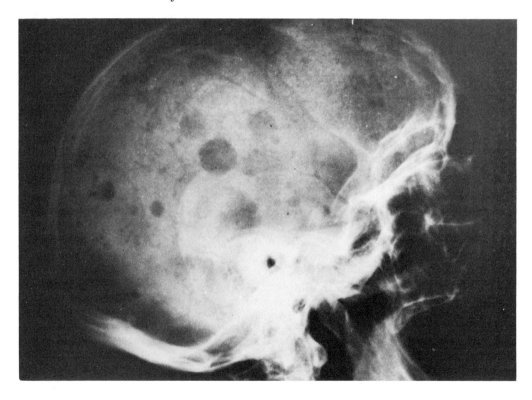

Figure 41-18 Lateral skull radiograph. Multiple regular, well-defined lucencies due to multiple myelomatosis.

Reticulum cell sarcomas are less common; they may give rise to diffuse intra-cranial mass lesions (microgliomatosis) producing headache, early personality change, seizures, dementia, and focal signs according to the areas involved.

Myeloma

The apparently well-demarcated or "punched-out" holes in the skull seen on some x-rays are usually due to venous lakes, but sometimes multiple translucent areas are due to secondary carcinoma or to multiple myeloma. Myelomatosis causes head-ache resulting from skull invasion (Fig. 41-18). Paraparesis or radicular pain may result from spinal collapse with compression of the cord or cauda equina. Multiple myeloma may be associated with the nonmetastatic syndromes of malignancy described later. Occlusive cerebrovascular disease, herpes zoster, seizures, cere-bellar ataxia, and uni- or bilateral carpal tunnel syndromes (probably here because of the presence of a paraproteinemia with abnormal protein deposition in the tissues) are less common manifestations.

MANAGEMENT

When you suspect an intracranial tumor on the basis of progressive functional dis-ability with or without localizing signs, or on the basis of evidence of raised intra-cranial pressure, refer the patient at once to a neurological center. Here, the investigations with the highest yield are the CT scan, x-rays of the chest and skull, and perimetry. Brain scan, EEG, and arteriography are useful screening tests.

Treatment is usually surgical if the tumor is at all accessible, followed in most cases by radiotherapy. The use of metronidazole as a radiosensitizer is under study. Chemotherapy is seldom of value, although the nitrosoureas are being test-ed in conjunction with radiation. Even in the most malignant cases, reduction in intracranial pressure can be effected using steroids, and a biopsy can be taken, at least to prove the diagnosis and to allow histological grading. A lumbar puncture with examination of CSF is dangerous (it may precipitate coning) and usually tells one little more than that the CSF pressure is raised and the protein level elevated. With a Millipore filter, malignant cells might be identified, but this is seldom done outside those major centers to which the patient must be referred anyway. Meth-ods of reducing raised intracranial pressure are described in Chapter 16.

NONMETASTATIC MANIFESTATIONS OF MALIGNANCY

Diffuse Polioencephalopathy

A clinical picture resembling encephalitis may be seen with carcinoma of the lung. Dementia, an amnestic syndrome, lability of mood, seizures, pyramidal weakness, and blindness are the main features.

Subacute cerebellar cortical degeneration caused by a diffuse loss of Purkinje cells causes progressive ataxia, while concurrent brainstem involvement leads to drowsiness, oculomotor palsies, vertigo, and dysarthria.

Metabolic Encephalopathy

With some tumors, hypercalcemia, hyperadrenalism, hypoglycemia, or hyperviscosity states may result in a diffuse encephalopathy. Each can be diagnosed clinically or biochemically by the usual features of these conditions because the nonmetastatic form mimics that resulting from primary endocrinopathy.

Raised levels of adrenal hormones lead to the usual signs of Cushing's syndrome, while the cerebral and muscular syndrome of hypercalcemia is the same as that seen with hyperparathyroidism. Hypoglycemia is more common with sarcoma than with other malignant tumors.

The syndrome of inappropriate secretion of antidiuretic hormone is best known in association with a carcinoma of the bronchus but also occurs after head injuries, with cerebral tumors and abscesses, and as a complication of the Guillain-Barré syndrome. Anorexia, nausea, and vomiting are the usual initial features, while later, when the serum sodium concentration has fallen below 125 mmol/L, delirium, seizures and coma supervene. In all such cases the serum sodium level is low but urinary excretion is high — the urine may be hypertonic with respect to the serum. Treatment is by fluid restriction, but successful treatment of the underlying disease is necessary for permanent relief.

Myelopathy

In some patients presenting with a combination of upper and lower motor neuron lesions, an underlying malignancy is found. Although the clinical features may be typical of motor neuron disease, the neurological course may be more benign than in the usual form and the symptoms may continue for years. A subacute necrotic myelopathy with a more rapid progression is also described. The clinical picture is that of an isolated severe transverse myelitis.

Neuropathy

A mixed sensory and motor polyneuropathy is often found among patients with terminal malignancy. The cause is unknown, but nutritional deficiency may be responsible. A pure sensory neuropathy sometimes complicates carcinoma of the bronchus. It is due to degeneration of the dorsal root ganglion cells, and it causes numbness and paresthesia, sensory ataxia, areflexia, and clumsiness.

Lymphomas associated with paraproteinemia may cause a demyelinating sensorimotor polyneuropathy. The many drugs, such as antineoplastic agents, that cause neuropathy are listed in Chapter 43.

Tumors that alter the patient's metabolic, endocrine, or nutritional status may induce secondary neuropathies as well; thus cachexia and prolonged bed rest are likely to lead to compression of the ulnar and common peroneal nerves.

Disorders of Muscle and of the Myoneural Junction

A *diffuse myopathy* with wasting is common in the late stages of malignancy. Its specific etiology is not known.

The *myasthenic syndrome* is usually associated with a bronchogenic carcinoma. The patients complain of weakness and fatigability in their legs, blurring of vision, and dry mouth. Bulbar symptoms, diplopia, and ptosis are unusual. The characteristic finding on examination is weak muscle contraction which becomes stronger

Table 41-4   Classification of Nonmetastatic Carcinomatous Neurological Disease

---

Encephalopathy

    Progressive multifocal leukoencephalopathy

    Diffuse polioencephalopathy
        with mental symptoms
        subacute cerebellar degeneration
        brainstem lesions

    Metabolic, endocrine, or nutritional encephalopathy
        hypercalcemia
        hyperadrenalism
        hypoglycemia
        inappropriate secretion of ADH
        hyperviscosity states (macroglobulinemia)

Myelopathy

    Chronic myelopathy simulating motor neuron disease

    Subacute necrotic myelopathy

    Nutritional myelopathy

Neuropathy

    Sensory neuropathy with dorsal column degeneration

    Peripheral sensorimotor neuropathy

    Metabolic, endocrine, and nutritional neuropathies

Disorders of muscle and myoneural junction

    Generalized myopathy

    Disorders of neuromuscular transmission
        myasthenic syndrome
        myasthenia gravis

    Polymyositis and dermatomyositis

    Metabolic myopathies (secondary to hyperadrenalism,
        hypercalcemia, hyperthyroidism, etc.)

---

with repeated exercise, although with prolonged use, the muscles become weaker again. On the EMG the initial action potential size is reduced, but subsequent stimuli evoke increasingly large action potentials, which only later diminish. These patients often respond temporarily to oral guanidine hydrochloride.

Myasthenia gravis is associated with a thymoma in many cases, particularly in males with a later onset of the disease. In such cases, the prognosis is poorer than in young women with myasthenia gravis who usually have thymic hyperplasia.

Polymyositis and *dermatomyositis* are associated with neoplasms in half of all cases over the age of 50 years. The response to therapy in these patients is poor compared with that seen in polymyositis unassociated with malignancy.

Proximal myopathies may occur because of metabolic or endocrine problems that result from some tumors. If the specific abnormality (hyperadrenalism, hyper-calcemia, hyperthyroidism) can be corrected, the myopathy improves.

Vascular Disease

Vascular complications of many carcinomas include arterial and venous thrombo-embolic disease that may be due to polycythemia, nonbacterial thrombotic endo-carditis, or consumption coagulopathy. All of these have potential for causing CNS disease.

BIBLIOGRAPHY

Duffy, P.E. *Tumors of the Nervous System.* Philadelphia, F.A. Davis Co., 1976.

Henson, R.A., Urich, H. *Cancer and the Nervous System.* Oxford, Blackwell Scientific, 1982.

Spillane, J.A., Kendall, B.E., Moseley, I.F. Cerebral lymphoma; Clinical and Radiological correlations. *J. Neurol. Neurosurg. Psychiatry* 45:199–208, 1982.

Thompson, R.A., Green, J.R. (eds.). *Neoplasia in the Central Nervous System.* New York, Raven Press, 1976.

42
Neurological Complications of Systemic Disease

HEPATIC DISEASE

In *acute hepatocellular failure* the most common neurological findings are confusion, with generalized hyperreflexia and signs of organic brain dysfunction (see Chap. 11) progressing rapidly to coma and brain death. Liver function tests are wildly abnormal. These symptoms result from increased CSF levels of ammonia and glutamine, from compeition for receptor sites on adrenergic neurons by "false" neurotransmitters not cleared by the liver, and from anoxia (Fig. 21-1). After some time, liver stores of glycogen will be greatly diminished, so hypoglycemia may exacerbate the encephalopathy. This acute delirium occurs in acute hepatic failure caused by toxic or viral hepatitis and may be worsened if excessive ADH is produced.

With portocaval shunts, either developing spontaneously in portal hypertension or created surgically, a picture of chronic *portosystemic encephalopathy* may be seen. It is not always detectable when mild because only the highest intellectual and emotional functions may be impaired. Patients with a high level of intelligence may complain of difficulties in concentration and in various intellectual functions such as decision making and judgment. The attention span is much reduced. As the condition progresses, former traits of personality may be accentuated and disorders of sleep rhythm occur. Emotions tend to be labile; euphoria, and later, apathy and inertia supervene. The patient's writing becomes ill-formed and one of the best clinical means of following the metabolic disorder of chronic liver disease is to have the patient draw simple designs such as stars or a maze to demonstrate this apraxia.

Neurological signs include the subacute development of *dysarthria, dysphasia,* and a flapping *tremor* with brief, almost twitching movements of the fingers and wrists known as *asterixis.* There may be a slow rhythmic tremor in the extended arms. *Myoclonus,* and very infrequently *epileptic seizures,* may occur. *Parkinsonism, cerebellar signs,* and evidence of *corticospinal tract* involvement occur at a

529

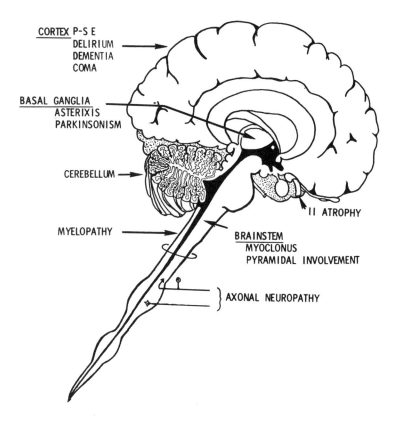

Figure 42-1   Neurological involvement in hepatic disease.

late stage. The plantar responses are frequently normal until the patient has a definitely diminished level of consciousness. The EEG may show reduction in frequency
of cortical rhythms and triphasic waves, and this again is a useful and almost immediate test in the day-to-day supervision of the patient's clinical state, because
abnormalities occur even when clinical signs are minimal.

   Wilson's disease is described in Chapter 46. Chronic peripheral *neuropathies*
of the demyelinating type occur in patient's with long-standing hepatic dysfunction,
but those caused by related factors, such as chronic alcoholism, are much more
common.

   A *myelopathy* has been described in patients with liver disease, particularly
those who have had portocaval shunting. These patients may also develop ataxia,
spastic paraplegia, dementia, and choreoathetosis. In *hemochromatosis* recurrent
encephalopathy with added brainstem signs have been described and probably result from raised serum ammonia levels.

   The pathological changes in the nervous system in liver disease include a loss
of neurons in the basal ganglia, cortex, and cerebellum, and an unusual increase in
the number and size of astrocytes in these areas.

RENAL DISEASE

Patients with kidney diseases of acute onset, such as acute glomerulonephritis, may
develop neurological syndromes because of the accompanying hypertension. In

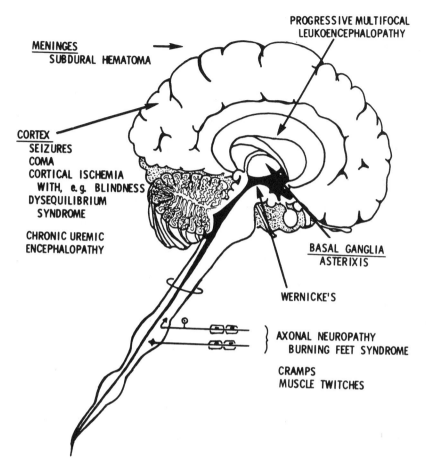

Figure 42-2   Neurological involvement in renal disease.

chronic renal disease however, a state of persistent failure of excretion of metabolic products gives rise to a number of more specific syndromes; others are associated with dialysis (Fig. 42-2).

The acute rise in blood pressure and marked fluid retention occurring in acute
renal failure may cause *raised intracranial pressure* because of cerebral edema. In
this acute phase, intracranial vascular spasm may lead to cortical blindness, and
the severe features of untreated chronic uremic encephalopathy (see the next
paragraph) may also appear. Since this is really a form of hypertensive encephalopathy, management will be directed toward reduction in blood pressure and restoration of artificial or natural renal function.

Chronic uremic encephalopathy is another complication. Diminished
awareness, shortened attention span, slurred speech, and apathy mark its onset,
but untreated it progresses to agitated delirium with tremor, asterixis, multifocal
myoclonic jerks, and eventually grand mal or focal motor seizures and coma. Accumulation of toxic organic acids has been suggested as the mechanism of this condition. Dialysis usually reverses it.

In chronic renal disease, *peripheral neuropathy,* which begins as an axonal type
but leads on to segmental demyelination, is extremely common; in fact, the nerve
conduction speed has been used as an index of the adequacy of dialysis in patients

with chronic renal failure. The symptoms are of chronic, distal, symmetric senso-rimotor neuropathy with mild diminution of sensation over the feet accompanied by diminution or loss of ankle reflexes and moderate peripheral weakness and mus-cle wasting.

The *burning feet syndrome* presents as distressing hyperesthesia with a burning sensation in the feet and lower leg. The patients dislike wearing socks or even hav-ing bed clothes touch their legs. If it is severe, they may refuse to walk. Adequate dialysis and treatment with B vitamins including pantothenic acid is sometimes ef-fective. This treatment also protects against the effects of thiamine deficiency (Wernicke's encephalopathy), which can be induced by dialysis. Such patients also suffer from *muscle cramps* and *twitching,* perhaps because of hypocalcemia in asso-ciation with phosphate retention, and the *restless legs syndrome* and *pressure palsies* from prolonged recumbency. Additional causes of neuropathy in uremic patients include diabetes, amyloidosis, collagen-vascular diseases, and myeloma. Aminogly-cosides, penicillin, and nitrofurantoin, often given to patients with kidney disease, are toxic causes.

If hemodialysis proceeds too quickly in a patient with a long-standing high urea level, then the cerebral urea level may remain high even though the plasma level is reduced by dialysis. The osmotic gradient produced may cause fluid to enter the brain producing raised intracranial pressure and seizures — the *dysequilibrium syn-drome.* After dialysis, symptoms such as faintness, dizziness, or asthenia are usu-ally due to hypotension and zinc and sodium depletion.

In patients on chronic dialysis, an irreversible syndrome of hesitant, stuttering speech disturbance (both dysarthria and dysphasia), gait disorder, myoclonus, sei-zures, and dementia signify the presence of *dialysis encephalopathy.* In this condi-tion, the EEG is always abnormal. Chronic aluminum toxicity has been suggested as the cause; proof is awaited.

Patients on dialysis therapy are also liable to *other CNS complications* includ-ing subarachnoid hemorrhage, ischemic infarcts, central pontine myelinolysis, and subdural hematomas, which must always be remembered in uremic patients who show alteration of personality of conscious level or who develop other neurological signs. Secondary hyperparathyroidism leads to bone pain and myopathy, mainly af-fecting the pelvic girdle.

Patients immunosuppressed after renal transplants are at increased risk of op-portunistic fungal and viral infections, of reticulum cell sarcoma (cerebral micro-gliomatosis), and of the slow virus disease, progressive multifocal leukoencepha-lopathy (Chap. 40).

THYROID DISEASE

Hyperthyroidism

There is an association between hyperthyroidism and both *myasthenia gravis* and *periodic paralysis* (Chap. 45). Patients with hyperthyroidism tend to be irritable, overactive, and anxious; they sometimes have a short attention span. An increased frequency of seizures and choreiform movements are both described in hyperthy-roidism, as are psychotic illnesses. In acute thyroid crisis, hyperthermia and coma may occur. Other mental changes range from anxiety and hyperactivity to psycho-sis (Fig. 42-3). Most of the physical signs of hyperthyroidism are those of excessive discharge and can be temporarily reduced by beta-blocking agents.

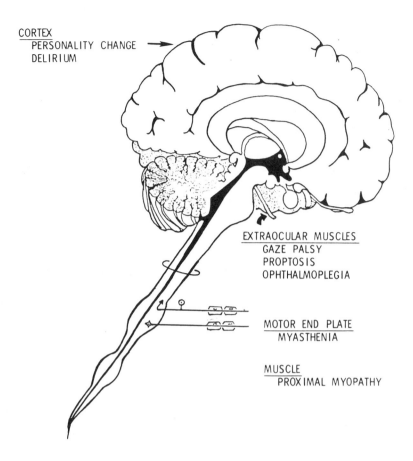

CORTEX
PERSONALITY CHANGE →
DELIRIUM

EXTRAOCULAR MUSCLES
GAZE PALSY
PROPTOSIS
OPHTHALMOPLEGIA

MOTOR END PLATE
MYASTHENIA

MUSCLE
PROXIMAL MYOPATHY

Figure 42-3   Neurological involvement in hyperthyroidism.

Three other features are found among these patients.

1. A fine rapid finger *tremor* is seen when the arms are outstretched, very much like the physiological tremor that occurs in many normal people, particularly when anxious. In this condition however, the hands will be warm rather than cold, with bounding pulses and increased sweating; *hyperreflexia* is also common.
2. Proximal weakness and wasting of muscles is common and is particularly noticed in the shoulder and pelvic girdles. This *thyrotoxic myopathy* is described in Chapter 45.
3. Limitation of upward gaze is the first of the *external ocular movements* to be affected in hyperthyroidism; later, proptosis, sometimes diplopia, and a failure of convergence and of conjugate movement of the eyes in other directions may occur. There may be chemosis of the eyelids. The eventual ophthalmoplegia may be marked. Occasionally papilledema is seen.

Hypothyroidism

Hypothyroidism is often accompanied by *pseudomyotonia,* best shown by the slow contraction and relaxation phases of the ankle reflex when it is elicited with the patient kneeling. Pseudomyotonia is not due to electrical abnormality of the muscle fibers but to mechanical difficulties affecting the ease with which the muscle filaments slide beside each other. *Organic mental changes* suggesting mild dementia or depression are frequent. *Decreased hearing* is common and is often mistaken for dementia. In advanced cases, *coma* with hypothermia may occur (Fig. 42-4). Because of some depression of pituitary function and the tendency to cerebral edema as the patients are warmed, treatment should begin with rapid warming of the patient up to 30°C, going on to *slow* rewarming when that temperature is achieved. Only steroids and very small doses of thyroxine should be employed and an ECG monitor utilized. Because such patients frequently secrete ADH inappropriately, IV fluids must be given only with great caution.

A slight to moderate increase in the *CSF protein* level is common in hypothyroidism.

Peripheral neuropathy is also recognized. The most common form is compression of the median nerve in the carpal tunnel. Symptoms of thyroid dysfunction must be sought in all patients with this syndrome. Some also have a mild symmetric peripheral neuropathy and complain of paresthesia in the legs and hands.

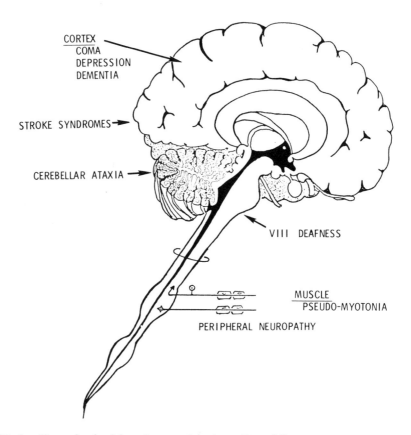

Figure 42-4   Neurological involvement in hypothyroidism.

The development of atherosclerosis is probably accelerated in patients with hypothyroidism, and another cause is morbidity in such patients therefore is *cerebrovascular accident.* Hypothyroidism is also associated with a previous history of hyperthyroidism and thus with pernicious anemia, myasthenia gravis, rheumatoid arthritis, carcinoma of the stomach, or diabetes mellitus, all of which have direct or indirect effects on the nervous system as well.

ADRENAL GLAND

In *hypoadrenocorticalism,* drop attacks, decreased energy, and generalized muscle wasting and weakness are common, but organic psychoses, memory deficits, and so on are rare. *Cushing's disease* is associated with alterations in personality, chronic tiredness, irritability, and sometimes paranoia. Proximal myopathies in Cushing's syndrome are uncommon and may be due to hypokalemia.

Seizures may be more frequent in these patients, probably in association with sodium and water retention. Pseudotumor has also been described. Although this may also occur with the use of steroids, it more commonly presents when they are withdrawn. If the fluorinated steroids are prescribed proximal *myopathy* may result.

Primary hyperaldosteronism may result in metabolic alkalosis with tetany or flaccid muscle weakness. Paroxysmal hypertension from a *pheochromocytoma* may be seen in association with neurofibromatosis or tuberous sclerosis: headache is a leading symptom.

FLUID AND ELECTROLYTE DISTURBANCES

Hyponatremia

Hyponatremia results in generalized apathy with weakness, headache, and sometimes delirium and coma. Muscle cramps are frequent complaints in the early stages. In an acute form, seizures and reduced conscious levels result from overhydration in association with the low serum sodium concentration.

A serum Na^+ less than 125 mmol/L may occur in cardiac failure, hepatic cirrhosis, cachectic states, and in the inappropriate ADH secretion syndrome. It may also complicate K^+ depletion and hypoglycemia, as well as treatment with barbiturates, thiazides, clofibrate, antineoplastic drugs, and acetaminophen. Central pontine myelinolysis (Chap. 48) is a possible complication of prolonged hyponatremia.

Hypernatremia

In infants given the wrong formulas or patients given hypertonic saline solutions intravenously, hypernatremia may occur leading to water retention with initial irritability and later delirium, seizures, and coma.

Hypokalemia

Hypokalemia is associated with ECG changes (ST segment depression, prominent U waves, and reduction in the amplitude of the T wave*) and *flaccid weakness* and hyporeflexia in the limbs. Reduction in consciousness is uncommon unless the

---

*No pot, no tea!

serum level is extremely low. The sudden onset of hypokalemia may result from the administration of potassium-losing drugs, particularly antihypertensives, and one must be aware that patients presenting with a picture resembling the Guillain-Barré syndrome (ascending bilateral motor weakness and hyporeflexia) may have a hypokalemic myopathy, rather than a postinfectious neuropathy.

Hyperkalemia

A similar flaccid muscle *weakness* may be seen in hyperkalemia, but the *cardiac changes* (decreased strength of contraction, arrhythmias, cardiac arrest) and ECG findings such as peaked T waves and QRS and PR prolongation assist in making the diagnosis.

Hypercalcemia

Forty percent of patients with raised serum calcium levels have neurological signs. Calcium maintains selective cell membrane permeability and controls the release of acetylcholine at ganglia and at end-plate. It is also concerned in sarcoplasmic contraction and appears to stabilize the membrane potential. The clinical features of hypercalcemia are largely mental or muscular.* The mental features are those of *encephalopathy* with headache, lethargy, drowsiness, delirium, hallucinatory states, cerebellar signs, and occasionally coma. *Muscle weakness,* mainly proximal, with reduction in tone and either increased or decreased reflexes may be seen, whereas wasting may occur at a late state. *Autonomic* involvement produces constipation and dysphagia. Nausea, vomiting, anorexia, and peripheral paresthesia are common. These patients may also have a slightly raised CSF *protein* level. Polydipsia and polyuria are commonly associated. Similar features occur with hyperparathyroidism.

Hypocalcemia

Symptoms are uncommon in hypocalcemia before the calcium level has fallen below 60-70 mmol/L (assuming the serum albumin level to be normal). When they occur, numbness, paresthesia, and weakness are the first symptoms but the later the later syndrome is mainly cerebromuscular. *Mental* fatigue, hypochondriasis, headaches, depression, and irritability (all sometimes presenting together as a retarded state mimicking dementia) may be seen. The dentate nuclei and basal ganglia may calcify but this seldom produces symptoms. Occasionally epileptic *seizures,* increased *intracranial pressure,* or x-ray evidence of *basilar impression* are found.

Neurologic signs include tetany with carpopedal spasms, cramps, and positive Chvostek's or Trousseaus's signs (Table 42-1). Chvostek's sign is facial muscle contraction on tapping over the facial nerve branches anterior to the ear. Trousseau's signs is a tetanic spasm of the hand muscles when the arm is made ischemic by inflating a blood pressure cuff. Spasm and contraction of the respiratory, laryngeal, and pharyngeal muscles may cause dyspnea, choking, stridor, and painful dysphagia. *Cataracts* may also occur. A *myopathy* often complicates hypoparathyroidism.

------

*"Stones, bones, and groans."

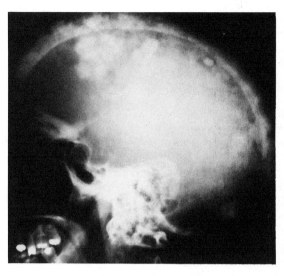 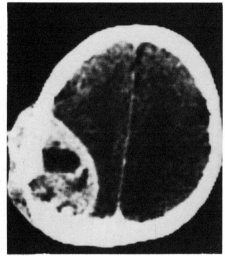

A   **B**

Figure 42-5   (A) Lateral radiograph of skull; Paget's disease, with the typical fluffy outline of the bones of the calvarium. (B) CT scan of the same patient. A sarcoma arises from the diseased skull bones.

Table 42-1   Causes of Tetany

Hypocalcemia
Low Ca^{2+} intake
Increased loss from GI tract
Increased loss in urine
Increased serum phosphorus
Hypomagnesemia
Alkalosis
Respiratory
Metabolic

PAGET'S DISEASE

The enlarged, softened bones in Paget's disease are responsible for most of its neurological complications (Fig. 42-5A, B). Bilateral compression of the *eighth nerve* is the most common of these, leading of course to deafness, while softening of the bones of the skull leads to *platybasia* with direct compression of the cerebellum, brainstem, and cord or vascular compression. Whichever obtains, the result is a syndrome of bulbar palsy with cerebellar features. At a lower level, the vertebral abnormalities cause low-back pain and further compression of the lumbar roots. Neurological signs occur in over half the patients with this condition.

ACID-BASE DISTURBANCES

In the presence of a low level of ionized calcium, excessive neuromuscular irritability can lead to seizures (grand mal or myoclonic), tinnitus, facial or distal paresthesias, tetany, or fasciculations. An absolutely reduced serum calcium concentration and both respiratory and metabolic alkalosis may all produce a low level of ionized calcium. *Respiratory* alkalosis is caused by overbreathing for any reason including anxiety, salicylate poisoning, brainstem disease, or pulmonary diffusion defects. It may also result from excessive mechanical ventilation. *Metabolic alkalosis* occurs with excessive intake of alkalis, loss of gastric acidity, and with severe hypokalemia, which causes excessive loss of hydrogen ions by the kidney.

Acidosis, again both respiratory and metabolic, may produce neurological features, but in different ways. *Respiratory acidosis* is due to carbon dioxide retention and is almost always a result of ventilatory failure. Carbon dioxide narcosis may develop rapidly but usually a rise in intracranial pressure occurs because of cerebral vasodilation, leading to headache, drowsiness, asterixis, subacute delirium, and at a late stage, coma. *Metabolic acidosis* has many causes, chiefly diabetes and acute or chronic renal failure. Again, delirium and coma are seen as a late result but without any rise in intracranial pressure.

It is most unusual however for any patient to present with *pure* signs of acid-base disturbance in the nervous system, particularly in the case of acidosis because other disturbances involving fluid and electrolytes are usually found, such as diabetes, renal failure, liver disease, or respiratory disorders. The picture is thus often mixed and confusing. It is not common to see confused patients in general hospital wards in whom four or five possible causes can be incriminated as contributing to their delirious state.

DISORDERS OF MAGNESIUM

Low serum magnesium levels produce symptoms rather like those of low calcium, including seizures, neuronal irritability, fasciculations, and athetosis. Peripherally, the manifestation is commonly tetany with a normal serum calcium concentration. More centrally, tremors, delirium, and depression may result. High serum magnesium levels result in drowsiness, hypotonia, decreased reflexes, and neuromuscular blockade.

HYPOGLYCEMIA

The effect of progressive reduction in blood sugar is similar to that of progressive hypoxia. Early psychological and cortical signs are replaced by evidence of subcortical dysfunction, as there ensues a depression of the nervous system at progressively lower levels.

The initial psychological symptoms include hunger, headache, malaise, and anxiety, coupled with alterations of personality and behavior. Cortical depression gives rise to restlessness and confusion, drowsiness, focal neurological signs such as dysphasia, and cortical blindness. Further cortical and subcortical depression, particularly frontal, results in sucking and grasping responses, and later stupor or coma with muscular twitching and focal or generalized seizures. When the mesencephalon is affected, tonic spasms or decerebrate rigidity with Babinski's signs supervene. In the final stages, medullary depression results in loss of brainstem reflexes. Patients who are treated with intravenous sugar will recover these functions in reverse order.

Patients with repeated hypoglycemic attacks may show evidence of mild chronic anterior horn cell damage, giving rise to a syndrome resembling progressive muscular atrophy and fasciculations and wasting of muscles, dementia, or seizures.

DISEASES OF THE CHEST

Chronic obstructive lung diseases are commonly associated with chronic and acute-on-chronic increase in pCO_2. Since CO_2 is a potent intracranial vasodilator, intracranial pressure will be increased. Initial symptoms of clouded consciousness, anxiety, and headache lead to a subacute delirium and eventual coma. In later stages, myoclonus and a flapping tremor much like that seen with chronic hepatic encephalopathy may occur. Papilledema is a *late* sign of CO_2 retention.

Lung abscesses and *bronchiectasis* may predispose to intracranial abscess formation. The effects of *carcinoma* of the lung on the nervous system are considered in Chapter 41.

VITAMIN DEFICIENCY SYNDROMES

Deficiency in vitamin A is said to cause night blindness and reduction in the sense of smell.

It is very unusual to get isolated deficiency of any one of the B group vitamins, with the exception of vitamin B_{12} (discussed later under Pernicious Anemia). Thiamine, nicotinamide, folic acid, riboflavin, pyridoxine, and pantothenic acid deficiencies usually occur together. In many instances however, there is more evidence of thiamine deficiency than of the other B vitamins.

Dry *beriberi* is a peripheral neuropathy due to thiamine deficiency and is distinguished from wet beriberi by the absence of cardiomyopathy and peripheral edema. The *neuropathy* in all forms of vitamin B deficiency is of chronic peripheral sensorimotor type with primary axonal damage and secondary demyelination. The *burning feet syndrome* may occur with a deficiency of pyridoxine and/or pantothenic acid (mentioned earlier).

Deficiency of all the B vitamins, but especially of niacin and pantothenic acid, is responsible for the syndrome of *pellagra* (derived from the Italian words for rough skin). The systems involved include the peripheral nerves, spinal cord, brain, skin, and gastrointestinal tract. Corticospinal tract and dorsal root ganglion cell involvement lead to a pyramidal syndrome and a sensory neuropathy. Retrobulbar neuritis may also occur. Patients with pellagra sometimes are demented but delirium or depression are more common. The clinical picture may closely resemble that of Friedreich's ataxia.

The *Wernicke-Korsakoff syndrome* is described in Chapter 43.

A lack of vitamin D produces rickets with bone deformity, tenderness, swelling, and myopathy. The hypocalcemia is probably responsible for tetany and the increased frequency of seizures. The same findings occur in hypoparathyroidism. A syndrome of retinitis, tongue fasciculations, sensory loss with areflexia, limb ataxia, disturbed gait, and abnormal SEPs has been attributed to vitamin E deficiency. We have never spotted it.

CARDIOVASCULAR DISEASE

Neurologists and cardiologists have very frequent interaction, not only through the medium of strokes, but because of many other vascular problems. Many patients with muscle diseases develop a cardiomyopathy: hypertension is responsible for some cerebrovascular catastrophies; ECG changes are seen in many electrolyte disturbances and intracranial lesions; and similar drugs are used by both specialists. Important neurological aspects of cardiac disease include the following.

Hypertensive Encephalopathy

If blood pressure is severely and persistently elevated, the resulting combination of intracranial arteriospasm and cerebral edema sometimes induces reversible focal and general ischemic damage leading to severe headaches with decrease in consciousness, visual disturbances, papilledema, fundal hemorrhages, and seizures. This syndrome can complicate malignant hypertension, eclampsia, and acute nephritis. The pathogenesis is most likely a failure of cerebral autoregulation in the face of a rapid and severe rise in blood pressure. Urgent reduction of the pressure is essential. Sodium nitroprusside or diazoxide intravenously are the most favored agents employed to achieve the goal of a diastolic pressure of 100 mmHg, any greater reduction being likely to cause further cerebral ischemia.

Myocarditis

Many bacteria and all viruses and fungi that cause myocarditis may also affect skeletal muscle. Autoallergic disease may cause myocarditis and varying neurological syndromes. Toxic myocarditis caused by arsenic, alcohol, and porphyria may be accompanied by neurological disease.

Cardiomyopathy

The myocardium may be infiltrated by amyloid, sarcoid, or glycogen deposits as may peripheral muscle or nerve. In Friedreich's ataxia, myotonic dystrophy, Duchennes dystrophy, and periodic paralysis, cardiac involvement is common. Alcoholic cardiomyopathy and neurological disease frequently coexist. Recently a mild or subclinical myopathy has been identified in patients with hypertrophic subaortic stenosis.

Fits or Faints

Acute reduction in available cerebral blood flow may be due to problems in the *primer* (postural hypotension, acute blood loss, and shock), the *pump* (cardiac arrhythmias, myocardial infarction), or the *pathway* (cardiomyopathy, subaortic or aortic stenosis, mitral stenosis, atrial mass lesions, coarctation, arterial stenosis, or occlusion), or to a reduction in the oxygen-carrying capacity of the *blood*. Seizures may complicate hypertension and dissection of the aorta. The subject of faints is discussed in Chapter 10.

ECG Changes

Ninety percent of patients with Duchenne's dystrophy and many with myotonic dystrophy have significant changes. Subarachnoid hemorrhage frequently produces U waves and nonspecific ST-segment changes. Symmetric T-wave inversion is also common and is possibly due to myocardial sympathetic stimulation. In Friedreich's ataxia, small-vessel disease in the branches of the coronary arteries leads to true myocardial ischemia and fibrosis with typical ECG changes.

Cardiac Surgery

Neurological changes follow cardiac surgery in up to a third of the patients. The most common are focal signs caused by embolism (hemiparesis, hemisensory deficits), cognitive problems, brachial plexopathy and Horner's syddrome, and peripheral nerve pressure palsies.

Polycythemia

Polycythemia is associated with an increased prevalence of stroke, headache, and brainstem symptoms such as tinnitus and vertigo. Venous infarctions also occur, and complaints of limb pain may be due to reduced venous flow as well.

Miscellaneous

Following myocardial infarction or in association with other intrathoracic or cervical diseases, reflex sympathetic dystrophy may occur *(the shoulder-hand syndrome)* manifested by shoulder pain and stiffness, swelling, and pallor of the hand. X-rays show osteoporosis of the hand bones and sometimes changes of calcific tendonitis at the shoulder. *Bacterial endocarditis* is considered in Chapter 40.

Propranolol, phenytoin, quinidine, procainamide, potassium, and calcium are just a few of the chemical agents and *drugs* used in neurology that have a direct effect on the heart.

GASTROINTESTINAL DISEASE

Pernicious Anemia

This is a state of vitamin B_{12} deficiency characterized by macrocytic anemia, megaloblastic hyperplasia of the bone marrow, gastric achlorhydria, and in the late stages, by subacute combined degeneration of the spinal cord. It was originally labeled "pernicious" because it was progressively debilitating and ultimately fatal before the discovery of ways of providing vitamin B_{12}.

Vitamin B_{12}, containing cobalt, functions as a coenzyme in nucleoprotein synthesis. A deficiency usually occurs because of a lack of intrinsic factor in normal gastric juices that promotes the transfer of vitamin B_{12} across the intestinal mucosa.

Rarely, pernicious anemia may result from a dietary deficiency of vitamin B_{12} and this has been reported in strict vegetarians (Fig. 42-6). It may also be seen in the "blind-loop syndrome" as a result of gastric surgery, in which it may result from abnormal bacterial growth in a loop of small intestine, impairing utilization of B_{12}. Pernicious anemia has also resulted from total gastrectomy, malabsorption syndromes, fish tapeworm infestation, and chronic use of tetracycline and colchicine.

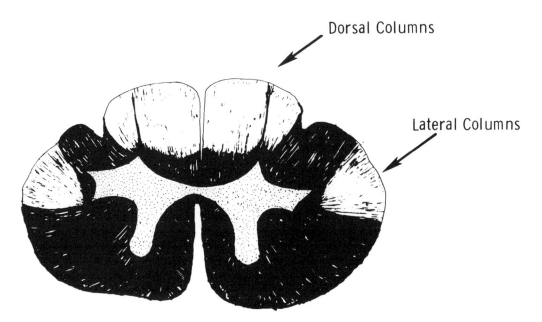

Figure 42-6   T/S thoracic cord. Demyelination in fasciculus gracilus and cortico-spinal tract on each side. Pernicious anemia. (Diagrammatic.)

Pernicious anemia occurs in all races. A family history of the same condition, of thyroid disease, or of rheumatoid arthritis can be obtained in 20 to 30 percent of cases. Although it *may* occur in young adults, onset is *usually* in later adult life.

Early symptoms include insidiously increasing weakness, anorexia, tongue sore-ness, and a yellowish skin color. Some patients complain of diarrhea and of abdomi-nal cramps. Eventually there supervenes a severe anemia which itself causes few symptoms. Neurological features usually develop at the same time but occasional-ly come on before the hematological abnormalities appear.

The neurological complications of pernicious anemia include *subacute com-bined degeneration of the cord, peripheral neuropathy, dementia,* and *optic atrophy.* The first symptoms are usually related to the axonal neuropathy with numbness, tingling, and burning in the feet and legs, with loss of vibration and position sense, and a positive Romberg's sign on examination. Further evidence of dorsal column involvement may include a positive Lhermitte's sign.

Involvement of the corticospinal tracts leads to weakness and stiffness in the legs, so gait may be both spastic and ataxic. The deep reflexes are decreased or absent because of the peripheral neuropathy but the plantar responses are usually extensor because of the pyramidal tract involvement.

Mental changes include confusion, irritability, memory loss, depression, and paranoid ideation. Slowly progressive dementia is sometimes seen, occasionally as the presenting problem.

Optic nerve involvement may include a retrobulbar neuritis with reduction in visual acuity and perhaps a centrocecal scotoma. It is thought that vitamin B_{12} deficiency will not alone cause optic atrophy, only in combination with tobacco smoking. It also has been noted that in tobacco amblyopia without pernicious anemia, defective absorption is the cause of the reduced serum levels of vitamin B_{12} observed.

The specific test for vitamin B_{12} deficiency is the measurement of serum levels. A Schilling test measures the patient's ability to absorb the vitamins. The most accurate test is the measurement of hepatic deposition of cobalt 57, but this takes a week to perform.

A blood smear will usually show macrocytes, and the bone marrow will how megaloblastic hyperplasia. In some instances, the peripheral blood smear is normal, although the bone marrow will still show megaloblasts. The achlorhydria can be detected by gastric aspiration with histamine stimulation.

To replace depleted body stores and maintain normal B_{12} levels, the patient is given 100 μg of vitamin B_{12} daily for 2 weeks, after which 100 μg IM monthly is sufficient.

The blood picture should return to normal within 4 to 8 weeks and the neurological symptoms begin to clear within the first month, continuing to improve over many months. Residua occur only in those whose neurological signs went untreated for a prolonged period.

The patient must understand the importance of maintenance therapy. All too often, patients are lost to follow-up because they feel fine and cannot see the need for continued injections, especially since they have had no symptoms after missing a few; only to present with further neurological difficulties many months or years later. Periodic upper gastrointestinal barium studies are important because carcinoma of the stomach is more common in patients with pernicious anemia.

Malabsorption Syndromes

The many vitamin and mineral deficiencies resulting from *adult celiac disease* may lead to a host of neurological problems, apart from B_{12} and the other deficiencies described previously. Loss of calcium causes osteomalacia with platybasia and tetany. Peripheral neuropathy and cortical, posterior column, cerebellar, and cord lesions are also described, as are depression and other mental symptoms, although their mechanism is not known.

In *Whipple's disease,* dementia, myoclonus, seizures, and gaze palsies are recognized, an important fact since the dementia may improve with antibiotic therapy.

PORPHYRIA

The porphyrias are a heterogenous group of diseases characterized by the excretion of porphyrins in the urine or stools. The type of greatest interest from a neurological point of view is acute intermittent porphyria, and our discussion will center around that.

Acute Intermittent Porphyria

The important finding in this illness is not the excretion of porphyrins but of large amounts of delta-aminolevulinic acid (dALA) and of porphobilinogen (PBG). The nature of the underlying defect is still uncertain however, because the substances present in excessive amounts are not in themselves toxic. The disease is inherited as an autosomal-dominant trait (Fig. 42-7), and presents in one of three ways: neurological, psychiatric, or acute abdominal. The *neurological* complications include a demyelinating peripheral neuropathy and vascular changes in the brain.

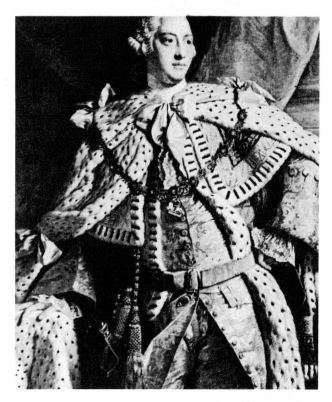

Figure 42-7   His late Majesty, King George III of England, a victim of porphyria and its attendant episodes of mental dysfunction.

The patients sometimes complain of limb pains, paresthesias, wrist- and footdrop, flaccid paraparesis or quadriparesis, and occasionally transient blindness. *Psychiatric* symptoms include agitation, depression, memory loss, delirium, and hallucinations. The *abdominal* symptoms include acute colic and constipation.

The peripheral neuropathy may progress rapidly in acute porphyria and a significant percentage of patients will die in the acute stage, usually from respiratory and bulbar involvement.

Characteristically, these patients have increased pigmentation of their skin, without which the diagnosis probably cannot be made. The urine will turn burgundy red on standing, particularly in sunlight, and some patients note this themselves. Many have had frequent laparotomies because of acute abdominal pain. Diagnostic laboratory findings include increased PBG and dALA in the urine. Porphyrins are excreted in the urine and feces in various forms. Coproporphyrins are *normally* present in urine and feces but may be *increased* in alcoholic cirrhosis, heavy-metal poisoning (lead or arsenic), polio, Hodgkin's disease, and acute intermittent porphyria.

Treatment consists of avoiding barbiturates, steroids, griseofulvin, and phenytoin (since these may precipitate attacks), and supportive care during an episode. Respiratory function must be monitored with frequent measurement of vital capacity. Vitamin B_6 should be administered in high dosages, because this vitamin is hypermetabolized during acute attacks of porphyria; this may be responsible for the neuropathy. The acute abdominal pains and psychotic symptoms respond to chlorpromazine. Guanethidine and propranolol have been reported as useful, both during acute attacks and as prophylaxis. The birth-control pill may suppress any attacks associated with menstruation. For seizures, bromides and clonazepam are probably the drugs of choice because they do not cause further porphyrin excretion.

COLLAGEN-VASCULAR DISEASE

The phenomenon of immediate hypersensitivity *(anaphylaxis)* is dependent upon the explosive liberation of histamine from mast cells. Because these are not present in the nervous system except in the meninges, choroid, and pituitary stalk, anaphylaxis does not involve CNS structures. The *Arthus phenomenon,* as examplified by serum sickness, depends upon the formation of antigen-antibody complexes, producing fibrinoid necrosis of blood vessels. The widely scattered intravascular lesions that result are examplified by those of polyarteritis nodosa, which does affect the nervous system. Such direct toxic effects of circulating antibodies depend upon complement to produce lysis of the cell surface antigens. This can occur experimentally in the brain, but *delayed hypersensitivity* (a cell mediated reaction by a specifically sensitized mononuclear cell) is the usual form of CNS involvement in collagen-vascular disease.

Patients with collagen-vascular diseases frequently have involvement of the nervous system. The syndromes that occur are surprisingly similar until one recalls that some patients begin their illness with, for example, polymyositis and later go on to develop features of systemic lupus erythematosus (SLE), finally terminating with the lesions of polyarteritis nodosa (PAN). The rheumatoid factor appears in over 30 percent of patients with systemic lupus and also in other conditions, including scleroderma, polymyositis, PAN, and Sjögren's syndrome. There is a similar lack of specificity in other tests designed to demonstrate autoallergic abnormalities.

It should also be mentioned that in the pedigree of the patient with one autoallergic disorder of this type, family members may be found to have others.

Systemic Lupus Erythematosus

Eighty-five percent of patients with systemic lupus erythematosus (SLE) are women in young- or middle-adult life. Occasionally it may be precipitated by the administration of anticonvulsants including phenytoin, the diones, primidone, and the succinimides. The neurological involvement is usually intracranial and develops eventually in two-thirds of the patients, a result of thrombocytopenic purpura, vasculitis, or steroid treatment (Fig. 42-8).

Seizures

Seizures occur in many patients with lupus and may result from vascular involvement, uremia, hypertension, or intracerebral hemorrhage. Chorea is also described.

Cranial Nerves

Forty percent of patients develop cranial nerve lesions, either because of specific involvement of nuclei and fibers within the brainstem or because of involvement of the cranial nerves themselves. Pseudobulbar signs may develop, and myasthenia occurs in association with lupus in about 5 percent of the cases.

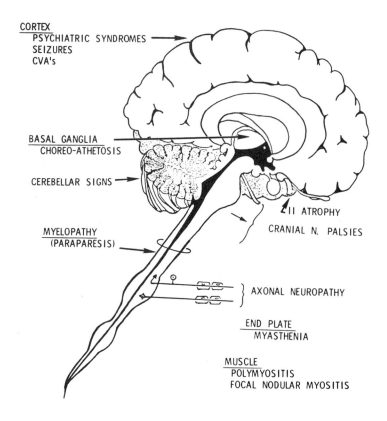

CORTEX
  PSYCHIATRIC SYNDROMES
  SEIZURES
  CVA's

BASAL GANGLIA
  CHOREO-ATHETOSIS

CEREBELLAR SIGNS

II ATROPHY
CRANIAL N. PALSIES

MYELOPATHY
  (PARAPARESIS)

AXONAL NEUROPATHY

END PLATE
  MYASTHENIA

MUSCLE
  POLYMYOSITIS
  FOCAL NODULAR MYOSITIS

Figure 42-8 Neurological involvement in systemic lupus erythematosus.

Hemiparesis

Transient ischemic attacks and small-vessel infarctions are not uncommon, and even large vessel occlusions may develop. Intracerebral hemorrhages are unusual, but any of these factors may result in hemiparesis, which affects 10 percent of patients with SLE.

The cerebrospinal fluid in SLE often shows a slight elevation of protein concentration even without evident CNS involvement. There may also be an increase in mononuclear cells and occasionally in pressure; with cerebral infarction or hemorrhage, blood may be found in the CSF.

Paraparesis

About 4 percent of patients develop significant arteritis of the spinal cord resulting in leg weakness. Spinal subdural hemorrhage is uncommon.

Peripheral Neuropathy

A symmetric sensorimotor neuropathy develops in about 8 percent of patients; some have a more dramatic illness which resembles the Guillain-Barré syndrome. Multiple mononeuropathy is not uncommon because of the vascular lesions of specific nerves.

Movement Disorders

Many forms of movement disorders are described in lupus including tremor, cerebellar ataxia, parkinsonism, and choreoathetosis. They are due to an arteritis involving specific CNS structures.

Autonomic Disorders

Raynaud's disease is quite common in all forms of collagen-vascular disease. Hypothalamic lesions can also occur and give rise to autonomic disturbances.

Mental Changes

About a third of patients with SLE will, at some time, develop an acute delirium with delusions and hallucinations, a dementing illness, functional affective disorders, or schizophreniform states.

The EEG is usually normal but may show focal or widespread changes, depending upon the degree of CNS involvement.

Most of the collagen-vascular diseases may be associated with the clinical picture of polymyositis, with or without skin involvement. However the picture of polymyositis does not differ in the various forms and is not significantly different to idiopathic polymyositis occurring by itself. Scleroderma, SLE, PAN, and Sjogren's syndrome all are described as accompanying the clinical features of polymyositis which is discussed more fully in Chapter 45.

There is a variable response of the neurological complications to steroids or immunosuppressants but these usually do improve the clinical picture, and the results are sometimes dramatic. Although uremia is the most common cause of death in SLE, CNS involvement is second to this.

Rheumatoid Arthritis

Rheumatoid arthritis (RA) affects some 3 percent of the population and, even though a comparatively small proportion of patients suffering from this condition have neurological disorders, this represents a large number of people. The abnormalities that are found are usually due to disorders of the cervical spine or of the peripheral nerves or are traceable to the presence of another autoallergic disorder.

Myelopathy

Subluxation of the cervical spine, particularly atlantoaxial dislocation, amy occur because of softening of the ligaments. As a result of this, the odontoid peg may be dislocated backward, pressing upon the anterior aspect of the cervical spinal cord. Far more common however is a true rheumatoid spondylitis with associated heaping-up of an hypertrophied ligamentum flavum. If associated with arteritis of the radicular vessels, an ischemic myelopathy can result.

Peripheral Neuropathy

Numerous nerve compression syndromes are described in RA but particularly the carpal tunnel syndrome. Usually in RA this is due to tenosynovitis of the long flexor tendons as they lie beneath the flexor retinaculum of the wrist, causing compression of the median nerve. Other ischemic neuropathies can occur in association with an underlying arteritis and theoretically could affect any peripheral nerve. Generalized peripheral neuropathies are usually of the thick-fiber type and involve mostly sensation, but combined sensory and motor neuropathies also occur.

Sjögren's Syndrome

Sjögren's syndrome is characterized by inflammation of the mouth and conjunctivae in association with raised gamma globulin levels and with evidence of a collagenosis, usually RA, but equally well SLE, PAN, or scleroderma. The usual neurological complication is a proximal myopathy, giving rise to clinical features similar to mild polymyositis, but cranial and peripheral neuropathies also occur.

Ankylosing Spondylitis

Ankylosing spondylitis bears certain similarities to rheumatoid arthritis and may also be associated with subluxation of the atlantoaxial joints and, because of the rigidity of the spine, with fractures. Because such patients are often treated with deep x-ray therapy, radiation myelopathy is a danger but is seldom seen now because of reduction in x-ray dosage. Most neurological damage is in the region of the cauda equina, but other neurological syndromes may occur, such as *vertebrobasilar insufficiency* caused by pressure upon the vertebral arteries, focal *epilepsy,* peripheral *neuropathy,* and *cervical myelopathy.*

Polyarteritis Nodosa

Polyarteritis nodosa is an autoallergic inflammatory disease affecting particularly the medium-sized and large blood vessels. Unlike rheumatoid arthritis and Sjögren's syndrome, but rather like ankylosing spondylitis, this condition particularly affects males. The vessels involved are very numerous and may include the aortic arch and its major branches and the coronary, pulmonary, and occasionally even the mesenteric vessels.

Polyarteritis occurs mainly between the ages of 20 to 40 years and produces a large number of nonspecific systemic features such as headache, fever, skin rash, arthralgia, nasal stuffiness and discharge, epistaxis, myalgia, cough and wheeze, weight loss, anorexia, fatigue, general weakness, chills, night sweats, and abdominal pain. Because of involvement of the intracranial arteries, almost any neurological structure may be affected; the most common single abnormality however is a *peripheral neuropathy* or multiple mononeuropathy.

The combination of asthma and a peripheral neuropathy should suggest this diagnosis. Almost any cranial or peripheral nerve can be involved, and the pattern of neurological dysfunction found with this type of ischemic neuropathy is very much the same as that seen in diabetes. In the CNS, headaches, focal seizures, organic syndromes, and all focal neurological disorders imaginable have been described. Involvement of the ophthalmic or retinal arteries may lead to blindness, while field defects are described in association with lesions more posteriorly, involving the occipital cortex or the internal capsule. The diagnosis is made by finding a raised ESR, abnormal gamma globulins, rouleaux formation in the blood, and characteristic changes in an inflammatory arteritis in muscle or renal biopsy specimens.

Details of steroid and immunosuppressant therapy will not be given here.

Aortic Arch Disease

Aortic arch disease (Takayasu's disease) causes ischemic symptoms in the territory of supply of the first and major branches of the aorta, producing strokes, ischemic pain, and loss of pulses. The disease occurs mainly in young women, and mesenteric vascular insufficiency or occlusion of the subclavian or carotid arteries are the usual presentations.

Giant Cell Arteritis

Also known as cranial arteritis, giant cell arteritis affects more females than males at a much later age (always over aged 50 and usually over 65). As in PAN, the coronary, pulmonary, and other systemic arteries may be involved, as well as branches of the external and internal carotids. The most important of the latter is the ophthalmic artery, involvement of which may lead to blindness in one or both eyes. The patients complain of fever, malaise, anorexia, weight loss, and fatigue and, in particular, continuous burning (or initially throbbing) *headache* and marked *scalp tenderness.* They may also complain of pain in the jaw muscles with chewing because of vascular insufficiency.

Examination reveals diminution or lack of pulsation in the superficial cranial arteries, which are red, swollen, and nodular (Fig. 42-9A). The patients are sometimes so uncomfortable they are not able to wear a hat, to brush their hair, or to lie comfortably on a pillow. Biopsy of a long stretch of the superficial temporal artery may reveal granulomatous giant cell arteritis (Fig. 42-9B); unfortunately, skip areas are not uncommon and so a small segment biopsy may be normal. The most important laboratory findings is a very high ESR, often above 100 mm/hr.

The vision is involved mainly through ophthalmic and posterior ciliary artery occlusion, producing a pale swollen optic disk and resulting blindness. *Stroke syndromes* and *oculomotor palsies* are also described.

If you see a patient who you think may have this condition, then you have an emergency on your hands. Sudden visual loss may occur at any time and any suspicion of the diagnosis requires that you obtain an emergency ESR and administer steroids even during that hour in which the test is being done. An initial dose of 100 mg of prednisone is not excessive. Arrange a biopsy as soon as possible and be prepared to continue the steroid treatment for at least 2 years, watching the patient clinically and with repeated ESRs because flare-ups can occur.

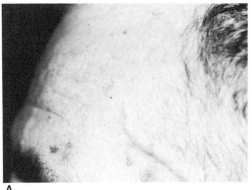 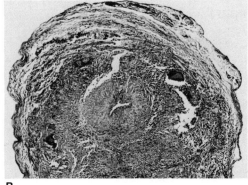

A   **B**

Figure 42-9   (A) Cranial arteritis causing thickened, cordlike, pulseless temporal arteries. (B) Cranial arteritis: arterial biopsy showing proliferation of arterial wall, giant cells and occlusion of the lumen.

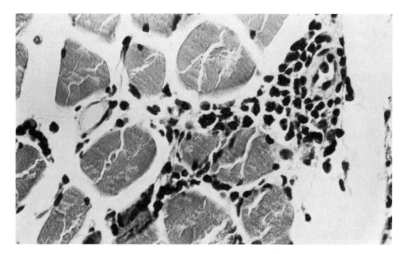

Figure 42-10   Polymyalgia rheumatica. Round cell infiltration between myofibrils and in the perivascular spaces.

Polymyalgia Rheumtica

A variant of giant cell arteritis, polymyalgia rheumatica is usually seen in patients over the age of 60 with nonspecific systemic symptoms and leading complaints of proximal muscle stiffness of the shoulder or pelvic girdles, *unassociated* with weakness. The muscles are tender, and other evidence of cranial arteritis may be detected. Biopsy of a temporal artery may show characteristic giant cell granulomas in 50 percent of the patients, even in the absence of symptoms referable to those vessels. A very high ESR and a normocytic, normochromic anemia may be expected. Muscle biopsy sometimes shows perivascular infiltration with inflammatory cells (Fig. 42-10). Striking improvement is seen with prednisone therapy. Although some reports suggest that only small doses need to prescribed, most patients require at least 40 mg/day to achieve maximal clinical benefit and a fall in the ESR.

Orbital Pseudotumor

In orbital pseudotumor (which may also be a form of arteritis) the retro-orbital tissues are infiltrated with edema and mononuclear cells, particularly in perivascular areas. It presents in elderly patients who complain of proptosis, ocular pain, and failure of eye movement. They may also notice proximal stiffness, as in polymyalgia rheumatica. Treatment is with steroids.

Wegener's Granulomatosis

In Wegener's granulomatosis, neurological features are seen in perhaps half of the cases. Here, an autoallergic granuloma is seen most frequently in the orbit producing exophthalmos, but associated polyarteritic manifestations include maxillary and frontal sinusitis, pulmonary disease, and multiple neuropathies affecting the occulomotor, optic, and peripheral nerves.

Systemic Sclerosis

Systemic sclerosis is an uncommon condition of vascular insufficiency, ischemic atrophy and fibrosis, and occurs most often in women in early adult life. It may appear in patients formerly diagnosed as having SLE or polymyositis, or it may present with neuropathy or seizures. The onset is insidious; Raynaud's phenomenon is the most prominent early clinical feature, while later, thickening and tightness of the skin, sometimes with trophic ulceration, are seen. Dysphagia is due to involvement of the esophagus with damage to the autonomic plexus in its wall. Such patients may show tenderness and atrophy of their proximal musculature. Because of reduced calcium absorption, hypocalcemia with carpopedal spasm or even seizures has been reported. Otherwise, CNS involvement is uncommon.

The syndrome that comprises features of SLE, polymyositis, and systemic sclerosis is called *mixed connective tissue disease* (MCTD). Half of these patients have neurological problems of many types — peripheral and trigeminal neuropathy, cerebellar syndromes, seizures, aseptic meningitis — as well as multisystem involvement.

Rheumatic Fever

Rheumatic fever is becoming an uncommon condition. In boys, it seldom produces any neurological dysfunction, while in girls, the picture of Sydenham's chorea is classic. The end results of cardiac valvular damage, atrial fibrillation, or early myocarditis may all predispose to the formation and liberation of emboli to the brain.

Thrombocytopenic Purpura

Ninety percent of patients with thrombocytopenic purpura have neurological involvement that may overshadow the picture of hemolytic anemia and purpura in association with fever, renal involvement, and small vessel occlusion elsewhere in the body. The signs of neurological disturbance are delirium and focal abnormalities such as hemiparesis or hemisensory loss, ataxia, dysphagia, or seizures. The EEG frequently shows generalized abnormality. If small-vessel lesions extend to many parts of the brain, coma, raised intracranial pressure, and focal signs may be expected.

SARCOIDOSIS

An uncommon disease, sarcoidosis causes CNS complications in only 5 percent of the cases. Most typical are seventh nerve palsy and hypothalamic involvement producing diabetes insipidus, sleep disturbances, endocrinopathy, and so on; but a chronic granulomatous basal meningitis occurs that may damage any of the cranial nerves, and sarcoid is also a cause of seizures, presumably through cortical infiltration, and of random focal CNS signs.

DIABETES MELLITUS

Almost every patient with diabetes, if carefully examined, will be found to have some evidence of neurological dysfunction because of the acute or chronic metabolic abnormality. Most commonly this is a peripheral neuropathy but vascular disease also frequently causes damage to the central and peripheral nervous systems (Figs. 42-11, 42-12). The neuropathies of diabetes are described in Chapter 44.

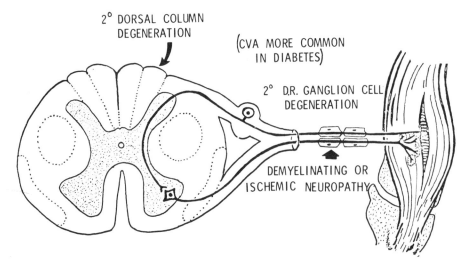

Figure 42-11   Neurological involvement in diabetes mellitus. Coma, optic atrophy, and vasculopathy are not shown in this diagram.

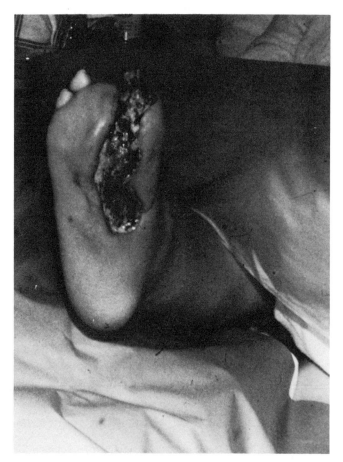

Figure 42-12   Diabetes mellitus. A huge perforating ulcer with massive local infection and sloughing of infected tissue.

Retinopathy

About 7 percent of the people who go blind each year do so because of diabetic retinopathy. Findings in the retina include the presence of microaneurysms, retinal or
vitreous hemorrhages, soft and hard exudates, neovascularization and gliosis, venous dilation and tortuosity, and degeneration of the vitreous. The first three of
these are the most frequent. The retina may behard to see because of diabetic
cataracts, but with experience one will be able to see around the edges of the cataracts in most cases, using the smallest spot on the ophthalmoscope.

Other Findings

Cerebrospinal fluid protein values are frequently raised to a maximum of about
1000 mmol/L. *Coma* may occur in diabetes for many reasons. Hypoglycemic coma
accompanied by sweating and signs of excess adrenergic activity (vasoconstriction,
tachycardia, dilated pupils) is probably the most common form, at least in patients
taking insulin or oral antidiabetic agents of the sulfonylurea type. Diabetic hyperglycemic coma with acidosis presents with gradually deepening coma in the presence
of dehydration, tachycardia, peripheral circulatory failure, dry skin, and hyperventilation. Nonketotic hyperosmolar coma and lactic acidosis are other causes of coma
in diabetic subjects.

    Cerebrovascular accidents are more common in diabetic patients than in non-
diabetic people because of the accelerated atherosclerosis in this condition. Diabetics have an increased susceptibility to *infections* involving the nervous system
as well as other areas. Tuberculous and fungal meningitis are uncommon diseases
that are nevertheless well recognized as occurring with much greater frequency in
diabetic subjects.

NEUROLOGICAL COMPLICATIONS OF PREGNANCY

The neurological complications of pregnancy can be grouped under two headings:
(1) disorders or complications that are virtually specific for pregnancy and (2) disorders wherein pregnancy either plays a part in etiology or else aggravates the
condition, although it does not actually cause it.

CNS Complications
Specific to Pregnancy (Table 42-2)

Eclampsia

In eclampsia, hypertension and ischemic necrosis of arterioles and capillaries result in vascular occlusion and hemorrhages. These are found in the kidneys, liver,
brain, lungs, and heart. Neurological features include convulsions, cerebral hemorrhage, and continuing coma. Pulmonary edema, cardiac failure, and renal cortical
necrosis also occur. Two-thirds of the patients who die have cerebral changes,
most often multiple small hemorrhages in the cortex or a large intracranial hemorrhage. Changes in the EEG parallel the severity of the condition but are of uncertain value in diagnosis or prognosis.

    Eclampsia occurs in about 1 of 1000 pregnancies and is most common in primi-
gravidae, twin pregnancies, and women with diabetes or chronic vascular or renal
disease. About half of the cases occur in the last trimester of pregnancy or close
to term and the remainder occur during labor or within 24 hr of delivery.

Table 42-2   CNS Complications Specific to Pregnancy

Eclampsia

Chorea gravidarum

Choriocarcinoma metastasis

Lumbosacral plexus injury (fetal head or forceps)

Sheehan's syndrome

Vena cava obstruction

Afibrinogenemia because of retained fetus

Hyperemesis gravidarum with Wernicke-Korsakoff
  syndrome

Preeclampsia is an important warning state that demands definitive steps in management before it becomes more serious. The patient may have had excessive weight gain, edema, hypertension, proteinuria, and sometimes spasm of retinal arterioles with retinal edema. Severe preeclampsia is characterized by blood pressures above 160/110 at rest, heavy proteinuria, oliguria below 400 ml in 24 hr, headache, generalized edema, severe epigastric pain, excitability and hyperreflexia, amaurosis, and retinal hemorrhages and exudates. These are probably on the basis of generalized, pregnancy-induced, noninflammatory vasculitides. Thrombotic thrombocytopenic purpura is another cause of an almost identical syndrome. The condition may be regarded as a variety of malignant hypertension with the possibility therefore of hypertensive encephalopathy. When seizures are added to the clinical features of preeclampsia as just given, the *eclampsia* is said to have occurred.

Grand mal seizures may lead to status epilepticus and coma; focal cerebral deficits and organic mental changes may be left as residua. Pulmonary edema with cyanosis is sometimes seen, particularly after convulsions.

The problems clear spontaneously within 24 hr of evacuation of the uterus but immediate management is that of status epilepticus (Chap. 15) and of malignant hypertension. Delivery of the fetus must be accomplished with extreme urgency.

Chorea Gravidarum

This condition may occur during the first trimester of pregnancy and can be accompanied by quite marked and exhausting choreiform movements. There may or may not be evidence of the effects of past rheumatic fever, but in many cases a past history of Sydenham's chorea can be obtained. The condition clears quickly after delivery but during pregnancy, specific drug treatment for chorea is not advisable, particularly early in the pregnancy.

Choriocarcinoma Metastasis

This tumor of placental tissue is preceded by a hydatidiform mole in 40 percent of the patients, missed abortion in 40 percent, and an otherwise normal pregnancy in 20 percent. It is more common in older primiparae and if a new conception rapidly follows the last pregnancy. Cerebral metastases from this tumor may hemorrhage with resulting hematomas. Symptoms and signs are of raised intracranial pressure with added focal deficits.

Lumbosacral Plexus Injury

This occurs particularly in patients with cephalopelvic disproprotion or following a difficult labor, when the lumbosacral plexus becomes pressed against the pelvis by the fetal head. This may result in transient footdrop or sciatic pain, but more extensive injury can result in weakness related to the obturator or superior gluteal nerves or to the fifth lumbar and first sacral roots. This results in weakness of the abductors and external rotator of the thigh, footdrop, and weakness of the gastrocnemius muscle. The disorder is usually a neurapraxia and can be expected to recover spontaneously in up to 3 to 4 months.

Sheehan's Syndrome

This unusual complication of pregnancy is due to infarction of the anterior pituitary. Initially, failure of lactation may be the only sign, but other signs of hypopituitarism may develop months or years later. The pituitary infarction appears to be related to hemorrhagic shock at the time of delivery or in the postpartum period.

Vena Caval Compression

In late pregnancy, the uterus may compress the inferior vena cava, reducing venous return to the heart, especially when the patient is on her back. Some patients develop faintness and swelling of the ankles, relieved by standing or lying on the side.

Afribrinogenemia

If the fetus dies after the 16th week and is not expelled, afibrinogenemia may develop, usually within a month. Widespread venous occlusions and small vessel hemorrhages may produce neurological illness.

Hyperemesis Gravidarum

Hyperemesis gravidarum is thought to have a major psychological basis, whether or not other factors are important in etiology. The continued vomiting may give rise to a deficiency of many vitamins and, in the presence of severe thiamine deficiency, even a small carbohydrate load may exhaust the remaining supplies and lead to the picture of Wernicke-Korsakoff syndrome (Chap. 44).

Nervous System Disorders
Aggravated by Pregnancy (Table 42-3)

Cerebrovascular Disease

Cerebral *ischemic infarction* is more common during pregnancy although the cause of this is unexplained: vascular changes, hypertension, or various alterations of clotting factors may underlie the problem.

It is possible for *air* to enter the venous circulation through the uterus particularly after cesarean section, abortion, vaginal insufflation, douching, or complicated deliveries. If the amount of air is large, it can enter the right side of the heart, forming a bubble trap obstructing blood flow to the lungs. Embolism may also occur because of thrombophlebitis in pregnancy, but the brain is thus involved only if one invokes the overused theory of paradoxical embolism. *Amniotic fluid* embolism may result in respiratory distress, pulmonary edema, cyanosis, shock, convulsions, or coma. *Fat* embolism is rare but may occur from the trauma of a difficult delivery.

**Table 42-3   Nervous System Disorders Aggravated
by Pregnancy**

Cerebrovascular disease

Peripheral nerve lesions

    Herniated lumbar disk

    Meralgia paresthetica

    Thoracic outlet syndrome

    Carpal tunnel syndrome

    Polyneuritis

Tetany

Epilepsy

Brain tumors

Other conditions

When *cerebral venous thrombosis* occurs, it is usually in the puerperium and may be due to vascular changes during pregnancy, alteration of blood clotting factors, or as an extension of venous thrombosis from pelvic veins through the paraspinal and intraspinal venous plexuses. The patient may have had previous brief episodes of neurological deficit that cleared quickly. In the more severe cases, there may be a progressive neurological deficit associated with headache, focal cerebral lesions, decreasing level of consciousness, convulsions, and coma. Cerebral edema may produce papilledema in such patients, and a lumbar puncture will show increased pressure. The CSF is often bloody, the EEG may show localizing abnormalities, and the CT scan is often positive early. Occasionally, the venous phase of an arteriogram may demonstrate obstruction if the vessels involved are large. Rupture of an *aneurysm* may cause cerebral hemorrhage during pregnancy. Presumably the aneurysm had been present for some time but ruptured because of hypertension, increased blood volume, vascular changes, eclampsia, or the use of oxytoxic or vasopressor drugs. The subarachnoid hemorrhage produced commonly occurs in the third trimester although seldom during labor. Twenty-five percent of cases occur in the immediate postpartum period. The mortality equals that of SAH unassociated with pregnancy. Cerebral *hemangiomas* may also bleed during pregnancy but these are rare.

Peripheral Nerve Lesions

In many women the first evidence of a *lumbar disk* syndrome appears during pregnancy, perhaps related to the abnormal posture and weight of the uterus or to the relaxation of ligaments that occurs at this time.

    Meralgia paresthetica is the term applied to an annoying syndrome characterized by pins-and-needles and burning over the lateral thigh in the distribution of the lateral femoral cutaneous nerve. It is due to entrapment of that nerve as it crosses the anterior pelvic brim below the inguinal ligament. If the symptoms are very distressing, the nerve can be injected with local anesthetic or hydrocortisone, but usually one may expect relief from the symptom after delivery.

Pressure upon the lower brachial plexus at the *thoracic outlet* is probably produced in pregnancy by ligamentous relaxation and poor posture. The usual symptoms are paresthesia in both hands, particularly at night or in the early morning. with associated stiffness of the hands and rarely weakness and atrophy (see Chap. 44).

About 10 percent of pregnant women complain of symptoms suggesting a mild *carpal tunnel syndrome.* This is often bilateral and clears after delivery. If the symptoms are severe, then injection with hydrocortisone is often effective. Even more simply, night splints can be made that maintain the wrist in slight dorsiflexion, and these are often sufficient to relieve the patient of paresthesia and pain during the early morning, which is the most common time for symptoms to occur.

Idiopathic facial paralysis *(Bell's palsy)* occurs more frequently during pregnancy, particularly in the last trimester and in the postpartum period. The prognosis is good and the patients should be treated as outlined in Chapter 23.

There is no specific form of polyneuritis in pregnancy but vitamin deficiency and diabetic neuropathies may occur with greater than usual frequency, as may the Guillain-Barré syndrome.

Tetany

Depletion of calcium stores during pregnancy and lactation may result in numbness or tingling in the circumoral areas and hands. Episodes of carpopedal spasm and rarely positive Trousseau's and Chvostek's signs, decreasing levels of consciousness, convulsions, or mental changes may occur.

Seizures

About one-third of patients with epilepsy will have an increase in the frequency of their seizures during pregnancy, particularly in the last trimester. This may be associated with increased blood volume, hypocalcemia, or occasionally hyperventilation. Seizures also occur in eclampsia.

Because of a 10 percent risk of fetal hydantoin syndrome in the children borne to mothers taking phenytoin, it is best to avoid this drug in young women. If a patient who is taking anticonvulsant drugs becomes pregnant, the risk of her having a deformed child is increased. Unfortunately, the risk of her having uncontrolled seizures and perhaps status epilepticus is great if her anticonvulsants are stopped, and they therefore should be continued in whatever dosages are required to control seizures for the whole of the pregnancy, although both the risks of *taking* and of *not taking* anticonvulsants should be carefully explained. It may also be suggested that another anticonvulsant drug replace the phenytoin, such as carbamazepine, but the risks to the infant on this drug are unclear and the change-over time may increase the risk of seizures. She can be reassured that the overall chance of her child having seizures is still low (about 1 in 15) although this figure is actually about 10 times the prevalence in the general population. The risk is greater with type I than with type II seizures.

Brain Tumors

Primary brain tumors may become clinically evident during pregnancy. We have had the experience of seeing women with cerebral neoplasms in whom there was a previous indication of an underlying neurological lesion 1 or 2 years before, also during a pregnancy. The symptoms and signs may vanish after delivery, giving one the mistaken feeling that the problem was purely transient. Management is complicated during pregnancy by the correct tendency to omit irradiation wherever possible.

Cerebral and spinal *hemangiomas* tend to increase in size during pregnancy, sometimes causing evidence of compression and occasionally hemorrhage.

Other Conditions

Porphyria can be precipitated or aggravated during pregnancy whether or not barbiturates have been prescribed.

It was once said that *multiple sclerosis* patients deteriorated during pregnancy, but other studies have shown that one-third improve, one-third remain the same, and one-third appear to worsen! There does seem to be an increase in attacks and of new symptoms in the 6 months following pregnancy, however.

Myasthenia gravis also has an unpredictable course during pregnancy but there is no change in most patients. About 25 percent of patients go into remission during the last half of their pregnancy, sometimes relapsing in the postpartum period.

Infections which formerly occurred with greater than usual frequency during pregnancy (cerebral or spinal abscesses, tetanus, meningitis, and tuberculosis) are seen less often nowadays in the Norther American population.

The *restless legs syndrome* is a peculiar "creeping, crawling" sensation deep in the lower legs with an irresistible need to move them. It occurs in 10 to 15 percent of pregnant women and clears after delivery. The paresthesias occur only at rest, particularly 10-15 min after retiring at night or after prolonged sitting (watching TV, movies, concerts). The same syndrome is seen in about 5 percent of the population at times, particularly in those who drink a lot of coffee, and it is also more common in patients who are anemic or uremic. The patient gets relief by walking around but the symptoms return when she goes back to bed. They can be helped by a nightly dose of chlorpromazine 25 to 50 mg, clonidine, or folic acid 5 mg daily. A small amount of brandy may be just as good.

BIBLIOGRAPHY

Aita, J.A. *Neurological Manifestations of General Diseases.* Springfield, Ill., Charles C. Thomas, 1964.

Donaldson, J.O. *Neurology of Pregnancy. Major Problems in Neurology.* Vol. 7. Philadelphia, W.B. Saunders Co., 1978.

Fauchauld, P. et al. Temporal arteritis and polymyalgia rheumatica. *Ann. Intern. Med.* 77:845, 1972.

Feinglass, E. et al. Neuropsychiatric manifestations of SLE. *Medicine 55:*323-338, 1976.

Lederman, R.J., Henry, C.E. Progressive dialysis encephalopathy. *Ann. Neurol.* 4:199-204, 1978.

Moore, P.M., Supps, T.R. Neurological complications of vasculitis. *Ann. Neurol. 14:*155-167, 1983.

Plum, F. (ed.). Brain dysfunction in metabolic disorders. *Assoc. Res. Nerv. Ment. Dis. 53,* New York, Raven Press, 1974.

Pruitt, A.A. et al. Neurologic complications of bacterial endocarditis. *Medicine 51:*329, 1978.

Raskin, N.H., Fishman, R.A. Neurologic disorders in renal failure. *N. Engl. J. Med. 194:*143–148, 204–210, 1976.

Williams, R. Hepatic encephalopathy. *Proc. R. Coll. Physic. Lond. 8:*63, 1973.

43
Toxic Damage to the Nervous System

Many chemicals, drugs, and other pharmaceutical agents may cause either permanent or reversible damage to the nervous system. When it is recalled that over 10 percent of patients in a hospital at any time have leading symptoms because of toxicity from treatment agents (as opposed to intrinsic disease), it will be understood that a knowledge of intoxications is of great importance.

Nobody expects the medical student or intern to *know* the contents of this chapter, but it is included to indicate the types of toxic damage known and to provide a source to which reference may be made when any clinical syndrome is encountered. Sometimes the CNS symptom results from the normal pharmacological actions of a drug, e.g., coma with sedative overdosage. Sometimes it will be due to direct damage to neurons, e.g., lead or carbon monoxide poisoning. Competition for enzymes in the nervous system or in the liver may also produce symptoms; thus phenothiazines may produce dyskinesias, phenytoin induces rickets, and isoniazid induces neuropathy through pyridoxine deficiency. Other methods include alterations in CSF secretion or drainage producing benign intracranial hypertension, and alterations in the membrane potential of the neurons with resultant epilepsy. Other toxic effects still cannot be explained, such as the production of glare photophobia with trimethadone (Tridione).

DRUGS DIRECTLY AFFECTING CNS FUNCTION

Encephalopathy

Many drugs and toxins can result in alteration in consciousness, personality change, delirium, seizures, lethargy, raised intracranial pressure, or coma with or without focal signs of neurological dysfunction and with evidence of intact brainstem function. They include

Alcohols
    Ethyl, methyl, propyl
    Ethylene glycol
Analgesics, narcotic
    All
Anticonvulsants
    Diphenylhydantoin
    Bromides
    Barbiturates
    Primidone
    Benzodiazepines
    Sodium valproate
Antidepressants
    Tricyclic drugs
    Lithium
Antineoplastic drugs
    L-Asparaginase
    Methotrexate
    Nitrogen mustards
    Procarbazine
    Vidarbine
    Vinca alkaloids
Diuretics
Miscellaneous
    Acetominophen
    Amantidine
    Aminophylline
    Amphetamines
    Arsenic
    Aspirin
    Atropine and belladonna alkaloids
    Baclofen
    Bismuth
    Bromocriptine
    Carbon disulfide
    Carbon monoxide
    Chloroquine
    Cimetidine
    Cycloserine
    Cyproheptadine
    Disulfuram
    L-Dopa
    Digitalis
    Gasoline
    Gold
    Heroin
    Isoniazid (INAH)
    Insulin
    Interferon
    Lead
    Methyl bromide
    Methyl mercury
    Metrizamide

Organophosphorus
Penicillin
Prajmalium
Propranolol
Rifampin
Steroids
Streptomycin
Strychnine
Sulfonamides
Sulfonylureas
Thallium
Toluene

Sedatives and Hypnotics
    All

Delirium also occurs in the dysequilibrium syndrome during dialysis, and a subacute encephalopathy occurs following cranial irradiation.

Seizures

Epileptic seizures may occur in patients taking a variety of drugs, sometimes in normal dosage; but in other situations, seizures only occur in the presence of toxic levels of the drug or if the patient has a preexisting low threshold for seizures. Usually, the manifestation is of generalized epilepsy, but if there is any preexisting brain disease that formerly had not produced seizures, the reduction of threshold because of the toxic agent may produce a focal seizure. Drugs that may be incriminated include:

Alcohol (and withdrawal from alcohol)
All analeptic agents
Aminophylline
Amiodarone
Amphetamines
Anticholinesterases
Birth-control pill
Camphor
Carbon monoxide
Chlorambucil
Cocaine, IV
Corticosteroids
Cycloserine
Deanol
Ergotamine
Furosemide
Heroin
Isoniazid
Insulin
Lithium
MAO inhibitors
Marijuana
Methyl bromide
Metrizamide
Nalidixic acid
Penicillin
Phenothiazines
Physostigmine, IV
Reserpine
Strychnine
Theophylline
Tolbutamide
Tricyclic drugs
Vincristine (perhaps because of excess ADH secretion)

Dementia

The clinical features of dementia are outlined in Chapter 12. Dementing syndromes are usually regarded as being irreversible, but this is wrong in drug-induced dementia. Focal neurological signs referable to the frontal lobes, the cerebellum, or the basal ganglia may also be present along with the altered mental state. It is even more common for patients with organic brain syndromes to have their condition worsened by drugs, particularly sedatives, hypnotics, and tranquilizers; dialysis is another cause. In recent years progressive dementia as a result of solvent sniffing has become an increasing problem. Glue, gasoline, and many other chemicals are used. Other responsible drugs include

Alcohol
Barbiturates
Benzodiazepines
Bromides
Carbon monoxide
Gasoline
Lead
Manganese
Mercury
Organic substances (e.g., CCl_4, CS_2, TOCP)
Phenytoin
Toluene

Reduction in Conscious Level

The management of coma is outlined in Chapters 7 and 10. Patients who are comatose as a result of drugs and toxins ingested show evidence of normal brainstem function thus, with retained doll's head movements and ice-water caloric responses and with normal pupillary reactions. This is not true with drugs that have an anticholinergic effect (see later discussion). Respiratory and/or cardiovascular depression may be marked and cause further brain damage because of hypoxia. In severe intoxication the EEG may be isoelectric; this is not a sign of brain death in this circumstance (see Chap. 10).
Causal agents include

Alcohol (ethyl and methyl)
All analgesics
All anticonvulsants
All antihistamines
All psychoactive drugs
All sedatives
Anticholinergic agents
Baclofen
Bromides, methyl bromide
Digoxin
Organophosphates
Orphenadrine
Phenylbutazone

In fact, almost *any* drug in sufficient quantity can cause coma. The syndrome also occurs as a complication of dialysis.

Extrapyramidal Syndromes

Chorea

Some patients who have had Sydenham's chorea in childhood, usually women, may again develop abnormal jerking movements (described in Chap. 29) if they are given

L-dopa or phenytoin. Choreic movements in parkinsonian patients treated with L-dopa are a common toxic manifestation. The birth-control pill may induce chorea.
Chorea may also be produced by

Amphetamines
Anticholinergics
Carbamazepine
CO_2 narcosis
Methylphenidate
Opiates
Phenytoin
Primidone

Parkinson's Syndrome

The four classic features of parkinsonism, (tremor, rigidity, akinesia, and postural changes) are produced by a number of agents. Tremor however is less prominent in drug-induced parkinsonism. Drugs may also induce oculogyric crises, which are otherwise seen only in the postencephalitic form of parkinsonism. The effects are reversible when the drug is withdrawn. Responsible agents include

Butyrophenones
Carbon tetrachloride
Diazoxide
Manganese
Mercury
Methyldopa
Metoclopramide
Phenothiazines
Reserpine
Tricyclic drugs

Following CS_2 or CO poisoning and with most other causes of severe hypoxia, a parkinsonian syndrome may occur, but without oculogyric crises, caused by permanent neuronal damage in the basal ganglia. Note that while tricyclic drugs may produce a parkinsonian syndrome rarely, they are also of value in treatment of depression in Parkinson's disease.

Acute Extrapyramidal Symptoms

The severe disorders of movement included under this heading include dystonias, facial tics and spasms, akathisia, and so on. The symptoms usually occur in young males given bromocriptine, butyrophenones, phenothiazines (with a piperazine ring), phenytoin, or metoclopramide, and also in people stung by insects. In older patients, methyldopa, tricyclics, and L-dopa produce severe extrapyramidal symptoms of this type. Akathisia and other dyskinesias may also occur with benztropine, which is otherwise a reasonable choice among synthetic anticholinergic agents used to treat parkinsonism and which can be given intramuscularly in dosage of 1-2 mg for acute extrapyramidal symptoms. Intramuscular diphenydramine or IV diazepam 10-20 mg given slowly usually stops the acute symptoms in these cases but must be coupled with withdrawal or reduction in the dosage of the drug. Intravenous diazepam is most safely given when respiratory support is available, should it be required.

Tremor

Regular and repetitive tremor, usually fast and of small amplitude and not very much like that of parkinson's disease, can be produced by amiodarone, lithium, metoclopramide, sodium valproate, thyroxine, tricyclics, and vidarabine.

The problem of *tardive dyskinesia* is considered in Chapter 46.

Cerebellar Ataxia

The usual cerebellar syndrome (see Chap. 49) with horizontal jerk nystagmus, limb or trunkal ataxia, and failure of motor control, may be caused by a number of agents including

Amiodarone
Benzodiazepines
Carbamazepine
Carmustine (BCNU)
Ethyl alcohol
5-Fluorouracil
Gasoline
Iodochlorhydroxyquin (clioquinol)
Lithium
Mercury
Perhexiline maleate
Phenobarbitone
Phenytoin
Procarbazine
Toluene

Nystagmus

Both horitontal and vertical jerk nystagmus may occur, without other evidence of a cerebellar syndrome, because of toxicity. Cerebellar connections are probably involved, but there may also be damage to the medial longitudinal fasciculus. Substances incriminated include

Amiodarone
Barbiturates
Carbamazepine
Glucose in vitamin B_1-deficient subjects
Phenytoin
Primidone

Myelopathy

Spinal diseases are discussed in Chapter 50. Upper motor neuron and long-tract signs, usually without a discrete cord level and with or without evidence of anterior horn cell or dorsal root ganglion cell involvement, can occur with

Deep x-ray therapy
Electric shock
Halogenated hydroxyquinolines (?), e.g., Entero-Vioform
Heroin

Mercury
Methotrexate (intrathecal)
Methylene blue (intrathecal)
Metrizamide
Organophosphorus compounds
Phenytoin
Tricyclic drugs
Vaccination

Tetracycline and colchicine may induce vitamin B_{12} deficiency with resulting myelopathy.

DRUGS AFFECTING OTHER
INTRACRANIAL COMPONENTS

Meningism

Still neck with positive Kernig's and Brudzinski's signs, fever, and photophobia may occur as a drug reaction. The CSF usually contains either no cells or only a few mononuclear cells, but the pressure may be slightly raised. The CSF should, of course, be sterile on culture.
Agents include

Air encephalopathy
Disulfuram
Heroin
Ibuprofen
MAO inhibitors (+ tyramine)
Sulfonamides
Tridione

Chemical Meningitis

The same picture of menigism may occur following intrathecal injection of a number of agents. Here the CSF contains many mononuclear cells, increased protein and sometimes reduced sugar levels. Responsible agents include

Amphotericin
Local anesthetics
Radioiodinated serum albumin
Steroids
Streptomycin
X-ray contrast media

Fungal Meningitis

The picture of acute or chronic meningitis with markedly raised protein level, low sugar level, mainly mononuclear cells, and also the presence of fungi (usually *Candida albicans)* may complicate treatment with immunosuppressive agents and steroids. Fungal meningitis may also be seen in patients with diabetes or with alcoholism.

Benign Intracranial Hypertension

Benign intracranial hypertension is described in Chapter 16. Papilledema is unaccompanied by focal neurological signs and investigations will be negative. The CT scan shows the ventricles to be normal or small in size. The patient's usual complaint is headache, sometimes with visual obscurations. The following substances produce this syndrome:

Birth-control bill
Carbon dioxide
Nalidixic acid
Organic insecticides
Perhexiline maleate
Steroids
Steroid withdrawal in children
Tetracyclines
Vitamin A

Migrainous and Other Vascular Headaches

The differential diagnosis and management of headaches are described in Chapter 17. Typical vascular headaches may occur *de novo* or preexisting migraine may be made more severe or more frequent if the patient takes

Baclofen
Birth-control pill
Chloroquine
Ergot derivatives*
Ethosuximide
Indomethacin
Nitroglycerin
Organophosphates
Perhexilene maleate
Verapamil

Headaches because of a sudden, marked rise in systolic blood pressure may occur in patients who eat foods high in tyramine while they are taking MAO inhibitors. Other causes of vascular headache include the ingestion of alcohol in patients who are taking disulfuram. Withdrawal from caffeine is a common but poorly recognized cause of headaches.

DRUGS AFFECTING NERVES

Cranial Nerves

Anosmia

Parosmia is a common result of the chronic use of nasal decongestant sprays and drops resulting in severe damage to the unmyelinated fibers of the first nerve. In time, loss of olfactory acuity supervenes. Toluene also causes hyposmia.

---

*With chronic use, ergotamine actually *causes* headaches.

Optic Atrophy

The clinical appearance of optic atrophy is described in Chapter 20. It may be caused by a number of agents, and from the following list it will be seen that many of these are either derivatives of the original sulfonamide drugs or are agents used in the treatment of rheumatoid arthritis. Visual acuity may not be greatly affected despite marked primary optic atrophy.
Toxic causes include

Alcohol (methyl and ethyl)
Arsenic
Carmustine
Chloramphenicol
Chloroquine
Chlorpropamide
Digitalis
Disulfuram
Ethambutol
Heavy metals: gold, mercury
Isoniazid
Methyl bromide
Para-aminosalicylic acid (PAS)
Penicillamine
Phenylbutazone
Quinine
Quinidine
Salicylates
Streptomycin
Sulfonamides
Tobacco
Toluene

Subacute Myelo-Optico Neuropathy: A virtual epidemic of a disease marked by optic neuropathy, encephalopathy, and transverse myelopathy has occurred in Japan and in the Western world in the past 10 years. The distinction from multiple sclerosis is hard to make, but the CSF is normal. Toxicity from halogenated hydroxyquinolines (iodochlorohydroxyquin; Entro-Vioform) and/or a herpes-related virus are both under suspicion as causes.

Miosis

Small pupils that do not appear to react, but that are not usually associated with any subjective complaint, may occur with the use of

Opiates
Organophosphates
Physostigmine
Pilocarpine
Sedatives

Mydriasis

Dilation of the pupils bilaterally, with subjective difficulty in accommodation and focusing and sometimes with photophobia, may occur as a drug effect. In such cases, pupillary constriction to light may be reduced. Drugs responsible include

    Amphetamines
    Antihistamines
    Atropine (all muscarinic blockers)
    Cocaine
    Disopyramide
    Glutethimide
    Haloperidol
    L-Dopa
    Phenothiazines
    Phenytoin
    Tricyclic drugs

Ophthalmoplegia

Carbamazepine and tricyclic drugs have been incriminated as causes of ophthalmo-plegia in cases of overdosage. Beta-blocking drugs may cause diplopia.

Trigeminal Sensory Loss

Trigeminal sensory loss is usually unilateral but can extend to both sides of the face in any of the three divisions of the nerve. Apart from the patient's subjective complaint of numbness, which is objectively verifiable, no motor signs and no other sensory changes are usually detected. The agents that are responsible include

    Stilbamidine
    Trilene (a solvent)

Seventh Nerve Palsy

Unilateral Bell's palsy is more common in women taking the birth-control pill.

Eighth Nerve Involvement

Different agents affect the cochlear and vestibular components of the eighth nerve to a different extent. The typical picture is of vestibular impairment with strepto-mycin, compared with the primarily cochlear damage caused by dihydrostreptomy-cin. However both divisions are involved to some extent with most of the following drugs.

    Ethacrynic acid
    Furosemide
    Heroin
    Lead
    Mercury
    Quinine
    Quinidine
    Salicylates
    Streptomycin and other aminoglycosides
    Toluene

Recurrent Laryngeal Palsy

This is an uncommon complication of the vinca alkaloids.

Peripheral Nerves

Most of the agents in the following have been shown to produce neuropathy. In some, the association is less certain. In almost all cases, the pathology is primary axonal degeneration with secondary demyelination but primary Schwann cell damage is a possible cause. The clinical picture produced is of distal, symmetic polyneuropathy. In patients with diabetes or rheumatoid arthritis and associated neuropathy, steroids seem to worsen the condition, perhaps by damaging the small vasa nervorum. Steroid withdrawal may be involved in the severe neuropathy occurring in some patients with rheumatoid arthritis. Sensory functions are almost invariably affected first, and motor involvement is less severe and is seen at a later stage.

Agents causing neuropathy include

All anticoagulants
All antineoplastic agents
Most antibiotics and antimalarials
Amiodarone
Arsenic
Antitetanus serum
Acrylamide
Bismuth
Butazolidine
Barbiturates
Carbon monoxide
CS_2
CCl_4
Chloral hydrate
Chloramphenicol
Chloroquine
Chlorpropamide
Clofibrate
Colchicine
Dapsone
Disulfuram
2-4, D
Electric shock
Emetine
Ergotamine
Ethionamide
Ethyl alcohol
Ethylene oxide
Gasoline
Glue
Glutethimide
Gold
Hydralazine
n-Hexane
Indomethacin
Industrial solvents
Ipecac
Imipramine
Isoniazid

Lacquer thinners
Lead
Lindane
Lithium
Mercury
Methaqualone
Metronidazole
Nitrofurantoin
Nitrous oxide
Organophosphates (TOCP)
Perhexiline
Phenylbutazone
PCBs
Phenytoin
Podophyllin
Procainamide
Procarbazine
Prophylthiouracil
Pyridoxine (high dose)
Stilbamidine
Sulfonamides
Thalidomide
Thallium
Trilene
Toluene
Tolbutamide
Tricyclic drugs
Vermouth
Vincristine
Prolonged cold

Autonomic Nerves

Impotence

Impotence is discussed in Chapter 34. Most drugs causing it are either ganglion blockers or specific parasympatholytics, but most antihypertensives including thiazide diuretics are causal. Other responsible agents include

Anticholinergic drugs
Some anticonvulsants, e.g., barbiturates
Ethyl alcohol
Ganglion-blocking agents
Guanethidine
Haloperidol
Primidone
Thoridiazine and other phenothiazines
Tricyclic drugs
Vasodilators

DRUGS AFFECTING MUSCLE

Myopathy

The usual features of primary, proximal muscle disease with atrophy and weakness, and usually without pain, can occur in patients who have taken

Amphetamines	Penicillamine
Bretylium	Pentazocine
Chloroquine	Phencyclidine
Cimetidine	Phenytoin
Clofibrate	Procainamide
Colchicine	Propranolol
Emetine	Quinidine
Epsilon-aminocaproic acid	Rifampin
Guanethidine	Spironolactone
Heroin	Steroids (especially if fluorinated)
Hydralazine	Succinylcholine
Imidazole	Triamterene
Immunosuppressants	Vincristine
Lithium	

Hypokalemia secondary to the administration of diuretics, licorice, carbenoxolone, or amphotericin B, may also be associated with severe proximal weakness, pain, and wasting. Intramuscular paraldehyde, phenytoin, and lidocaine give rise to local pain, muscle fibrosis, and atrophy. Clofibrate and the other drugs just listed may cause elevation of serum CK levels. Phenytoin may cause metabolic bone disease, associated with proximal myopathy.

Neuromuscular Blockade

The cardinal symptom of myasthenia is fatigability, particularly seen in the ocular, bulbar and proximal limb muscles as described in Chapter 45. Patients with myasthenia may have an exacerbation of their symptoms, or a myasthenia-like syndrome may occur in patients without previous evidence of that condition in the presence of hypokalemia from any cause, such as steroids, muscle relaxants, or ether, or after enemas or wasp stings. The following drugs tend to increase neuromuscular block and should not be given to patients with myasthenia gravis.

Aminoglycoside antibiotics	Polymyxin B
Chloroquine	Propranolol
Clindamycin	Quinine*
Colistin	Quinidine
Lidocaine	Tetanus antitoxin
Lincomycin	Tetracyclines
Lithium	Thyroxine
Penicillamine	Trimethaphan
Phenytoin	

---

*In myasthenic patients, toxic water isn't.

In the event of myasthenic symptoms being produced or exacerbated when these agents are administered, intravenous calcium may reverse the immediate severe weakness and fatigability.

Acute Muscle Necrosis

Acute muscle necrosis, an uncommon complication of a number of drugs, produces a rise in serum CK and myoglobinuria with pain and proximal weakness. It is more likely to happen in patients who are dehydrated. Agents incriminated include

Alcohol
Amphetamines
Amphotericin
Barbiturates
Carbenoxolone
Diazepam
Epsilon-Aminocaproic acid
Heroin
Isoniazid
Methadone
Phencyclidine

Muscle Cramps

Muscle cramps are discussed in Chapter 30. Responsible drugs include

Cimetidine
Clofibrate
Diuretics
Lithium
Nifedipine
Salbutamol

Hypoglycemia

Propranolol may mask the signs and symptoms of hypoglycemia and must be carefully used in diabetics. The usual symptoms and signs of hypoglycemia (Chap. 42) may be induced by

Alcohol
Insulin
Sulfonylureas (especially if used with phenylbutazone or salicylates)

Alterations in Blood Pressure

The clinical manifestations of hypo- and hypertension will not be described here, nor shall we attempt to list any of the huge range of drugs that have effects upon blood pressure. Any patients with abnormal blood pressure readings, or even symptoms of postural hypotension, should be questioned carefully about all drugs taken, because these are often responsible, at least in part, for the abnormality. The dangers of taking sympathomimetic drugs (including cold remedies), meperidine, phenothiazines, methyldopa, and numerous foods at the same time as MAO inhibitors should be mentioned again in this context, because headaches, subarachnoid or intracerebral hemorrhage, delirium, or severe hypertension may result. Carbamazepine may cause Stokes-Adams attacks with loss of consciousness.

Hypercoagulability

The increased susceptibility to venous (and possibly to arterial) thrombotic occlusions in women taking the birth-control pill has been noted in Chapter 37.

Vasculitis

The hematological manifestations of polyarteritis nodosa are considered in Chapter 42. The condition may complicate ingestion of

Organic arsenicals
DDT
Gold
Hydantoins
Iodides
Mercurial diuretics
Phenothiazines
Sulfonamides and derivatives

The same agents, and

Carbamazepine
Griseofulvin
Hydralazine
Isoniazid
Methyldopa
Para-aminosalicylic acid
Phenylbutazone
Phenytoin
Procainamide
Streptomycin
Tetracycline

have been incriminated in the production of the syndrome of SLE.

MISCELLANEOUS ASSOCIATIONS

Neoplasia

Lymphoma has been described in patients who have been given immunosuppressive agents following renal transplantation and in patients taking phenytoin. Although lymphoma is an uncommon neurological malignancy, lymphomas may present with features of chronic basal meningitis, of scattered demyelination, and rarely of intracranial mass lesions.

Photophobia

Complaints of pain in the eyes and of excessive glare may be heard in any patient with dilated pupils because of the use of mydriatics and in patients taking lithium.

Glare photophobia is commonly associated with the use of trimethadione, an anti-epileptic drug of slight value in true petit mal epilepsy.

INTERACTIONS INVOLVING
DRUGS USED IN NEUROLOGY

Enzyme Induction

Through enzyme induction, warfarin and phenytoin may be mutually antagonistic and less effective clinically. Phenytoin, phenobarbitone, and valproic acid induce hepatic microsomal enzymes. Although a reduction in the availability of each drug would be expected, serum levels nevertheless usually change but little. Drugs that inhibit oral anticoagulants include

Barbiturates
Meprobamate
Tranquilizers
Tricyclic drugs

Interactions between anticonvulsants are many, involving increased or decreased metabolism, substrate competition and reduced absorption. In addition, serum phenytoin levels may be markedly increased or decreased by other drugs, as may other drug levels be reduced by phenytoin, phenobarbital, or carbamazepine.

EMERGENCY TREATMENT
OF POISONED PATIENTS[*]

The basic treatment of "mild" overdosages (for instance, the patient is conscious and has taken drugs such as aspirin or barbiturates), is gastric lavage with a wide-bore stomach tube (not a nasogastric tube) passed through the mouth, the instillation of activated charcoal, and the observation of vital signs for at least 6 hr. The object of treatment is to remove any intoxicant in the stomach and to reduce absorption of that remaining in the small bowel. Observation is necessary as some patients who appear alert will later become unconscious because of absorption of that quantity of the drug that had already passed into the small bowel before the instillation of charcoal. Once through the observation period and after being cleared by the casualty officer (and the psychiatrist in appropriate cases), the patient may leave.

The passage of a stomach tube is dangerous and inappropriate if there is any doubt about the nature of the intoxicant or if the ingested agent is corrosive or caustic. Lavage is not indicated if the time interval since ingestion is long or if the quantity involved is trivial. However awake patients frequently give a false account of the quantity of drugs they have ingested and some will subsequently lapse into coma, so you must treat confessions of having taken trivial quantities of drugs with suspicion, trying to get independent evidence on the quantity of pills available for ingestion.

---

[*]The authors are most grateful to Dr. Martin Tweeddale for his advice and assistance in the preparation of this section.

There is no place for the routine use of emetics in adults. There is a very real danger of a decreased level of consciousness developing before an oral emetic works, with consequent aspiration of gastric contents when vomiting does occur.

Once vital functions are assured, and if the patient's condition permits it, gastric lavage with instillation of charcoal may be undertaken, but the risks of aspiration in a patient with depressed reflexes are great so intubation with a cuffed endotracheal tube is usually indicated. The use of charcoal in such patients (in whom absorption is often complete) is to prevent reabsorption of the appreciable quantities of many drugs that are excreted in the bile. This will help to shorten the time during which blood levels are excessive. All such patients must be admitted to the hospital until they are fully recovered.

In cases of "severe" intoxication (patients who are unresponsive or respond only to intense stimulation, whose protective reflexes are blunted, or whose vital functions are depressed), initial therapy should be directed to the maintenance of respiration and tissue perfusion. Almost all will need intubation, certainly if lavage is to be performed. Blood samples for gas analysis, BUN, electrolytes, and sugar concentrations are obtained before or immediately after the institution of emergency therapy.

The conscious level and physical signs may change rapidly during the observation period. Accurate recordings of pulse, blood pressure, respiratory rate and quality, pupillary responses, muscle tone, and reflexes should be made repeatedly. In such patients, gastric absorption of drugs is much reduced, so slow absorption may continue for a long time.

Fluid replacement is an integral part of the treatment of drug intoxication, but one should beware of giving a large volume of fluid to those whose myocardium is affected by age, disease, or the intoxicating agent. Similarly, renal function may be abnormal in a poisoned patient and fluid overload is easy in such cases. Forced diuresis, with or without alkalinization, is potentially hazardous and is seldom indicated; hemodialysis is far superior.

Blood, urine, and gastric washings can be analyzed for toxic agents but the assays are tedious and complicated. Such assays should seldom be undertaken routinely, but save blood samples, urine, and gastric washings for 48 hr, or until the patient is discharged, in case they are required later. An exception to this statement is the measurement of acetaminophen concentrations, since a knowledge of the time of ingestion and of the blood concentration helps in deciding whether or not treatment with acetylcysteine is indicated in an attempt to prevent liver damage.

Specific anitdotes are few; oxygen for CO narcosis, naloxone for opiate poisoning, atropine and pralidoxime for organophosphorous poisoning, and physostigmine for anticholinergic drug poisoning are available, if early identification of the agent is possible.

Barbiturates and ethanol together cause two-thirds of all drug-induced coma incidents; tricyclics, lithium, and benzodiazepines are next in frequency. Fifty percent of all cases of coma in an emergency room are drug-induced, and half of these patients have ingested more than one drug. The most common agents causing death are barbiturates, acetaminophen, and dextropropoxyphene, but the combination of alcohol and diazepam is also dangerous. Intravenous naloxone has been suggested as a diagnostic test if drug coma is suspected.

The Anticholinergic Syndrome

Numerous drugs used for treating depression, Parkinson's disease, and psychosis and also the antihistamines and antispasmodics, atropine itself, potato leaves, and jimson weed all produce a very typical syndrome. The patient is initially anxious, febrile and dry, with tachycardia, arrhythmias, and mydriasis; later on, delirium, hallucinations, and seizures occur. Finally, coma and medullary paralysis super-vene. If the diagnosis is made, IV physostigmine 1-4 mg is a specific antidote and may awaken the patient.

THE NEUROLOGICAL COMPLICATIONS OF ALCOHOL

The complications of alcohol abuse have been classified as those caused by acute intoxication, by withdrawal, and by nutritional disease in chronic alcoholism (Table 43-1). There is another large group of CNS disorders that occur in alcoholics resulting from unknown causes (Fig. 43-1). A chronic alcoholic is a person whose dependence on alcohol interferes with his health, interpersonal relationships, social adjustments, job, or economic efficiency. About 5 percent of the adult population are so classifiable, constituting one of the major health problems of our country.

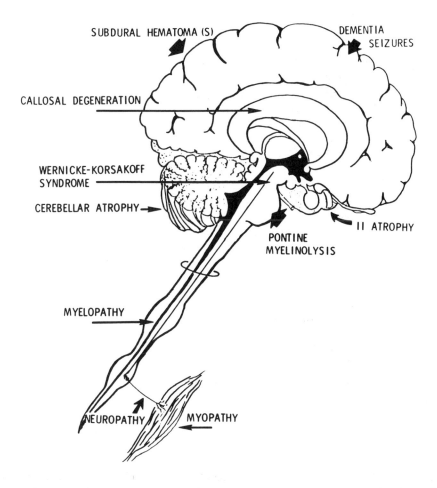

Figure 43-1   Lesion diagram of neurological involvement in chronic alcoholism.

Table 43-1   The Complications of Chronic Alcoholism

Intoxication

    Acute drunkeness
    Pathological intoxication
    Alcholic coma

Withdrawal

    Tremors
    Hallucinations
    Seizures
    Delirium tremens

Nutritional

    Wernicke-Korsakoff syndrome
    Polyneuropathy
    Amblyopia
    Pellagra

Uncertain causes

    Cerebellar degeneration
    Marchiafava-Bignami syndrome
    Central pontine myelinolysis
    Cerebellar cortical atrophy
    Myelopathy
    Hypoglycemia

Other associations

    Enlarged sella turcica
    Pressure palsies
    Subdural hematoma
    Hepatic encephalopathy (cirrhosis)
    Carcinoma of the stomach
    Vitamin B_{12} deficiency
    Dupuytren's contracture
    Cardiomyopathy
    Venereal disease
    Tuberculosis
    Spastic paraplegia
    Hypernatremia

Intoxication

Acute Drunkeness

The symptoms of acute alcoholic intoxication have undoubtedly been learned at first hand by many medical students. Initial exhilaration, relaxation, and excitement are followed by signs of decreased inhibition, slurred speech, ataxia, irritability, combativeness, and drowsiness. After very heavy drinking, the person may pass into a state of stupor and possibly even to coma. Because 90 percent of the ingested alcohol is oxidized by the liver at a fairly constant rate, the time taken to recover from the bout is variable. However the next morning the ghost of the evening past may return in the form of a vascular headache with its accompanying irritability, nausea, hyperacusis, photophobia, and anorexia. Although eating increases the metabolism and slows absorption of alcohol somewhat, most methods of treating a hangover are probably ineffective.

Pathological Intoxication

Occasionally a person may develop a marked excitatory response to even a small amount of alcohol. Symptoms of this acute psychosis include excessive excitement, combativeness, destructive behavior, and motor restlessness. The patient should be sedated and protected until the episode has passed, usually in a few hours.

Alcoholic Coma

Because alcohol depresses both subcortical (brainstem) and cortical structures in the same way as anesthetics, a patient who ingests a large amount may pass through a state of stupor to actual coma. With high blood levels of ethanol (300 mg/dl) reduction in consciousness is usual, but this may occur at lower levels. A comatose patient with alcohol on his breath may have any number of different problems, and the coma may have nothing to do with drinking. He could be comatose from alcohol, but also from a seizure, a head injury, a subdural hematoma, hypoglycemia, or a cerebral infarction. He may have ingested other drugs with the alcohol in a suicide bid. Occasionally a well-meaning bystander tries to revive an unconscious person with brandy or whiskey, so he arrives in the emergency room with the smell of alcohol on his breath.

When the patient is seen, management follows the outline in Chapter 10, with the added caution that a head injury, subdural hematoma, meningitis, pneumonia, liver failure, or gastrointestinal hemorrhage may be present in an alcoholic who has a decreased level of consciousness.

The patient will require IV glucose and saline, always covering glucose with thiamine because the Wernicke-Korsakoff syndrome can be precipitated by glucose infusion in someone who is thiamine deficient. Gastric lavage is not helpful because the alcohol is absorbed too rapidly from the gastrointestinal tract. The patient should be nursed in a semiprone position to avoid aspiration: failing that, intubation may be needed.

Alcohol Withdrawal Symptoms

Alcoholic Tremulousness

In a chronic alcoholic, even a night without alcohol may produce the early symptoms of withdrawal, including tremulousness, irritability, headache, anorexia, sweating, depression, and anxiety. He quickly learns that another drink in the morning will relieve "the shakes." If he is unable to obtain alcohol, the tremulousness increases to a peak at 24 hr and is associated with general irritability, nausea, and vomiting. His face is flushed and the conjunctivae injected. He appears generally weakened with a rapid pulse. An irregular gross tremor involves the hands and forearms but can be generalized and so marked that he has difficulty walking, speaking, or feeding himself. He is extremely susceptible to startle and tends to remain preoccupied with his own misery and relatively inattentive to those around him. He should be encouraged to eat and drink fluids and should be given moderate doses of chlordiazepoxide or chlorpromazine. A multivitamin preparation should be given, particularly to provide vitamin B_1.

If kept in hospital for a few days he will get over the most uncomfortable period of withdrawal and may be able to accept long-term help, but to discharge him from the emergency room will almost certainly send him back to alcohol as a form of relief.

Alcoholic Hallucinosis

The tremulous patient will often develop fearful visual or auditory hallucinations. These are similar to "bad dreams," and there is evidence that they result from rebound after the deprivation of REM sleep that occurs while drinking. This state is treated like acute tremulousness.

An unusual variant of the foregoing is a more chronic *auditory hallucinosis.* The hallucinations are of voices, often those of his family which are reproachful, critical, or threatening. The episode usually lasts about 6 days but occasionally goes on much longer. Although initially he lacks insight, the patient begins to question the voices' reality as the episode ends and afterward understands and can discuss his former abnormal thought content.

Alcoholic Seizures

The withdrawal seizures of alcoholism are of generalized type. Ninety percent of these seizures occur within 48 hr of the last drink. Usually there is only one seizure. Tremulousness and hallucinosis also occur and may be followed by delirium tremens (DTs), but they do not follow the appearance of delirium.

Seizures caused by the withdrawal of alcohol have been termed "rum fits" but it is important to remember that people with a low convulsive threshold for other reasons may have seizures provoked by alcohol or its withdrawal. Thus some epileptics may have seizures when they drink a little alcohol, or a lot. If the seizure is focal, then a focal lesion is present and the patient does not have "rum fits." Respiratory alkalosis and a low serum Mg^{2+} level may be factors in the production of withdrawal seizures. Alcohol can also induce hypoglycemia in 6 to 12 hr, possibly because of a reduction in the amount of glycogen stored in the liver through a reduction in the capacity for hepatic gluconeogenesis; this may be another cause of seizures.

Anticonvulsants are not usually required after a single withdrawal seizure, and long-term anticonvulsants are neither logical nor practical, because both cause and prevention lie in the alcoholism, but prophylactic carbamazepine may prevent their occurrence and decrease withdrawal symptoms. In rare instances status epilepticus develops and this should be treated as described in Chapter 15.

Delirium Tremens

After 12 to 24 hr without alcohol, the chronic alcoholic may become irritable, nauseated, sweaty, restless, sleepless, and tremulous, entering a state of delirium tremens with the dramatic appearance of delusions, confusion, irritability, vivid hallucinations, and marked agitation. Other evidence of increased autonomic activity includes dilated pupils, hypertension, tachycardia, and fever. It becomes difficult to keep the patient calm. His agitation partly reflects fear of his delusions and hallucinations. An irregular tremor involves the hands, face, and tongue in all of these patients, increasing with activity. A tendency to tug at the clothes and bedclothes is also characteristic. His speech becomes more difficult to understand as he screams, whimpers, or mumbles garbled sentences. The DTs may clear after a week, almost as quickly as they developed, leaving little memory of the delirious period. Occasionally, patients die during the acute stage, probably because of hyperthermia, hypokalemia, and peripheral circulatory collapse, but the cause of death in some is uncertain.

The management of these cases includes a search for other underlying problems including infection, subdural hematoma, and meningitis. Correction of fluid and electrolyte imbalance and the addition of thiamine are vital steps. Shock should be treated immediately with fluids and vasopressor drugs, and if hyperthermia develops, ice packs, fans, and a cooling mattress should be used.

The patient's room should be well lighted, as he will be fearful of every shadow. Sound is kept to a minimum and he requires continuous reassurance. Family members are sometimes helpful in keeping him calm. High dosages of chlordiazepoxide (25-50 mg q6h) or chlorpromazine are helpful in reducing agitation and consequent exhaustion. Steroids have no place except in the event of shock but propranolol may be very useful in the agitated, tremulous patient with autonomic overstimulation. Small doses of alcohol have been used as a temporary measure with success.

Nutritional Disorders

Wernicke-Korsakoff Syndrome

Wernicke's syndrome comprises ophthalmoplegia, ataxia, and mental disturbance associated with edema, petechiae, and demyelination in the walls of the third ventricle, aqueduct, and fourth ventricle, and in the medial dorsal nucleus of the thalamus and mammillary bodies (Fig. 43-2). The disorder can occur with any chronic cause of thiamine deficiency but is more common in alcoholism.[*] Korsakoff's psychosis refers to the loss of ability to record new data, sometimes seen in (mainly male) chronic alcoholics. Korsakoff also described a peripheral neuropathy accompanying the memory loss. Korsakoff's syndrome is a residue from an episode of Wernicke's encephalopathy, which may not have been evident clinically in its acute stages, and one designates the picture *Wernicke-Korsakoff syndrome* to encompass both the acute syndrome and its residua.

The odd distribution of the demyelination and petechiae is probably because the oligodendroglia in these areas contain thiamine-dependent transketolase enzymes.

The clinical features are first of delirium, which may be a typical agitated and excited delirium tremens or a quiet confusional state occurring with a decreasing level of consciousness, even amounting to coma. Headache, nausea, vomiting, and depression may precede this state. The involvement of the brainstem around the third and sixth nerve nuclei give rise to both *ocular muscle* and gaze palsies, but the pupils are normal. Nystagmus and poor caloric responses probably result from lesions around the vestibular nuclei. Truncal *ataxia* results from involvement of the cerebellum or vestibular nuclei.

---

[*]In 1881 Carl Wernicke described three patients with this syndrome. Two were alcoholics and one was a young woman with chronic vomiting following a suicide attempt in which she ingested sulfuric acid. He thought that this was inevitably a fatal disease because his patients died, as indeed yours may if you miss the diagnosis.

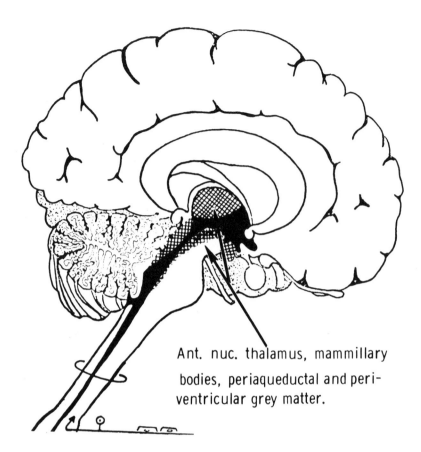

Ant. nuc. thalamus, mammillary
bodies, periaqueductal and periventricular grey matter.

Figure 43-2 Wernicke-Korsakoff syndrome. Involvement of the anterior nucleus of the thalamus, mammillary bodies, and fornix is shown, but other sites in the limbic system are also affected.

Most of the patients have a peripheral neuropathy because of a thiamine deficiency, but beriberi heart disease is unusual. Complications in the acute stage include hyperthermia, seizures, and a syndrome of inappropriate ADH secretion.

The picture of *Korsakoff's psychosis* becomes apparent as the patient recovers. The ataxia and eye signs improve relatively quickly in the first few days or weeks, but the memory abnormality becomes more evident and may never entirely clear. It may be so bad that the patient remembers nothing that happened more than 45 sec ago, although he retains his previously learned skills. Confabulation is usual — i.e., there is a tendency to answer with incorrect statements any question put by the examiner. The patient is not lying to cover up his poor memory, but rather his answers are disjointed memories from the past which are out of temporal sequence. Confabulation is not always present in Korsakoff's syndrome and it clears fairly rapidly, so one should not depend upon it to make the diagnosis. The lesion responsible is probably in the medial dorsal nucleus of the thalamus, rather than the mammillary bodies.

Blood pyruvate is elevated in the thiamine-deficient alcoholic, indicating interference with glucose metabolism through the Krebs cycle, but this test is of little clinical value. Transketolase activity in red cells is markedly reduced in patients with Wernicke-Korsakoff disease prior to the administration of thiamine, but again this has little clinical relevance.

Wernicke's disease is an emergency because the patient can die if untreated, or he may be left at least with serious memory loss. Initial treatment should be 50 mg of thiamine intravenously and 50 mg intramuscularly. Larger doses of thiamine are unnecessary. The patient should be made to eat a balanced diet. Sedation with phenothiazines or diazepam may be necessary during the early stages. Oral thiamine must be continued.

Treated as outlined, the eye signs begin to improve within 12 hr.

Alcoholic Peripheral Neuropathy

The neuropathy of chronic alcoholism affects both sensory and motor functions because of chronic deficiency of thiamine. There is degeneration of peripheral nerves distally with destruction of both the myelin sheath and axon. Although sensory symptoms are common, the chronic alcoholic usually does not complain unless motor changes are marked or a "burning feet syndrome" develops.

Examination shows a distal loss of all modalities of sensation with mild motor weakness or atrophy in most cases. The reflexes are absent distally. Treatment (alcohol withdrawal, vitamins) leads to a very slow improvement; residual sensory and sometimes motor losses are common.

Alcohol Amblyopia

Some alcoholics develop blurring of vision with decreased acuity because of central scotomas. Examination shows mild hyperemia of the disk or, later, optic atrophy. There may be a relationship with tobacco amblyopia in these patients, but alcoholic amblyopia is due to nutritional deficiency and is not a toxic effect of alcohol or tobacco. Treatment is by a balanced diet and administration of B vitamins.

Pellagra

Nicotinamide deficiency results in mental changes, insomnia, irritability, and depression. Neurological signs include posterior and lateral column involvement and peripheral neuropathy (see Chap. 42).

Alcoholic Cerebellar Degeneration

Some chronic alcoholics develop bilateral cerebellar incoordination and instability in the legs. There is little abnormality in the arms, and evidence of nystagmus or cerebellar speech difficulty is rare. This involvement is due to selective degeneration of the anterior lobe or vermis. A CT scan may show characteristic atrophy of the folia in this region. Occasionally the syndrome can be reversed by stopping the intake of alcohol; in the chronic form this is not so, but at least it will not get worse. This chronic cerebellar degeneration may represent a residuum from a previous Wernicke-Korsakoff syndrome, suggesting that it is due to a nutritional deficiency.

Complications of Alcoholism, of Uncertain Origin

Marchiafava-Bignami Disease

Marchiafava-Bignami disease is a rare complication of alcoholism characterized by degeneration of the corpus callosum. It is seen more commonly in Italian males who drink homemade red wine and is characterized by a progressive decrease in mental function, convulsions, tremor, rigidity, paralysis, akinetic mutism, and coma. There is evidence of bilateral frontal lobe and more generalized cerebral disease, as well as the pathological appearance of degeneration of the corpus callosum. Some contaminant in the alcohol or a nutritional deficiency may be the cause.

Central Pontine Myelinosis

Central pontine myelinosis is characterized by rapidly progressing demyelination in the central pons which results in pseudobulbar palsy and spastic quadriplegia with a decreasing level of consciousness, coma, and death. Although usually seen in alcoholics, it also occurs with underlying malignancy, chronic renal disease, and other debilitating disorders.

This syndrome is usually due to inappropriate rehydration of patients at risk, with a prolonged perriod during which the serum sodium level is low. The syndrome of inappropriate ADH secretion and hyponatremia for any reason are other causes.

Cerebral Cortical Atrophy

Many chronic alcoholics show evidence of diffuse cortical atrophy, especially of the frontal lobes, with enlargement of the ventricles. This is evidenced by an organic mental deficit, even long after they have stopped drinking.

Alcoholic Myopathy

Three myopathies are associated with alcoholism. The acute syndrome is characterized by painful, swollen, and tender muscles, occasionally with myoglobinuria and renal damage. Another type shows subacute girdle weakness and atrophy with aching pains; and a third resembles McArdle's disease, with muscle cramps and a flat lactic acid curve after ischemic exercise. Alcoholic cardiomyopathy, sometimes associated with hyperkinetic heart failure, is probably part of a deficiency syndrome, but an outbreak in Quebec was traced to the use of cobalt as a preservative in beer.

Other Complications of Chronic Alcoholism

Chronic alcoholics who develop *hepatic insufficiency* may show evidence of encephalopathy or coma.

Pressure palsies are common in alcoholics. A common one affects the radial nerve when the drunk person falls asleep with his arm hanging over the back of a chair ("Saturday night palsy").

Half the patients in any large series of *subdural hemorrhages* will be alcoholics. The hematomas may be bilateral. Occasionally, chronic alcoholics may show an *enlarged sella turcica* on skull x-ray. Nobody knows why. They also have an increased prevalence of *carcinoma of the stomach* and some show evidence of B_{12} *deficiency* resulting from chronic gastritis, gastrectomy for ulcers, or poor dietary intake. Dupuytren's contractures in the hands, chronic infections, *venereal disease,* and *tuberculosis* are all much more common in alcoholics than in the general population.

BIBLIOGRAPHY

Argov, Z., Mastaglia, E.L. Drug-induced peripheral neuropathy. *Br. Med. J. 1:* 663–666, 1979.

Dreisbach, R.H. *Handbook of Poisoning,* 7th Ed. Los Altos, CA, Lange Medical Publications, 1971.

Ehle, A., Homan, R. In *Neurology,* R.R. Rosenberg (ed.). New York, Grune & Stratton, 1980.

Goodman, L.S., Gilman, A.H. *The Pharmacological Basis of Therapeutics,* 6th Ed. New York, Macmillan, 1980.

Victor, M., Adams, R., Collins, G. *The Wernicke-Korsakoff Syndrome. Cont. Neurol. Ser.* No. 7. Philadelphia, F.A. Davis Co., 1971.

44
Disorders of the Peripheral Nerves

Any of the four components of peripheral nerves may be the site of primary damage; the *cell body* and its axon, the *Schwann cell sheath,* the *supporting tissue,* and the *vascular supply* (Fig. 44-1). To classify neuropathies as primarily caused by damage of one of these four components is of diagnostic value, although the differences between the four are not always easy to determine clinically. Nerve conduction studies and nerve biopsies however do assist greatly in determining which type of pathology is present. The patterns of motor and sensory involvement in peripheral nerve lesions were described in Chapters 9 and 26.

Classification of the neuropathies by clinical presentation alone is somewhat fallacious as the same pathological process may give rise to different manifestations. Clinical evaluation helps one toward pathological diagnosis, so long as it is done methodically. Starting with the question of neuropathy being raised, decide whether this is a polyneuropathy with a symmetric (usually distal) pattern of involvement; a mononeuropathy (the symptoms being confined to the distribution of a single nerve), or a multiple mononeuropathy (discrete nerves being involved in various sites). The latter two groups are usually due to nerve compression or infiltration and are discussed later (see p. 599). Polyneuropathies may be predominantly motor or sensory (Table 44-1), but in acquired forms they are usually eventually both. The speed of progression of symptoms, nerve enlargement, and the presence or absence of pain are further diagnostic points.

In practice however, a neurologist relies more upon the family and past medical histories and upon evidence of toxic exposure to make the pathological diagnosis; if these do not help, studies of nerve conduction usually determine whether the neuropathy is neuronal or demyelinating.

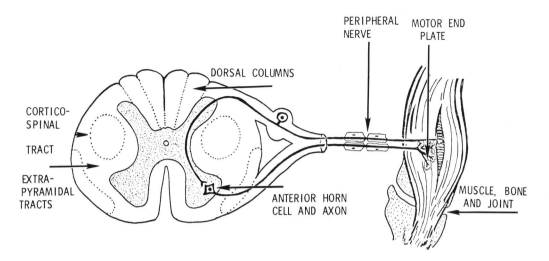

Figure 44-1   The components of the reflex arc. This may be broken centrally, in the cord; or peripherally in the muscle or in the efferent or afferent neural pathways.

Table 44-1   Motor and Sensory Neuropathies

Predominantly Motor	Predominantly Sensory
Guillain-Barré syndrome[a]	Vitamin B group deficiency
Lead[a]	Carcinoma (paraneoplastic)
Porphyria[a]	Uremia
Diphtheria[a]	Myelomatosis
TOCP, acrylamide poisoning[a]	Amyloidosis
Anterior horn cell disease, e.g., polio[a], ALS	Drug-induced/toxic
Diabetic girdle neuropathy[a]	Hereditary dorsal root ganglion diseases
Compressive lesions[a]	Herpes zoster[a]

[a]Neuropathies often having an acute onset.

VARIETIES OF NEUROPATHY
(Table 44-2)

Neuronal (Axonal) Neuropathy

In neuronal neuropathies the damage is to the cell body or to the axon itself. On the motor side, damage to the anterior horn cell is manifested clinically as motor weakness with wasting and fasciculations. If the process is severe or long-standing, diminution or loss of deep tendon reflexes occurs; this is seen at an *early* stage if the reflex arc is interrupted on the *sensory* side. Anterior horn cell damage indicates that the pathology is really operating at a spinal cord level, but the condition is still referred to as a neuropathy because the clinical effects are almost entirely related to peripheral nerve dysfunction.

Motor Type

Examples of disorders affecting the *anterior horn cell* include poliomyelitis, hereditary motor neuropathies, motor neuron disease, syringomyelia, and other cord diseases such as trauma, meylitis, and tumor.

Hereditary Motor Neuropathies (HMN): Hereditary motor neuropathies have too many names and not enough treatments; HMN is the fashionable term, but "spinal muscular atrophies" and the eponymous terms Werdnig-Hoffmann and Wohlfarht-Kugelberg-Welander disease refer to the same problems.

These disorders are reasonably common, have varied modes of inheritance, and share degeneration of the lower motor neuron as their common primary pathology. The severity of the disorder varies with the age of onset. Infantile onset presages rapid progression and early death; the later the onset, the more benign the course. Eight percent of cases present before the age of 4 years.

Clinical Features

Evidence of the condition may appear before birth. Mothers of infants with HMN often comment on reduced fetal movements in the last trimester of the pregnancy. The infant will show proximal or distal symmetric weakness and wasting with hypotonia and anergy, respiratory and feeding problems being marked. Fasciculations are seen in only half the babies, the fat layer obscuring them. Reflexes are depressed. Muscle contractures and aspiration pneumonitis are common complications.

When the onset is in childhood, pelvic girdle weakness causes a waddling gait and problems in climbing stairs; arm weakness is due to involvement of the shoulder girdle muscles, and scoliosis to trunk weakness. In adults girdle weakness and wasting with fasciculations and hyporeflexia produce similar features but progress slowly.

Diagnosis

Diagnostic confirmation depends upon muscle biopsy (Fig. 44-2); EMG is of confirmatory value and serum CK levels are mildly elevated. Only supportive treatment is available.

Without muscle biopsy, HMN is easily misdiagnosed as limb girdle dystrophy. Uncommonly, other patterns of weakness and wasting in HMN mimic facioscapulohumeral or distal myopathies. In all adult cases, differentiation from motor neuron disease is only possible with time and detection of corticospinal tract signs.

Table 44-2   Causes of Neuropathies by Clinical Type

Cause	Pure Motor	Pure Sensory	Mixed
Genetic	Proximal HMN infantile juvenile adult	HSN I (AD) II (AR) Freidreich's etc.	HMSN I demyelinating II neuronal Other forms
	Distal, scapulo- peroneal, and facioscapulo- humeral forms		leukodystrophies
Malignancies	Lymphoma		Macroglobulinemia Cryoglobulinemia Myelomatosis
		Carcinoma Lymphoma Paraneo- plastic Gammopathy	Carcinoma Lymphoma Leukemia
Other degenerative	Multiple system atrophy Motor neuron disease (Multiple radiculopathies)		Multiple system atrophy
Infective	Guillain-Barré and variants Diphtheria Poliomyelitis	Herpes zoster Leprosy	Guillain-Barré Diphtheria Herpes simplex Leprosy
Metabolic	Diabetes Porphyria	Diabetes Amyloid Beriberi B_{12} deficiency Hypothyroisism Acromegaly	Diabetes Amyloid Beriberi Porphyria Hypothyroidism Acromegaly Sprue Hepatic insufficiency Uremia

Table 44-2 (cont'd)

Cause	Pure Motor	Pure Sensory	Mixed
Autoallergic		Rheumatoid arthritis	
		Polyarteritis nodosa	Polyarteritis nodosa
		Systemic lupus (SLE)	SLE
		Wegener's granuloma-tosis	
		Sjögren's syndrome	
Toxic	Organo-phosphates	Acrylamide	Alcohol
	Dapsone	Vinca alkaloids	TOCP
	Gasoline	Glutethimide	CS_2
		Thalidomide	n-Hexane
	Lead	Ethionamide	Carbon monoxide
	Mercury	Mercury	PCBs
		Chloram-phenicol	DDT
		Iodochloro-hydroxyquin	Methyl bromide
		Phenytoin	2,4-D
		Metronidazole	Perhexilene
		Trilene	Thallium
		Pyridoxine	Arsenic
		Cisplatinum	N_2O
		Isoniazid	Isoniazid
			Disulfuram
			Nitrofurantoin
			Vinca alkaloids
			Gold
Vascular neuropathies	Small aa		
	Arteritis		
	Diabetes		
	Amyloid		
	Infective typhus		
	Abnormal viscosity	Macro/cryo-globulinemia TCP, sickling, polycythemia	

Table 44-2 (cont'd)

Cause	Pure Motor	Pure Sensory	Mixed
Vascular neuropathies (cont'd)	Clotting hemophilia Cold trench foot Large *AA* Emboli Compression (and anterior tibial syndrome) Infections Volkmann's ischemic contracture Buerger's disease Atherosclerosis		

The other neuronal neuropathies of motor type mentioned earlier are considered elsewhere in this book. The history or accompanying evidence of CNS dysfunction allows a reasonable chance of making the correct diagnosis clinically.

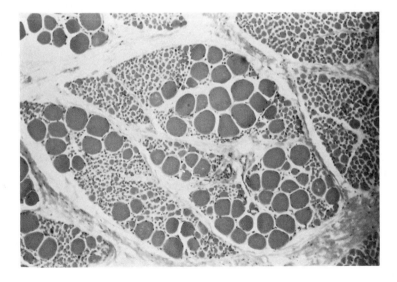

Figure 44-2   Neurogenic atrophy of muscle. There are numerous small, angulated muscle fibers occurring in groups.

Sensory Type

Four syndromes will be mentioned.

1. When the *dorsal root ganglion cells* are primarily involved one must consider tabes dorsalis, subacute combined degeneration of the cord, Friedreich's ataxia, and certain hereditary syndromes characterized by diminution or loss of pain sensation (Figs. 44-3; 44-4A,B). The same picture may be seen as a nonmetastatic syndrome of malignancy (usually an oat-cell carcinoma of the bronchus, lymphoma, or carcinoma of the breast).

2. In the uncommon hereditary sensory neuropathies (HSN), either pain or temperature loss develops insidiously in the second decade, or all forms of sensation are absent from birth. The loss of pain and position sense lead to terrible mutilation. Obsessive care of the feet and hands is the only prophylactic measure that can be taken.

3. A third syndrome in this category is dysautonomia, in which autonomic failure leads to postural hypotension, anhydrosis, pupillary abnormalities, and sphincter disturbances.

4. Finally, a mixed sensory and motor neuronal neuropathy (neuronal form of HMSN, which is described later, is also recognized.

In most of these conditions, mild but progressing centripetal sensory loss, especially affecting thick-fiber functions, brings the patient ot the doctor. Complaints of girdle pains, atrophic changes in the feet, and imbalance are also common.

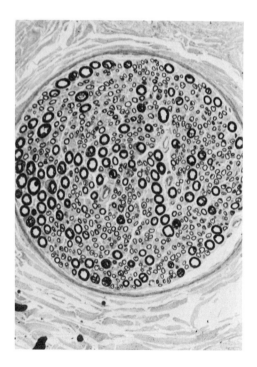
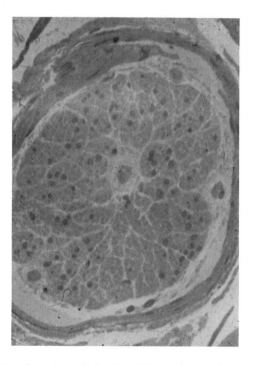

Figure 44-3   Transverse sections of peripheral nerve, stained with osmium tetroxide to show myelin. On the left is a normal nerve and on the right that from a patient with hereditary sensory neuropathy. In the latter, the myelinated fibers are almost all destroyed.

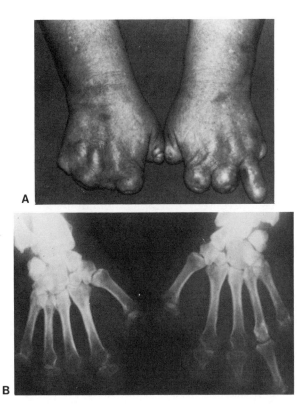

Figure 44-4A, B   Hereditary sensory neuropathy. The loss of the distal parts of the digits is due to infection following painless trauma and leading on to necrosis. This has earned for this and other conditions such as syrinogmyelia the designation of "mutilating acropathy."

Acute inflammation of *dorsal root ganglion cells* occurs with herpes zoster, when it affects the fifth nerve or a few dermatomes at most, or as a toxic effect of penicillin, doxorubicin (Adriamycin), mercury, or a remote carcinoma. In the latter instance, generalized profound sensory losses occur with little improvement.

Damage to the *axon* can follow trauma to the nerve. With mild compression or stretching, function may be only temporarily interrupted. Because there is no damage to the anatomical integrity of the nerve, pressure having produced only local ischemia and edema, recovery occurs over minutes, days, or a few weeks, depending upon the severity of the pressure. With more severe but briefly applied trauma, such as a severe stretch or a heavy blow to the nerve, the axons may be interrupted, but the Schwann cell sheaths remain in continuity. Wallerian degeneration will occur distally and for one or two segments proximally, after which axonal sprouting occurs. Sprouts will grow down the still-present Schwann cell tubes to reach their end-plates or sensory receptors, growing at about 1 mm daily. With yet more severe trauma, the whole anatomical nerve may be lacerated and divided, again producing distal wallerian degeneration. This leads to inefficient axonal sprouting because some motor nerve fibers may grow down tubes leading to the wrong muscle or, for example, into tubes formerly occupied by sensory nerves.

Apart from trauma, many metabolic and toxic neuropathies (particularly those caused by exogenous chemicals or drugs) produce major damage both to the axons and to the cell body. Examples include deficiency of vitamin B (beriberi, pellagra) and B_{12}, sprue, alcohol ingestion, uremia, and many toxins (see Chap. 43). Neuropathy from glue sniffing is progressive, primarily affecting motor functions and caused by the organic solvents n-hexene and toluene in the glue, but most other toxic agents affect sensory function more than motor, and the clinical presentation is more frequently a subacute or chronic symmetric and distal sensorimotor neuropathy. The nerves are not thickened in these cases and the legs are affected more than the arms. The likely reason for this is that because of the effect of the toxin, metabolism of the cell body is impaired to the extent that it cannot easily pump axoplasm to the most distant points along its axon. The process of "dying back" then occurs, and it is the "Outposts of Empire" rather than the regions close to the nerve cell body that are first affected, at least as seen clinically.[*] Afferent fibers in the legs can be over 3 ft long, whereas in the arms the distance is a good deal less; thus the first symptoms usually appear in the lower limbs. By the same token, the face is seldom affected, although stilbamidine and trichloroethylene do particularly impair fifth nerve sensory function.

Demyelinating Neuropathies

Both wallerian degeneration and dying-back neuropathies lead to secondary redundancy of Schwann cells which may disappear or become markedly reduced in numbers. This secondary demyelination must be distinguished from primary demyelination in which the major damage is caused to the Schwann cells in the first place. The cells of Schwann perform the same function vis-a-vis the axon as the oligodendroglia perform in the CNS; that is, they have nutritive and insulating functions. In the peripheral axon, their presence with interspersed nodes of Ranvier allows saltatory conduction to occur and their absence causes a marked reduction in the speed of passage of the nerve impulses.

If there is significant Schwann cell damage, the first axons to have their function impaired will be those that rely most on the insulating action of these Schwann cells, namely those with the thickest layer of myelin, the fastest-conducting fibers. Clinically, the first and most severe modalities of sensory loss will be those of vibration, joint position sense, and tactile discrimination, although there usually will also be a diminution in thin-fiber function. In axonal sensory neuropathies, different sensory modes tend to be affected to the same extent.

Demyelinating neuropathies lead to loss of tendon reflexes early on. Both motor and sensory nerves are involved, although in most instances the sensory overshadow the motor findings. Spontaneous pain is not uncommon but is not a strong diagnostic indicator of any particular type of neuropathy (nor indeed of neuropathy itself because spontaneous pain and tenderness in muscles may occur with both neuropathy and primary muscle disease).

Hereditary Demyelinating Neuropathies

Most hereditary motor and sensory neuropathies (HMSNs) are of the demyelinating type. The prototype is *Charcot-Marie-Tooth disease,* also known as *peroneal muscular atrophy.* This may be inherited in any way, autosomal-dominant, autosomal-recessive, or sex-linked recessive, and it may occur sporadically.

---

[*]Even a cursory study of history shows that empires recede from their furthest points, served by the longest lines of communication.

Clinical Features

In youth, the patient complains of foot deformity (high arches), difficulty in getting shoes to fit, hammer toes, dropfoot, and the insidious progression of wasting and weakness of the distal musculature of the leg and much later of the arms (Fig. 44-5A & B). A family history of "arthritis," or various hereditary neurological syndromes is common.

Atrophy of the lower one-third of the thigh and in the calf is said to give the leg an "inverted champagne bottle" appearance.* The deep tendon reflexes are usually lost in the legs but present in the arms until a late stage. Minor sensory symptoms and signs (diminution of vibration and light-touch sensation and of joint position sensation) maybe found at a later stage. Other signs sometimes found include optic atrophy, cerebellar signs, scoliosis, and retinal changes. Circulatory insufficiency is common and thickened nerves may be visible or palpable. Pes cavus is caused by this condition in about a third of cases, and occurs alone as frequently. The remaining cases are associated with a wide range of upper and lower motor neuron lesions, spinal dysraphism or spinocerebellar degenerations.

---

*Although this is the classic description, connoisseurs will immediately protest that the leg shape resembles more that of a hock bottle.

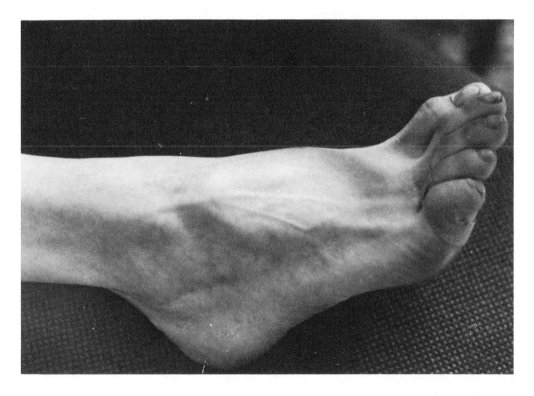

Figure 44-5A   Pes cavus in a patient with hereditary motor and sensory neuropathy.

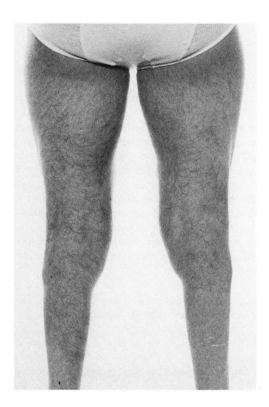

Figure 44-5B Distal atrophy of the legs in the same condition.

Diagnosis and Management

The family pedigree frequently contains evidence of similar neuropathies and of
spinocerebellar degenerations of one kind or another, which is a great help in diagnosis. The disease is slowly progressive but there is extreme variability in this,
and while sometimes patients die with cardiac conduction defects in the fourth
and fifth decades, others are still working at the ordinary age of retirement.

The neurogenic atrophy of muscles that results from denervation can be confirmed by EMG and by muscle biopsy, if necessary. Motor nerve conduction
velocities are markedly slowed and sensory nerve action potentials are diminished
or absent. Nerve biopsy shows a hypertrophic neuropathy with characteristic
"onion-bulb" laminations of Schwann cells resulting from episodes of de- and re-
myelination.

No specific treatment is possible, but physiotherapy may delay contractures
and assist the patient in using his remaining motor skills in the most efficient way.
Bracing, special shoes, and orthopedic procedures to improve mobility or stability
of the ankle may be helpful.

Another form of HMSN is accompanied by pyramidal and cerebellar signs with
choreiform movements, nystagmus, miosis, raised CSF protein levels, kyphoscloio-
sis, and marked enlargement of the peripheral nerves. In a third form, *Refsum's
syndrome,* anosmia, nerve deafness, retinitis pigmentosa, cerebellar signs, raised
CSF protein, icthyosis, and skeletal abnormalities such as kyphoscoliosis and pes

cavus are associated. In this condition, a high level of circulating phytanic acid is found, which can be reduced (and to some extent symptoms also reduced) by restricting the amount of animal fats and foods containing chlorophyll that the patient is allowed to eat.

Many of the hereditary demyelinating neuropathies fall within the spectrum of the spinocerebellar degenerations. *Porphyria* and some of the *leukodystrophies,* producing in childhood symptoms of optic atrophy, seizures, amentia or dementia, and various motor signs, are also associated with a hypertrophic demyelinating neuropathy.

Acquired Demyelinating Neuropathies

Distal and symmetric motor, sensory, or mixed neuropathies also result from acquired damage to the Schwann cells. Causes include *rheumatoid arthritis,* particularly if treated with steroids, *diphtheria,* and uncommonly *lead poisoning* and acute intermittent *porphyria,* in which the signs are almost entirely motor and also often proximal. In association with *carcinoma,* usually of the bronchus or ovary, a sensorimotor neuropathy can also occur. But far more common are two other conditions that deserve discussion in some detail.

Diabetes: In diabetes mellitus a number of types of neuropathy may be found. The most common neurological problem is a subacute or chronic peripheral, symmetric, *sensorimotor demyelinating neuropathy* that is probably related to the duration (but not to the degree of control) of the diabetes. Rarely, evidence of the neuropathy precedes clinical or significant biochemical evidence of diabetes. Signs include a diminution of vibration, touch, deep pain, and joint position sensation and reduction of distal reflexes. Some distal wasting occurs at a later stage.

This neuropathy is seldom a major problem for the patient, but when it is severe, an autonomic component may result in poor healing and the lack of deep pain sensation and unawareness of trivial trauma may in time produce skin ulcers and disorganization of joints — the Charcot joints also described in patients with syringomyelia, HSNs, and tabes dorsalis.

As a result of *pure sensory neuropathy,* diabetes is also a cause of mutilating acropathy, with damage to the distal parts of the body because of cumulative trauma and lack of care of the relatively painless denervated areas. Unfortunately, control of diabetes is usually unrelated to the severity of the neuropathy and no effective treatment is known.

Ischemic diabetic neuropathies are described later. They are multiple mononeuropathies and are more amenable to treatment. Diabetics with nerves "at risk" because of metabolic factors are unusually prone to pressure palsies.

A syndrome of proximal, asymmetric pelvic girdle wasting and weakness may occur in diabetes because of *lumbosacral plexopathy.* This usually happens only when control has been poor. In such cases thigh pain is often severe and quadriceps and adductor wasting marked, with loss of the knee jerk. Recovery occurs slowly with improved control — which almost always means insulin. The pain is best treated with a combination of amitryptyline (up to 75 mg at night) and fluphenazine 1-2 mg t.i.d.

The *autonomic nervous system* may be involved, producing postural hypotension, nocturnal diarrhea, acute gastric dilation, impotence, disturbance of bladder function, lack of sweating (anhidrosis), and a loss of vasomotor and axon reflexes in the skin. Argyll Robertson pupils may be seen in diabetes because of involvement of the parasympathetic fibers to the eye.

Acute Inflammatory Polyneuropathy (Guillain-Barré Syndrome): The other important demyelinating peripheral neuropathy is that described by Landry and later by Guillain, Barré, and Strohl, which is known as the *Guillain-Barré syndrome,* *postinfectious polyneuropathy,* or *acute inflammatory polyneuropathy* (AIP).

Etiology: This condition commonly follows a viral or mycoplasmal illness affecting the upper respiratory or alimentary tracts; vaccination or surgery, or it may complicate an underlying malignancy such as Hodgkin's disease. Because infections seem to have occurred in the preceding 2 weeks in about the half the cases seen the term *postinfectious polyneuropathy* is preferred by some. Increased titers of antibodies to Epstein-Barr virus and cytomegalovirus have been reported, which makes that name a reasonable choice.

The sexes are equally involved. This condition occurs at any age but most commonly in adults aged over 40. It is a polyradiculopathy, which means that the brunt of the acute allergic response is seen in the spinal (or cranial) nerve roots. Here, intense round cell infiltration is seen, extending distally in the nerves with accompanying demyelination because of Schwann cell damage.

Clinical features: The onset is acute or subacute over a week or two. Complaints of paresthesias, numbness, muscle tenderness, and weakness appear in that order, initially in the legs. There is no fever. Weakness may be markedly asymmetric, although it is nearly always bilateral; and it may progress to any degree of severity from minimal weakness in the legs to profound quadriparesis with respiratory and bulbar failure, which occurs in about 10 percent of the patients.

The distal muscles are usually involved first, and the disease normally spreads centrally, although rarely the reverse is the case. The bladder is never much affected, and although facial involvement is common, the eyes are seldom involved.

Examination shows predominant motor findings, consisting of flaccid weakness peripherally, without fasciculations but with areflexia. Power also may be lessened or lost proximally in the girdle muscles, trunk, bulbar muscles, and face, or these areas may escape entirely. Wasting occurs early in the affected limbs. Sensory findings are minimal, but pain may be severe. Autonomic features represent a dangerous complication. Tachycardia, postural hypotension, pupillary disturbances and lack of variation in the interbeat interval (measured by the RR intervals on an ECG with deep breathing) signify autonomic disturbances which require further ECG and blood pressure monitoring.

In a malignant form of AIP, there is early involvement of the cranial nerves and trunk with bulbar palsies and respiratory failure. In all, up to 20 percent of patients develop some degree of ventilatory inadequacy because of involvement of the diaphragm and intercostal muscles. Because one cannot predict who is, or who is not, going to progress to this severe form, all patients with AIP must be admitted to the hospital until at least the first signs of recovery appear.

A variant of AIP produces a combination of ophthalmoplegia, ataxia, and areflexia with little systemic weakness (Miller Fisher syndrome).

Investigations: The CSF protein is initially normal but rises as the disease progresses. Protein values are seldom above 2 g/L and the cell count is normal, a fact serenaded by the euphonious French term *dissociation cyto-albuminologique.* Occasionally, the protein level exceeds 10 g/L, producing a Froin's syndrome (xanthochromic acellular CSF that clots spontaneously). Early electrodiagnostic studies show slowing or loss of late responses; later in the illness there is marked slowing of motor nerve conduction velocities.

Course: The recovery period is prolonged; over half the patients are completely better by 6 months and three-quarters within a year, but continuous weakness, malaise, and easy fatigability trouble the remainder and in a few, recurrent attacks occur. Those patients who begin to recover in the first 2 weeks after onset usually do so completely.

The syndrome of AIP is the most important cause of acute severe progressive motor peripheral neuropathy. Other causes include acute porphyria, diphtheria, and some form of toxic exposure.

Fatalities occur in 5 percent of cases because of ventilatory failure, pneumonia, cardiac arrhythmias, or autonomic failure. These deaths should be preventable with intensive nursing and medical care; one must be vigilant for any hint of respiratory involvement during the early stages, intubating with a soft tube immediately when the vital capacity drops below 1 L. In any patient whose diagnosis is AIP, the vital capacity should be repeatedly measured.

Treatment: Subcutaneous heparin injections to prevent deep vein thrombosis, frequent limb movement for the same purpose and to prevent contractures, and oral quinine 300 mg/day for pain are useful therapeutic agents. Steroids are not of proven benefit in acute cases (they may be harmful), although there are reports of improvement with plasma exchange in some acute cases. It is not possible to predict which patient might benefit. Ventilatory support, attention to fluid and electrolyte status, and monitoring for such complications as cardiac arrhythmias and inappropriate ADH secretion are vital for the severely affected patient. Feeding is best done with a nasogastric tube. Psychological support is essential — some of these patients are "locked-in" and unable to move at all. Successful management of such a case is a triumph of medical and nursing care. Protection from pressure palsies of the *ulnar, peroneal,* and *sciatic* nerves is necessary; otherwise the patient recovers from AIP only to be left with a dropfoot or hand weakness from secondary compression. Similar care must be taken to maintaining the feet in dorsiflexion to prevent permanent contractures.

Chronic relapsing dysimmune polyneuropathy can only be differentiated from AIP by its course over months. Unlike AIP, this condition responds well to immunosupression with azathioprine and steroids; some patients have shown a good response to plasma exchange.

Infiltration of nerves with *myeloma, amyloid, sarcoid, xanthoma,* or *carcinoma* may also cause Schwann cell dysfunction and visible and pathological enlargement of the nerves. In *leprosy* (Hansen's disease) excessive amounts of collagen produce ischemia and Schwann cell damage in both the lepromatous and tuberculoid forms. In the former a distal, symmetrical, sensory neuropathy or a multiple mononeuropathy is seen, and many acid-fast bacilli will be detected in the hypertrophic skin lesions. In the tuberculoid form the skin atrophies, loses pigment, and becomes anesthetic. The nerves are nodular and thickened. This form usually presents as a slowly progressive multiple mononeuropathy. Leprosy is probably the most common cause of neuropathy in the world, although rare in North America. Various demyelinating neuropathies such as HMSN, described earlier, and those caused by diabetes or leukodystrophies, also show increased amounts of connective tissue or abnormalities of the composition of myelin. Abnormal amounts of connective tissue may also be found in relapsing forms of AIP.

Ischemic Neuropathy

Schwann cells tolerate ischemia badly, having a high metabolic rate and being dependent upon the vasa nervorum for their blood supply. If this supply fails, the insulating capacity of the Schwann cell is damaged as it becomes metabolically embarrassed, leading to conduction block. Such failure of blood supply may occur because of occlusion of the vasa nervorum from compression (see following section), or in diabetes, collagen-vascular diseases, atheroma, or paraneoplastic vasculitis, producing ischemic mononeuropathies that may affect multiple nerves. The diabetic forms are typical of them all.

In diabetes, the sixth, third, and fourth cranial, and the femoral and obturator nerves are most often affected. Diabetic femoral neuropathy (which is really a lumbosacral plexopathy), was described previously. Diabetic third nerve palsies frequently spare the pupil,[*] perhaps because the parasympathetic fibers are situated around the outside of the nerve, where they can receive some blood supply from the local pia-arachnoid vessels. The initial complaints are of eye pain, headache, and diplopia that have sudden onset but usually clear after weeks or months. In diabetes, such ischemic neuropathies are often superimposed upon a preexisting metabolic polyneuropathy.

Compression Neuropathies

Although nerve compression produces dysfunction partly through the mechanism of ischemia, compression neuropathies will be described separately because of their great frequency. Any superficial nerve in the body may be stretched or compressed; even comparatively minor pressure will give rise to long-lasting symptoms if the nerves have been damaged already and are thus at risk. Such may occur in the presence of any subclinical neuropathy and also when a lesion is situated proximally (such as cervical spondylosis) where it is already damaging the nerve fibers at a higher level. Patients with generalized wasting diseases and loss of fat will have less of a subcutaneous buffer between nerves and external objects. Because they may be lying in bed for long periods, compression neuropathies are also common in such cases.

The *upper fibers of the brachial plexus* may be compressed by fibrous tissue after radiation therapy, when lymphedema is commonly found but pain is seldom present. Weakness and wasting of the deltoid, spinati, biceps and other shoulder-girdle and upper-arm muscles are found (Erb's palsy). For some reason, myokymia in the proximal muscles is common in this situation. However a stretching injury to the *C5-6 roots,* rather than compression, is the usual cause of Erb's palsy, in which weakness of shoulder abduction and external rotation, elbow flexion and supination, and wrist and finger dorsiflexion give rise to the classic "porter's tip" appearance (Fig. 44-6).

The *lower fibers* may be infiltrated by malignant tissue; this produces a Horner's syndrome, pain, and mainly distal signs, such as wasting and weakness of the thenar and hypothenar muscles, and reduced sensation in the distal upper limb. Damage to these fibers also occurs with abduction injuries of the shoulder (Klumpke's palsy) which stretch *C8 and T1 roots.*

The *thoracic outlet syndrome* is more a vascular than a neurological entity; although the diagnosis is often made, objective neurological or electrical signs are rare. Symptoms of the condition include pain in the arm, especially with heavy lifting or carrying; coldness, color change and pain in the hands; and weakness of the forearm and hand. Symptoms may be produced or exacerbated by downward traction on the arm and sometimes by hyperabduction at the shoulder, when a diminution of the radial pulse may be found which may be the key to the whole matter if the problem is venous or arterial compression rather than stretching of the lower fibers of the brachial plexus. Objective physical signs such as C8-T1 sensory loss or small hand muscle wasting are rare; but many of these patients have long necks and droopy shoulders, suggesting that this is sometimes purely a disorder of posture.

---

[*]But so do aneurysms sometimes. The Golden Rule is that there are no Golden Rules.

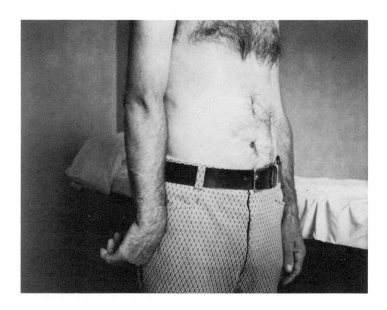

Figure 44-6 Erb's palsy following injury to the C5-6 roots in a motor vehicle accident. The "porter's tip" position of the hand is shown.

When physical signs are actually found, even if x-rays do not show cervical ribs, a fibrous band may be present between the (often large) C-7 transverse process and the first rib. The scalenus anticus muscle is inserted into the first rib, just anterior to the subclavian artery and the lower trunk of the brachial plexus, and it has been suggested that hypertrophy or abnormal contraction of this muscle causes compression.

The differential diagnosis is from all the conditions listed under *Distal Weakness and Wasting* in Chapter 26. In the presence of even minor vascular changes, the potential damage to the subclavian artery (dilatation or thrombosis) makes surgical exploration advisable.

Resection of the scalenus anticus or of the first rib, a cervical rib, or a band between them have all been advocated as effective treatments. But we advise those of our patients who have neither vascular nor neurologic signs on examination (a huge majority) to practice shoulder-girdle strengthening exercises, and we seldom refer anyone for surgery.

The *axillary* (circumflex) nerve may be damaged when the head of the humerus is dislocated posteriorly, and less often by direct trauma. The same nerve is severely involved in the condition of neuralgic amyotrophy (see Chap. 36). Weakness and wasting of the deltoid, with a small patch of sensory loss over the outer part of the shoulder, are the only signs resulting from selective axillary nerve damage. This condition must be differentiated from a C5 root lesion, in which there will also be signs of a lower neuron lesion affecting the rhomboids and the supra- and infraspinati, as well as other muscles supplied in part by C5.

Some other nerves may be damaged in isolation. The nerve to the *serratus anterior* is one such, causing winging of the scapula in healthy, young people who have been exercising heavily (Fig. 44-7), and the *suprascapular nerve* is cometimes compressed or traumatized locally.

The most common nerve to be affected by compression is undoubtedly the *ul-*

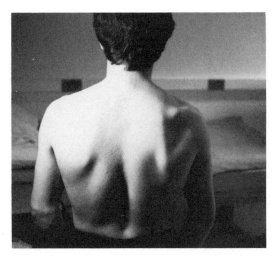

Figure 44-7 (A) Serratus anterior palsy. This young man took a summer job haul-
ing lumber and developed his muscular bulk; but then complained of shoulder weakness. The palsy is probably caused by pressure on the nerve by strongly contracting
hypertrophied muscles of the chest wall; (B) Wasted spinati in a man with a traumatic suprascapular nerve palsy.

nar. Its involvement in lesions affecting the lower trunk has already been mentioned, but the most frequent site of damage is the cubital tunnel, behind the medial
epicondyle of the elbow where it passes under the common origin of the flexor
muscles. Probably every medical student has experienced the disagreeable pain
and electric shock sensation of banging his "funny bone" and the paresthesias in
his hand when leaning on the elbows while burning the midnight oil over his studies
(Fig. 44-8A-C).

When the elbow is flexed, the nerve is partially stretched and rises superficially, where it may well be damaged when the elbow rests on a hard surface. Symptoms of ulnar nerve weakness (involving the ulnar half of flexor digitorum profun-
dus, all the interossei, the hypothenar muscles, and adductor pollicis) and sensory
symptoms (diminution of common sensation in the little finger and the ulnar half
of the ring finger) may be expected and Tinel's sign will be positive at the elbow.
Striking wasting of the dorsal and palmar interossei may be seen. (Fig. 44-9.)

In carpenters and shoemakers using palm pressure on screwdrivers and awls,
or in heavy equipment operators and truck drivers who push gears with the palm
of the hand, the deep palmar branch of the nerve may be compressed just medial
to the pisiform bone at the wrist. This is below the origin of the superficial sensory branch to the fingers and that of the motor branch of the hypothenar eminence, so the effect is of interosseous wasting and weakness of adductor pollicis
only.

Median nerve compression in the carpal tunnel is another classic, occurring
in healthy people and in those with any abnormal degree of fluid retention, e.g.,
hypothyroidism, pregnancy, or chronic renal disease. It is also seen in Paget's
disease, myelomatosis, acromegaly, obesity, and in local conditions involving the
flexor tendons lying, with the nerve, under the flexor retinaculum of the wrist.
Thus synovial herniation or tenosynovitis, a simple ganglion, or a lipoma may be
present.

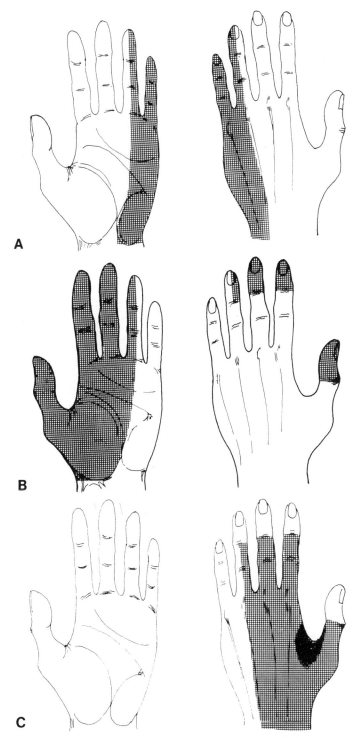

Figure 44-8 (A) Distribution of the sensory loss because of an ulnar nerve lesion anywhere below the mid-upper arm; (B) Distribution of the sensory loss because of a median nerve lesion anywhere below the brachial plexus; (C) Distribution of the sensory loss because of a radial nerve lesion anywhere below the upper arm.

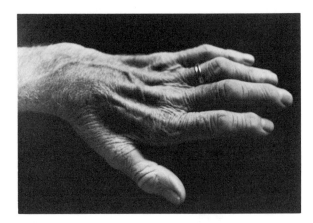

Figure 44-9   Ulnar nerve palsy; cubital tunnel syndrome. The wasting of the adductor pollicis and interossei is marked.

Clinical Features

Patients are more frequently women than men. They complain of pain in the hand that rises up the arm even as far as the shoulder and characteristically awakens the patient at night; in association with paresthesias of at least three-and-a-half fingers (but sometimes patients do not remember their anatomy and complain of tingling throughout the whole hand; Fig. 44-8B). When the patient does wake up early in the morning, she tends to rub or flick the hand to try and restore it to life. Any heavy exertion during the day tends to bring on the symptoms, especially gripping a steering wheel or carrying a suitcase. Weakness of the thumb is manifested as clumsiness and difficulty with some fine movements. Examination reveals weakness of the thenar muscles (not the adductor) and possibly of the two radial lumbricals so that extension at the interphalangeal joints of the second and third fingers is impaired.

Diagnosis and Management

Precise electrophysiological criteria for the diagnosis of carpal tunnel syndrome have been defined and most surgeons prefer to operate after the diagnosis has been confirmed by nerve conduction studies. The best long-term results are achieved by incision of the flexor retinaculum under local anesthesia, to relieve the pressure on the nerve. Alternatively an injection of 20 mg of prednisone under the flexor retinaculum may produce temporary relief. Conservative measures are correctly used in pregnant women because the condition often clears after delivery.

The *radial nerve* may be involved in the upper arm if the arm is allowed to hang over the back of a chair for a long period, for example in the common Saturday night palsy. With damage at that site, the branches to the triceps are spared, so that the patient can still extend the elbow. There is, however, a marked wristdrop and failure of finger extension (Fig. 44-10). A small patch of sensory loss can often be detected between the thumb and first finger on the dorsum of the hand (see Fig. 44-8C). The condition is common among alcoholics, in whom there is often the added factor of preexisting alcoholic neuropathy.

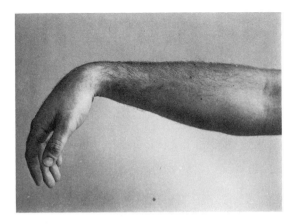

Figure 44-10   Radial nerve palsy, following trauma to the nerve above the elbow. The triceps was spared but weakness and atrophy of all the forearm extensors has led to wristdrop.

The nerve may also be involved at a lower level, where it passes underneath the origin of the extensor carpi radialis longus and supinator. Here it may be compressed by a fibrous band or by a posterior dislocation of the radial head. The *posterior interosseous nerve* (the continuation of the radial) may be damaged with forearm fractures more distally.

In the legs, pressure may cause trouble at a number of sites. *Lumbosacral plexopathy* is most often due to diabetes, but retroperitoneal tumors, aneurysms, abscess, or a vasculitis in elderly patients can produce the same picture. Patients with this last problem will complain of severe root pain and focal deficits in the distribution of the femoral, obturator, and/or sciatic nerves. The diagnosis is seldom possible without the aid of EMG and CT scanning, but a clue may be obtained from the high ESR generally found.

The *sciatic nerve* may be damaged by a posterior dislocation of the hip or by a misplaced IM injection. The initial result will be paralysis of all the muscles in the leg except for those innervated by the obturator and femoral nerves. Sensory loss will be complete below the knee.

The *lateral femoral cutaneous nerve* is sometimes compressed as it passes through the outer edge of the inguinal ligament. This is common in pregnancy and in obese people, in whom the nerve is compressed by a pad of fat. Pain, burning paresthesias in the lateral part of the thigh, and a small area of local sensory loss characterize this condition , known as meralgia paresthetica (Fig. 44-11). Treatment comprises weight loss, local injection of the nerve with hydrocortisone and local anesthetic, and if necessary, surgical decompression.

The *obturator nerve* is occasionally damaged in the obturator canal, usually by the fetal head during·parturition, or after the imprecise application of forceps. The main features are pain in the inner side of the thigh, with some sensory loss in that area and weakness of the adductors.

Damage to the *common peroneal nerve* as it winds around the neck of the fibula is a common problem. Perhaps because of the anatomical arrangement of its fibers, those that pass in the deep peroneal to form the anterior tibial nerve (which innervates the space between the hallux and the second toes) are sometimes spared. Those running in the superficial peroneal nerve, carrying sensation from the outer

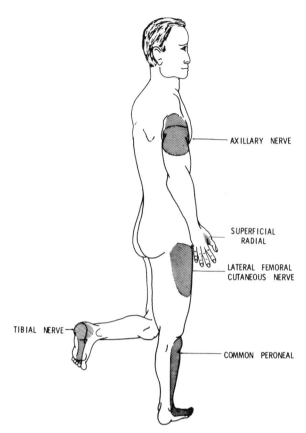

Figure 44-11   Distribution of sensory loss with lesions of a number of peripheral nerves.

edge of the calf and the dorsum of the foot, are usually involved, with diminution or loss of sensation in that area. The motor fibers running to the peronei and the anterior tibial muscles are also affected, producing a footdrop and failure of eversion of the foot. Tinel's sign will be positive, initially at the neck of the fibula, when regeneration begins. Patients placed in stirrups in the Trendelenburg's position, those who have ill-fitting plaster of Paris casts or braces applied, those who are wasted and who lie long in bed, or especially those who sit with their legs crossed for a long time, are likely to develop peroneal nerve palsy.

The *posterior tibial* nerve may be compressed when it runs behind the medial malleolus under the flexor retinaculum to supply the small foot muscles (as the medial and lateral plantar nerves) and the skin of the sole of the foot on the medial side. Apart from these motor and sensory changes, pain may also be predominant feature. Surgical decompression is effective treatment.

Rather more distally, a *lateral plantar* nerve may be compressed by a neuroma between the heads of the third and fourth metatarsals, producing very little in the way of clinically definable sensory loss or motor weakness but causing a lot of discomfort. The patient has a characteristic pattern of pain in the foot while walking, often stopping to take off the shoe and rub the foot. This condition, known as Morton's metatarsalgia, is also helped by surgery.

Because all the *cranial nerves* leave the skull through foramina, they are also prone to compression, e.g., the seventh as in Bell's palsy, the eighth in a cerebello-pontine angle tumor or Paget's disease, and the third with a temporal lobe expanding lesion producing the uncal herniation syndrome. Pressure on the lower cranial nerves from inflammatory, neoplastic, or vascular lesions may occur as well. Pressure on *spinal nerve roots* by tumors, disks, or osteophytes, etc., could also be regarded as compression neuropathies but these are considered in Chapter 30.

Autonomic Neuropathy

In diabetes, tabes dorsalis, multiple sclerosis, myelopathies, AIP, Wernicke's, amyloidosis, and certain rare degenerative diseases, the autonomic nervous system (ANS) is markedly involved. In elderly patients also, mild ANS degeneration is seen. The drugs affecting the ANS are considered in Chapter 43. Such patients may complain of the symptoms of postural hypotension, diarrhea, especially nocturnally, impotence, and the consequences of incomplete bladder emptying. Demonstration on the ECG of a lack of "overshoot" tachycardia on standing up, of variations in pulse rate with the Valsalva maneuver or in the cold pressor test, and of a blood pressure increase of less than 10-mm systolic with sustained hand grip, all suggest autonomic involvement.

Treatment of postural hypotension and the other features of autonomic failure is difficult. One may try getting the patient to eat more salt than usual and if necessary may prescribe fludrocortisone, but this is seldom very effective. Elastic stockings are often prescribed, again seldom with great help to the patient. An anti-G suit may however be useful, but if the postural blood pressure fall is extreme, even this will be inadequate. Cholinergic drugs may reinforce bladder contraction. In the Shy-Drager syndrome (idiopathic hypotension plus basal ganglion and cerebral degeneration), fludrocortisone, indomethacin, and occasionally propranolol may be helpful, although the course is progressive.

APPROACH TO THE PATIENT WITH NEUROPATHY

Given the clinical diagnosis of peripheral neuropathy, i.e., not a mononeuropathy, one has then to decide what is its pathology and pathogenesis. Some clinical clues, such as the extent of motor or sensory involvement or the type of sensory loss, have already been mentioned. Here is another way.

Start by assessing the rapidity of onset of the condition. *Acute* neuropathies, developing in less than a week, are almost all motor. With distal involvement and slowed motor nerve conducting velocity (MNCV), consider diphtheria, AIP, lead poisoning, and porphyria. Distal involvement and normal MNCVs may be caused by the same condition, but at an early stage, or may be due to toxic agents or to poliomyelitis. Proximal motor neuropathies are probably diabetic, but AIP can present thus sometimes.

Acute sensory neuropathies are usually due to toxic agents, but sometimes occur in association with underlying malignancy.

Chronic neuropathies, taking more than a week to become symptomatic, are much more common. With more motor than sensory involvement, and distal distribution, think first of HMSN, AIP, and toxic causes. If the distribution is proximal, diabetes, motor neuron disease, and HMN are the most likely causes.

With more sensory than motor involvement and distal distribution, demyelinating neuropathies caused by diabetes, uremia, myelomatosis, dysproteinemia, and HSN should be considered first. Axonal neuropathies (less slowing of conduction velocities) may be due to toxins, including alcohol, vitamin B deficiency, or HSN. Look also for clues to the presence of CNS disorders, such as a spinocerebellar degeneration, in such cases.

If no cause for a chronic polyneuropathy is found initially, about 40 percent will turn out to have some medical illness (diabetes, malignancy, collagen-vascular, organ failure, B_{12} deficiency, alcoholism, etc.) and in 30 percent, an HMSN or spinocerebellar degeneration will be found. Inflammatory disease will be the cause in another 20 percent. Adults with a chronic, slowly progressive sensorimotor neuropathy usually have axonal damage and both sensory and motor deficits; they must be followed carefully for development of the evidence of the causal illness which will some day appear.

Investigation

It will be obvious that for the patients in whom no causative pathology can be found, and in those in whom more than one cause may be operating, investigations are best carried out by a neurologist with access to EMG because nerve conduction studies are an extension of the clinical examination.

Obviously, a full family history must be obtained as it may indicate at the outset whether this is hereditary or an acquired disease. In hereditary neuropathies, examination of serum proteins, lipoproteins, and an estimation of such substances are phytanic acid and porphyrins is wise.

Depending upon the clinical findings already discussed, the usual battery of screening tests in hematology and biochemistry and a glucose tolerance test, urine microscopy, renal and liver function tests, serum folic acid and B_{12} estimations and serum protein electropheresis might be of value in acquired neuropathies. If there is any suggestion of previous infection, viral studies and examination of CSF for protein and cells will also be required, whereas in diphtheria, bacteriological proof must be obtained. A suspicion of general medical conditions, such as carcinoma, myeloma, reticulosis, amyloidosis, collagen vascular disease, ingestion of toxic chemicals and drugs, will direct other appropriate investigations.

In acute forms, serum lead and porphyrins and urinary dALA should be requested if the neuropathy is mainly proximal and motor.

It will already have been seen however that a good start in the differentiation of neuropathies can be made if the pathological basis can be determined. Electrodiagnostic studies are helpful here; they are called for in the case of any peripheral neuropathy of which the diagnosis is not absolutely clear. In primary axonal disorders, one can obtain an indication of severity, e.g., partial vs complete axonal interruption, by conduction studies, which are also of great value in localizing the precise site of nerve compression in the entrapment neuropathies and in giving an early indication of reinnervation of denervated muscles. In selected patients, nerve biopsy will give direct information about the pathological process involved. In infiltrations, such tests may be diagnostic.

TREATMENT

Because there is no specific treatment which can be given to the nerves (except when they are compressed), but only to the causes leading to their dysfunction, therapy is really dependent upon the diagnosis and treatment of the causative disease. Patients whose neuropathy is of the Guillain-Barré type, must be observed intensely in case they should pass into a stage of respiratory inadequacy, as described earlier. Management in or close to an intensive care unit is also essential in patients with diphtheria or botulism, in whom bulbar paralysis may be life-threatening, and ventilatory support essential.

The management of patients with hereditary neuropathies was discussed in the appropriate section.

Patients with symptomatic compressive neuropathies need decompression if the site of the lesion can be determined accurately by clinical and electrodiagnostic methods. A search for other causes of subclinical neuropathy should be instituted in all such patients.

In all of the remaining types of neuropathy, treatment is determined by the cause. Thus replacement of vitamin deficiencies, removal of toxic agents, and treatment of such medical conditions as diabetes, collagen-vascular disease, and cancer, will often lead to improvement in the neuropathic symptoms. Rehabilitation must not be omitted; even if the cause is untreatable, walking aids, braces, splints, and limb or gait training may improve function to the patient's great relief.

BIBLIOGRAPHY

Asbury, A.K. Diagnostic considerations in Guillain-Barré syndrome. *Ann. Neurol.* Suppl. 1, 1-5, 1981.

Bannister, R. *Autonomic Failure.* New York, Oxford, 1983.

Brown, M.J., Asbury, A.K. Diabetic neuropathy. *Ann. Neurol. 15:*2-12, 1984.

Dawson, D.M. et al. *Entrapment Neuropathies.* Boston, Little, Brown & Co., 1984.

Dyck, P.J., Thomas, P.K., Lambert, E.H. (eds.). *Peripheral Neuropathy,* 2nd Ed. Philadelphia, W.B. Saunders Co., 1984.

Peet, R.M. et al. Thoracic outlet syndrome; Evaluation of a therapeutic exercise program. *Mayo Clin. Proc. 31:*281-287, 1956.

45
Diseases of Muscle

The main disorders of muscle may be divided between those having some *genetic* basis and those *acquired* later. In the former group are the progressive dystrophies, myotonic disorders, congenital myopathies, and some metabolic myopathies. In the latter are inflammatory diseases of muscle, myasthenia, and various metabolic, endocrine, or toxic myopathies with no known genetic basis.

The terms *dystrophy* and *myopathy* are confusing. The former term is reserved for certain genetically determined and progressive disorders such as Duchenne's, myotonic dystrophy, and so forth. All other disorders of muscle are generally termed myopathies, although because dystrophies are disorders of muscle, they might equally well be called myopathies too. This is another idiosyncrasy of medical terminology that is regrettable but probably by now irreversible.

HEREDITARY DISEASES OF MUSCLE

The Genetic Dystrophies

These disorders (Table 45-1) are all progressive to a greater or lesser extent. At one extreme, Duchenne's dystrophy is usually lethal before the age of 25, while at the other, ocular dystrophies may not alter life expectancy at all. Not all of the muscular dystrophies are congenital, as the facioscapulohumeral type may not develop until the teens and myotonic dystrophy may first manifest at any time up to age 60.

Duchenne's Dystrophy

Duchenne's dystrophy (DMD) is a severe genetic dystrophy that occurs at a rate of 1 case in every 3000 live male births. It is inherited as an X-linked recessive; however there is a high mutation rate, so isolated cases are common.

610

Table 45-1   Classification of Muscular Dystrophy

Duchenne's

    Sex-linked recessive

        severe

        benign

Limb girdle

Facioscapulohumeral

Distal

Ocular/oculopharyngeal

Congenital

Clinical Features: Affected boys may have normal milestones up to the age of 1 year, but they learn to stand and walk somewhat late and speech may be slow in developing. They exhibit progressive weakness over the next few years and seldom if ever are able to run, although trying their hardest with flailing arms and fast-moving, waddling legs; but weak hip flexors prevent them from getting both feet off the ground at the same time when they try. They walk uneasily with abdominal protruberance and marked lumbar lordosis.

Initial involvement is of the proximal muscles of the pelvic girdle, only later of the shoulder girdle, and terminally of the face. Apparent hypertrophy of the calf muscles (and occasionally of other muscles) may be seen in about 90 percent of cases; this hypertrophy is due both to infiltration of the muscle with fat and to an increase in the size of some of the remaining myofibrils. (Fig. 45-1.)

Sir William Gowers described a sign of proximal weakness that typically appears at about the fourth year; the child who is lying prone, rises by making a four-point stand on both feet and both hands and then "climbs up" his legs with his hands gripping and resting upon his shins, knees and thighs before he finally attains the upright position (Fig. 45-2).

Despite their large size, the muscles are weak. Eventually they atrophy and develop contractures. Atrophy affects the pelvic girdle muscles, the quadriceps, hamstrings and glutei, and later the shoulder girdle muscles (Fig. 45-3A, B), but it is often hidden by fat. Involvement of the face occurs only late in the disease. Deep tendon reflexes are depressed or absent in the arms and at the knees, but the ankle reflexes may be retained for a long time. No abnormality of sensation, signs of anterior horn cell disease, and no long-tract signs occur. Skeletal deformities, such as kyphoscoliosis and contractures of the gastrocnemius and other muscles, are common. Intelligence is slightly below normal in many boys with DMD; this is not explained by deprivation arising from their enforced isolation from school and friends.

The course of the disease is progressive, the boys becoming dependent upon a wheelchair by age 10 to 12 and bedridden perhaps 5 to 10 years after that. Death is due to respiratory insufficiency because of thoracic muscle weakness or to cardiac complications, because the changes in voluntary muscles also affect the heart.

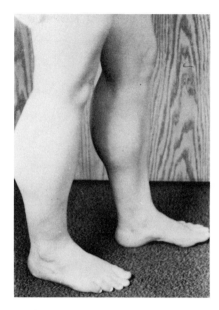

Figure 45-1   Pseudohypertrophy of calves in muscular dystrophy.

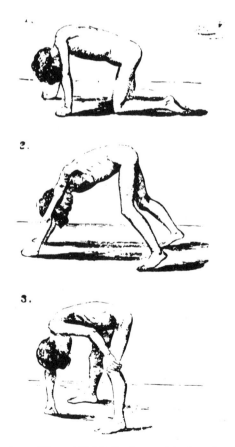

Figure 45-2   Gower's sign. The child "climbs up his legs" to compensate for weakened hip extensors. This illustration was used by Sir William Gowers in his original paper.

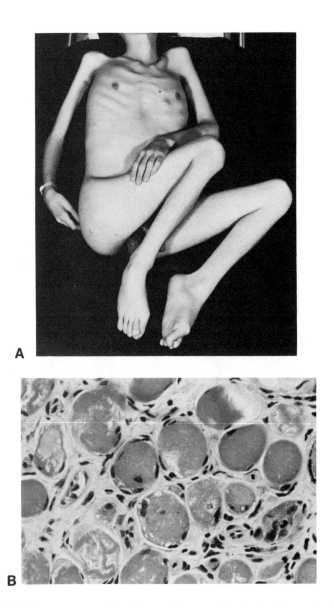

Figure 45-3   (A) Severe generalized muscle atrophy in Duchenne's muscle dystrophy. (B) Muscle biopsy (H & E stain) in Duchenne dystrophy. Many central nuclei, the variable size of the myofibrils, and increased amounts of fibrous tissue are visible.

Investigations: On the ECG, tall R waves are seen in the *right* and deep Q waves in the *left* ventricular leads, accompanied often by tachycardia and occasionally by conduction defects.

Serum CK values are high, even before clinical involvement is obvious. Levels sometimes reach a value of 300 times normal. Both EMG and muscle biopsy show features of a primary myopathy.

Management: While there is no treatment for this condition, there are a few points in management that should be known to every practitioner. First, these children must *not* be put to bed or allowed to get off their feet unless it is absolutely essential because they will never again regain their previous functional ability if they have enforced rest for any period. Second, despite the eventual necessary isolation of the boy in a wheelchair or in bed, all forms of intellectual and similar stimulation are required. Third, false hopes of cure are all too frequently raised in parents by journalistic trash. There is no cure; when there is it will be publicized in an appropriate place. Meanwhile, sympathetic counseling and continued support by the family physician are always needed.

Last, genetic counseling is vitally important.* If the mother has a son and other relatives on the female side with Duchenne's dystrophy, she is definitely a carrier of the disease. If she has two sons with Duchenne's dystrophy by different fathers, again she is definitely a carrier. Moreover, not only is she a carrier, but there is a 50 percent chance that each of her daughters will also be a carrier. Women should all understand that they have at least a good chance of knowing whether their sons will have muscular dystrophy if they are investigated with repeated serum CK estimations and perhaps EMG, muscle biopsy, and serum pyruvate kinase levels, which will allow diagnosis of the carrier state in most women.

Diagnosis of DMD sometimes requires admission to a neurological unit, but it is usually obvious clinically. Management, including that of contractures, may require time spent at a rehabilitation center. Muscular dystrophy associations exist in the United States, Canada, and most European countries, and parents should be informed of this and directed to the local chapter.

A benign form of muscular dystrophy with similar but far less severe signs also occurs (Becker's muscle dystrophy). This disorder is slowly progressive and there is no cardiac involvement.

Limb Girdle Dystrophy

Limb girdle dystrophy is a traditional but suspect diagnosis because in the past many patients with proximal muscle weakness who did not conform to the other well-known syndromes were given this diagnosis. As more precise pathologic methods developed however, many of them were found to have, for example, adult onset hereditary motor neuropathies, acid maltase deficiency, or one of the heterogeneous group of "congenital" or "morphologically distinct" myopathies.

Clinical Features: Limb girdle dystrophy is recessively inherited and may begin at any time up to the age of 30 years. Involvement of the pelvic musculature (particularly of the quadriceps) occurs first, later spreading to involve other trunk muscles and the shoulder girdle, often asymmetrically; when the deltoids are relatively spared and stand out against the wasted shoulder girdle muscles, this is a useful diagnostic pointer. Pseudohypertrophy of the calves may be seen.

The process continues slowly; cardiac involvement is seldom a feature. Although the usual onset of the disease is in young adult life, childhood forms and "congenital" muscular dystrophy presenting with hypotonia and joint contractures probably fall into this category (although many such patients have a course that is more typical of the congenital myopathies).

Facioscapulohumeral Dystrophy

Facioscapulohumeral dystrophy (Fig. 45-4) is dominantly inherited, may occur at any age, and may be of any degree of severity. Initially the facial muscles are

---

*If properly employed, a third of pregnancies now ending in the birth of a boy with DMD would not have occurred.

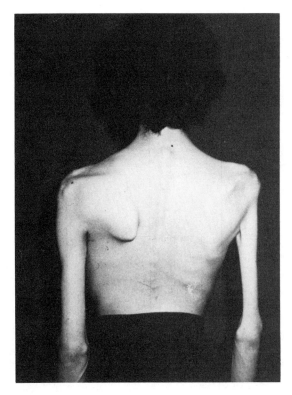

Figure 45-4   Gross wasting of the shoulder girdle muscles in facioscapulohumeral muscle dystrophy.

involved so that it is hard for the patient to whistle, drink through a straw, or pucker the lips, and he produces a transverse smile when trying to laugh. Wasting of the temporalis, masseter, and facial muscles follows. After that, obvious wasting of the scapula and thinning of the shoulder girdle and arm muscles proceeds slowly and asymmetrically, going on to involve the pelvis only after many years. The external ocular muscles and the heart are unaffected in this condition. The reflexes are depressed early on in the arms, but are retained in the legs. As in the other forms of muscular dystrophy, there are no clinical signs of corticospinal tract nor of anterior horn cell damage. However some workers contend that this and many other myopathies, even DMD, are actually a result of neurogenic dysfunction and are not primarily myopathic.

  Scapuloperoneal dystrophy is a similar condition, inherited in an autosomal-dominant manner, but it is milder and lacks facial involvement. Characteristically the wasting and weakness are seen proximally in the shoulder girdle (scapula) and distally in the legs (peroneal). It may occur apparently on either a myopathic or a neuropathic basis.

Distal Myopathy

Distal myopathy is a rare condition manifest by weakness and wasting of the small hand and foot muscles at any age. There is some involvement of more proximal muscles later, but the disease progresses very slowly. The differential diagnosis from a neuropathy is made by EMG and muscle biopsy.

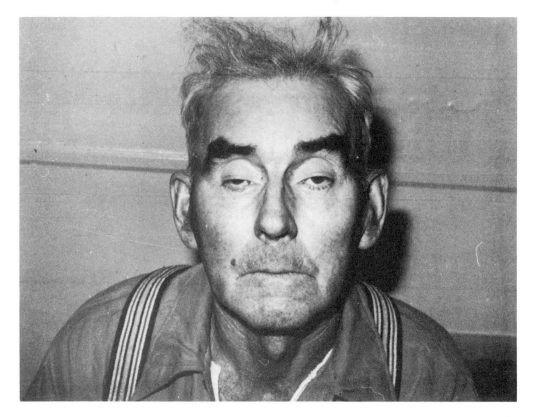

Figure 45-5 Oculopharyngeal dystrophy. There is bilateral ptosis and the face is impassive and unlined. The forehead is not furrowed to correct for the ptosis.

Ocular and Oculopharyngeal Dystrophies

It is not known for certain if these progressive external ophthalmoplegias are primarily neurogenic or myopathic; the findings on biopsy and EMG of the external ocular muscles are confusing.

The major clinical features include progressive ptosis and failure of external ocular movements, initially upward but later in all directions. The eyes are symmetrically involved so diplopia is not a symptom. The pupils are normal.

The disease progresses very slowly with increasing weakness and wasting of facial and later bulbar and girdle muscles, producing dysphagia, dysphonia, dysarthria, and proximal weakness (Fig. 45-5). The whole syndrome has been termed *ophthalmoplegia plus* because a huge range of apparently distinct neurological syndromes have been associated with the essential finding of progressive external ophthalmoplegia (see Chap. 21). This suggests that there is a neurogenic basis for the condition.

Management of Genetic Dystrophies

Despite the progressive loss of function and the poor prognosis in most of these genetic dystrophies, something can always be done to help. Management should be under the control of a pediatrician or neurologist, with advice from a geneticist,

Because there are a number of ancillary services that may be able to help, supervision is often best carried out from a rehabilitation center where there will be facilities for schooling, physiotherapy, and occupational therapy, where wheelchairs may be fitted, braces ordered and made, orthopedic evaluation carried out, and social services mobilized; and where there is usually a concentration of experience, skill, and understanding such as is seldom found in offices or outpatient departments. The role of the family physician is not to search for a cure but to support the family much as he supports that of a child with cerebral palsy. He must open up the available services to the family which, in every case, needs all the help — emotional, economic, educational, social — that it can get. It is a huge psychological burden to nurse a close relation through a terminal illness for a few weeks. In the case of DMD, the illness lasts perhaps 20 years before death. Unless they know that they have available our profession's interested advice and empathetic support, the parents die a little every day.

Congenital Myopathies

Most congenital myopathies present in a way similar to the dystrophies, with proximal muscle wasting and weakness of the face, neck, and limbs, causing delayed motor milestones. Representative types are *central core disease* and *nemaline* and *centronuclear* myopathies.

Most of these conditions are dominantly inherited and have a slow or nonprogressive course. The main clinical features are the poor muscle bulk throughout the body with mild or moderate weakness. Proximal muscles are most affected, the cranial muscles sometimes also being involved. Contractures are common. Deep tendon reflexes are either normal or depressed. Congenital dislocation of the hip, pes cavus, scoliosis, signs reminiscent of Marfan's syndrome, seizures, and reduced mental ability can occur alone with congenital myopathies.

The EMG features are those of myopathy but do not enable differentiation between the various kinds.

The diagnosis is made by muscle biopsy (which must include histochemical study) and electron microscopy. The findings have allowed definition of a number of morphologically (but not chemically or clinically) distinct subtypes. The trouble is that hardly any typical clinical pattern of disease is linked with any of the "specific" morphological appearance identified, and indeed some microscopic changes "typical" of congenital myopathies have been found in the genetic dystrophies, in unrelated muscle disorders, e.g., after tenotomy, and in CNS diseases such as parkinsonism.

Myopathies characterized by mitochondrial abnormalities on biopsy have been found associated with a host of disorders, in most of which progressive external ophthalmoplegia is also present. Many workers are currently laboring in the rich soil of this unclassified vineyard.

Myotonic Disorders

Almost all disorders in which myotonia occurs are dominantly inherited. Three major forms exist.

Myotonia Congenita

Myotonia congenita affects all of the muscles of the body and is present at birth. The muscles are large, and when the patient is active and warm, they are strong. Deep tendon reflexes are normal, but with coldness and after an initial strong

voluntary contraction, delayed relaxation occurs because of instability of the sar-
colemmal membrane, producing continued contraction of the fibers. When the
patient makes a strong voluntary contraction, such as gripping an object, he may
have difficulty letting go. Because the muscles are often large the patient's slowness gives him the appearance of being "musclebound." He may "freeze" and fall
if he has to do something suddenly (intention rigidity). With exercise, muscle activity becomes normal so he can play sports, limited only at the start of activity but
becoming normal in a few minutes after "warming-up" the limbs by exercise.

Myotonia is shown by asking the patient to close his eyes very tightly, to
clench his teeth or to grip something with his hand. He will have trouble relaxing
to command and this is markedly increased in coldness and decreased by exercise
and warmth. Percussion of the involved muscles produces a rising-up of the area
of muscle percussed, with slow settling.

In myotonia congenita this can be seen in almost any muscle, for exmaple the
thenar or forearm muscles. Quinine (0.3-0.4 g t.i.d.), procainamide (0.25 g t.i.d.),
or phenytoin (100 mg t.i.d. or q.i.d.) effectively reduce the myotonia.

Myotonic Dystrophy

Myotonic dystrophy is the most prevalent dystrophy of all. It is dominantly inherited and makes its appearance usually before the age of 40. The most typical features include myotonia of the tongue and forearm muscles (Figs. 45-6; 45-7A-C):
wasting and weakness of the facial, neck, distal hand, and latterly limb girdle muscles; bulbar weakness; and involvement of smooth muscle that gives rise to problems with swallowing and intestinal motility.

This is a multisystem disease; apart from muscle signs, CNS changes lead to
striking apathy and lack of insight. In the eyes, lens changes (especially posterior
polar star-shaped cataracts) or low intraocular tensions are invariable. In the
initial stages the weakness may not be marked and progression is slow, but other
abnormalities later appear, including the lens changes just mentioned, testicular
atrophy, frontal baldness, and a tendency to hypoventilation.

In addition, there is an increased prevalence of diabetes, hypothyroidism, thyroid nodules, and cardiac abnormalities among these patients. About two-thirds
of them have arrhythmias or cardiac conduction defects; hypotension and syncope
commonly result. The ECG is usually abnormal in some respect. A reduced metabolic rate may be found even in the presence of normal thyroid function. Women
with myotonic dystrophy often bear hypotonic, myotonic infants, and their obstetrical records are frequently appalling; hydramnios, miscarriages, and postpartum
hemorrhages figure prominently. A maternal nongenetic factor is possibly partly
responsible. Interestingly, affected babies who survive the neonatal period often
improve for years before the more typical features of myotonic dystrophy appear.

A common feature of this disease is an increased turnover of IgG and measur-
ably low serum gamma globulin levels. It can thus be seen that myotonia is only
part of the syndrome. Unfortunately, it is the only aspect that is treatable; again,
quinine, procainamide, and phenytoin are all effective in diminishing the excessive
sensitivity and after-discharging tendency of the muscle fibers, but the former
two drugs may exacerbate any cardiac conduction defect and only phenytoin should
be used. Both the depression and anergia should respond to tricyclic drugs. Even
if little can be done to treat the patients' other symptoms, genetic counseling may
put a brake on the progressing tragedy within the families. Because new mutations
seldom occur, meticulous ophthalmolegic and neurologic evaluations, with EMG
(Fig. 45-8), are necessary to detect cases in a kinship.

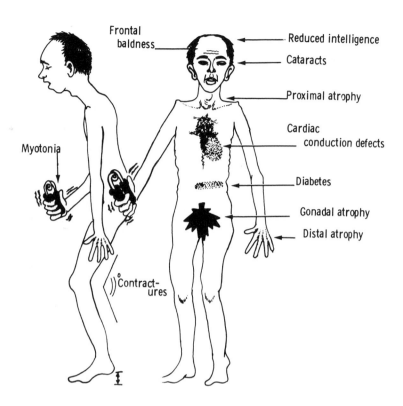

Figure 45-6 Myotonic dystrophy. Some of the areas affected by this multisystem disease are shown in this diagram.

Paramyotonia

Paramyotonia may be identical with hyperkalemic periodic paralysis (see following discussion). Although unassociated with other evidence of primary muscle disease, myotonia may occur in these patients in the cold, affecting particularly the exposed areas of the face and hands.*

Myotonia also occurs when the patient is resting after exercise and may result in attacks of profound muscular weakness of the limbs and trunk. The onset is usually before the age of 10; the duration of the attacks of weakness varies between 2 and 4 hr. Potassium, infections, cold, hunger, general anesthetics, and rest following exercise are typical precipitants. After many years, fatigability, permanent muscle weakness, and mild wasting result.

---

*Inability to eat ice cream because of the myotonia produced in the throat and tongue is a symptom occasionally described.

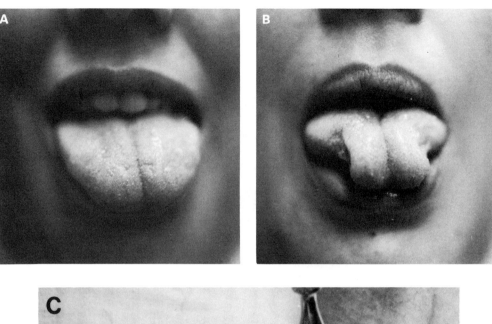

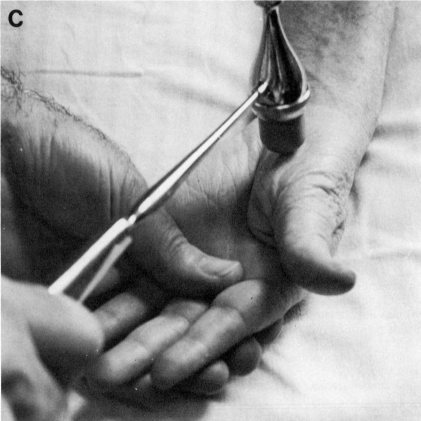

Figure 45-7   Percussion myotonia of the tongue; (A) Before and (B) after percussion; (C) Percussion myotonia of the thenar muscles.

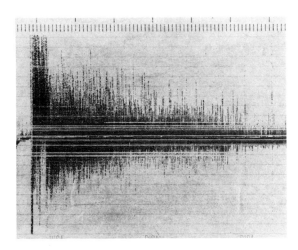

Figure 45-8   The EMG appearance of myotonia; a high-frequency burst of abnormal activity diminishes over a few seconds after percussion of the muscle.

Periodic Flaccid Paralysis

Familial periodic paralysis is characterized by recurrent attacks of weakness or paralysis of the skeletal muscles, accompanied by loss of deep reflexes and failure of muscle to respond to electrical stimulation. The disease has hypokalemic, hyperkalemic, and normokalemic forms, all dominantly inherited. *Paramyotonia congenita* is probably related to the hyperkalemic form.

Hypokalemic Periodic Paralysis

This disorder is most common in males around the age of puberty, but it may begin at any age. It is characterized by attacks of muscle weakness, associated with potassium levels usually below 3 mmol/L. Attacks (which may last from 2 hr to 2 days) can be precipitated by general anesthesia and by the injection of insulin, adrenaline, fludrocortisone, or glucose; or they may follow the ingestion of a meal high in salt or carbohydrates. They usually follow a period of rest (e.g., in the morning after a night's sleep) and vary from slight weakness to total paralysis. The bulbar muscles are usually involved, but the diaphragm is spared. If the patient can remain mobile, the weakness may decrease. Bradycardia and cardiac arrhythmias often occur and may be equally dangerous.

In some cases attacks seem to have been precipitated by hyperthyroidism or malaria. The frequency of attacks diminishes after some years, and they may stop after the age of 40 or 50.

The diagnosis is made by the clinical features, the family history of such problems, and by the low potassium and high serum sodium levels during an episode. Acute treatment involves the oral administration of potassium. Prophylactic management includes the restriction of carbohydrates and sodium intake and the administration of oral potassium and spironolactone or acetazolamide.

Hyperkalemic Periodic Paralysis

Hyperkalemic periodic paralysis is characterized by an onset under the age of 10 years, and shorter, less severe attacks of paralysis, occurring after rest or during a rest after exercise; for instance, hard exercise followed by half an hour of rest may result in increasing weakness of the low back, thighs, calves, hands, and arms. In severe attacks the neck and trunk muscles may be involved and coughing impaired. The facial muscles usually escape, but ptosis is common. Myotonia may be demonstrable.

The paralysis develops over 30 to 40 min and lasts 1 to 2 hr, followed by mild residual weakness. Attacks may be aborted by exercise but his may cause painful muscle cramps that last for days.

The serum and urinary potassium levels are elevated, at least during severe attacks. Symptoms can be precipitated by oral potassium. It is thought that potassium leaks from muscles during the attacks, but its concentration in muscle is low even in the interval between them.

If treatment of an attack is needed, oral calcium gluconate or oral glucose with parenteral insulin are effective. Prophylaxis is with a thiazide diuretic or acetazolamide.

Normokalemic Periodic Paralysis

Normokalemic periodic paralysis looks like the hyperkalemic form but attacks occur mainly at night, are more severe, and may last for weeks. In these patients potassium is retianed even though the serum level is normal. Potassium administration will worsen the symptoms but sodium chloride improves them.

Muscle biopsy shows vacular and chronic myopathic changes similar to those seen in other forms of periodic paralysis.

Therapy is with acetazolamide, 250 mg daily. Steroids and a low potassium diet may also be helpful.

Glycogen Storage Diseases

Glycogen is normally stored in myofibrils, where it is broken down by a series of enzyme degradations to glucose-1- or glucose-6-phosphate, lactate, and pyruvate. The pyruvate is then metabolized through the TCA cycle, yielding energy available for muscle contraction and relaxation. In the event of failure of this glycolytic pathway, glycogen will accumulate and energy will not be available. A number of types of glycogen storage disease lead to similar features including enlargement of muscles and the early appearance of cramp contractures during exercise. Shortly after commencing any activity the muscles may go into painful spasm that wears off slowly over the course of an hour or more. Many types of glycogen storage disease have been identified.

The *type II* (Pompe's disease), acid maltase deficiency causes glycogen deposition in the heart, the tongue, and the anterior horn cells, as well as in muscle, so that the patient may present with cardiac failure, generalized muscle weakness or proximal muscular atrophy. In infants the cause is malignant and death often occurs. An adult form looks like a limb girdle muscle dystrophy or polymyositis, but respiratory muscle weakness is unusually severe.

In *type III* (limit dextrinosis or Cori's disease), the liver, heart, and muscles are the sites of deposition but the disease is milder, hence children with the condition improve and adults complain only of moderate weakness.

Type V (McArdle's disease) is characterized by muscle pains, weakness and stiffness, and sometimes myoglobinuria resulting from damage to muscle fibers with exercise. The disorder is inherited as an autosomal-recessive trait, with onset in the teenage years. Permanent damage to proximal muscles is likely; it causes weakness, wasting, and contractures. This disorder is due to deficiency of muscle phosphorylase, which normally catalyzes the breakdown of glycogen to glucose-1-phosphate. As a result of the deficiency, the muscle cannot produce sufficient energy for contraction and relaxation.

Type VII, caused by phosphofructokinase deficiency, presents also with cramps, weakness, and occasional myoglobinuria.

The diagnosis of glycogen storage muscle diseases is confirmed by an ischemic lactic acid test, EMG, and muscle biopsy. If a blood pressure cuff is inflated around the upper arm of a normal subject and the forearm exercised, there will be an increase in lactic acid in the venous blood from that arm. Becaue the arm performs the exercise without available oxygen, the anaerobic metabolism of glycogen normally results in an increase in lactic acid. If however the glycogen cannot be mobilized through these pathways, the lactic acid level will stay constant.

The EMG studies will show that muscles in contracture show no electrical activity because the muscle shortening is due entirely to a local chemical reaction.

Muscle biopsy with histochemical staining will show abnormal deposits of glycogen in crescents around the muscle fibers. The CK levels will be markedly raised after exercise in these patients, which is a nonspecific but important diagnostic test.

Some enzyme deficiencies may also be detected by examination of their levels in leukocytes. Milder syndromes resembling McArdle's syndrome are also seen, caused by failure of enzymes apart from muscle phosphorylase. The detection of such conditions will be possible only in a unit with sophisticated biochemical and histochemical facilities available.

Lipid Storage Myopathies

Lipid storage myopathies are rare enzyme-deficiency diseases in which triglycerides accumulate in muscles and white blood cells. Thus because of lack of carnitine palmityl transferase, fatty acids cannot be used as energy sources, and patients complain of easy fatigability, recurrent cramps, and muscle pain and weakness on exertion, especially if they are fasting. Myoglobinuria may occur after heavy exercise. Plasma free fatty acids and triglycerides and the serum CK levels are raised, providing a diagnostic screening test. Muscle biopsy assists greatly in making the diagnosis. Less often, progressive weakness is the only evidence of lipid metabolic disorders. Propranolol has been found effective in reducing symptoms of pain and muscle damage.

Arthrogryposis

Arthrogryposis is an uncommon condition in which children are born with rigid joints, particularly of the hands and feet. The contractures may be the result of primary joint, nerve, and/or muscle disease; the cause is not yet known.

Malignant Hyperthermia

In recent years much attention has been paid to malignant hyperthermia, a hypermetabolic muscle state in which there occur insidious or fulminating crises of fever, tachycardia, tachypnea, cyanosis, chest pain, muscular rigidity, and intense metabolic acidosis. The attacks are usually precipitated by general anesthetics, succinylcholine, or overdosages of drugs such as tricyclics or codeine.

Autosomal-dominant transmission occurs in half the patients. The disorder is probably due to a failure of the sarcoplasmic retinulum to rebind calcium, which then remains in the myoplasm, causing continuous activation of myosin-ATPase.

As a result of this failure, myofibrils that have contracted remain locked in contraction leading to intense hypermetabolism. Some of these patients have had prior evidence of musculoskeletal disease, for example ptosis, kyphoscoliosis, muscle weakness, or cramps. When the families are studied, some members are found with abnormal muscle biopsies, raised serum CK and serum pyrophosphate levels, or an abnormal EMG, suggesting that they are also at risk. Definitive diagnosis can be made by exposing muscle taken at biopsy to halothane and caffeine; abnormal muscle contracts, normal muscle does not. The test is complicated and available in only a few centers.

Some people may have no problems despite repeated operations, until they have an acute attack of malignant hyperthermia with a fourth or fifth procedure. Thus an uncomplicated operation does not mean that the disease will not occur in the future. Identification of the risk is important because the anesthetist must be aware of the possibility so that he can avoid the anesthetics and muscle relaxants known to precipitate the syndrome and can monitor the patient's temperature during surgery. If the patient develops a change in temperature, tachycardia, or tachypnea during anesthesia, all drugs must be discontinued and urgent treatment begun.

The treatment to correct the acidosis with IV sodium bicarbonate, to correct hyperthermia with cooling, to allow rebinding of calcium by IV administration of dantrolene sodium or procainamide in high doses repeated under ECG control until relaxation occurs, and to prevent renal damage with mannitol and furosemide. Following this, a major investigation of the family should be undertaken and the family counseled and educated regarding the problem. Those at risk should wear Medic-Alert bracelets in case of accident or emergency surgery.

ACQUIRED DISEASE OF MUSCLE

Inflammatory Disease (Table 45-2)

Myositis Associated with Infection

Viral myositis causes acute localized pain with tenderness. A benign form in children is associated with influenza. In *Bornholm disease,* inflammation of the intercostal muscles is due to coxsackievirus which leads to a syndrome resembling pleurisy, accompanied by fever, malaise, tachypnea, and intestinal complaints. The chest pain may be severe and dramatic ("Devil's grippe"). Except for the myalgia, cramps, and fatigability commonly associated with upper respiratory infections, infective causes of myositis are relatively uncommon, but when they do occur symptoms may last for a year or more.

Inflammatory destruction of muscle may also occur caused by herpes zoster, toxoplasmosis, cysticercosis, trichinosis, or clostridial infections. *Trichinosis* (Fig. 45-9) is associated with localized acute tenderness and swelling of muscles, frequently with a skin rash, generalized allergic edema, and eosinophilia. It occurs following the ingestion of inadequately cooked, contaminated pork.

Polymyositis (Idiopathic Inflammatory Myopathy)

Clinical Features: Polymyositis occurs more commonly in females, especially in later childhood and in the fifth decade. They complain of proximal muscle weakness of acute, subacute, or chronic onset with (usually) symmetric involvement of the neck and bulbar muscles and those of the pelvic and shoulder girdle. The

Table 45-2   Classification of Inflammatory Myopathies

Isolated polymyositis (without skin involvement)		30%
Polymyositis complicating other collagen-vascular disease or sarcoidosis		20%
Dermatomyositis	childhood or adult onset	40%
	with underlying malignancy	10%

Infective myositis

Viral	coxsackie
Metazoal	toxoplasma
Bacterial	clostridia, staphylococci, leptospira
Protozoal	trichinosis, cysticercosis, schistosomiasis

Myositis complicating myolysis

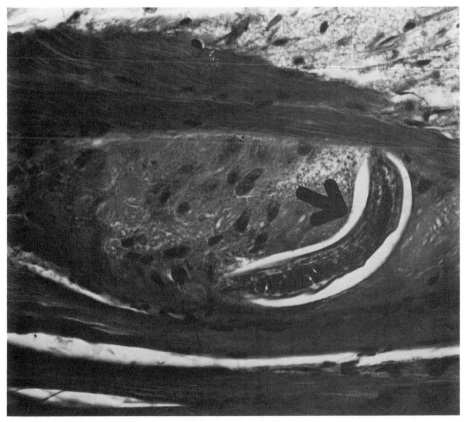

Figure 45-9   Trichinosis. This muscle biopsy shows an encysted parasite.

muscles are stiff, tender, weak, and sometimes obviously swollen, but distal power is usually well maintained, and the reflexes are not depressed. Later the swelling gives way to atrophy and sometimes contractures form. In acute cases, myoglobin is released from the damaged myofibrils, leading to renal damage. Both cardiac and pulmonary inflammation may occur as well.

In half the cases there is involvement of skin as well as muscles, in the form of hyperemia of the nailbeds, a bluish discoloration of the eyelids, scaly erythema of the face, upper trunk, extensor surfaces, and knuckles, and edema of the skin. Also, in half of all cases associated diseases are present, mainly autoimmune or less often malignant. The latter is more likely if skin involvement is present and if the patient is over the age of 50.

Childhood dermatomyositis probably represents a different disease, the vasculitic component being more marked. Symptoms however are much the same; only the prognosis for recovery after steroid or immunosuppressive treatment is substantially better.

In chronic cases, telangiectasias over the face and Raynaud's phenomenon are commonly seen. When the condition occurs in adults aged over 60, an underlying malignancy should be excluded, particularly of the lung or stomach or of the breast or ovaries in females. When the underlying disease is a collagen-vascular disease (SLE, rheumatoid arthritis, scleroderma), joint pain, sclerodactly, and Raynaud's phenomenon are common.

Investigation: Serum CK and LDH levels and the ESR are high. The EMG shows evidence of a myopathic process with irritable muscle fibers. Biopsy will show inflammatory changes, often with small cell infiltration and muscle fiber necrosis (Fig. 45-10).

Treatment: Physiotherapy, aimed at maintaining the full range of motion of the affected limbs, is always necessary. Specific therapy consists of steroids given for 6 months to 2 years. Patients are started on a high dosage (80 to 100 mg of prednisone daily) and decreased to a maintenance dosage of alternate-day therapy, the amount depending upon the clinical picture and response. Serum CK levels, the ESR values and the clinical findings govern the level of steroid therapy. Azothioprine, methotrexate, and whole-body irradiation have all been successfully used as treatment as well.

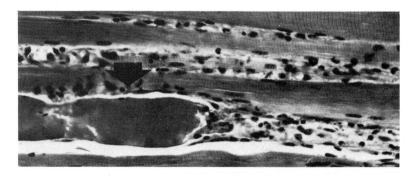

Figure 45-10   Muscle biopsy in polymyositis. There are many inflammatory cells present and a necrotic fiber is arrowed.

Myopathies Associated with
Collagen-Vascular Disease

Because the varieties of collagen-vascular disease blend into a spectrum, features seen in one disorder may be seen in others. Myopathy is an example. Polymyositis can probably be regarded as a collagen-vascular disease on its own, but a similar if milder picture can be seen in association with lupus erythematosus, scleroderma, rheumatoid arthritis, or thrombotic thrombocytopenic purpura.

Polyarteritis nodosa may be associated with myopathy resulting from widespread vascular disease. Other vasculitides, including giant cell arteritis, aortic arch arteritis, and polymyalgia rheumatica, may also induce myopathic symptoms. They are described in Chapter 42.

In many cases of collagen-vascular disease without gross muscle involvement, biopsy may nevertheless show focal areas of inflammatory and mononuclear cell accumulation (focal nodular myositis), and a distinction between polymyositis occurring alone and in association with other collagen-vascular disease may be impossible.

Myasthenia Gravis

Myasthenia is an autoimmune neuromuscular disease characterized by excessive skeletal muscle fatigability on continued exercise, caused by a disorder in transmission at the neuromuscular junction. This disorder is due to a decreased availability of receptor sites for acetylcholine (ACh) on the postjunctional membrane because of their blocking or destruction by antibodies produced by B lymphocytes.

Clinical Features

The disease most commonly begins between the ages of 15 and 25 but can occur at almost any age. It is more frequent in women. Symptoms vary in severity from mild ptosis lasting for many years to acute and fulminating weakness with respiratory and bulbar failure and death.

The key symptom of the disorder is variable *fatigability*, fluctuating from hour to hour. Initial movements may be perfectly strong but power quickly declines, either with repetitive activity or as the day progresses. This may be seen first or most prominently in the *ocular* muscles, with complaints of increasing ptosis or diplopia. *Bulbar muscle* involvement leads to a weakening voice, dysarthria, facial weakness, and dysphagia. *Skeletal muscle* involvement causes more proximal than distal involvement so that small finger movements are relatively strong but the arm may be lifted only with difficulty. Despite this, tendon reflexes are preserved until late in the course of the disease, when muscle damage with atrophy and permanent weakness may occur.

Congenital myasthenia affects about 10 percent of the children born to mothers with myasthenia gravis, but only lasts for about 6 weeks and responds to anticholinesterase therapy. At birth the infants cry weakly and suck feebly. Their motor movements are diminished in strength and number. The immediate need to treat these infants at birth must be anticipated in myasthenic women who are pregnant.

Concurrently with myasthenia there may also occur collagen-vascular diseases, Hashimoto's disease and other thyroid abnormalities, atrophic gastritis, pernicious anemia, and even multiple sclerosis. Fifteen percent of patients have a tumor of the thymus gland (thymoma). Although histologically thymomas often look benign, they can extend outside the capsule of the gland into the surrounding tissues and involve the mediastinum, lungs, and heart by direct extension. Thymomas are more commonly seen in older males and carry a bad prognosis; the patients tend to die of poorly controlled myasthenia rather than from the thymoma. Eighty-five percent of patients with myasthenia have thymic hyperplasia with abundant germinal centers in the gland, rather than thymoma. Antibodies to various muscle components are often present in the blood but are neither of diagnostic nor of prognostic value, except for anti-ACh receptor antibodies. Drugs and toxins causing pre- or postsynaptic failure are listed in Chapter 43.

Differential Diagnosis

Depression is the disease that most commonly presents with fatigability and requires care in diagnosis. Myasthenia must, of course, be differentiated from the fatigability that may be seen with primary muscle disease such as the dystrophies, polymyositis, and with muscle weakness secondary to neuropathies. In these patients, the other clinical features should allow the diagnosis to be made; their fatigue is usually due to tiredness in permanently weak muscles. In motor neuron disease (Chap. 47), a "pseudomyasthenic" syndrome may confuse the situation; such patients may even have a false-positive response to edrophonium. Some MS patients have a form of fatigue that sound "myasthenic" in that it is present much of the time but worsened by activity and improved with rest.

Diagnostic Tests

The clinical diagnosis is confirmed with EMG, using repetitive stimulation techniques (Fig. 45-11) or by the use of edrophonium chloride (Tensilon). For the latter test, the patient should have the appropraite muscles fatigued by exercise so that any change can be noted when the injection is given. Thus he is asked to look upwards for 60 sec so that ptosis can develop, to count continuously up to 100 to note

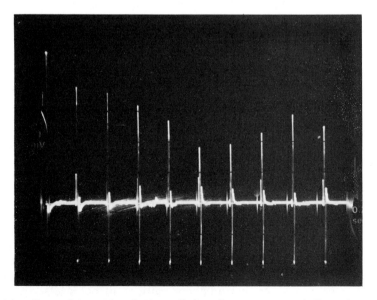

Figure 45-11   Repetitive stimulation of the ulnar nerve at 2 Hz, with recording from the hypothenar muscles in myasthenia gravis. There is a reduction in size of the evoked potential during the first six stimuli, followed by a slight increase, but to a level smaller than the first potential.

a decrease in voice, or to elevate or carry out repetitive motions with his arm until weakness develops. Then 2 mg (0.2 ml) of edrophonium is injected intravenously and the patient is asked if he feels any untoward reaction occurring.* If he does not, then 8 mg (0.8 ml) is injected as a bolus and the patient observed. The return of strength following myasthenic weakness can be dramatic. A nonmyasthenic patient will usually develop fasciculations from this dose, but myasthenics do not. This can be a useful (but soft) clinical sign that myasthenia gravis is not present.

If weakness could be on a hysterical or functional basis, the patient can be given an IV injection of normal saline first to test for any placebo response.

In doubtful cases, the edrophonium test can be combined with repetitive stimulation on EMG, or the EMG tests can be performed after regional injection of a very small dose of curate, to which myasthenic patients are particularly sensitive. Serum ACh receptor antibody levels are increased in up to 90 percent of myasthenic patients.

Investigations should also include a search for other autoimmune diseases. A chest x-ray should be done, as should tomograms of the mediastinum, but a thymoma is most likely to be shown by CT scanning.

Treatment

Treatment of myasthenia usually requires the use of anticholinesterase drugs such as neostigmine or the longer-acting pyridostigmine. The use of these drugs can be hazardous in high doses, particularly in patients with bulbar or respiratory involvement because excessive doses may result in a *cholinergic crisis* with increasing muscle weakness, and may actually damage the muscle receptors. Another problem may be that of differing responses in different muscle groups, so that some muscles remain weak because the dose is not enough, while others become even weaker because the dose for them is too much. Thus the limb muscles may be developing cholinergic block from the high anticholinesterase dosage while the bulbar muscle are still showing myasthenic weakness.

Anticholinesterases may have more effect on the limb than on the eye signs and, like edrophonium, can produce parasympathetic side effects such as diarrhea, urinary frequency, sweating, miosis, and bradycardia. To some extent, these can be controlled by a small dose of atropine. Oral is better than parenteral administration in all cases. Pyridostigmine bromide (Mestinon) 60 mg or neostigmine bromide (Prostigmin) 15 mg is the drug usually used, in a dosage of one tablet every 3 to 4 hr initially. This dosage however must be varied with the patient's needs, and indeed the patient is the best person to decide how much to take and when. Pyridostigmine can also be given in a long-acting form at night. Only one type of anticholinesterase should be given at a time. Atropine tablets (0.4 mg) may be given in the mornings to diminish muscarinic side effects. Such agents as oral potassium, calcium, and ephedrine are of very little practical value in myasthenia.

Except for those patients whose myasthenic symptoms are entirely confined to the eyes and are well controlled by anticholinesterase medications, all patients should be considered for thymectomy. This operation has a negligible mortality and may be expected to produce remission or marked improvement in symptoms within 5 years in at least two-thirds of the patients. The results are best in the 70 percent of cases in which the gland shows hyperplasia, and less so in the 10 to 20 percent of cases (usually older males) with a thymoma.

---

*Nausea, sweating, bradycardia, wheezing, abdominal cramps.

Many patients, especially those with purely ocular myasthenia, are greatly benefited by the use of oral prednisone. This suppressive treatment may induce remissions lasting months or years even without thymectomy. One favored regimen entails taking prednisone on alternate days, starting with a low dose (25 mg) and increasing slowly until a maximum of 100 mg is reached, after which a decrease to between 20 and 40 mg should be possible. This gradual increase in dosage avoids the acute and profound weakness sometimes seen when treatment was begun with high dosages, but for safety should be started in the hospital.

Azothioprine is being used increasingly as an adjunct with useful steroid-sparing effects. It is best reserved for older patients because of the increased risk of teratogenesis.

Myasthenic weakness may be worsened by many drugs (listed in Chap. 43). In a case of antibiotic-induced weakness, calcium is the most effective emergency treatment; give 10 ml of 10% calcium gluconate IV.

A *myasthenic crisis,* caused by worsening of the disease process itself, has to be differentiated from a *cholinergic crisis* resulting from depolarization block caused by excessive anticholinesterase medication. If atropine is given routinely, then the cardinal differentiating sign (namely, miosis in the cholinergic crisis group) will be lost. Although theoretically the IV edrophonium test can be used to differentiate between the two conditions (the myasthenic crisis should improve but the cholinergic crisis worsen), the response is seldom clear-cut, and further depression of respiration must be anticipated when the test is carried out.

In the event of rapidly progressive weakness, the best therapy is to assist ventilation using a soft endotracheal tube. All agents are withdrawn for 2 to 3 days, the patient is ventilated in an intensive care unit, and then therapy is restarted, either with a course of steroids or by restarting administration of the anticholinesterase medication. The response to these agents is often increased by a period off all medication.

In patients with severe or progressive weakness (e.g., those in myasthenic crisis, or who are being prepared for thymectomy), anti-ACh-receptor antibody removal by repeated plasma exchange has been successful in restoring power in the short term; treatment with high dosage steroids and azathioprine must be continued, otherwise rebound overproduction of receptor antibodies may make the patient weaker still. In some cases, long-term beneficial responses to steroids and azathioprine have been achieved only after plasma exchange.

Myasthenic (Eaton-Lambert) Syndrome

The myasthenic syndrome, usually occurring in association with an oat-cell carcinoma of the lung, is due to a presynaptic deficit consisting of a reduction in the release of ACh quanta from the nerve terminal, rather than from receptor blockade as in myasthenia gravis.

In this condition the patient may actually increase his strength for a short time with activation of his muscles, as is well seen when a weak grip increases on repeated exercise, or the knee jerk that is initially reduced becomes brisker on repeated testing. The decreased deep tendon reflexes, sparing of the bulbar muscles, and the poor response to anticholinesterase drugs are three points of value in differentiation of this syndrome from myasthenia gravis.

The diagnosis is made on EMG where, despite a diminution in potential size with slow rates of stimulation (as in myasthenia gravis), an increase in amplitude occurs with high rates of stimulation of the appropriate nerve (Fig. 45-12).

Treatment employs oral guanidine, 3,4-diaminopyridine, and phenytoin. If a carcinoma can be removed, then the long-term prognosis is better, but this is seldom the case.

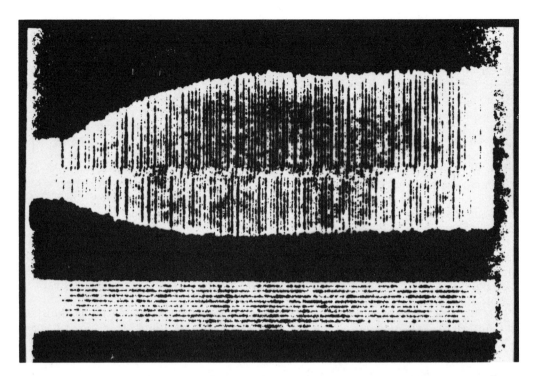

Figure 45-12   Myasthenic syndrome. Stimulation at 20 Hz leads to an increase in the size of the evoked potential. This man had a carcinoma of the bronchus.

Two other unusual disorders that also affect the neuromuscular junction presynaptically are *botulism* and *tick paralysis* (described in Chap. 40), but the onset is acute and severe in these conditions, hence they can usually be differentiated from both myasthenia gravis and the myasthenic syndrome. Some spider and scorpion venoms can also cause acute presynaptic block of neuromuscular transmission.

Metabolic, Toxic, and Endocrine Myopathies

In most of these myopathies the patient complains of painless proximal muscle weakness with little wasting. In such conditions the serum CK level is usually minimally raised if at all, but muscle biopsy usually shows abnormalities of diagnostic value.

Endocrine Myopathies

Proximal weakness and wasting are common in *Cushing's syndrome* and with the continued administration of fluorinated steroids. The weakness may involve all skeletal muscles, but it is initially seen in the pelvic girdle.

In *Addison's disease* weakness and generalized reduction in muscle bulk occur without any selective involvement.

In *hyperaldosteronism,* hypokalemia leads to intermittent weakness with diminution of deep tendon reflexes. The clinical picture is entirely dependent upon the low serum potassium level.

In *hyperthyroidism,* proptosis with chemosis and diplopia may progress to failure of eye movements in all directions. Steroids may be of value, but surgical decompression of the orbit is sometimes required. Although the condition tends to burn itself out after 2 or 3 years, irreparable harm may be done to the optic nerve and to the cornea if decompression is not carried out in those who fail to respond to steroid therapy and correction of the thyrotoxicosis.

Hyperthyroidism is associated with other muscle diseases, including a nonspecific myopathic weakness, myasthenia gravis, myopathy associated with mitochondial abnormalities, and periodic paralysis. Most of these will respond to treatment of the hyperthyroidism, but 5 percent of patients with myasthenia gravis have associated thyrotoxicosis, treatment of which does not improve the myasthenia, which has to be treated in the same way in any other case.

In *hypothyroidism* the best known feature is pseudomyotonia (delayed contraction and relaxation of muscles) because of a mechanical impediment to the sliding of muscle filaments over each other. This is best seen in the "hung-up" ankle reflex. Mild muscle pain and swelling are also described. Occasionally generalized proximal weakness with a rise in the serum CK level are found.

Primary and secondary *hyperparathyroidism* and other causes of hypercalcemia associated with *metabolic bone disease* cause excessive stabilization of postsynaptic membrane potentials, decreasing neuromuscular transmission. This causes generalized painful weakness, especially of the pelvic girdle muscles, producing a characteristic waddling gait.

Mild generalized weakness occurs in *acromegaly* but the myopathy has neither characteristic EMG nor muscle biopsy findings. These patients often look rather powerful, and one is surprised to find that they are not.

Myopathies Associated with Malignancy

Rarely, polymyositis complicates malignancies in either sex, an oat-cell carcinoma of the lung being the most common tumor. Loss of muscle bulk and power is also seen in most terminal malignancies, with cachexia, hypokalemia, or inappropriate secretion of ADH or ACTH. Carcinomas may also be complicated by both the myasthenic syndrome and myasthenia gravis.

Toxic Myopathies

Many drugs (see Chap. 43) produce a myopathy marked by muscle weakness, pain, and wasting. Chloroquine may produce a myopathy by its interference with muscle carbohydrate metabolism. Alcohol produces at least three forms of myopathy (Chap. 43).

Myoglobinuria

Myoglobinuria results from diverse causes, all of which produce acute breakdown of muscle cells. It can occur as a primary (genetic) disease or as a secondary result of other diseases.

Genetic (Idiopathic)

Most patients with the inherited form are male; they present with pain and cramps in the muscles and fever, weakness, and leukocytosis. The urine is dark red or brown during the acute stage of the attack. In some primary types of unknown cause (but presumably on a genetic basis) and occurring in both children and adults, there may be recurrent mild episodes; in 10 percent, acute, sometimes fatal episodes occur. After recurrent attacks, contractures and muscle atrophy are common.

Acquired

There are many secondary causes of myoglobinuria. They include crush injury to muscle in acute trauma and prolonged immobile coma, muscle infarction, status epilepticus, and the infective and metabolic disorders already considered. The clinical features are the same as in the inherited form.

Localized damage to muscle occurs in the *anterior tibial syndrome*. This occurs in people who have taken unaccustomed heavy exercise, such as military recruits during training. Pain, footdrop, and minor sensory changes in the distribution of the anterior tibial nerve result from entrapment of the overworked and now swollen anterior tibial musculature beneath the overlying fascia. Urgent surgical decompression of the muscle is essential to prevent necrosis of the muscles leading to fibrosis and permanent footdrop.

Whatever the cause, renal damage because of tubular obstruction by myoglobin leading to renal shutdown is a feared complication. The urine contains protein and "hemaglobin" although no red cells are present — in fact spectroscopy shows that the pigment is myoglobin. Pathological examination shows rhabdomyolysis with waxy degeneration, vacuolization, necrosis, and liquefaction of the muscle fibers. Nonsurgical treatment includes a high fluid intake and the use of mannitol and diuretics. Dialysis may be required.

Myositis Ossificans

Myositis ossificans is a disorders in which bone is laid down in muscle. This can be secondary to old trauma, with bony organization within a hematoma, or it may be a primary phenomenon inherrited as an autosomal-dominant trait. In these rare primary cases, children progressively develop hard, tender lumps in their muscles. Marked muscle contractures and deformities result. Involvement of chest and abdominal muscles causes ventilatory impairment. No treatment is available. When bone formation occurs in old muscle hematomas, surgical removal may be successful.

In any patient seen with focal areas of muscle calcification, hemophilia must be excluded.

Benign Muscle Fasciculations

Because of their training in the observation of such phenomena, physicians and medical students sometimes complain to neurologists of fasciculations, fearful of serious disease. The muscle twitches are usually noticed following exercise, may be associated with muscle cramps, and are unassociated with any other signs of neurological disease. These factors help to differentiate them from the fasciculations of, for example, motor neuron disease.

Athletic people who become sedentary, body builders, people who are very fatigued, and those taking mercurial diuretics may also have fasciculations. Any muscle, but chiefly those of the shoulders, thighs and calves can be affected. When patients are reassured about the benign nature fo the condition, they usually manage to ignore it.

Myokymia is a brief, rippling, involuntary contraction of part of a muscle, probably resulting from hyperexcitability of intramuscular nerves. It is uncommon, usually benign, and occurs chiefly in the face, in the small hand muscles, or in the calves. Fatigue and excessive loss of salt may be associated. Multiple sclerosis is an occasional cause when the myokymia involves the face.

Benign and pathological fasciculations cannot be differentiated by EMG. In myokymia, abnormal motor unit discharges may be recorded which may confirm the presence of the condition but does not diagnose its cause.

Neuromyotonia was described in Chapter 47.

BIBLIOGRAPHY

Bohan, A., et al. A computer-assisted analysis of patients with polymyositis and dermatomyositis. *Medicine 56:*255-286, 1977.

Brooke, M.H. *A Clinician's View of Neuromuscular Disorders.* Baltimore, Williams & Wilkins, 1977.

Carpenter, S., Karpati, G. *Pathology of Skeletal Muscle.* Toronto, Churchill-Livingstone, 1984.

Layzer, R.B. *Neuromuscular Manifestations of Systemic Disease. Contemporary Neurology Series No. 25.* Philadelphia, F.A. Davis Co., 1985.

Rowland, L.P. Controversies about the treatment of myasthenia gravis. *J. Neurol. Neurol. Neurosurg. Psychiatry 43:*644-659, 1980.

Rowland, L.P. Myoglobinuria 1984. *Can. J. Neurol. Sci. 11:*1-13, 1984.

Taft, L.T. The care and management of the child with muscular dystrophy. *Dev. Med. Child Neurol. 15:*510-518, 1973.

Walton, J.N. (ed.). *Disorders of Voluntary Muscle,* 4th Ed. London, Churchill, 1981.

46

Parkinson's Disease and Other Diseases of the Basal Ganglia

Parkinson's disease is a disorder of the basal ganglia and its connections, character-ized by tremor, rigidity, bradykinesia (poverty of movement), postural disorders, and autonomic abnormalities (Fig. 46-1).

Parkinsonism is a pathophysiological state resulting from degeneration or dys-function of the dopaminergic nigrostriatal system. This system includes the sub-stantia nigra, caudate nucleus, putamen, and globus pallidus. The cell bodies are in the substantia nigra and their axons run to the upper basal ganglion structures where dopamine normally acts as an inhibitory neurotransmitter, balancing an excitatory cholinergic system. Loss of the neurons in this system leads to the de-pigmentation of the substantia nigra so typical in Parkinson's disease (Fig. 46-2). The disorder may be more complex than this, as other biochemical changes are apparent in Parkinson's disease, and neuronal degeneration occurs not only in the substantia nigra but also more widely within the basal ganglia and sometimes dif-fusely in the cerebral cortex (see Fig. 46-2).

Etiology

Parkinson's disease can be classified as idiopathic or secondary. The idiopathic form, sometimes called paralysis agitans, may eventually be shown to be due to a viral infection as now suggested by the presence of inclusion bodies in the de-generating neurons of the substantia nigra (Lewy bodies); however the exact repli-cation of the pathology and clinical features in subjects poisoned with a narcotic derivative has led to the hypothesis of a toxic cause.

The secondary causes of parkinsonism are many, but all affect the neurons involved in basal ganglion function. The classic secondary cause was the world-wide pandemic of influenza beginning in 1917 that often resulted in von Economo's encephalitis. Many of these patients developed parkinsonism even years later with typical degenerative changes in the basal ganglia and substantia nigra.

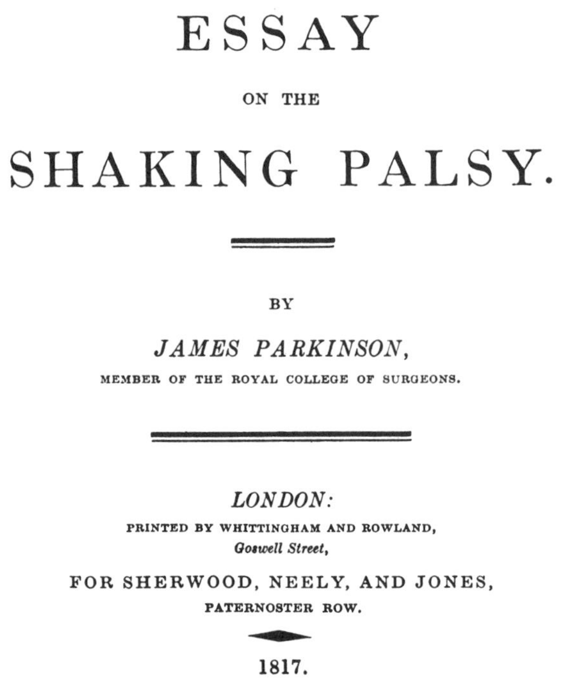

ESSAY

ON THE

SHAKING PALSY.

BY

JAMES PARKINSON,

MEMBER OF THE ROYAL COLLEGE OF SURGEONS.

LONDON:

PRINTED BY WHITTINGHAM AND ROWLAND,
Goswell Street,

FOR SHERWOOD, NEELY, AND JONES,
PATERNOSTER ROW.

1817.

Figure 46-1   The original description of the syndrome.

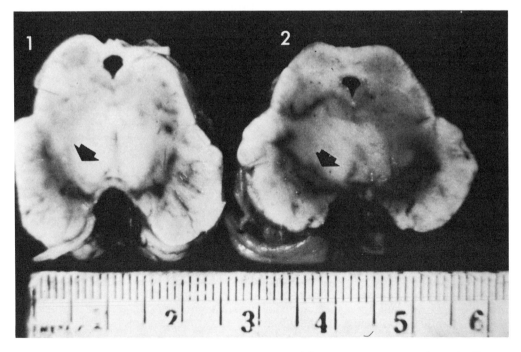

Figure 46-2   Transverse section of midbrain. (1) Patient with Parkinson's disease; (2) Normal control. Note the lack of pigment in the substantia nigra in the abnormal brain.

Parkinsonism may also result from brain trauma and from carbon monoxide, manganese, and other heavy-metal poisoning, and may be due to drugs (see Chap. 43). It may also be associated with diffuse cerebral degenerative processes causing various neuronal losses, the *multiple system atrophies*. Parkinsonian features may be seen in GPI but are hardly found in association with multiple sclerosis or cerebral tumor. Cerebral anoxia from any cause, including "successful" resuscitation after cardiac arrest, repeated hypoglycemic attacks, and repeated head injuries (as in boxers) also produce parkinsonian signs. Rigidity and akinesia, but not true Parkinson's disease, may follow multiple cerebral infarcts and have been seen in patients with normal pressure hydrocephalus and Wilson's disease.

Epidemiology

Parkinson's disease seems to be distributed evenly throughout the world. The prevalence is about 100 cases per 100,000 population; it is estimated that 1:40 people will eventually develop parkinsonism. On the theory that many cases have resulted from the influenza pandemic of 1917, it might have been expected that the prevalence of parkinsonism would diminish, but as yet there is no sign of this.

Symptoms and Signs

There is some variability in the pattern of clinical features of parkinsonism, according to the cause. Thus in postencephalitic and phenothiazine-induced forms, severe autonomic disturbances and *oculogyric crises* are seen, but the latter do not occur in other types. Rigidity is severe in postencephalitic patients, but it is not particularly marked in idiopathic Parkinson's disease until a late stage. Tremor is prominent in idiopathic and postanoxic forms but may not be at all marked in postencephalitic parkinsonism nor in that caused by phenothiazine drugs, in which bradykinesia is the most striking of the four major features.

Development of *symptoms* in the idiopathic variety is often slow, and their insidious onset may make patients unaware of exactly what has happened to them. The early picture may also confuse the physician, particularly if the characteristic tremor is not yet present. Early symptoms are often related to rigidity of muscles and include complaints of slowness of movements and vague heaviness, stiffness, or aching in the limbs. As time goes by, postural disturbances appear, e.g., generalized flexion and a loss of associated movements such as arm-swing while walking.

In the earlier stages, most patients have normal intellectual abilities and are in effect functioning within a body that responds poorly or slowly to their own drives, but dementia eventually occurs in at least one-third of them.

Examination of the cranial nerves shows a masklike faces with a blank stare and infrequent blinking. Voluntary and emotional facial movements are both limited and slow. If the bridge of the nose (the glabella) is tapped repeatedly, blinking continues, whereas normally, adaptation to the tapping will stop blinking after three or four taps. However this abnormal response also occurs with other causes of diffuse cerebral dysfunction and is not at all specific (Fig. 46-3).

Speech is low, monotonous, and in time, hard or impossible to understand: the problem is compounded by the drooling of saliva.

Motor examination shows that strength is normal but voluntary and spontaneous tasks are made difficult by the rigidity and slowness in initiation of movements. The patient may sit motionless, even if in an uncomfortable position, not making those minor postural adjustments that normal people make automatically. When he does move, each action is performed in a series of separate steps rather than in

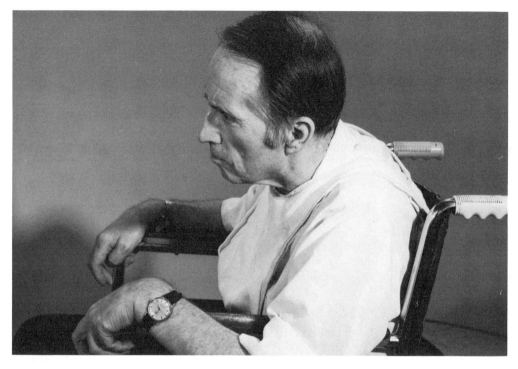

Figure 46-3   Patient with Parkinson's disease. Note the generally flexed posture and the resigned, impassive facial expression.

a smooth continuum. *Handwriting* changes are often useful diagnostic early signs; the writing is shaky and small, tending to get even smaller as the sentence continues (Fig. 46-4). Micrographia is later seen; the writing may not be read without a magnifying glass in some instances. *Rigidity* is found in most muscles, although the initial appearance of rigidity may be confined to one limb. At first, only a slight increase in tone may be felt within the muscles on movement, but eventually a ratchetlike jerking is felt (cogwheel rigidity). It is brought out by having the opposite arm perform rapid alternating movements or the opposite fist clenched while tone is tested in the first limb. In the trunk, the increase in tone can be felt over the paraspinal muscles if the patient flexes and extends his back.

Parkinsonian *tremor* is characteristic when present. At first confined to one hand, it may spread to all limbs. It is commonly a four to six per second alternating flexion-extension or rotatory movement most noticeable in the thumb and index finger. This last characteristic led to the old term *pill-rolling tremor,* ascribed to it from the days when pharmacists rolled pills by hand. It rarely occurs in the head, and significant head tremor usually indicates essential tremor rather than parkinsonism; but it may be seen in the closed eyelids, in the tongue, or the chin. It is characteristically best seen when the limb is maintaining a posture, and it is absent when the limb is at complete rest, e.g., during sleep. At a later stage, there is sometimes an added action component, so the tremor occurs during the whole range of a voluntary movement and the leverage effect from extending the arm may make it appear that the tremor is actually worse during movement. Any form of emotional stimulation will increase tremors of all types.

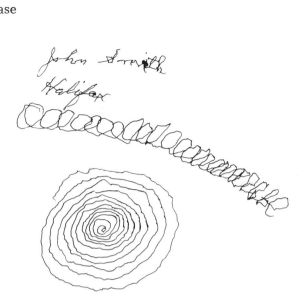

Figure 46-4   Typical handwriting in Parkinson's disease.

Apart from the stooped, flexed, and shuffling *gait* disturbance, propulsion and retropulsion may be found. When these are present, the patient who managed to start walking forward or backward finds himself unable to stop so that it is as if he were chasing his own center of gravity (festinating gait). This inability to halt may be extremely dangerous.

Sudden "freezing" of movements occurs at a later stage; the patient may be unable to walk through a doorway without a brief involuntary stop, and on sitting down may hold himself suspended just above the seat for a few seconds before "plumping" down into the chair. All actions are performed slowly and with effort — so to get ready in the morning, patients may need an hour or two of time for toilet, shaving, and dressing.

There are no sensory changes but patients often complain of stiffness and aching in the muscles. Reflexes, including the plantar responses, are normal unless there is other evidence of generalized brain disease.

Abnormalities of the *autonomic nervous system* result in excessive sweating, oily skin, abnormal gastric motility, and slight bladder disturbances in some cases. Impotence is probably due to the motor disabilities as much as to autonomic changes.

Most patients have relatively normal *intellectual* function despite their appearance, which must be remembered in dealing with them, because there is a tendency to talk down to them or about them as if they were children or retarded. As a result of their encasement within a body with high inertia, and undoubtedly because of primary biochemical disturbances, most patients are *depressed*. In the later stages of disease, intellectual involvement occurs in one-third of cases.

Diagnosis

Diagnosis is not always easy and can require perception and acumen in the early stage when signs are minimal and symptoms vague. Early signs of value include infrequent blinking, the lack of arm swinging, and cogwheel or plastic rigidity accentuated when the opposite side is stressed. The history must concentrate on those possible causes of secondary parkinsonism mentioned earlier, in particular, recent anoxia or drug ingestion; a family history is sometimes of value (though more commonly in cases of essential tremor).

The disorder has to be differentiated from *Wilson's disease* (discussed later), but this disorder occurs in children and young adults. *Striatonigral degeneration* should be suspected when a patient with parkinsonian features has predominant rigidity, a poor response to L-dopa, and rapid deterioration. *Essential tremor,* especially in the elderly, is often mistaken for Parkinson's disease, but the other features of parkinsonism are not present and these tremors frequently involve the head, are more rapid, and tend to occur when a limb is maintained in an antigravity posture or during movement rather than, as in true parkinsonism, when a limb at rest is maintaining a posture, but supported.

Treatment

Physiotherapy is of value to maintain mobility and optimal activity. Massage, exercises, and posture and gait training have been found helpful, the latter particularly so if propulsion or retropulsion are present.

Drug therapy of parkinsonism, at present, is based on the observation that dopamine is depleted in the nigrostriatal tracts and that the excitatory cholinergic effects are relatively increased. *Anticholinergic drugs,* such as trihexyphenidyl (Artane), benztropine (Cogentin), and orphenadrine (Disipal) and antihistamine drugs such as diphenhydramine (Benadryl) are used with variable results but have more effect upon the tremor than upon rigidity or akinesia. If these drugs are used for any length of time, they must not be stopped abruptly or a rebound effect with increased symptoms may occur. Cerebral stimulants such as dextroamphetamine have been used with only occasional improvement.

Amantadine hydrochloride (Symmetrel) is less effective than L-dopa in improving the symptoms of parkinsonism but is relatively free of serious side effects. It may be used alone or in conjunction with L-dopa. It was originally developed and prescribed as an antiviral agent, and its method of action in Parksinson's disease is as yet unclear.

Although L-dopa coupled with a decarboxylase inhibitor is at present the most popular agent, *tricyclic agents,* e.g., amitriptyline, may increase activity as well as lightening the frequently added depression; and nocturnal antihistamines, e.g., diphenhydramine, are sedative, dry up secretions, and reduce tremor. The dopa-receptor stimulator, *bromocriptine* (dosage 2-40 mg/day), has shown good success against many parkinsonian symptoms. *Propranolol* diminishes the tremor and some of the psychological effects of anxiety. All of these agents should be considered before L-dopa is given and may be given concurrently.

A combination drug such as Sinemet (L-dopa plus carbidopa) is the most effective agent but should not be administered until symptoms have become serious enough to impair mobility and function. It is best to begin with a small dosage (100/10 mg combination tablet twice a day) and slowly increase. When the patient begins to respond, maintain that dosage level. The average dosage is two or three 250/25 capsules, daily. If the effect is variable during the day, give divided doses every 2 to 3 hr.

Long-term results over the years also have not been encouraging as the symptoms progress despite continued therapy. It has been suggested that the prescription of L-dopa should be delayed and *not* given on diagnosis because it appears to lose its effect after a few years. It has also been observed that many patients on long-term L-dopa develop significant mental changes, which may be due either to the therapy or to the natural history of the disease.

The most common early complication of L-dopa are nausea caused by stimulation of the vomiting center in the brain and possible direct gastric irritation; postural hypotension; anorexia; depression and confusion; abnormal movements such as retrocollis, dystonic postures, and akathisia; and cardiac arrhythmias. After long-term therapy with L-dopa, an "on-off" effect with variability in the signs and symptoms throughout the day may be seen, whereby abrupt increase of all symptoms — freezing, rigidity, etc. — occurs as the serum levels of L-dopa decline. End-of-dose deterioration, fatigue, and loss of efficacy of the drug also occur, usually after 3 to 5 years of use, emphasizing that L-dopa should not be used until it is really needed. It has been estimated that L-dopa loses a third of its effect in two-thirds of patients within 3 years. A less common complication is hip fracture resulting from overenthusiastic resumption of physical activity as the benefits of L-dopa therapy appear. The formerly publicized aphrodisiac effect of the drug is probably mainly due to an increase in physical freedom rather than to stimulation of sexual appetites.

Bromocriptine (Parlodel) may be used in addition to L-dopa or used alone. It may reduce some of the long-term complications of L-dopa, but when bromocriptine is used, the dosage of L-dopa may need to be reduced by 10 to 50 percent over many weeks, or toxicity may occur to L-dopa.

Initial dosages should be low (1.25 mg twice a day), slowly increasing by 2.5 mg weekly to a maintenance dosage of 5-10 mg three times a day.

Amantadine is given in oral dosages of 100 mg one to two times daily. Its action is rapid but decreases over a few months. Depression, confusion, hypotension, and cardiac failure are the main unwanted effects.

Thalmotomy in the treatment of Parkinson's disease is primarily beneficial for tremor and rigidity but does not affect the bradykinesia, which is the single most disabling symptom of all. Although safe and effective in an experienced neurosurgeon's hand, thalamotomy is accompanied by significant morbidity, especially when done bilaterally, and it has been performed much less frequently since the advent of L-dopa.

Variants of Parkinson's Disease

Juvenile Parkinson's disease is a rare familial variety of the disease now seldom seen. The earlier cases may have been postencephalitic in origin.

Jakob-Creutzfeidt disease is characterized by parkinsonian and pyramidal signs, myoclonus, dementia, and atrophy of the hand muscles. It is discussed in Chapter 40.

Parkinsonism-plus is a term useful in reminding us that many other signs of CNS dysfunction, e.g., autonomic insufficiency hypotension, and ocular palsies, dementia, cerebellar signs, and lower motor neuron lesions, may accompany the clinical features of Parkinson's disease, perhaps as examples of "multiple system atrophy," in which parkinsonism represents only the basal ganglion component of a process involving many areas and levels of the nervous system.

HUNTINGTON'S CHOREA

Huntington's chorea is a dominantly inherited disease of the basal ganglia and cerebral cortex characterized by the development in adult life of chorea and progressive mental deterioration.

Pathology

Pathologically, there is widespread degenerative change in all cortical areas, with marked atrophy of the caudate nucleus, the putamen, and the globus pallidus. Although prominent, atrophic changes are seen elsewhere including the thalamus, other basal nuclei, and the brainstem. There is widespread dropout of neurons with lipoid pigmentation in many of the remaining nerve cells, in the glia, and around the small blood vessels. In the region of degeneration there is often loss of myelin and an increase in glial cells.

Clinical Picture

The disease begins at any time between childhood and old age, most often between ages 30 and 40. Although it is an autosomal-dominant condition, inheritance is quite irregular in some families. Normally it passes directly from one generation to another and does not skip generations. Each offspring of a patient with Huntington's chorea has a 50:50 chance of being affected. Because of the late onset of the disease, many of these patients have had children by the time they develop symptoms. Thus another generation of Huntington's cases begins.

The characteristic *features* of the disease are the chorea and the progressive mental deterioration. If onset is early in childhood the picture is often that of rigidity, but more commonly the first symptoms appear in the late teens and 20s. Sometimes, chorea is an early symptom, but more often neurotic illness, alcoholism, or depressive symptoms appear first, or the picture may resemble Parkinson's disease. However the typical onset in the 30 to 40 age group is characterized by the development of abrupt and jerky choreic movements of the face, tongue, arms and hands, legs, and trunk. Mental deterioration follows the onset of the chorea sometimes years later in this group of older patients.

When the disease first begins the patient often hides his chorea by transferring a sudden jerky movement into a purposeful one. Thus as his arm jerks upward he continues the movement and scratches his ear, or as his head jerks to the side he continues the movement and looks out the window or at the wall. A sudden choreic movement in his legs is hidden by either crossing or uncrossing of the legs to another position. An early sign of the disease is often the inability to keep the tongue protruded. As the disease progresses, the chorea becomes marked and the patient develops a grotesque dancelike gait with an appearance of repeated involuntary jerking of all muscle groups.

The progressive mental deterioration is noted as the patient becomes more and more withdrawn, impulsive, and forgetful. Initially episodes of depression alternating with violent behavior may also be seen. Alcoholism is extremely common. As time goes on the patient becomes quite apathetic. Seizures are unusual. At the end-stage the patient is often rigid and the chorea may give way to severe akinesia. Death usually results from intercurrent infection in a bedridden state.

The only *investigation* that is helpful is the CT scan that shows cerebral atrophy, enlargement of the ventricles, and a characteristic "butterfly" appearance of the lateral ventricles due to the atrophy of the caudate nucleus (Fig. 46-5).

Diagnosis is easy if the family history is known, but many patients either deny the family history or are unaware of it. The initial symptoms then can be very difficult to clarify. Occasionally one notes "hysterical" chorea in a young person who is aware of the family's disease.

Huntington's chorea is progressive and ultimately fatal. The duration of life is variable but averages 20 years from diagnosis. Because of the dread of the disease in many affected families, alcoholism, psychiatric disease, and suicide are common even among unaffected members. As the disease continues, institutional care is almost always necessary.

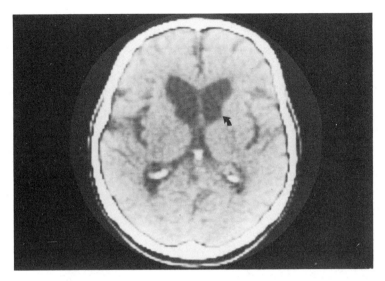

Figure 46-5   CT scan in Huntington's disease. Atrophy of the caudate nucleus (arrowed) produced an indentation in the sides of the lateral ventricles.

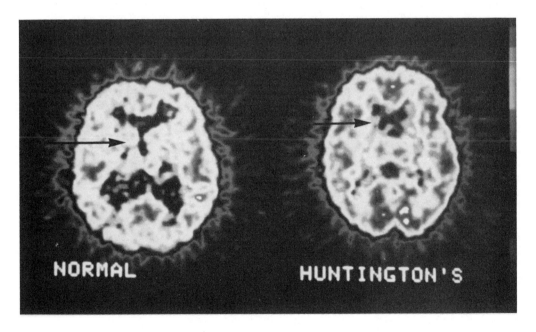

Figure 46-6   PET scan in Huntington's disease. The metabolism of glucose is mapped here, with the highest levels showing as white areas on the scan. Compare the caudate nuclei (arrowed) in the two pictures; the grayness of the diseased caudate indicates a reduction in its metabolic activity. By courtesy of Dr. W. R. Wayne Martin and Dr. M. Hayden.

Although there is no cure and no treatment can stop the disease from progressing, medications may alleviate some of the symptoms. Fluphenazine, dimethylaminoethanol, reserpine, and haloperidol all may reduce the abnormal movements. but nothing prevents the progressive mental deterioration. Most of the medications that benefit Huntington's chorea cause parkinsonism as a side effect, while the drugs that benefit parkinsonism cause deterioration in the Huntington's patient. Thus L-dopa worsens the signs so frequently that it was once suggested as a method of making the diagnosis early. The ethics of producing Huntington's symptoms to make presymptomatic diagnosis may seem questionable, because we are unable to offer any effective therapy, but it may be very important for the purpose of genetic counseling. An abnormal gene has been located on chromosome 4. The new and exciting work on gene markers may allow predictive tests to identify the subclinically-affected family members before they have children.

Counseling of these families regarding the hereditary aspects of the disease is extremely important; referral to a geneticist is advisable. All members of the family must have an intelligent understanding of the disease, because it is only through this type of education that they will be able to take steps to eliminate it in future generations. A Huntington's Disease Society exists as a community service to provide information to patients, families, and physicians.

OTHER FORMS OF CHOREA

Movements simulating those of Huntington's chorea but perhaps less severe and more rapid and tending to spare the trunk and proximal girdle muscles occur in a wide range of other conditions. Usually, they are not accompanied by the dreaded mental concomitants of that disease. In such patients, chorea is incidental, usually transient, and seldom requires treatment on its own account.

Sydenham's chorea, perhaps the most common cause of chorea overall, is probably due to a vasculitis affecting the basal ganglia. It mainly occurs in girls who have rheumatic fever. Chorea also is seen in *pregnancy* and with administration of the *birth-control pill.* Vasculitis may also account for the appearance of choreiform movements in *SLE,* viral *encephalitis, pertussis,* and *diphtheria.* Cerebral *anoxia,* e.g., CO poisoning, cerebrovascular occlusion, or other causes of *ischemia* such as polycythemia and purpuric states, account for a few more cases but are not common. Unilateral ischemia produces contralateral hemichorea as an uncommon stroke syndrome. Intoxication with *manganese, mercury,* and *L-dopa* have been described as producing choreiform movements.

Chorea has been described in cases of *portosystemic encephalopathy, hypo- and hyperthyroidism, Tay-Sachs disease,* Lesch-Nyhan syndrome, and *cerebral palsy.* It is seen in *old age:* this so-called "senile" chorea is a state resembling Huntington's but with a negative family history and only mild or moderate dementia of slow onset.

If chorea does need treatment, aspirin in the Sydenham's form, and chlorpromazine 25-50 mg t.i.d. or haloperidol 1 mg t.i.d. in other forms, are sometimes

ATHETOSIS

The slow, writhing movements characteristic of athetosis were described in Chapter 29. Undoubtedly, most cases are due to cerebral palsy, usually as a result of kernicterus.

Kernicterus results from markedly elevated bilirubin levels in the newborn usually because of Rh or ABO incompatibility. It may also result from prematurity or the use of antibiotics. Because unconjugated bilirubin will pass the blood-brain barrier easily in the infant, there is bile staining of the basal ganglia and olives with secondary degenerative changes. Modern methods of identifying and managing Rh and ABO incompatibility and prematurity have resulted in a marked reduction in the number of cases over the last decade.

Double athetosis refers to a group of disorders affecting the basal ganglia which results in bilateral athetosis and dystonias of the face, trunk, and limbs. Changes of marbling and mottling of the basal ganglia are visible macroscopically and caused by large bundles of abnormally situated myelinated fibers. The onset is usually in the first year of life, often following *perinatal anoxia* and the disease tends not to be progressive. Onset in adolescence or later is very unusual. Most of these children have evidence of hypotonia, mental deficiency, and other neurological abnormalities as well. Familial cases are known. Generalized *anoxia, cerebrovascular disease,* and *Wilson's disease* are much less common causes. Therapy of athetosis with carbamazepine, trihexyphenidyl, or L-dopa has been variably successful.

DYSTONIC STATES

Dystonia Musculorum Deformans

Dystonia musculorum deformans is a disease of the basal ganglia characterized by twisting, turning, and writhing movements of any or all somatic muscles. They occur particularly in the trunk and proximal limb muscles and the contractions are extremely strong and sustained in character. They resemble athetosis but are slower and stronger and cause wider excursions. Although dystonic movements may occur in the other diseases mentioned previously and with drug toxicity (Chap. 43), dystonia musculorum deformans is a separate entity.

The pathological changes are not clearly known because of the limited number of autopsy cases, but degenerative changes have been reported in the cerebral cortex and all areas of the basal ganglia.

The disease is uncommon. It usually develops between the ages of 5 and 15 years and gradually worsens until the torsion spasms interfere with walking and with the use of the arms and hands. Eventually the distortions of the neck, trunk, and limbs may interfere with purposeful movements and disable the patient. While awake, the patient's muscles may be in continuous contraction causing excessive fatigue, interference with speech, difficulty in eating, and pain. They are often truly hypertrophic. Mental deterioration is sometimes seen in the end stages but as a general rule no other motor, psychological, or sensory signs are to be found.

The disease is slowly progressive and the patient often becomes disabled within 10 years with death later resulting from intercurrent infections. Remissions are uncommon but may occur. Ventrolateral thalamotomy has been successful in some patients.

When dystonia or any other involuntary movement disorder develops in a young person, Wilson's disease must be excluded. Phenothiazine and L-dopa may induce dystonia. Hysteria may manifest as abnormal twisting movements.

L-dopa, carbamazepine, diazepam, haloperidol, and cerebellar stimulation by implanted electrodes have all been tried, with variable success.

Spasmodic Torticollis

Children may consistently rotate their heads to one side owing to the presence of a *hematoma* in the sternomastoid muscle, to *ocular* muscle imbalance, or to *cervical anomalies,* and torticollis may develop after rheumatic fever. Torticollis is also seen in *Wilson's disease* or as a sign of a *posterior fossa tumor* and is sometimes hereditary. In adults it occasionally develops as a sequel to epidemic *encephalitis,* in *multiple sclerosis,* or *syphilis,* or due to *painful cervical muscles.* In most patients, however, intermittent spasmodic movements or distortion of the head and neck toward one side occur for no apparent reason. Initially it was thought that the problem might be psychogenic, but there is increasing evidence that it has an organic basis, although many of these patients do have psychopathology as well. The CNS lesion producing the problem is thought to be in the basal ganglia, and the condition is properly regarded as a focal dystonia.

It is an uncommon disorder that may develop at any age, most often between 20 to 40 years. Initially, patients develop minimal jerky turning of the head toward one side and the chin may be rotated towards the shoulder. The muscles involved are usually the sternomastoid on the side opposite the deviation of the head, and the trapezius and lateral cervical muscles on the same side. In a few patients contraction in other muscles of the shoulder girdle and face may be seen. As in most organic movement disorders, tension and anxiety worsen the symptoms, and the patients note aggravation of the problem when they become self-conscious about it.

As time goes by, the symptoms progress until the jerky nature of the head-twisting decreases and the head becomes permanently deviated to one side, except in sleep. A partial or complete remission may be seen in some patients, but it tends to remain as a chronic problem in most.

Many forms of therapy have been tried, usually without significant effect. Destructive surgery to the cervical muscles, accessory nerve, or cervical roots has not been helpful because it may produce so much weakness that the head becomes unstable. Better results have been achieved by thalamotomy and more recently tricyclic drugs, diazepam, haloperidol, and L-dopa have given fair results. In some centers, biofeedback has been used with marked symptomatic relief. Occupational cramps (e.g., writer's cramp, Chap. 37) are also examples of focal dystonia.

WILSON'S DISEASE

Wilson's disease (hepatolenticular degeneration) is a recessive inherited disorder of copper metabolism characterized by damage to the basal ganglia and cirrhosis of the liver. Although an unusual disease, it is important because excellent methods of detection of subclinical cases and carriers are available and therapy is highly successful.

Pathogenesis

Copper ingested in the normal diet totals about 20 mg/day, of which 75 percent is not absorbed. Most of the 25 percent that *is* absorbed is bound to an alpha globulin, ceruloplasmin. The normal serum level of ceruloplasmin is 158–538 mg/L. Only a small amount of copper is bound to albumin which transports it from the gastrointestinal tract to the body tissue. In this state it is metabolically active, while ceruloplasmin-bound copper is not.

Copper is widely distributed, with the highest amounts found in the liver, kidney, muscles, CNS, and bone. Excretion is by the gastrointestinal tract, with only 0.1 mg/day being lost in the urine.

The biochemical defect is characterized by a low serum ceruloplasmin, perhaps because of a deficient enzyme that results in decreased production. The ceruloplasmin-bound copper concentration is low and urinary copper excretion is increased. Normally albumin-bound copper would be transported to the liver and the copper transferred to ceruloplasmin, but in Wilson's disease, the copper remains bound to albumin until it is deposited in the tissues in high concentrations. Such deposits in the brain, liver, and kidney cause destructive lesions that result in the clinical abnormalities.

The pathological changes in the nervous system are widespread and involve chiefly the basal ganglia. In advanced cases there is cavitation in the putamen and globus pallidus. There is loss of neurons in the involved areas, and very large astrocytes (Alzheimer's cells), large phagocytes, and patchy demyelination are seen. The liver shows nodular cirrhosis. The spleen is usually enlarged and congested. Examination of the cornea reveals a ring of fine yellow granules in Descemet's membrane.

Symptoms and Signs

The symptoms and signs of Wilson's disease are due to damage to the liver, nervous system, and eyes. Evidence of liver disease (jaundice, hypersplenism, abnormal enzymes) may appear early or late in the disease, but death caused by liver failure is not uncommon. The neurologic manifestations are extremely varied but the common patterns of presentation are tremor, rigidity, ataxia, athetotic or choreiform movements, or a parkinsonian syndrome. Difficulties with writing and speech are common and intellectual failure or psychiatric disorders are the presenting problems in 20 percent. A peculiar upper arm tremor, called *wing-beating,* is sometimes seen when the arms are held extended. The abnormal movements may involve the trunk, limbs, and head. Patients may show spasticity and the tendon reflexes are usually increased with bilateral extensor plantar responses. The sensory examination is usually normal.

Brown-green rings around the cornea (Kayser-Fletcher rings) are diagnostic, but may only be visible through a slit lamp.

Diagnosis

When suspected, the diagnosis of Wilson's disease can be made without much difficulty in most cases. This is often aided by a positive family history. The diagnosis
should be suspected in *any* young person presenting with a progressive neurological
problem characterized by spasticity, rigidity, dystonia, tremor, choreoathetosis,
dysarthria, or ataxia. The detection of the Kayser-Fleischer ring is quite diagnostic.
The diagnosis may be suggested by a low ceruloplasmin level, increased urinary
excretion of copper, low serum copper, and an abnormal liver biopsy. One can also
often see a gray lunule in the fingernails and increased melanin pigmentation of
the shins in these patients. About 25 percent of the cases present with evidence of
liver disease before neurologic symptoms appear.

Even if the family history is negative, all family members should be assessed
for evidence of subclinical disease or of the carrier state. Early diagnosis is extremely important so that therapy can be instituted before permanent brain and
liver damage occur. Serum ceruloplasmin concentration and urine copper excretion
following penicillamine are useful screening tests, but liver biopsy may be omitted
unless there is clinical or biochemical evidence of hepatic dysfunction.

Treatment

Therapy is based on the assumption that tissue destruction results from excessive
copper deposition. Patients are put on a low-copper diet (no nuts, chocolate, dried
beans, broccoli, corn, mushrooms, peas, shellfish, lamb, pork, dark chicken meat,
or liver) and must take potassium sulfide 20 mg with each meal to minimize copper
absorption. The major therapeutic agent is penicillamine, 1-4 g daily in divided
doses taken on an empty stomach, which increases the urinary excretion of copper.
It must be continued for life.

The unwanted effects of penicillamine include skin rashes, gastrointestinal disturbance, leukopenia, and optic neuritis. Symptoms often worsen when penicillamine therapy is started owing to the mobilization of tissue copper, although this is
only a temporary setback. If the patient develops an allergy to penicillamine the
drug triethylenetetramine dihydrochloride (Trien) can be used. Recently zinc has
been used to treat Wilson's disease and may be the only therapy needed in some
cases.

Course and Prognosis

The onset of the disease is insidious but the neurological manifestations are usually
seen first. The disorder is often not recognized because it is not considered by
those assessing the patient. The long-term results depend upon how much permanent damage there has been before the institution of therapy, but with early treatment the patient's quality and duration of life need not be greatly impaired.

OTHER CONDITIONS

The syndrome of *Gilles de la Tourette* is characterized by muscle twitching, coprolalia (literally, filthy speech), and convulsions; multiple tics affect the face, head and limbs. It begins in childhood, is seldom progressive, and does not affect intelligence.[*] There is a family history of similar problems in 50 percent of the cases. Treatment with clonidine or luphenazine may be successful, as may be the use of haloperidol in low and intermittent doses.

Hemiballismus is a condition characterized by wild, flinging movements on one side of the body, so bad that the patient may become exhausted. It results from a lesion (usually ischemic, sometimes inflammation or tumor) in the contralateral subthalamic nucleus. Although rare, it is most likely to be seen in the first few weeks after a small hemorrhagic (lacunar) stroke, disappearing spontaneously even if the patient is not treated. Very occasionally, hemiballismus occurs in the late stages of a generalized degenerative or dementing disease.

The most effective drugs are haloperidol and perphenazine. The dosage will have to be titrated against the patient's response, but in each case a 1 mg initial dose given IM would be reasonable. Intravenous diazepam may be useful until the haloperidol takes effect. In refractory cases, thalamotomy may give excellent results.

Essential tremor is a condition inherited in an autosomal-dominant manner or occurring sporadically. It is also known as benign, heredofamilial, or senile[†] tremor. The patient complains that the distal parts of his arms shake when he maintains them in a certain position (positional tremor); when he moves them (kinetic tremor); or when his arms are stretched out in the final part of the movement (terminal or intention tremor). There may also be a side-to-side or to-and-fro shaking of the head, which is known as titubation. Tremulous speech and jaw tremor may be present. Handwriting is sometimes very much impaired by the intention element of the tremor. As with all other types of tremor, attention, anxiety, and arousal all increase its severity.

If the symptoms warrant therapy at all then the drug of choice is propranolol. The beta-adrenergic-blocking effect of propranolol is exerted both centrally and peripherally and if the patient has no cardiac conduction disorder or bronchospasm, 10-40 mg may be given up to four times daily. It is most effective among patients who showed symptoms early in life and who were treated for them at an early stage. Alcohol, even when taken in moderate amounts, may markedly diminish the severity of the tremor, but it is not recommended as a form of therapy becuase the tremor may worsen after the alcohol wears off, and chronic alcoholism is a definite danger. Primidone may be used if propranolol is not effective enough, and thalamotomy may be helpful but is rarely recommended because a bilateral procedure is necessary and the surgery is a very major therapy for a benign, although embarrassing condition.

---

[*] Dr. Samuel Johnson, the eighteenth century literary genius, undoubtedly suffered from this syndrome.

[†] The term *senile* means belonging, or incident to, old age. Because this condition, as well as many others with the same prefix, may occur at any age, and because the term is one frequently used as a pejorative by journalists when writing about the Senate or the House of Lords, the term is best left to them and deleted from the medical vocabulary.

All the major antipsychotic agents and L-dopa are capable of inducing abnormal movements (see Chap. 43). In both children and adults, acute dystonias, akathisia (motor restlessness), or parkinsonian features, including oculogyric crises, may occur and will require reduction or omission of the drug. *Tardive dyskinesia* is the name used for a syndrome of repetitive choreic movements, frequently affecting the face, eyes, lips, tongue, and the trunk, and coming on after some months of treatment with phenothiazine, butyrophenone, promethazine or metoclopramide. Omission of the drug seldom relieves the dyskinesia, which often occurs only weeks or months after stopping it in the first place (thus the term "tardive"). Reserpine and many other agents have been used with partial success.

BIBLIOGRAPHY

Calne, D.B. *Therapeutics in Neurology,* 2nd Ed. Oxford, Blackwell Scientific, 1981.

Faldridge, R., Faldridge, A. (eds.). Dystonia. *Adv. Neurol.* Vol. 14, New York, Raven Press, 1976.

Godwin-Austin, R.S. The treatment of the choreas and athetotic dystonias. *J. R. Coll. Physicians Lond.* 35-38, 1979.

Lang, A.E., Blair, R.A.B. Parkinson's disease in 1984: An Update. *Can. Med. Assoc. J. 131*:1031-1037, 1984.

Symposium. Current Concepts and Controversies in Parkinson's Disease. *Can. J. Neurol. Sci. 11*:1-233, 1984.

47
Motor Neuron Disease

In motor neuron disease (MND) the anterior horn cells and corticospinal tracts are usually affected at many levels, although a few patients have clinical manifestations of involvement at only one level. According to the pattern of involvement, different names have been employed; e.g., anterior horn cell degeneration only (progressive muscular atrophy), pyramidal tract degeneration only (primary lateral sclerosis), brainstem motor nuclear degeneration (progressive bulbar palsy), and pseudobulbar palsy. The most common picture however in a mixture of these features (amyotrophic lateral sclerosis, ALS), the patient having both upper and lower motor neuron signs and symptoms often with bulbar involvement as well (Table 47-1). Because the separation of types is based only on clinical presentation, many authors use the term *amyotrophic lateral sclerosis* for all forms. We retain the differentiation because some patients continue to show only one form of involvement and because the prognosis does vary according to the type.

PATHOLOGY

The pathological features are primarily degeneration of motor cells in the spinal cord, brainstem, and, to a lesser extent, cerebral cortex, with secondary degeneration of pyramidal tracts. The anterior horn cells and pyramidal tracts are more or less severely affected; the cellular destruction is greatest in the cervical and lumbar regions of the cord (Fig. 47-1). There is some diffuse loss of myelin in all areas of the spinal cord except the posterior columns, but striking loss occurs in the pyramidal tracts, giving the cord a characteristic picture on myelin staining.

In the brainstem, degeneration occurs in the motor nuclei of the cranial nerves but the three oculomotor nuclei are always spared; this feature is worthy of careful investigation, as we might learn more about this enigmatic disease from the few nuclei that are never involved than from the many that usually are.

651

Table 47-1   Names for the Different Forms of Motor Neuron Disease

	LMNL	UMNL
Bulbar	Progressive bulbar palsy	Pseudobulbar palsy
Spinal	Progressive (spinal) muscular atrophy	Primary lateral sclerosis
	Amyotrophic lateral sclerosis	

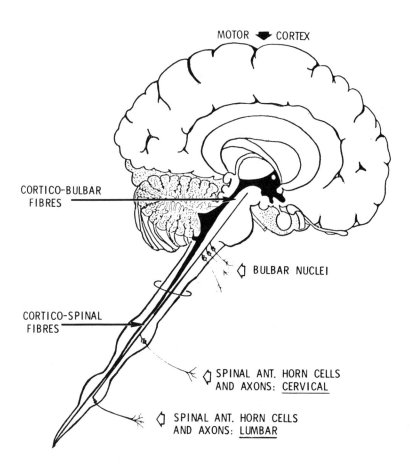

Figure 47-1   Sites of the lesions in motor neuron disease.

Degeneration is found in the pyramidal tracts and sometimes in other fiber tracts in the brainstem. Pyramidal degeneration can be traced into the internal capsule in about one-half of the cases, and one-third can be shown to have a decreased number of Betz cells in the motor cortex and a variable loss of medium-sized motor cortical cells.

CLINICAL FEATURES

The prevalence of all forms of MND is 5:100,000. The onset is usually between the ages of 50 and 70 years and twice as many men develop the disease as women. The disease appears as a dominant character in some families. It accounts for 1 in 1000 deaths.

Although this is a disease of the motor neurons and the findings are entirely motor, secondary degeneration in the nerves and muscles may give rise to vague pains and paresthesias particularly at the onset of the disease. Most first notice weakness in their legs or arms, sometimes mentioning atrophy or fasciculations. Bulbar symptoms are unusual at the onset.

The classification of motor neuron disease into four types based on the predominant clinical features is somewhat artificial in that many patients classified as having one will later develop features of other types. Other patients at the time of death will have clinical evidence of degeneration at one level, but will have pathological changes at other levels that were not evident clinically (Fig. 47-2).

In *progressive muscular atrophy* the clinical features are those of degeneration of the anterior horn cells of the spinal cord. The patient notes weakness in the hands and legs, and on examination is found to have atrophy of the small muscles of the hands and of the more distal muscles of his arms and legs. Fasciculations can be seen not only in these areas but often over the shoulder girdle, trunk, tongue, and face as well.

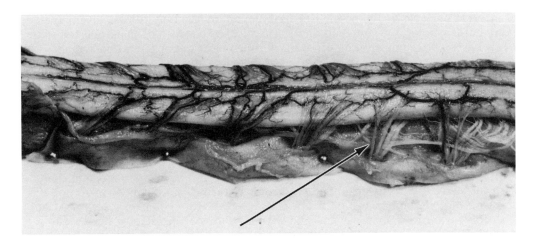

Figure 47-2 The spinal cord in advanced motor neuron disease. The anterior roots are atrophied (arrow) while the posterior roots are normal.

In *primary lateral sclerosis* the manifestations are of pyramidal tract degeneration, with weakness and spasticity of the legs and later of the arms. Hyperactive deep tendon reflexes, palmomental reflexes, increased jaw jerk, Hoffmann's and Babinski signs and a pouting reflex are commonly found. This is a difficult diagnosis however, as many more common causes of paraplegia must first be excluded (Chap. 50).

In *progressive bulbar palsy* the degeneration is primarily of the motor nuclei of the brainstem. The patient complains of slurred speech and later difficulty in swallowing and coughing, so aspiration is a constant danger. There are atrophy and fasciculations of the tongue, poor palatal movement, and sometimes fasciculation or weakness of the facial muscles. Although less than 10 percent of cases have pure progressive bulbar palsy, most MND patients eventually have some degree of bulbar involvement.

Amyotrophic lateral sclerosis is the term correctly applied to the most common form, in which there is evidence of both anterior horn cell and pyramidal degeneration. Seventy-five percent of cases will eventually show bulbar or pseudobulbar signs, the latter indicating degeneration of the supranuclear fibers. On examination, patients with ALS have atrophy, weakness, and fasciculations in their limbs, indicating a lower motor neuron lesion, combined with hyperactive reflexes and Babinski signs. It is this combination of upper and lower motor neuron signs in all limbs that is the hallmark of ALS (Fig. 47-3).

ASSOCIATED DISEASES

The picture of MND has been described in association with many diseases including hypoglycemia, hyperthyroidism, poliomyelitis, and carcinoma. It has also been reported with pregnancy and following gastrectomy. With most of these conditions, the association is rare and may be coincidental. However malignant tumors, particularly carcinoma of the lung, have been noted in about 10 percent of the patients. There is also evidence for the unusually frequent occurrence of a condition resembling MND many years after an attack of poliomyelitis. This association has been of interest because of the possibility that the poliovirus may remain latent for years before damaging motor neurons. The disease has also been associated with a few cases of acromegaly, electric shock injury, and heavy-metal poisoning. Parkinsonism and dementia are associated in the illness prevalent in Guam; some features of MND are present in Jakob-Creutzfeldt disease (Chap. 40).

COURSE AND PROGNOSIS

The course in motor neuron disease is variable, but the average life expectancy is 3 years from onset and only 20 percent survive over 5 years. To some extent survival depends upon the type of MND, but there is great variation among patients with the same type. Although bulbar palsy is regarded as an ominous form of the disease, some patients survive for up to 15 years, while in contrast, other patients with this form of the disorder may die within months of developing brainstem symptoms. In general, those with bulbar palsy have a more rapid course than those with primary lateral sclerosis, in whom the prognosis is markedly better.

DIFFERENTIAL DIAGNOSIS

Motor neuron disease must be differentiated from other conditions that produce a combination of upper and lower motor neuron lesions. The most obvious of these are disorders of the cervical cord, such as skull base deformities, syringomyelia, cord tumors, and cervical spondylosis. Here however, there should not be any evidence of anterior horn cell involvement in the legs and trunk, but only in the upper limbs, and any signs of disease because of a lesion above the foramen magnum (bulbar signs, fifth, or seventh nerve involvement) would rule out a cervical cause. Lower motor neuron lesions may be predominant with spinal arachnoiditis (usually syphilitic), cervical ribs, and peripheral nerve lesions, and with spinal radiculitis. Weakness and wasting, although without fasciculations, also occur in primary muscle disease and with rheumatoid arthritis and myotonic dystrophy. If there is doubt about evidence of anterior horn cell disease in the trunk or legs, EMG may be able to demonstrate that which cannot be seen clinically. The causes of bulbar and pseudobulbar palsies are discussed in Chapter 25 and of distal weakness in Chapter 26. Fasciculations were discussed in Chapter 9.

LABORATORY STUDIES

Although the diagnosis is usually evident clinically, there are a few investigations that can be used to confirm the diagnosis or to rule out other disease or an associated condition.

Nerve conduction studies yield results that are normal or only slightly below, making demyelinating neuropathies unlikely. An EMG shows evidence of denervation and reduced numbers of motor unit potentials among which are giant units and polyphasic potentials, as well as fasciculations.

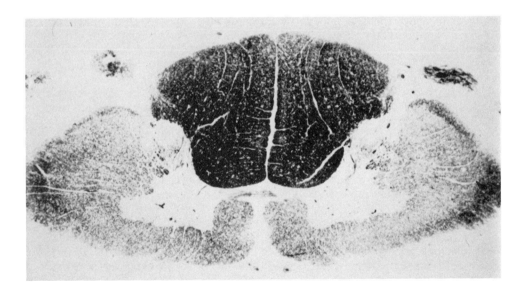

Figure 47-3 Spinal cord, stained for myelin. The posterior columns are well preserved but there is demyelination in the anterior and lateral funiculi and wasting of the anterior horns.

The CSF protein level is elevated in the range of 45-95 mmol/L in one-third of cases. Decreased urinary creatine and increased urinary creatinine levels are found but are not useful diagnostic tests.

There have been reports of abnormal pancreatic enzyme secretion in MND; but this has not been consistently confirmed and no laboratory tests of any value are based on this observation. Abnormal glucose tolerance curves and insulin curves after glucose loads have also been described.

Muscle biopsy will demonstrate the characteristic features of a neurogenic muscular atrophy but is seldom needed.

Investigations should be undertaken in motor neuron disease to rule out underlying malignant tumors if there is any atypical feature on examination or investigation, such as marked slowing of motor nerve conduction velocities. Most of the associated conditions mentioned before can be excluded by history (prior gastrectomy, polio, or electrical injury) by examination (hyperthyroidism, acromegaly), or by laboratory tests (lead or other metal poisoning, recurrent hypoglycemia).

Treatment

Some dementing diseases, some muscular dystrophies, and all motor neuron disease (ALS) share this characteristic; that neurologists can do nothing either to prevent or even to slow down their relentless course to death. In every other area of neurology we can expect that our interventions will at least buy time during which a life can be lived; here we cannot even offer that.

But we can offer relief from the major symptoms of ALS so well documented by Newrick and Langton-Hewer (see Bibliography). Here is what we think we should do when there is nothing to be done:

Slurring, Choking, and Drooling

Use anticholinergics to dry secretions; or (a paradox) neostigmine to increase muscle power temporarily. The patient will decide how liquid his food should be, and how large the mouthfuls. Cricopharyngeal myotomy can be performed to aid swallowing.

Involuntary Limb Jerks

Use phenytoin or carbamazepine; clonazepam may work but can reduce respiratory power.

Cramps and Aching Limb Pains

Try quinine, phenytoin, or carbamazepine. When pain is a real problem do not hesitate to use opiates in doses that work.

Insomnia and Problems Turning in Bed

There are special beds that can be leased or borrowed; otherwise try to organize a roster of people to sleep over, sparing the spouse from waking every 3 hours to turn the patient.

Frustration and Boredom

Mobilize the family and volunteers, from neighborhood church or social groups, etc., to visit in order to talk, listen, play cards, turn over pages or read, or just

to be there for a while. Occupational therapists can advise on a number of communication aids — the fear of choking without anyone present, for example, is a
terrible burden for the patient, and a means of summoning assistance that he can
use will be a boon.

Motility

Arrange OT assessment of the house, providing rails, hoists, or supports, eliminat-
ing stairs where possible, and advising on gadgets for feeding, shaving, dressing,
recreation, and ambulation.

Leg Swelling

Elevate the legs and use elastic stockings, not diuretics.

Posture

This may be improved with a collar, brace, or spring-loaded splints.

Cachexia

Improve swallowing as far as possible as recommended earlier; consider a nasogastric tube. We advise against gastrostomy because of the added misery it
induces.

Constipation

This is due to weak abdominal muscles and reduced activity. Use bulk purgatives,
laxatives, and enemas. Try to avoid the need for manual evacuations.

Sexual Frustration

This is common and we never seem to talk about it. Do so freely and without embarrassment to both the patient and spouse; the problems are mainly matters of
method.

Pneumonia

Treat this complication as you would in anybody else.

Respiratory Failure

Do not embark upon measures that will only prolong disease. With a tracheostomy
and ventilator you may sentence the patient to a year of passive, uncommunicating
agony. Is that what he really wants?

Management of these problems demands a team approach, but the team has to
be led by somebody in charge who will identify the needs, prescribe for them, and
coordinate their delivery. That person should be a physician, but cannot always be
a rehabilitation specialist. The patient's personal doctor is perhaps best of all for
he is available, he knows all of the family, and he will probably take the final responsibility for guiding the patient gently and with minimal suffering, into harbor.

The recent observation of transient improvement with thyroglobulin has
sparked new interest in mechanisms for cell change in ALS and possible new
chemicals for therapy, but no effective treatment is yet available.

BIBLIOGRAPHY

Brooke, M.H. *A Clinician's View of Neuromuscular Disorders.* Baltimore, Williams & Wilkins, 1977.

Mulder, D.W., (ed.). *The Diagnosis and Treatment of Amyotrophic Lateral Sclerosis.* Boston, Houghton Mifflin, 1980.

Newick, P.G., Langton-Hewer, R. Motor neuron disease: Can we do better? *Br. Med. J. 289:*539-542, 1984.

48
Diseases of Myelin

MULTIPLE SCLEROSIS

Although many diseases affect the nervous system by causing demyelination, the only common primary demyelinating disease is multiple sclerosis. Multiple sclerosis is an acute, subacute, or chronic disorder of the central nervous system characterized by attacks and remissions, ultimately with a progressive course of neurological impairment caused by scattered plaques of demyelination of the brain, brainstem, and spinal cord.

Pathology

The *plaques* of demyelination within the central nervous system are characterized by breakdown of myelin, perivascular edema and inflammation, and gliosis (scarring) (Figs. 48-1, 48-2A, B). The axons are usually preserved but may be involved in the late gliotic stage of demyelination. Although regarded a random process, there is a predilection for the brainstem and periventricular regions and within the thickly myelinated areas of the brainstem such as the medial longitudinal fasciculi. Various abnormalities of enzymes, lipids, platelets, protein chemistry, lymphocytes, and capillaries are involved in the process of demyelination, but which ones are primary and which ones are secondary is uncertain. The lesions may occur suddenly and then apparently heal. It would seem that some of the apparent disappearance of demyelinating lesions is due to compensation, and various situations such as a hot bath, fever, or exercise may unmask a lesion that clinically had disappeared.

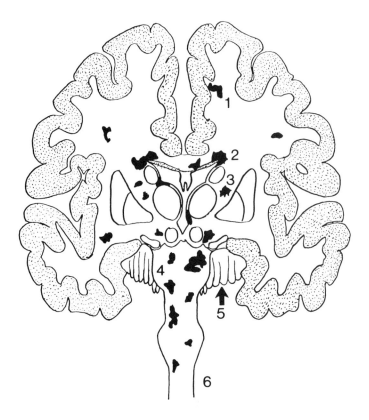

Figure 48-1   Diagram of coronal section of the brain, with multiple scattered plaques in subcortical white matter (1); corpus callosum (2); internal capsule (3); pons (4); cerebellum (5) and spinal cord (6).

Epidemiology

There are probably 25,000 patients with this condition in Canada. It has an incidence of 1:20,000/year, but because it is so chronic, prevalence is high, perhaps about 1:1000 of the population.

Multiple sclerosis occurs only rarely in childhood and in the elderly. Most patients develop their first symptoms between ages 20 and 40, and the disease is slightly more common in women.

Family

There is good evidence that multiple sclerosis is more common in families than one would expect in the normal population. About 10 to 20 percent of patients with multiple sclerosis have a family history of this disorder. It is likely that there are inherited immune factors that predispose the individuals and their families to whatever multiple etiological factors result in myelin breakdown.

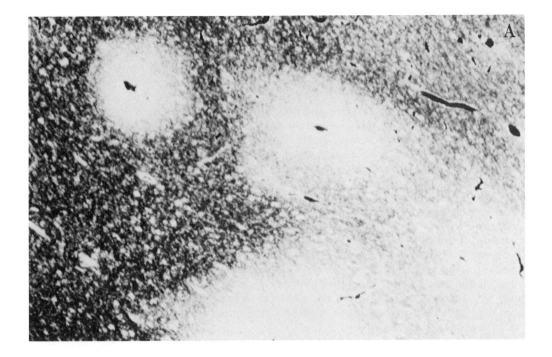

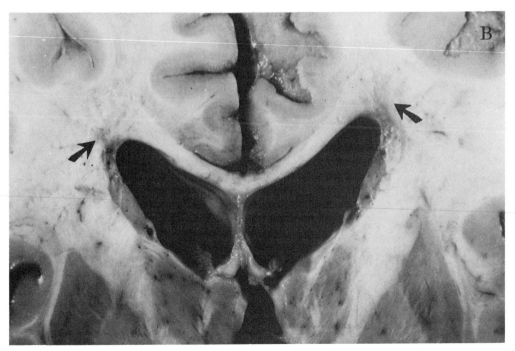

Figure 48-2   (A) Scattered plaques of perivascular demyelination. (B) Periventricular plaques of demyelination beside the lateral ventricles (arrowed) in multiple sclerosis.

Latitudes

The most intriguing finding in the epidemiology of multiple sclerosis is the increasing prevalence rate at latitudes farthest from the equator both north and south (Fig. 48-3). Thus it is almost an unknown disease at the equator but is one of the more common serious neurological disorders in the northern United States, southern Canada, Great Britain, and central Europe. More recently, isolated areas of increased prevalence have been found in New England, the Orkney Islands, Washington State, Nova Scotia, and Alaska.

Migration studies have demonstrated that whatever the risk factor is in multiple sclerosis, it is carried if a person goes from a high to a low incidence area of the world. Also, if one moves from an area of low incidence to an area of high incidence, one takes on a greater risk, but this is age-related to a great extent and a critical age of 15 years has been calculated. This suggests that whatever the risk factor is for developing multiple sclerosis it is acquired around the age of puberty. Studies of migration to Israel have further demonstrated that there is probably a 3- to 23-year incubation period before developing the disease. This is unlikely to be the only factor that is relevant however, because high-risk areas are also characterized by a tendency to provide a diet high in saturated fats, and this may also have a part to play in causation, as a low unsaturated fat intake is associated with a greater likelihood of developing experimental allergic encephalitis in laboratory animals.

Many theories to explain multiple sclerosis have been put forward suggesting a vascular (thrombotic or embolic) cause; other explanations have invoked biochemical change, infections, and allergies. Some more recent observations are beginning to tie together some of the older observations that led to isolated theories. The current leading theory is that of a slow virus infection with a long incubation period, resulting in a progressive neurological deficit many years later.

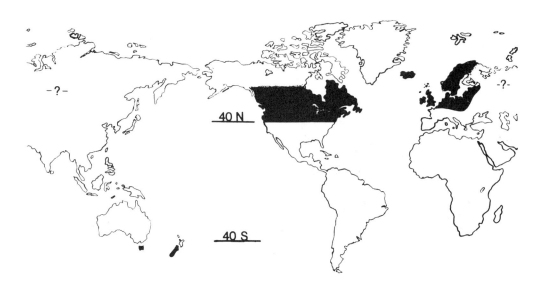

Figure 48-3   The areas where multiple sclerosis is known to have its highest prevalence.

The virus responsible has not been isolated, and there is some suggestion that perhaps a number of viruses may initiate a similar demyelinating disease in a predisposed patient. The leading suspect is a morbillivirus, because repeated studies have shown the antibody levels in MS patients to be higher than those of the rest of the population. In MS patients HLA typing has shown a preponderance of the A3,B7 Dw2 haplotype.

Further strong suspicions relate to a possible immunological basis for MS. It was noticed many years ago that the gamma globulin fraction was increased in the cerebrospinal fluid, and this appears to be the active antibody produced within the nervous system. It appears as oligoclonal IgG bands on CSF immunoelectrophoresis.

Various laboratories have reported myelinotoxic and cytotoxic circulating antibodies. Recently a clearer demonstration of cellular hypersensitivity to the basic A protein in myelin has been shown by macrophage migration inhibition, indicating a disturbance of cell-mediated immunity. Because there are certain resemblances between the clinical and pathological signs of MS and the experimental allergic encephalomyelitis (EAE) produced by injecting myelin and Freund's adjuvant into laboratory animals, it may be seen that a disturbance of immunological function is likely to be a part of the pathogenesis of this condition.

Clinical Course

While frequently an attack will occur without any obvious precipitant, exacerbation of the disease may occur following physical, or more often, emotional stress, in the puerperium, following vaccination or serum injections, and following infections.

The course varies in individual patients. An occasional patient will have an acute onset with a rapidly progressive course to disability within a few years. Others will have a much more benign course and may remain functioning normally 30 years later. The most common patterns are those of acute attacks and remissions (which are more common in those with an early onset) or a slowly progressive neurological deficit, more common in patients with onset at a later age. It is very common for the first attack to be followed by complete remission. However as attacks recur, more and more deficit is left. Despite this, about one-third of the patients with multiple sclerosis have a benign course. The prognosis is much better than had been previously thought, and the average duration of illness is over 30 years. Thirty-two percent of patients are functioning well at work 10 years after the onset of the disease and at 25 years, 75 percent of patients were alive in one study and two-thirds of the original group were still ambulant.

Symptoms and Signs

Multiple sclerosis is a condition with a multiplicity of lesions and a course that is classically relapsing. Nevertheless, a monosymptomatic onset is well recognized, even though other sites are affected within the nervous system as time progresses.

Initial events that cause difficulty in diagnosis when they occur alone include the appearance of retrobulbar neuritis, vertigo, facial myokymia, facial numbness, extraocular palsy, or facial weakness resembling Bell's palsy. Internuclear ophthalmoplegia, long-tract motor or sensory signs, and the presence of a Lhermitte's sign are other presentations, which may occur entirely alone and recover spontaneously only to be replaced in time by combinations of symptoms which allow that diagnosis to be regarded as probable, which may not have been even considered before.

The scattered plaques of demyelination may affect most nerve fiber pathways in the spinal cord, brainstem, or hemispheres. The common patterns of deficit are seen in the motor and sensory systems, the brainstem nuclei, and optic nerves.

Involvement of the *pyramidal tract* anywhere along its course will result in spasticity with the characteristic findings of hyperreflexia, clonus, loss of abdominal reflexes, and Babinski signs. The limbs may eventually become progressively weaker and paralyzed. *Cerebellar* involvement is common and the patient will demonstrate marked incoordination, dysarthria, and ataxia.

Numbness and altered *sensation* are common symptoms in multiple sclerosis and at the onset often have a peripheral distribution similar to a peripheral neuropathy, but the reflexes are usually increased. Involvement of the *posterior columns* leads to a common diagnostic symptom of an electric shock-like sensation down the back and in the limbs on flexion of the neck (Lhermitte's sign). This can occur with any involvement of the posterior columns but the commonest cause is multiple sclerosis.

Occasionally the patient may experience pain in the face with all the features of trigeminal neuralgia. Multiple sclerosis should always be suspected in any young person who presents with that symptom.

Any *brainstem nuclei* may be involved by the plaques of multiple sclerosis. Ocular muscle weakness is common, causing diplopia. Mild facial numbness or weakness and fine rippling of the facial muscles (myokymia) may occur. Involvement of the vestibular system results in vertigo and unsteadiness. It is common on examination to find nystagmus, but one should particularly look for an ataxic nystagmus, greater in the abducting eye and associated with poor adduction of the other eye. This is called an intranuclear ophthalmoplegia and results from demyelination in the medial longitudinal fasciculi which coordinate the movements of all the oculomotor muscles. It is a common finding in MS and is almost diagnostic in young people, particularly when bilateral.

The *optic nerves* are commonly involved, resulting in blurring of vision and alteration of visual fields. A common problem is acute retrobulbar neuritis (RBN) with pain on eye movement, blurring or loss of vision, decreased visual fields, or large scotomas. Forty percent of patients with MS develop RBN at some time; at least 50 percent of those with BUN have or will later develop signs of MS on careful examination. After one attack of RBN, one must examine the patient for evidence of any other neurological signs, and he must be kept under watchful review in case other signs develop even years later.

Mental changes are not of diagnostic value but sometimes do occur. Euphoria was once said to be the most common emotional abnormality, but depression is more common in our experience. The development of marked emotional changes in a patient with MS should always make one suspicious of demyelivation involving the periventricular areas and the frontal lobes.

Stress is intimately involved in the production of symptoms in MS, and many of the patients who perform worse than one feels they should in view of the extent of their lesions are tense and without confidence. Conversion symptoms may occur and may be hard to differentiate from another attack of demyelination. Indeed, a mistaken diagnosis of "hysteria" is commonly made in these patients because the fleeting signs of MS are not recognized for what they are. Some patients do show evidence of intellectual impairment late in the course of the illness.

It is not commonly recognized that grand mal *seizures* occur in about of 5 percent of MS patients.

In the presence of bilateral corticospinal lesions, a spastic bladder may be expected. This leads to complaints of urgency, frequency, and incontinence. Although this was understood to be due to a "spastic" bladder, it may be due to detrusor muscle spasticity, sphincter spasticity, dysynergia of these, or some other change, and a full urological assessment is required to choose appropriate therapy.

Impotence occurs in about half the males with MS, either becaise of para-paresis or occasionally on a psychogenic basis.

Cerebrospinal Fluid Findings

There is no pathognomonic test for multiple sclerosis but a number of tests are found to be useful in helping the clinician confirm his diagnosis. It should always be remembered that the most specific diagnostic method is a clear history and examination. Although the laboratory tests are valuable in confirming the diag-nosis, some patients show normal results regardless of the stage of the disease.

There is seldom any increase in CSF cell counts. About half the patients will have a slight elevation in total protein, but this is seldom above 0.70 g/L. An elevation of the amount of gamma globulin above 13 percent of total protein is not uncommon, but this test has been supplanted by examination for a few bands stain-ing in the gamma globulin region on electrophoresis of concentrated CSF. Such *oligoclonal banding* is a useful piece of supportive evidence in favor of the diagno-sis of MS, but it also occurs in neurosyphilis, collagen-vascular diseases, and encephalomyelitis.

Evoked Responses

Lesions of MS which are not clinically apparent may be revealed with the aid of visual, auditory and somatosensory evoked responses (see Chap. 8). These tests are painless and noninvasive; since they may demonstrate that the patient has lesions in many parts of the CNS, they may make unnecessary other tests which one might have wished to perform if one were trying to characterize a single lesion.

Scanning Techniques

The delayed, enhanced CT scan (Fig. 48-4A) may show up MS plaques which were unsuspected clinically, but the NMR scan is better (Fig. 48-4B).

Treatment

There is at present no specific cure for multiple sclerosis. Therapy is aimed at possible etiological mechanisms, at symptoms, and at complications.

Corticotropin (ACTH) Therapy

After many years of observation it has been concluded that ACTH therapy will marginally improve the symptoms and signs of an acute attack more rapidly than could be expected alone, so long as the disease is obviously active. There is no evidence that increased benefits result from long-term therapy because ACTH does not improve chronic, long-standing neurological deficits. Many patients have developed marked complications from excessive use of these drugs used long-term,

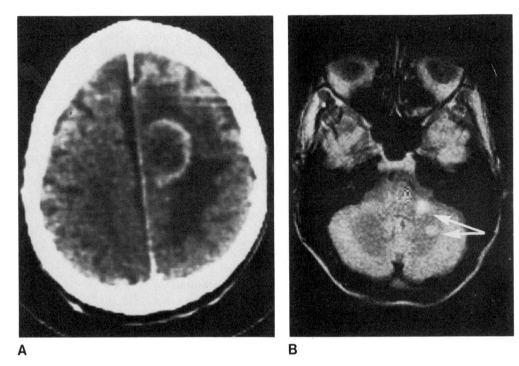

A   **B**

Figure 48-4   A. Enhanced CT scan. The mass is not a tumor but a plaque of multiple sclerosis as proved by biopsy. B. NMR (MRI) scan. MS plaques are seen in
the pons and middle cerebellar peduncle. Courtesy of Dr. David Li and Dr. William
Robertson.

but the sensation of well-being on steroids convinces them they are benefiting
from the therapy; and this is emphasized when they try and stop it. Intrathecal
steroids have been used, but the effects are transient and the procedure is aban-
doned because of the complications of arachnoiditis from repeated treatments.

High-Dosage Steroids

High-dose methylprednisolone has been used to treat acute attacks of MS and this
treatment is simple and well tolerated. Doses of 1000 mg intravenously are given
over 10 min every 2 days ("pulsed therapy") for five doses.

Immunosuppressants

The use of immunosuppressants, with or without plasma exchange is at present
under research study; early results hold some promise, but the potential side
effects and complications of these drugs are a concern. Almost total immuno-
suppression using antilymphocytic serum with cyclophosphamide, steroids, and
thoracic duct drainage has shown that acute attacks may be aborted by this

treatment and the frequency of relapse may be reduced, but such therapy is still experimental. Long-term, low-dose azathioprine and total lymphoid irradiation are also under study. There are as yet only early reports of their effectiveness and safety.

Treatment of Spasticity

A number of muscle relaxants have been used with variable results and probably the most useful drug has been diazepam, but even this drug has to be used in dosages that induce drowsiness before one can demonstrate significant reduction of spinal reflexes. Recently developed antispasticity drugs (dantrolene sodium and baclofen) are probably more specific and useful but should only be used in patients who have significant strength in the spastic limbs. Otherwise, removal of the spasticity makes the limbs even weaker and the patient will often have less function than before. Our results with these drugs have been disappointing because of the side effects and the limited benefit in all but a few patients. They are, however, useful (particularly baclofen) for spasms that often occur in patients with spasticity.

Many patients have noticed that sitting in front of a hot fire or taking a hot bath causes them to be very much weaker and sometimes spasticity or spasms increase. Conversely, treatment with ice packs sometimes markedly reduces spasticity and allows the patient 2 or 3 hr of painless increased mobility and strength, far outlasting the cooling effect of the ice.

Surgery

A number of surgical procedures have been carried out for contractures, spasticity, and deformities. The major thrust has been in reducing spasticity and muscle spasms by various destructive procedures on nerves, roots, and spinal cord, or by phenol or alcohol injections into the intrathecal space.

Bladder Management

Urological assessment is needed to clarify what type of bladder dysfunction is present when the MS patient begins to complain of frequency, urgency, or incontinence (see Chap. 33).

Mild degrees of upper motor neuron bladder dysfunction may respond to anticholinergic drugs such as propantheline bromide. The patients should try to schedule their fluid intake and activities in relation to bladder function. If necessary, when a more significantly spastic bladder causes incontinence, a condom drainage system can be used. A catheter should be avoided if at all possible because of the great danger of infection. If a catheter *has* to be used, intermittent self-catheterization is preferable. The patient should have a high intake of fluid, urine cultures must be performed regularly, and appropriate antibiotics must be used if significant infection develops. In some cases an indwelling catheter is needed. In the male, the penis should be taped to the abdominal wall to avoid a penile-scrotal junction fistula.

Management of Pain

Complaints of pain are common in MS. Patients may have trigeminal or segmental neuralgias, probably due to plaques at the dorsal root entry zones, and may have painful muscle spasms. Carbamazepine is effective for trigeminal pain and other lancinating pains that occur in MS, and the spasms in the back and limbs are often relieved by local cooling, massage, hydrotherapy, and exercise. Limb spasms may respond to baclofen.

Management of Psychological Problems

Multiple sclerosis patients should know and understand their disease and be re-assured about many of the fears that they have about it. They often have many unsolved conflicts and problems related to their families, income, and future, and many of these profound and long-standing frustrations can be resolved by a sensitive and understanding physician who will take the time to talk. Tranquilizers and antidepressants are effective when used in appropriate situations, but they should not be used to replace the personal impact the physician can make. Stress is an extremely important factor in the management of these patients, because acute exacerbations are often related to episodes of emotional trauma. Patients cannot possibly avoid all these situations, but they should recognize the importance of avoiding physical and physiological stress where possible and the family should understand the implications of stress as well.

Multiple sclerosis societies are active in North America and in Europe and chapters are to be found in almost all of the larger towns. They are able to pro-vide information, expertise, companionship, reassurance, social benefits, and health care aids. As well as having an important function in research funding, these societies offer much for the MS patient who would be well advised to con-tact them.

Diets

There have been many diets used in MS with various rationales, but none has yet proved to benefit patients permanently. The diet currently undergoing most care-ful evaluation is one that is low in cholesterol and that is supplemented by linoleic acid (sunflower seed, evening primrose oil, or corn oil). It has been suggested that linoleate may be immunosuppressant or is necessary to maintain the integrity of myelin against immunological challenge. Although the preliminary results of this diet are promising, it does remain to be proved that it is of permanent value.

OTHER DISEASES OF MYELIN

Although multiple sclerosis is the classic demyelinating disease, there are many other diseases that are characterized by a breakdown of myelin. It should be re-membered that demyelination is one of the relatively few ways that the nervous system can react to pathological stimuli. Thus many diseases that affect the nervous system, both peripherally and centrally, produce this effect. Diseases such as metabolic peripheral neuropathies, pernicious anemia, and tabes dorsalis, all produce much of their pathology by the process of demyelination. Many of the inborn areas of metabolism cause disruption of myelin.

Because they are mentioned elsewhere in this book and are not generally re-ferred to as demyelinating diseases, we will not discuss diseases such as post-infectious encephalomyelitis, central pontine myelinolysis, Marchiafava-Bignami disease, and progressive multifocal leukoencephalopathy, but it should be stated that these diseases cause their CNS signs and symptoms by the process of demyelination.

The diseases of myelin are divided into two large categories. The *first* includes disorders that cause disruption of normally formed myelin (at least we assume that the myelin has been normally formed; we are not sure in diseases such as multiple sclerosis and Schilder's disease). The *second* group comprises the disorders of abnormally formed myelin in which the breakdown of myelin results from a defective formation of the protein and lipid concentric layers of myelin around the axon. These are referred to as leukodystrophies. The general classification of diseases of myelin is shown in Table 48-1. There are numerous subtypes not mentioned in this list, particularly in the leukodystrophy group, that have been differentiated because of their pathological appearances, staining characteristics, or biochemical derangements. Most of these are rare and as yet untreatable, so they will not be discussed here.

Disorders of Normally Formed Myelin

Multiple Sclerosis

Multiple sclerosis is the typical demyelinating disorder and has just been fully discussed.

Adrenoleukodystrophy

Adrenoleukodystrophy is a sex-linked recessive disease and has been known by many confusing terms, the confusion initially precipitated by Schilder's original report. He described three patients, but retrospective evaluation suggests that the three had different diseases. The disorder now referred to as adrenoleukodystrophy is characterized by the onset in childhood of a slowly progressive CNS disorder with personality and behavioral changes, apathy, dullness, loss of energy and interest, headaches, dizziness, and weakness. Seizures and focal neurologic signs, especially field defects, follow. Extrapyramidal signs and progressive intellectual deterioration are common. Laboratory testing shows decreased adrenal function in most cases. In the final stages the patient is blind, agnosic, apractic, decerebrate, rigid, contracted, emaciated, and epileptic. These children usually

Table 48-1   Diseases of Myelin

Disorders of normally formed myelin (demyelinating disorders)
    Multiple sclerosis
    Neuromyelitis optica (Devic's disease)
    Adrenoleukodystrophy (Schilder's disease)
    Balo's concentric sclerosis

Disorders of abnormally formed myelin (leukodystrophies)
    Metachromatic leukodystrophy
    Krabbe's globoid cell type
    Miscellaneous types

---

die within 5 years of the onset. Occasionally a similar disease is seen in early
adulthood with primarily psychiatric symptoms to start with. The CSF examination shows high gamma globulin levels and brain biopsy or autopsy examination
shows diffuse demyelination in the white matter of the brain.

Neuromyelitis Optics (Devic's Disease)

Neuromyelitis optics is characterized by optic atrophy and a transverse myelitis.
Although there is no doubt that the condition does exist, it may just be a variant
of multiple sclerosis and there is probably no reason to discuss it as a separate
entity.

Balo's Concentric Sclerosis

In Balo's concentric sclerosis, a very strange pattern of demyelination occurs in
both hemispheres, in which there are concentric bands of demyelination radiating
out from the basal ganglia. The clinical picture is like that of progressive multiple
sclerosis, and the diagnosis is really pathological.

Disorders of Abnormally Formed Myelin (Leukodystrophies)

Metachromatic Leukodystrophy

Metachromatic leukodystrophy results from a deficiency of the enzyme arylsulfatase A which is required for the metabolism of sulfatide to cerebroside. Sulfatide
is a constituent of normal myelin, and because of the enzyme defect here, it accumulates and eventually disrupts it. Although the main site of this is the CNS,
peripheral nerve myelin is also affected with the production of a neuropathy.

Children show severe mental deterioration, optic atrophy, and pyramidal signs;
some have seizures as well. Neuropathy is more obtrusive in the adult form but
otherwise the features are similar. Death usually occurs within 3 to 5 years in
the affected children, while the course is slightly slower in young adults.

Because the sulfatide accumulates also in the testes, gallbladder, renal
tubules, and pituitary gland, diagnosis may be possible by nerve or renal biopsy, but
the most satisfactory method is the estimation of leukocyte arylsulfatase A levels.
This technique is also applicable to amniocentesis.

Krabbe's Globoid Cell Leukodystrophy

In Krabbe's globoid cell leukodystrophy, a rare disease, there is widespread CNS
and PNS demyelination with the accumulation of large, multinucleated giant cells
within white matter and Schwann cells. These "globoid cells" contain excess
cerebroside. The enzyme defect is either of beta-galactosidase or sulfotrans-
ferase, both substances concerned in the metabolism of cerebroside.

The disease develops in the first year of life, with irritability, slowing and
later cessation of psychomotor development, tonic spasms, seizures and myoclonus,
blindness, spasticity giving way to flaccidity as the neuropathy develops, and
eventual death.

Other Leukodystrophies

Many other enzyme defects are known or may be suspected to lead to abnormalities of myelin metabolism. All are now untreatable and most resemble the two disorders described earlier, so they will not be described here. If you should run into the terms *spongy sclerosis, Canavan's* or *Alexander's* disease, familial idiocy with spongy degeneration, or *Merzbacher's* disease, they belong here.

BIBLIOGRAPHY

Hallpike, J.F. et al. *Multiple Sclerosis.* Baltimore, Williams & Wilkins, 1983.

Noseworthy, J.D. et al. Therapeutic trials in multiple sclerosis. *Can. J. Neurol. Sci. 11:*355-362, 1984.

Rose, A.S. et al. Criteria for the clinical diagnosis of multiple sclerosis. *Neurology 26:*20-22, 1976.

Sanchez, J.E., Lopez, V.F. Sex-linked sudanophilic leukodystrophy with adrenocortical atrophy (so-called Schilder's disease). *Neurology 26:*261-269, 1976.

Scheinberg, L.C. *Multiple Sclerosis: A Guide for Patients and Their Families.* New York, Raven Press, 1983.

49
Diseases of the Cerebellum

Although it is common for the brain to be likened to a computer, probably the only part of the nervous system that functions really similarly is the cerebellum. For a fascinating review of the computerlike physiology of the cerebellum the student should refer to the writings of Eccles. The cerebellum is of increasing interest because of its role in the control of the autonomic nervous system, emotions, and seizures, functions not widely recognized a few years ago.

It will be recalled that the oldest part of the cerebellum, the flocculonodular lobe, is closely connected with the vestibular nuclei and is concerned with the position of the body in space (equilibrium). The anterior lobe of the cerebellum is part of the paleocerebellum and is concerned particularly with posture, gait, and to some extent, muscle tone. The cerebellar hemispheres are part of the neo-cerebellum and are concerned with the smooth performance of voluntary movements. It is seldom possible however to localize a lesion to one or the other part of the cerebellum, although midline lesions may produce only truncal ataxia (see Chaps. 2 and 9). The clinical manifestations of cerebellar lesions are primarily in terms of its control over motor coordination.

TYPES OF CEREBELLAR DISEASE

Congenital Diseases

Developmental abnormalities of the cerebellum are not uncommon. In the *Arnold-Chiari syndrome,* unusually long cerebellar tonsils are displaced downward into the upper cervical canal. There is associated downward displacement of the medulla and perhaps even of the pons (Fig. 49-1). Spina bifida often accompanies this defect and such children may present with hydrocephalus, as well as cerebellar and

672

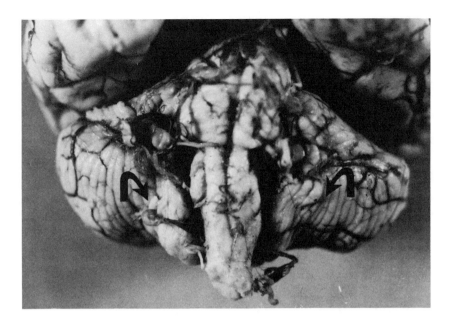

Figure 49-1   The cerebellar tonsils (arrowed) are unduly long and in life they projected through the foramen magnum. Arnold-Chiari malformation.

lower cranial nerve signs and evidence of pyramidal involvement. Less commonly the syndrome first presents in adult life (Fig. 49-2) when the signs mimic those of myelopathy, motor neuron disease, multiple sclerosis, or syringomyelia. Basilar impression of the skull and fusion of the cervical vertebrae are sometimes visible on skull x-rays.

In the *Dandy-Walker syndrome,* hydrocephalus is associated with a posterior fossa cyst (really a huge enlargement of the fourth ventricle) and hypoplasia of the cerebellar vermis. *Agenesis* of the cerebellum can occur, although this does not necessarily give rise to any symptoms. In the rare condition of *ataxia telangiectasia* (Louis-Bar syndrome), telangiectasias of the conjunctivae and face are associated with a cerebellar syndrome and sometimes choreic movements. The condition is of interest because of the associated low IgA and IgE levels, leading to repeated respiratory and sinus infections and bronchiectasis. These children usually die of chronic pulmonary disease. This disease is recessively inherited. Finally, *perinatal hypoxia* may produce severe cerebellar cortical atrophy, but the signs of cerebellar disease are usually overshadowed by evidence of cerebral cortical atrophy and of damage to the deep regions of the brain (Fig. 49-3).

Inflammatory Disease

Cerebellar signs, often unilateral, may occur with signs of raised intracranial pressure and otitis media, indicating that mastoiditis has spread to cause thrombophlebitis of the lateral sinus and that the infection has spread into the cerebellum, where an *abscess* may form. *Tuberculomas* of the cerebellum are common in countries of the Third World but are rare in Canada.

Involvement of the brainstem in *viral encephalitis* may induce cerebellar and brainstem signs and those of raised intracranial pressure and meningeal irritation.

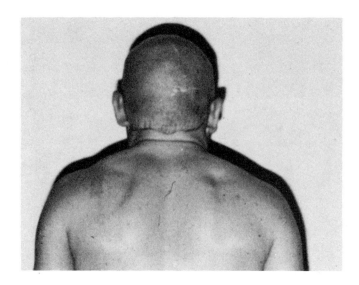

Figure 49-2   The short neck in Arnold–Chiari malformation.

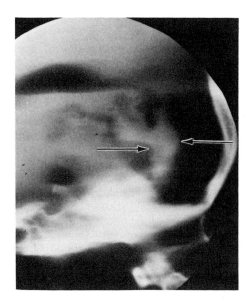

Figure 49-3   Cerebellar atrophy. Arrows indicate the small atrophic cerebellum.

This is a postinfectious, autoallergic disorder with myelin destruction. Some children with presumed viral infections also show isolated acute cerebellar signs (*acute cerebellitis*) as well as mild meningism.

Cerebellar signs may also be seen as part of the CNS involvement in *tertiary neurosyphilis*.

Neoplasms

Cerebellar signs may occur with tumors of the cerebellum itself or with those arising in the fourth ventricle or brainstem. Patients so affected develop progressively increasing intracranial pressure, cranial nerve signs, and a decreasing level of consciousness. Posterior fossa tumors are more common in children and in young adults. Four types occur: astrocytomas, medulloblastomas, fourth ventricle ependymomas, and brainstem gliomas.

Cerebellar astrocytomas (Fig. 49-4) make up a third of the posterior fossa tumors in children. The onset of symptoms is usually between age 2 and 15 years. The tumors are cystic and slow growing with a subacute course producing signs of raised intracranial pressure and cerebellar ataxia. If diagnosed early, surgery may allow a good prognosis.

Another third of the posterior fossa tumors in children are *medulloblastomas* that usually present before the age of 20. They produce features of a midline cerebellar lesion with severe truncal ataxia and early raised intracranial pressure.

Fourth ventricular *ependymomas* form less than 10 percent of posterior fossa tumors and are clinically indistinguishable from medulloblastomas.

Brainstem *gliomas* are about twice as common as ependymomas and produce dysfunction of any of the cranial nerves in association with long-tract signs and hydrocephalus.

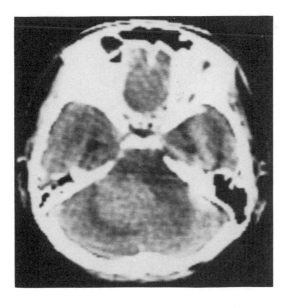

Figure 49-4   Cerebellar astrocytoma.

In adults, *secondary carcinomas, hemangioblastomas,* and tumors of the cerebellopontine angle are more likely neoplastic causes of cerebellar signs. *Schwannomas* of the eighth nerve, *meningiomas,* and *cholesteatomas* are the most common tumors to be found at the cerebellopontine angle. The patient will show signs of involvement of the fifth, sixth, seventh, and eighth nerves on the same side. Posterior communicating artery *aneurysms* may produce the same picture, damaging the inferior cerebellar peduncle and producing homolateral cerebellar ataxia in two-thirds of the cases. Raised intracranial pressure occurs at a much later stage. The usual angle tumor is an *acoustic neuroma (schwannoma),* a benign tumor arising from the vestibular portion of the eighth nerve. This is quite operable with a good prognosis, particularly in the early stages. Some patients will have loss of hearing on that side, and there is a risk of facial paralysis or a lateral medullary syndrome associated with surgery. Early referral for investigation and treatment is imperative.

In association with an underlying malignancy, *subacute degeneration* of the cerebellar cortex may be seen with ataxia, dysarthria, dysmetria, etc. (see Chap. 9). Although half the associated neoplasms are bronchogenic carcinomas, carcinoma of the breast or ovary or Hodgkin's disease may also be responsible.

Metabolic and Endocrine Disease

Hypothyroidism can produce striking signs of neocerebellar abnormality. The *Wernicke-Korsakoff syndrome* may also be associated with cerebellar signs in addition to the usual features of alcoholism and thiamine deficiency. A number of *chemical agents* produce cerebellar syndromes (see Chap. 43) (Fig. 49-5).

Hartnup disease and *pellagra* are two similar deficiency disorders of tryptophan metabolism that may present with ataxia. So may *Wilson's disease* in adults. Patients with *benign essential tremor* may have an intentional component augmenting the postural tremor.

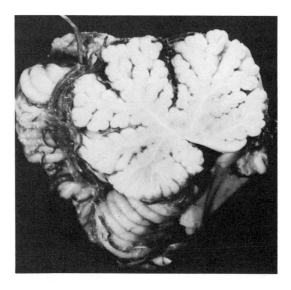

Figure 49-5   Saggital section of cerebellum, showing atrophy of the folia of the vermis in a chronic alcoholic.

Vascular

Occlusion of the superior, anterior-inferior, or posterior-inferior cerebellar arteries gives rise to major cerebellar signs. The vermis is supplied by the superior and posterior inferior cerebellar arteries, while all three vessels give a contribution to the lateral lobes. Signs of lateral pontine or medullary involvement should be expected in such cases, in which the cerebellar signs develop acutely and primarily on one side (Chap. 37).

Cerebellar hemorrhage presents with persistent vomiting and headache in hypertensive patients usually over the age of 60. Such people frequently have past histories of transient neurological symptoms. Examination may reveal signs of subacute delirium with small or unequal pupils, conjugate lateral deviation of the eyes away from the affected side, homolateral cerebellar signs, facial weakness, and early evidence of raised intracranial pressure. It is vitally important to recognize this condition and to differentiate it from a primary pontine hemorrhage because the early surgical removal of a cerebellar clot may be followed by an excellent recovery. An emergency CT scan is the fastest way to confirm this diagnosis.

Mechanical

With *basilar impression* from any cause, such as rickets, osteomalacia, osteoporosis, Paget's disease, or congenital malformations, the cerebellum can be damaged by direct pressure or ischemia with the production of both central and lateral lobe disturbances.

Demyelinating Diseases

Multiple sclerosis frequently involves the cerebellum. Charcot originally defined a diagnostic triad consisting of nystagmus, ataxia, and scanning speech, but all of those signs occur with any of the diseases mentioned above. Today we do not regard this combination of signs as specific for any particular cerebellar pathology, and they are often late findings in the course of MS. Cerebellar signs in multiple sclerosis may not be very severe when they are present, but the incoordination and ataxia can be disabling and seldom respond to treatment.

Spinocerebellar Degenerations

The term *abiotrophy* refers to the premature degeneration and functional failure of a group of cells within the nervous system; the specific cause not known. These cells might be in the dorsal root ganglion and its associated dorsal columns; the cerebellum with its afferent or efferent connections; the basal ganglia and their efferent systems; or the upper or lower motor neurons. Examples of cellular degeneration include Huntington's chorea, Parkinson's disease, spinocerebellar degenerations, Alzheimer's disease, and some muscular dystrophies. In all of these, the subject may seem perfectly normal at birth but structures that at first function normally later fail, with the production of the classic symptoms and signs associated with that failure. It is as though the subject lives to grow older but certain of his cells die young.

It is highly unusual for a single system of cells to be involved and there is much overlap between the different conditions described. Not only the nervous system, but others too may be involved in the same process. In Friedreich's ataxia, cardiomyopathy with hypertrophic subaortic stenosis and myocardial fibrosis or lipid infiltration is seen in about a third of the patients. Diabetes may also occur in this and other spinocerebellar degenerations, as also in myotonic dystrophy. Again, apart from the nonneurologic symptoms and signs, it is often hard to label a patient's disorder because frequently there is a family history of other degenerative diseases. Sometimes even in a single family, different members may present with different presentations of the same disorder. Often the pedigree of a patient with any form of spinocerebellar degeneration contains patients who have juvenile diabetes, cardiomyopathy, progressive external ophthalmoplegia, or syndromes of loss of reflexes, deafness, optic atrophy, paraparesis, or pure cerebellar or peripheral nerve disturbance.

Therefore it is hard to escape the conclusion that the disorders are due to many genes of small effect, usually inherited recessively, as opposed to a single factor responsible for all the manifestations of a disease entity. Just how many genotypes and how many phenotypes exist is not yet known, and the literature still contains case reports of hitherto undescribed patterns of neurological dysfunction reported, it seems, for their rarity value.*

Depending upon its severity, the condition may be apparent at birth and be regarded as a congenital familial disease or may not appear until e.g., the fourth or fifth decades. Most of the syndromes are, in part, clinically similar and tend to involve the cerebellum and its connections with or without other major areas of the nervous system. The overlap is extensive and Table 49-1 selects a few degenerations and shows how certain recurrent combinations of deficits closely resemble each other but are known by specific names. Thus in hereditary spastic paraparesis (which is only distinguishable from that form of motor neuron disease called primary lateral sclerosis by a positive family history and its slower course), signs of corticospinal tract damage are found in isolation. In Biemond's ataxia, a pure posterior column syndrome is seen; a hereditary cerebellar degeneration may also occur in isolation.

Obviously, one is going to investigate patients presenting with such syndromes for other disorders unless a clear family history is defined, which is seldom the case, most spinocerebellar degenerations being recessively inherited. To complicate classification and diagnosis still further, such conditions as peroneal muscular atrophy and progressive external ophthalmoplegia may exist in association with fragments of Friedreich's ataxic syndrome. Current views are that many of these syndromes, even though dissimilar in biochemical defect, genetic transmission, and clinical expression, should be lumped together as *multiple system atrophies.*

Fortunately, only Friedreich's ataxia is common enough to warrant description in this book. Others may be regarded as variants upon the same theme, but for complete assessment and family study, referral to a neurological center is advisable, so it is not necessary for most practitioners to be aware of the subtle differences among them.

Friedreich's Ataxia

Friedreich's ataxia is the classic prototype disorder and is usually recessively inherited, although dominant transmission has been described. The onset is usually before the age of 15 years, and the pathology is essentially neuronal death with replacement gliosis and secondary demyelination in the cerebellum, spinal cord and dorsal roots. It may be secondary to a defect in membrane transport of taurine and

---

*Other people collect stamps.

Table 49–1 Patterns of Involvement in Spinocerebellar Degenerations

	Post. col/DRG cell	Schwann cells	Cerebellum	II	Retina	Corticospinal tract	Anterior horn cell	Basal ganglia	Cortex	Myoclonus
Biemond's ataxia	+									
Pes cavus and areflexia	+	+								
Peroneal muscular atrophy	+		+	+/−						
Pure cerebellar degeneration			+							
Ramsay Hunt syndrome	+		+							+
Olivoponto-cerebellar atrophies			+			+		+	+/−	
Friedreich's ataxia	+		+	+	+	+	+/−	+/−	+/−	+/−
Hereditary spastic paraplegia	+/−		+/−			+			+	

beta-alanine or a defect in pyruvate oxidation. A deficiency of platelet lipoamide dehydrogenase has been described. Half of those affected have an abnormality of glucose tolerance.

Clinical Features

The classic features relate to degeneration in the cerebellum, posterior columns, corticospinal tracts, and dorsal root ganglia. Cortical involvement occasionally gives rise to some reduction in intellectual capacity. Optic atrophy is common, pigmentary degeneration of the retina less so. The most obvious findings are those of cerebellar disease. Upper motor neuron lesions and posterior column sensory loss also combine to produce a hyperactive jaw jerk but limb areflexia. Together they give rise to a syndrome of progressive incapacity leading to a wheelchair existence, frequently by age 20. A third of these patients have cardiomyopathies, among which group life expectancy is appreciably shortened. The legs are always much more affected than the arms, and most people who later develop evidence of Friedreich's ataxia may have had pes cavus from infancy.

Differential Diagnosis

Differential diagnosis includes conditions that affect particularly the cerebellar system, the upper motor neuron, the dorsal columns, and the optic nerve. Multiple sclerosis and pellagra do this, but in such cases the absence of a family history, the course of the disease, or a history of nutritional deficit should be enough to suggest the correct diagnosis. Charcot-Marie-Tooth disease with cerebellar signs (called the Roussy-Levy syndrome) is a *forme fruste* of Friedreich's, and hereditary spastic paraparesis also may show evidence of cortical, corticospinal, and dorsal column involvement (see Table 49-1).

Many other problems occur in patients with spinocerebellar degenerations or in their family members. A practitioner who has a patient with one of these conditions in his practice may expect to find these in his patient's family; thus Table 49-2 is included for reference purposes only.

Although the precise genetic abnormality and biochemical cause of this and other forms of ataxia are unknown, the disease can be mimicked by other conditions with a known biochemical defect. For example, Refsum's syndrome (Chap. 44) may show ataxia, and low or absent beta-lipoproteins have been found in the serum of other patients, so this test is a routine requirement. Investigation otherwise will probably seek to quantitate deficits, to demonstrate decreased speed of conduction in peripheral nerves to exclude demyelinating processes, and to seek for evidence of cardiac involvement.

Treatment

Treatment is disappointing. No specific treatment is possible as yet, but physiotherapy may delay contractures and assists the patient to utilize his remaining motor skills in the most efficient way. Bracing, special shoes, weights on the limbs to reduce the intention tremor, and sedation to reduce any anxiety, which may increase abnormal movements, may be helpful.

Drugs seldom reduce the severity of the ataxia or intention tremor but lecithin and isoniazid have been somewhat effective in a few patients. Thalamotomy may reduce the most severe cerebellar tremors, but it is seldom indicated.

Major social changes may be necessary; they include the provision of special schools or work environments, retraining, and the provision of pension or other

Table 49-2   Defects Associated with the Primary Spinocerebellar Atrophies

II	Primary optic atrophy Choroidal sclerosis	Retinitis pigmentosa Cataract
III	Ptosis Abnormal pupils	EOM palsies Color blindness
VII	Deafness	
Bulbar	Degeneration of brainstem motor nuclei	
Skeletal	Spina bifida occulta Syndactyly	Sacralized L5 Polydactyly
Muscle	Muscular dystrophy	
Brain	Epilepsy Mental defect	Myoclonic epilepsy Dementia
Other	Paranoia Diabetes Infantilism	Mongolism Cryptorchidism Hypogenitalism and obesity
	Hyperthermia	

Adapted from Tyrer, J. H., *Brain* 84:289–300, 1961, with permission.

benefits. Physiotherapy may help in gait training. Genetic counseling is advisable in all families.

Treatment for any signs of cardiomyopathy is best handled by a cardiologist, because pacemakers are sometimes needed. In a patient who has seen the progression of the disease in family members, depression is common and although entirely reasonable, if not actually predictable, may nevertheless be responsive to tricyclic drugs. Finally, a wheelchair may be either a prison or the basis of a whole new vista on life. It is damaging to offer a wheelchair too early, but as soon as the patient has recognized his difficulty in mobilization and seeks help, then the time for a wheelchair may have arrived. Never offer a wheelchair until the patient really wants it.

BIBLIOGRAPHY

Eccles, J.C. *The Understanding of the Brain.* Toronto, McGraw-Hill, 1973.

Gilman, S., Bloedel, J.R., Lechtenberg, R. *Disorders of the Cerebellum.* Cont. Neurol. Ser. No. 21. Philadelphia, F.A.Davis Co., 1981.

Refsum S., Skre H. Neurological approaches to the inherited ataxias. In *The Inherited Ataxias.* R.A.P. Kark et al. (eds.). New York, Raven Press, 1980.

50
Spinal Diseases

The clinical features of the different diseases that affect the spinal column or the cord and its roots are very similar (see Chap. 9). In brief, damage to the cord may produce signs of long-tract damage, both motor and sensory, and bladder dysfunction. There may also be evidence of damage to the entering sensory fibers or to the emerging motor roots and of pain and spinal deformity resulting from disease of the vertebral column. Depending upon the level of the lesion, a quadriparesis, a paraparesis, or only root lesions may result.

The characteristics of each clinical syndrome are also related to the speed of onset and progression of the lesion and to its site in the spine. Lesions may be inside or outside the dura, and those inside may be *intrinsic,* arising from the cord itself, or *extrinsic,* arising beside the cord and distorting or compressing it.

The most common spinal diseases caused by spinal arthritis, spondylosis, or the protrusion of intervertebral disks are discussed in Chapter 30. The conditions to be described here are included because they demand urgent management; others, although relatively uncommon, may have to be considered for exclusion or because effective treatment is available.

Symptoms of myelopathy may present acutely over hours or days or in a subacute or chronic manner, developing over weeks or months. *Acute transverse myelopathy* often follows a febrile illness. The patient complains of paresthesias, pain at the affected level (which is usually thoracic), and weak legs. With both intrinsic and extrinsic cord lesions, Lhermitte's sign is a valuable diagnostic pointer. On examination, meningeal signs, local tenderness, flaccid weakness with reduced or absent reflexes, and sensory loss with a definable upper level are found, and loss of sphincter control is also common. The CSF is abnormal in most cases, and the swollen cord may cause a block on myelography. The more common causes are post- or parainfectious myelitis, demyelination, vascular insufficiency, and remote carcinoma. Tuberculosis and vascular malformations are rare.

Chronic transverse myelopathy presents as a slowly progressive spastic para-paresis and affects mature adults most often. Sensory symptoms and signs, pain, and evidence of anterior horn cell disease, cord compression, and multifocal CNS disease are seldom found. Most of these patients have multiple sclerosis or cervical spondylosis; motor neuron disease, syphilis, neoplasms, arachnoiditis, or the Arnold-Chiari malformation are the cause in the remainder. This syndrome may occur in the year following radiation to the neck or chest.

CAUSES OF MYELOPATHY

The various causes of myelopathy will now be discussed in greater detail.

Congenital Lesions

Fusion of vertebrae may occur in the cervical region (i.e., Klippel-Feil syndrome). Other congenital lesions, such as winging of the scapula with wasting of serratus anterior, basilar impression, and other skeletal abnormalities may coexist with it.

Basilar impression is an anomaly of the skull base whereby the foramen magnum is distorted and invaginated upward. It may be associated with abnormal flattening of the base of the skull (platybasia). Although most often congenital, it may also occur as a result of bony softening in osteogenesis imperfecta, osteoporosis, Paget's disease, rickets, or osteomalacia. It is also sometimes associated with the Arnold-Chiari malformation, in which the medulla oblongata is unusually long and projects down into the cervical canal in company with the cerebellar tonsils. Compression of these structures and of the brainstem results because they all try to fit within a small foramen magnum. The most common symptoms are pain in the arm, neck, or suboccipital area, paresthesias in the arm, arm weakness, and ataxia. Findings may include weakness, hyperreflexia, poor rapid alternating movements, and pain and temperature loss in the arms with nystagmus and ataxia. Skull x-ray abnor-malities are seen in over half of all cases but a myelograpam is abnormal in all.

Cervical anomalies usually present in adult life, except for severe Arnold-Chiari malformations which may produce symptoms in childhood. The syndromes that result from these conditions are numerous. If the major effect is upon the flow of CSF, raised intracranial pressure and hydrocephalus follow. Distortion of the vertebral arteries occasionally may cause symptoms of brainstem ischemia (see Chap. 37). If the only problem is compression of the cerebellar tonsils, then natu-rally bilateral cerebellar signs will be all that can be detected. In other cases, a picture resembling syringomyelia is produced (discussed later). Because of pressure on the cord, any combination of long-tract signs may occur, often intermittently, giving rise to a picture not unlike multiple sclerosis. Sometimes the pyramidal tracts bear the brunt of the disorder with or without slight evidence of anterior horn cell disease in the upper cervical regions; this picture may mimic hereditary spastic paraparesis or motor neuron disease.

When a cervical anomaly is suspected, a careful clinical and radiological examination of the base of the skull and the upper cervical spine is required. Clin-ically, slight diminution of cervical movement, a short neck, and sometimes an abnormally shaped head are the only features likely to give rise to a suspicion of basilar impression. Radiologically, the odontoid peg may be seen on the lateral skull x-ray to project upward, above the level of a line drawn straight back from the hard palate. If that appearance is seen in the presence of any neurological syndrome, the patient should be referred for further study because surgical decom-pression may result in marked improvement.

Diastematomyelia is a condition of congenital origin that seldom makes its clinical appearance until after the age of 4 or 5 years. At lumbar or thoracic levels the spinal cord is split in two by a central bony spur or by cartilage or a fibrous band. The two halves of the cord may have their own dura and arachnoid. A tuft of hair is usually seen over the spine at the affected level. The splitting usually occurs over only the space of a few segments. Although initially asymptomatic, as the child grows the spinal cord lengthens more slowly than the vertebral bodies and the midline spur then causes traction upon the cord and roots. This may result in mild paraparesis and long-tract sensory impairment with a spastic bladder, and there may be early evidence of a lower motor neuron lesion at the site of the splitting of the cord. Surgical intervention is always required as soon as the diagnosis is made, whether or not there are any symptoms at the time.

Dysraphism refers to a condition of incomplete fusion of the neural arch or of the underlying neural structures. The most minor degree of this is a *dermal sinus* in which a small track leads from a dimple in the skin down into the dural space. Although usually asymptomatic, it may provide a pathway for infection to reach the nervous system, and any patient who has meningitis more than once should be examined most carefully from the sacrum up to the vertex of the skull (if necessary shaving the head) to search for the opening of such a sinus.

Spina bifida occulta is a radiological diagnosis in which there is a failure of fusion of the two halves of the vertebral arch posteriorly. The condition is not associated with any clinical symptoms itself, although an accompanying lipoma or dermoid cyst may cause cord or root compression. It is *not* a cause of enuresis.

A *meningocele* is a further development of spina bifida, in which a skin-covered sac protrudes backward through the open neural arch. The sac contains meninges and CSF but no neural elements. Unlike spina bifida occulta, which is very common (10 to 20 percent of the population have it in some degree) and which is usually lumbosacral, meningocele is uncommon and can occur at any level of the spinal canal.

Meningomyelocele occurs at the rate of 3:1000 live births (perhaps 800 a year or more in Canada). In this very serious condition, which usually occurs in lumbosacral regions, skin does not cover the protruding sac and neural tissue is covered only by a thin membrane. Rupture of the sac leads to escape of the CSF and almost invariably infection occurs. In association with meningomyelocele, hydrocephalus is extremely common (Fig. 50-1). The problems raised by meningomyelocele are numerous. *Neurological deficits* include permanent flaccid paraparesis below the level of the lesion, usually with complete sensory loss; although not progressive, such complete cord involvement is not improved by surgery. *Hydrocephalus* has been mentioned earlier and is often of such a degree that the child's mental development is markedly impaired. This leads to social and educational problems. It must be stated however that with early treatment of hydrocephalus many children now are able to grow up with only minimal, if any, evidence of mental retardation. *Locomotor disorders* include growth failure of the legs, equinovarus deformity of the feet, and muscle contractures involving mainly the adductors of the thigh and the gastrocnemii. These are amenable to surgical release but unless the level of the lesion is very low so that only sacral roots are involved, it is unlikely that, even with such surgical procedures, the child will be able to walk.

Bladder involvement is common; both motor and sensory supplies are involved, leading to a denervated bladder that is highly prone to infection. Pyelonephritis, hypertension, and renal failure often follow. Abnormalities of *renal* development such as double ureters and hydronephrosis also predispose to infection. Catheterization must be avoided if possible, and an ileal bladder may have to be constructed in these cases. *Rectal* incontinence may also be expected. The *spinal lesion*

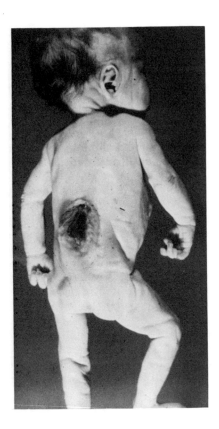

Figure 50-1   Myelomeningocele with hydrocephalus.

associated with the defect may give rise to kyphosis or scoliosis, again demanding careful orthopedic follow-up.

The presence of those degrees of dysraphism that cause neurologic symptoms should be obvious at birth and warrants emergency referral to a pediatric neurosurgical unit. Here, the child will be investigated for hydrocephalus and a shunt may have to be inserted between the ventricles and the right atrium or peritoneal cavity. The defect in the spine will be explored and the presence of absence of neural contents noted. The defect will then be closed by mobilizing skin for this purpose, and the child will then require further renal, neurological, and orthopedic assessment and follow-up.

Inflammatory Disease

Spinal epidural abscess, acute disseminated encephalomyelitis, tetanus, syphilis, and *tuberculosis* are described in Chapter 40.

The term *myelitis* signifies an inflammatory disorder of the spinal cord that may be infective or can occur in association with certain *toxic agents.* It is most commonly a complication of viral infectious mononucleosis, mumps, herpes zoster, and enterovirus infections (the latter sometimes producing a picture indistinguishable from poliomyelitis). *Pyogenic infections* of the cord itself are fortunately very uncommon. Whey they do occur, the patient usually shows signs of local infection, e.g., osteomyelitis, or of general disease such as bacterial meningitis.

The clinical features of myelitis from all causes are more or less similar and usually include fever and local spinal pain, sometimes radiating in girdle distribution; the patient may show exquisite local tenderness of the spine at the site of the inflammation. Depending upon the severity and extent of the condition, rapidly progressive long-tract signs, both sensory and motor, will appear with loss of bladder control and of sensation. Meningism is common. There may be evidence of accompanying local, cardiac, or systemic infection. Examination of the CSF may show a raised protein level (which will be very high if the condition has caused expansion of the cord and spinal block) and increased numbers of lymphocytes, or of polymorphonuclear cells if a bacterial infection is present.

A transverse myelitis with an upper sensory level and both motor and sensory long-tract signs below it, associated with current or previous optic neuritis, also occurs as a variant of *multiple sclerosis* (neuromyelitis optica or Devic's disease). Rarely a similar picture may occur in association with *remote carcinoma* as a non-metastatic syndrome. *Spinal anesthetics* may produce acute demyelination, sometimes at a single level, thus mimicking myelitis from infective causes. *Vascular occlusion* at a single level, usually affecting the lumbar cord, may occur after aortography as a result of the patient's sensitivity to the contrast medium used, to the ischemic effect of the medium itself, or to the dislodgment of atheromatous or cholesterol emboli from the intima by the catheter.

The prognosis with most of these conditions is poor, but following myelitis resulting from acute fevers, full recovery usually does occur. Myelography is needed if a noninfective lesion is suggested because these conditions may lead to spinal block, requiring surgical decompression. In most cases however, myelography is inadvisable, and treatment will be merely symptomatic unless an infective agent can be isolated.

Vascular Disease of the Cord

With one anterior and two posterior spinal arteries running the length of the cord and radicular vessels supplying it at various levels, the spinal cord might seem to be luxuriously vascularized, but this is not so (Fig. 50-2). The anastomoses between the anterior and posterior spinal arteries are relatively sparse; the vertebral artery supplies blood to the anterior spinal artery only down to about C-3 level; and the radicular vessels may number no more than six or seven down the whole length of the cord. In the cervical region only one or, at the most, two or three radicular arteries supply much blood to the anterior spinal system, and between there and the large artery of Adamkiewicz at about L-1, there may be very few segmental vessels supplying the cord. The artery of Adamkiewicz itself may supply the cord high up into the thoracic regions and right down to its termination. The third and fourth thoracic segments are particularly vulnerable to ischemia because they are a watershed area, comparatively far removed from any large radicular artery.

The anterior spinal artery is most peculiar, in that it contains blood flowing in both directions at the same time, making it an anastomotic channel rather than an artery. Blood supplied by a radicular artery perfuses the cord both upward and downward so that at some places, where the perfusion pressures from above and from below are equal, there will be no flow at all. If any of the major radicular supplying vessels are occluded, severe cord ischemia may result. Because anastomoses are better in the posterior than in the anterior spinal artery territory, major damage is felt in the anterior two-thirds of the cord, the so-called anterior spinal artery syndrome.

Despite this precarious state of affairs the spinal cord does seem to be relatively free from vascular disease. Thrombosis of the anterior or posterior spinal

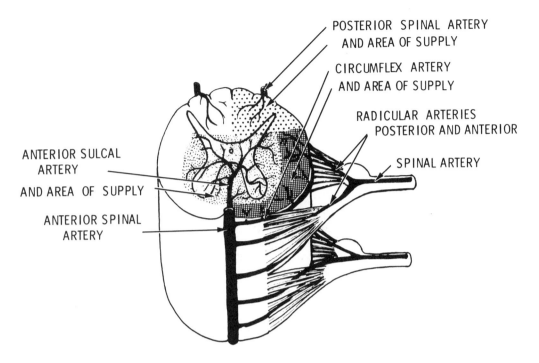

Figure 50-2   Blood supply of the spinal cord.

arteries is rarely, if ever, demonstrated pathologically. Infarction in the distribution of the anterior spinal artery is usually due to atheroma in the aorta, to aortic or thoracic surgery, or to compression of the radicular arteries.

In the *anterior spinal artery syndrome,* acute girdle pain leads to flaccid (later spastic) quadriparesis or paraparesis depending upon the level of the lesion, with dissociated anesthesia below the infarct because of the damage to the spinothalamic tracts on either side without ischemia of the posterior columns. Fasciculations and atrophy will occur in the muscles supplied by anterior horn cells at the level of the infarction and bladder dysfunction is likely because of the bilateral damage to corticospinal tracts. A slowly progressing presentation with flaccid paraparesis or paraplegia in extension and evidence of a spastic bladder is also recognized.

The brain is far more susceptible to embolization than the spinal cord, perhaps because the vessels supplying the cord usually take off from the aorta or subclavian artery branches more or less at right angles and thus tend to escape the emboli. However in the presence of aortic aneurysm, during aortic surgery, and with severe aortic atherosclerosis, emboli may make their way into the radicular vessels.

Although embolism is the usual cause, the same picture can occur from arteritis caused by collagen-vascular disease, syphilis, or diabetes. The development of nitrogen bubbles in the vessels during rapid surfacing from a deep or prolonged underwater scuba or compressed-air dive may produce vascular insufficiency and tissue damage to the cord ("the bends"). Similarly, with severe *systemic hypotension,* as with myocardial infarction or acute gastrointestinal hemorrhage, spinal blood flow will be markedly diminished, particularly in the watershed areas, which may become severely ischemic. Again, corticopinal damage and a sensory level to pinprick and temperature will result.

The late-onset *radiation myelopathy* is primarily a vasculitis of the cord that can develop 6 months to 3 years following high-dose radiation (4800 rad or more, especially if administered over a short period). The clinical picture is of a slowly progressive but relentless cord involvement at the level irradiated. (A more benign radiation myelopathy consists of Lhermitte's sign only; it develops within months of the radiation and clears with time.)

Traumatic dislocation of the spine may produce ischemic damage to the cord because of compression of an important radicular artery. Chronic vascular insufficiency resulting from compression of radicular arteries may occur in association with severe *spondylosis* with osteophytes and an hypertrophied ligamentum flavum.

Hemangiomas of the spinal cord are most uncommon but sometimes present in elderly men. They usually occur at thoracic or lumbar levels, causing progressive cord damage. There is rarely an audible bruit over the spine. The malformations consist of large arteries and veins with intervening sinuses and are usually sited in the thoracic regions. Unless there is some vascular lesion of the overlying skin or a bruit is heard, it is almost impossible to make the diagnosis from any other cause of chronic cord disease. The condition will be detected at myelography when the enlarged vessels will show up as negative shadows against the positive contrast, and may be confirmed by spinal angiography. Surgical treatment is of definite value.

Spinal Tumors

Both primary and secondary tumors may involve either the spine or the cord. Primary tumors may be situated either outside or inside the dura; the intradural tumors may be within the cord itself or beside it, i.e., intrinsic or extrinsic.

Primary *extradural* tumors are uncommon. Lipomas, meningiomas, and chordomas may occur. Meningiomas are usually found in thoracic regions, lipomas in thoracolumbar areas, and chordomas sacrally. The latter are tumors derived from the primitive notochord (and also occur in the region of the clivus at the base of the skull). As pointed out in Chapter 9, extradural tumors produce early root symptoms of pain and paresthesia; long-tract signs are asymmetric, and bladder involvement is late.

Extrinsic intradural tumors are not uncommon. meningiomas occur in the thoracic region (and occasionally around the foramen magnum). Neurofibromas occur at any level, on sensory roots only.

Intrinsic intradural tumors include astrocytomas (usually thoracic); ependymomas (usually cervical and occasionally in the filum terminale); and, far less commonly, angiomas, cysts, lipomas, or epidermoid tumors. Rarely, intracranial malignant tumors "seed" down the spinal cord. Painless progression of any combination of motor and sensory signs, sometimes including dissociated anesthesia, and usually involving the bladder at a comparatively early stage, are the major findings, all naturally depending upon the cord level involved.

Secondary tumors of the spine are most frequently extradural carcinomas derived from primary tumors of the breast, lung, prostate, or kidney; myelomatosis and reticulosis are also important causes. With all these secondary tumors, bony involvement occurs first, compression or infiltration of the nerve roots and cord (most often at thoracic levels) following later. Secondary invasion of the spinal cord itself is extremely uncommon.

With prostatic carcinomas, the progression of neurologic symptoms is slow, while with carcinoma of the bronchus it may be extremely fast, over hours or days. Local and radicular pain, upper motor neuron weakness (paraparesis), bladder dysfunction, and a sensory level are the main findings.

Plain x-rays of the spine are of vital importance in the diagnosis because with osteolytic and osteoblastic lesions, they will be abnormal at an early stage. Lucencies in the vertebral bodies, vertebral collapse, or widening of the transverse diameter of the cord with flattening or loss of pedicles are typical findings. Myelography will help to delineate the lesion more exactly and may also show the presence of spinal block. In Figure 50-3, the various myelographic appearances are shown schematically. A bone scan should also be performed.

Laminectomy and decompression of the cord or deep x-ray therapy relieves some of the pain and may preserve bladder function if performed early enough, but the 1-year survival is still less than 5 percent when a secondary tumor compresses the cord (Fig. 50-4). Primary tumors will always be removed but the patient may

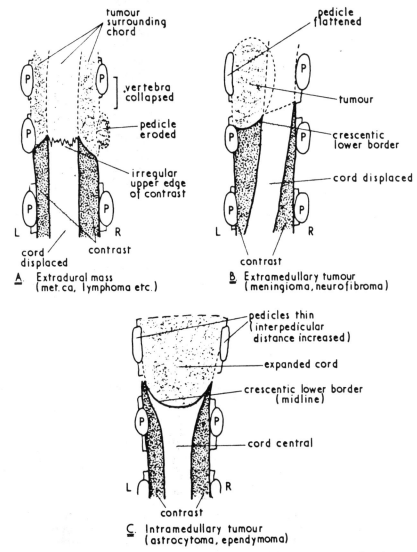

Figure 50-3 The myelographic appearances of different types of spinal cord compression. (By courtesy of Mr. Bernard Harries and the Editor of the British Medical Journal.)

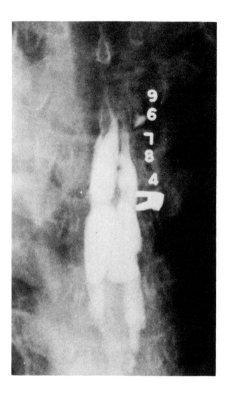

Figure 50-4   Myodil myelogram, showing the tapering cutoff of the dye column above an extradural mass causing spinal cord compression.

be left with some deficit, depending upon the duration and severity of the condition before operation.   Steroids must be given in high dosages upon diagnosis of spinal metastatic disease.

Syringomyelia

The term *syringomyelia* refers to a dilation of the central canal of the spinal cord or to the presence of any large cavity in the cord, whether or not it is connected to the central canal.   *Hydromyelia* is a term that is not used much these days; it denoted dilatation of the central canal only.   *Hematomyelia* refers to the same condition when a cavity is formed by extravasated blood; it is usually an acute lesion.

Syringomyelia is of two types, communicating and noncommunicating.   In the first form, the cavity is in direct continuity with the CSF in the fourth ventricle, while in the latter it is not, there being either a well-demarcated cavity within the cord or obstruction of the path between the cavity and the CSF in the ventricles. The symptoms and signs of the two conditions are almost identical.

Communicating syringomyelia is the most common condition, and its most probable cause is partial obstruction to the outlet foramina in the roof of the fourth ventricle.   As a result of this, pressure waves are transmitted through the CSF down the central canal of the cervical cord (Fig. 50-5).   At some point, and for some reason unknown, the ependyma lining the canal ruptures under these stresses and fluid tracks out along the lines of least resistance, usually posterolaterally beside

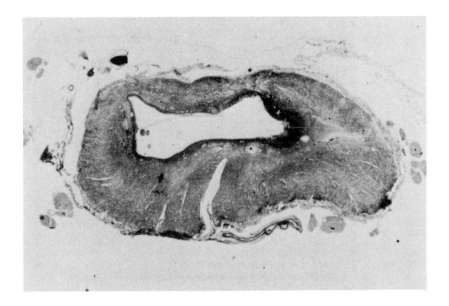

Figure 50-5   T/S cervical cord. A syrinx replaces much of the cord.

the dorsal horn of gray matter. The cavity so formed continues to enlarge and may track both upward, reaching the medulla, or downward, passing into low cervical or high thoracic regions. Hydrocephalus, the Arnold-Chiari malformation, basilar impression, or other skeletal abnormalities may be present in such cases.

Because the cavity is almost always in the cervical regions, the clinical features will include evidence of lower motor neuron lesions in the arms and long-tract signs below the midcervical cord. The enlarging cavity interrupts the crossing fibers (running from the dorsal root entry zone anteriorly and laterally to the ascending spinothalamic tract on the opposite side) and also those fibers entering the dorsal roots and running forward to make monosynaptic connection with anterior horn cells. The most prominent signs therefore will include diminution or absence of deep tendon reflexes in the arm and *dissociated anesthesia,* uni- or bilaterally, below the level of the lesion, often in the distribution of a cape or shawl (Chap. 35).

The cavity continues to expand, damaging the corticospinal tracts, the motor neurons in the anterior horns, and the ascending spinothalamic tracts, but usually does not involve the dorsal columns until very late. If entering root fibers are involved, paresthesias and pain will be felt in girdle distribution. Otherwise, weakness, atrophy, and fasciculations at the level of the lesion, with loss of pain and temperature uni- or bilaterally below it, and a pyramidal syndrome may be found.

Almost always, the signs are bilateral but asymmetric. Because of the loss of pain and temperature in the hand and the inner aspects of the forearms particularly, painless ulcers may follow trauma that the patient did not feel, giving rise to whitlows, ulcers, burns, or osteomyelitis. None of these are felt as painful. Horner's syndrome may result from interruption of the cervical sympathetic pathways.

Although a clinical diagnosis is usually possible, this must be confirmed by the appropriate x-rays of skull and cervical spine which may show marked widening of the spinal canal or basilar impression (Fig. 50-6A-C). Positive contrast myelography will outline an enlarged spinal cord while negative contrast (air) myelography may show that the cord in the same area collapses. The changing width of the cervical cord with these two techniques is diagnostic of syringomyelia (Fig. 50-7A, B). The NMR scan is very useful in this situation, since it shows the soft tissues well with marked reduction in bone shadows.

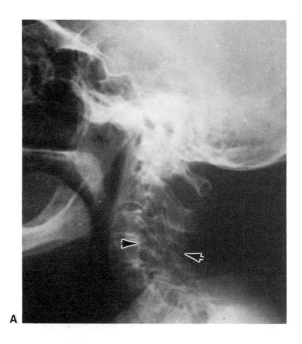

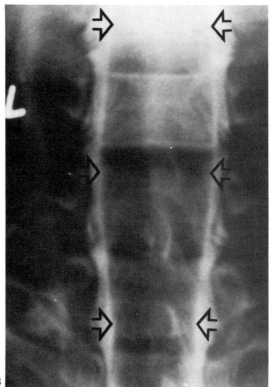

Figure 50-6   Syringomyelia. (A) Radiograph of lateral cervical spine showing increase in the AP diameter of the canal; (B) Metrizamide myelogram showing widening of the cervical cord; (C) In this myelogram, the dye has actually entered the syrinx.

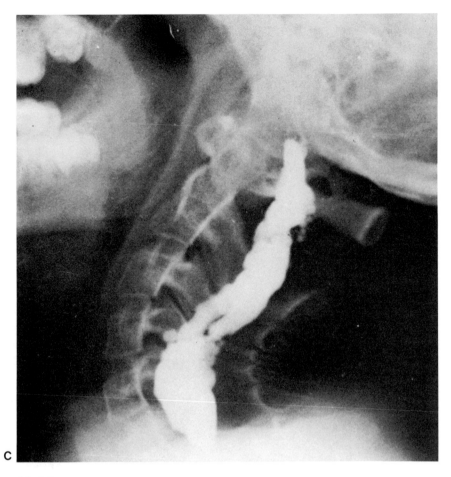

Figure 50–6C.

Following the demonstration of the importance of the abnormalities in the roof of the fourth ventricle, surgery has aimed at this area rather than at the syrinx itself. The surgeon tries to reestablish functional continuity between the subarachnoid space and the fourth ventricle and central canal and to dissect out the foramen of Magendie to allow normal CSF passage, thus damping the pressures formerly transmitted down the central canal. Ventriculocisternal shunts have also been used. In cases of noncommunicating syringomyelia or hematomyelia, the cyst can be aspirated percutaneously or at open operation. No other treatment seems to be of benefit. Obviously, surgery is not going to restore the patient to normal, but patients are frequently much benefited by an operation, indicating that their former functional deficits were partly due to reversible damage as well as to irreversible atrophy of cord structures.

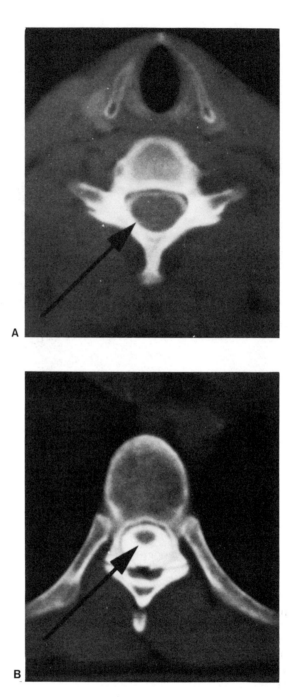

Figure 50–7   At these levels the varying size of the cervical cord is seen, the dilatation being due to a cervical syrinx. (A) cervical syrinx; (B) Thoracic cord.

BIBLIOGRAPHY

Barnett, H.J.M., Foster, J.B., Hudgson, P. *Syringomyelia. Major Problems in Neurology 1.* Philadelphia, W.B. Saunders Co., 1973.

Harries, B. Spinal cord compression. *Br. Med. J. 1:*611, 673, 1970.

Hughes, J.T., Brownell, B. Spinal cord ischemia due to arteriosclerosis. *Arch. Neurol. 15:*189, 1966.

Wilkinson, M. (ed.). *Cervical Spondylosis; Its Early Diagnosis and Treatment.* Philadelphia, W.B. Saunders Co., 1971.

51
Depression and Anxiety

"The Tower of Babel never yielded such confusion of tongues as
this chorus of melancholy doth variety of symptoms."

(Robert Burton—*The Anatomy of Melancholy*)

It has been remarked that psychiatry is concerned with neurology at its highest
level: neurology without physical signs. In the case of depressive illnesses, however, physical signs often abound, at least when the depression has attained sufficient severity. Such signs are as important in diagnosis and prognosis as are the
content of the patient's complaints. Even the symptom of sadness may be denied
by a patient with florid depressive state. Although psychiatrists talk about the
"somatization of painful mental content," there are very real reasons for supposing
that if a biochemical basis exists for depressive symptoms, such a basis may also
account for the bodily changes detected in a depressed patient.

It is a great pity that we call the illness *depression* because this name tends to
make one reluctant to make the diagnosis unless the patient appears unhappy. Such
is not always the case, however; in the following pages many manifestations of
depressive illness will be described that may merit that diagnosis whether or not
the patient complains of depression of mood. We urge students to get to know the
somatic symptoms of depression and to note that many of them sound "neurological."
In our experience 20 percent of the patients referred to a neurologist are depressed
and in one-third of them the depression is their primary problem.

GENERAL SIGNS AND SYMPTOMS OF DEPRESSION

Some symptoms of depression, taken in isolation, could be regarded as either neurological or psychiatric. The patient might present with any one as the chief complaint, but usually other symptoms surface on functional inquiry.

Insomnia

Difficulty going to sleep usually is due to pain, noise, or anxiety; *interrupted sleep* to similar conditions; while *early waking* remains as a traditional sign of depressive states. It has been suggested that increased cerebral arousal or hyperexcitability is the cause of the greater difficulty in falling asleep, the decreased duration of sleep, and the increased number of spontaneous awakenings in depressed patients.

Anergia

Coupled with such symptoms as *listlessness, indecision,* and *vacillation* are frequently *loss of energy,* easy *fatigue, heaviness* of limbs or head, and weakness. Analysis of that weakness, however, quickly demonstrates that it is neither particularly proximal nor distal and that, in fact, motor power is normal; but the patient's feeling about his ability to perform tasks with his usual energy is his real complaint. The diurnal variation and the general, not localized, distribution of these symptoms may lead one to suspect a genetic, endocrine, or inflammatory myopathy, but clinical examination shows no other evidence of nerve or muscle disease. *Isometric* contraction strength in such patients is frequently greater than *isotonic,* i.e., they may be able to maintain a position against resistance, while attainment of that position against a similar force seems much more difficult. Myasthenia-like weakness may be produced if motivation fails, and EMG studies may be necessary to rule out disease at the myoneural junction.

Psychomotor Retardation

Retardation of movement naturally produces less movement in unit time, bradykinesia or akinesia thus being the signs requiring differential diagnosis. Neurological disorders presenting similarly include almost any disturbance of motor system function including drug-induced or idiopathic parkinsonism, dementia, or stillness simply because of reduced awakeness. Because both plastic and cogwheel rigidity and *gegenhalten* (a peculiar, seemingly voluntary resistance of the patient's limbs to passive movement) may occur in severely depressed patients, and because increased deep tendon *reflexes,* a *palmomental response,* and *tremors* are also common, particularly in depression with an agitated component, the exclusion of structural brain disease can be difficult.

Agitation

Restlessness in association with anxiety is usually manifest as the frequent interruption of tasks, poor concentration, or the performance of repetitive, nonpurposive movements. The differentiation of general restlessness from *akathisia* (a basal ganglion disturbance usually seen in cases of phenothiazine toxicity) is hard; it is all a matter of degree. Localized *tremors, tics, habit spasms,* or repeated twisting, drumming, tapping, or jerking *movements* should be observed carefully over a period of minutes. The tremor of agitation is commonly distal and bilateral, affecting the arms more than the legs, and lacking the rhythmic and rotatory pattern seen in parkinsonism. Eyelid tremor or blepharospasm is common among patients with agitation superimposed upon their depression.

Somatic Anxieties, Headache and Other Pains, Dizziness

Headache is the most common neurological symptom in depression. One may encounter several types of headache as presenting depression symptoms such as the typical tension type, the combined headache, and migraine headaches. These are all described in Chapter 17.

Atypical facial pain is another reflection of underlying depressive illness in some cases. A series of patients with severe facial pain not of lancinating nature nor of split-second duration and usually without trigger spots (thus not diagnosable as trigeminal neuralgia) contained a high proportion of subjects who had enough somatic and psychological symptoms such as fatigue, agitation, sleep disorders, psychomotor retardation, melancholy, weight loss, and self-reproach to warrant a diagnosis of depressive illness. Women are particularly commonly affected by atypical facial pain.

This variety of pain is sharp, burning, or continuous in character; of moderate or severe intensity; well localized; and sited in teeth, maxilla, cheek, preauricular, or ocular regions. It may be unilateral or bilateral, often in the center of the face.

It lasts minutes or hours at a time, sometimes seeming to be almost constant over weeks or longer. Though seldom aggravated or relieved by external factors it may be worse during those periods of the day at which the depression of mood is most severe. Tearing and a dry mouth may be present but associated symptoms are otherwise rather few. On examination, local tenderness may be present, but objective signs are absent. Treatment of the underlying depressive illness may relieve the pain but may have to be continued for months before all complaints of facial pain are silenced; not all patients respond even then.

Dizziness is another somatic complaint frequently voiced by people who are depressed. The presentations of this symptom, its analysis, and diagnosis are outlined in Chapter 24. The symptom of "dizziness" caused by depression will not be accompanied by evidence of labyrinthine disease nor by neurological signs. Rotational vertigo or faintness, possibly with temporary visual loss, transient loss of consciousness, falling or nausea with pallor, sweating, and tachycardia is certainly not uncommon in depression and may be due to relative hypotension.

Other indices suggesting *reduced autonomic activity* include complaints of visual blurring because of impaired accommodation; constipation, and dry mouth, the latter of which may well be responsible for symptoms of difficulty in speaking. Perhaps because of retardation of thought or of movement, some patients with depression may lose their facility in spontaneous *speech* and even when they do speak may only use words of the highest substantive content, leading one to suppose that a degree of expressive (motor) dysphasia is present unless one is aware that the patient is depressed.

Depressed patients often have an increased reaction to painful stimuli, but this is not specific for them because muscle tenderness without muscle disease is also found in other psychiatric disorders, particularly those associated with increased muscle tension. *Pain* in other parts of the body are often accentuated during depressive swings or may arise *de novo*. Apart from muscle pain, both somatic (lumbar disk or joint) and visceral pains (cardiac, gastrointestinal, or renal) may be prominent and therapy that had once been effective may be of little value when recommended again. Depression can be, at least in part, the cause of pain as well as its consequence.

Somatic Symptoms, General

Myokymia, although seen sometimes in diseases such as multiple sclerosis, is more often caused by fatigue, anxiety, or depression. Paresthesias, usually distal and symmetric, are commonly associated with the hyperventilation of fear. In these cases carpopedal spasm and a positive Chvostek's or Trousseau's sign may be noted. Deep tendon *reflexes* may be exaggerated in both retarded and agitated depressive states.

Complaints of numbness or *sensory loss* are subjective and not objective on clinical examination and nerve conduction velocities in depressed patients are normal.

Body image disturbances include subjective complaints of change of shape, mass, size, or position of limbs and occur to a mild degree in perhaps 50 percent of depressed patients, but these are seldom, if ever, their presenting complaints.

Depersonalization and Derealization

These symptoms are common in patients with agitated depression. The differentiation from similar symptoms in temporal lobe epilepsy is made on the basis of their prolonged rather than paroxysmal nature and because of the absence of other evidence of abnormal electrical discharges such as change in consciousness or EEG features of epilepsy (see Chap. 15).

The Parkinsonian Symptom Complex

Patients with parkinsonism are usually unhappy and sometimes clinically depressed. The depression may become so severe that it becomes the presenting problem.

Thus the reduction of energy expended in both conditions is manifest as *bradykinesia,* e.g., facial impassivity and retardation of motor responses. Reduced peripheral *parasympathetic* activity shown by the dry mouth, constipation, and impaired accommodation are common to both, as are the slumped, flexed *posture* and the slowed and shuffling gait. In retarded depression, semivoluntary resistance to passive stretching of muscles may be hard to differentiate from parkinsonian rigidity. *Tremor* occurs in both conditions, although it is less regular and rotatory in depression. Some apparent reduction in *awareness* of, or response to environmental stimuli is a further common factor, reflecting the almost invariable if mild depressive state or dementia in Parkinson's disease.

The metabolic disorders underlying the two diseases probably overlap, which would explain why the clinical similarities between them are so strong. The physician will often need to treat depression among his parkinsonian patients and should be prepared for the frequent appearance of signs of basal ganglion disturbances among his depressed patients, whether or not they are under treatment.

Stupor, Arousal, and Dementia

The syndrome of absent motor responses with intact eye and ventilatory movements and with some degree of preservation of consciousness called *stupor* or akinetic mutism may be due to lesions of the basis pontis, of the frontal lobes, or of the area around the third ventricle, but a similar picture can be seen in depression. We tend to think that stupor is due to metabolic or structural lesions, but only 20 percent of such cases have a structural lesion, while a quarter of this group are actually depressed, the remainder being classified as schizophrenic, neurotic, and so forth. Whether structural or metabolic in origin the likely pathogenesis must include depression of ascending RAS activity in all cases.

The disorientation, defects in acquisitive skills, in retentive memory, in calculation and in judgment, and clouded consciousness, all reported in a small proportion of depressed patients, may be an expression of decreased cerebral arousal.

Epileptic Disturbances

The symptoms of many neurological diseases are intensified in depression. This is certainly true in epilepsy where escape from control of fits can be a sign of depression in formerly well-controlled epileptic patients. The depressive illness is at times relieved by a succession of seizures if they "break-through" despite medication, but otherwise it is usually relieved by tricyclic drugs. The form and content of the depressive state are identical with those in other depressed subjects.

Hallucinations of smell occur in depressive diseases of even moderate severity, particularly if they are long-standing. Hallucinations of foul personal body odor, generating secondary delusions or at least overvalued ideas of reference, and other olfactory perceptions interpreted as if from external objects or passively put upon the patient, appear with approximately equal frequency. Long-lasting, unaccompanied by features of temporal lobe epilepsy, and varying with external circumstances, the characteristics of these malperceptions allow accurate diagnosis in the office. True- and pseudohallucinations, both visual and auditory, also occur, particularly in the hypnogogic state when they too may be mistaken or epileptic manifestations. Their content is usually of a single voice, scene, or face, often recognizable and capable of producing strong emotional feeling, as when the voice of a long-dead parent seems to speak to the patient or call his name.

Fear, anger, depression and joy can all be produced as epileptic *emotional experiences* entirely apart from any internal or external stimuli. The possibility that the depression has an epileptic origin must be recalled when one sees depressed patients with abnormal EEGs; this is one of the many symptoms, including hallucinations, memory disturbances, compulsive behavior, depersonalization, and polyphagia, that strongly indicate temporal lobe involvement. Among epileptic subjects, depression occurs between the attacks in a third of those with focal and one-quarter of those with generalized epilepsy. Psychoses affecting patients with focal epilepsy last days or weeks. Their onset is not related to any particular seizure, but they are often terminated by one.

To summarize, depression in epileptic patients may be coincidental, reactive, the result of drugs directly or indirectly, caused by continuing subclinical electrical discharges affecting limbic system function, or because of seizure suppression (possibly again related to drug therapy). Depression worsens epilepsy and epilepsy encourages depression.

Other Associations

Drugs used in neurology and reported to produce symptoms of depression include sulfonamides, steroids, ACTH, phenobarbital, primidone, L-dopa, reserpine, tetrabenazine, propranolol, and phenytoin.

Either reactively, because of retention of insight, or primarily because of the basic disease process, depressive reactions are common complications of many neurological diseases. Multiple sclerosis, GPI, and traumatic frontal lobe damage are associated with depression in many cases; depression is more common in MS than is euphoria. Strokes are very often complicated by a depressive reaction that is often unrecognized.

The referring physician most often sends the patient to get an opinion about the significance of a *symptom* and not a *localizing sign*. The lesson to be learned is that when a patient presents diffuse complaints but has no typical signs to accompany them, when a patient who should be recovering from a neurological disease fails to do so, and when unusual signs appear that you feel may be out of the context of the patient's complaints, then remember depression, a disease that is common even among those who deny sadness.

ANXIETY

All people experience anxiety, some more often than others or with unusually slight provocation. Anxiety normally follows any threat to one's own or one's loved ones' values, self-image, or safety, but it is abnormal when provoked by unrealistic or minor circumstances, or when the response is so excessive or prolonged that it interferes with the person's normal functioning.

We are concerned here with the anxiety responses that suggest underlying "neurological" problems. These may color the patient's presentation of other problems, may precipitate or aggravate certain conditions, or may interfere with his management of them.

Anxiety Symptoms

The patient may complain of *nerves, tension,* or *worries* and describe sensations of tiredness, restlessness, dizziness, and malaise. Minor complaints that everyone experiences may be perceived with greater seriousness and thus compound the tension. He may not complain of the anxiety itself, but of its associated symptoms, and often states that these are his basic complaints, from which the anxiety results.

Behavioral Responses to Anxiety

Patients responding with excessive anxiety to certain circumstances often alter their life patterns to avoid them. Those with acute anxiety or panic attacks related to specific circumstances (elevators, crowds, being alone) rearrange their lives to eliminate their symptoms: logically, feeling that the crowds are the cause, they believe that if they avoid them they will be fine. This attitude prevents them from understanding why they are anxious and realizing that their fears have been displaced onto the crowds.

Chronic anxiety results in many more subtle changes in behavior and life patterns that are equally serious. Anxiety symptoms include restlessness, uncertainty, lack of productivity, and decreasing self-confidence; such patients gradually restrict their activities, social contacts, hobbies, and other endeavors. They complain of poor concentration and faulty memory and feel that they are mentally and physically unable to do the things they formerly did. Chronic tiredness and exercise intolerance are common complaints. Sleep is disturbed, with intermittent insomnia. Sexual interest wanes. As time goes on, most chronically anxious individuals become increasingly depressed.

Physical Symptoms of Anxiety

Increased muscle tension involves the whole body, often giving rise to muscle contraction headaches, low-back and limb pain, temporomandibular pain, and chest tightness. If anxiety is discussed with patients, they often respond in a hurt voice, "Then it's all in my mind," but it is vitally important that the patient understands that these are bodily accompaniments of tension and anxiety and that the doctor does not believe that the patient is "making up" the symptoms.

Excessive perspiration, shaky voice, sighing, habit spasms, tremor, motor rest-lessness, and weight gain or loss are common physical signs of anxiety. Anorexia, abdominal distension, diarrhea, constipation, belching and aerophagia, mild nausea and even vomiting, abdominal pain and cramps; sighing, mild or dramatic hyper-ventilation, shortness of breath and symptoms of chest pain and faintness; tachy-cardia, bounding pulse, increased blood pressure, premature systoles, frequency, nocturia, impotence, pelvic pain, dyspareunia, and frigidity are common symptoms.

The Acute Hyperventilation Syndrome

This syndrome will be emphasized because it is so common in neurological practice. Patients present complaining of attacks of dizziness, of blackouts, or of acute "spells" suggestive of epilepsy. Unfortunately, the diagnosis is often missed if such complaints are not examined in depth. Attention must be devoted to any precipitating factors, and to the whole constellation of other symptoms often present as well.

Thus the patient may complain of faintness but will admit that he also has had an overwhelming sense of panic or of impending doom, tachycardia, air-hunger, tightness in the chest, dry mouth, light-headedness, generalized weakness, shaki-ness, paresthesias around the mouth and in the hands, or even tetany. Some say that they pass out, but this is seldom so: usually they feel that they are "fading away," but they can still hear people around them and they do know what is going on.

Although patients with acute hyperventilation may not recognize that they are breathing deeply, it is usually obvious to observers who see it begin long before the attack happens. The acute hyperventilation syndrome can be thought of as the result of repressed anxiety from unrecognized or unsolved conflicts that break-through, often with minimal precipitation, and result in sudden and rapidly in-creasing anxiety. Adrenergic stimulation effects such as tachycardia, sweating, and hyperventilation follow. The resulting respiratory alkalosis causes the light-headedness, faintness, dizziness, paresthesias, and tetany. The hyperventilation syndrome is one of the most common causes of episodic dizziness (Chap. 24) and of the complaint of fainting (Chap. 10).

The precipitating factors are often minor or unrecognized, but anxiety is often displaced onto ordinary things such as elevators, crowds, darkness, and so on, which thus become the usual precipitant. In some patients a more chronic, free-floating anxiety state may occur, the hyperventilation syndrome extending over longer periods and with milder symptoms.

Differential Diagnosis

Most of the signs and symptoms that allow a diagnosis of anxiety result from ad-renergic stimulation, but these can also be seen in thyrotoxicosis, hypoglycemic attacks, pheochromocytoma, sedative drug withdrawal, or delirium tremens. Anxiety is also common in association with acute asthmatic attacks and with problems related to the face or the genitourinary system, both of which have great psychological significance. Thus patients with Bell's palsy may become extremely upset about the distortion of their facial features. Males who think they are be-coming impotent often become very anxious (which, needless to say, aggravates it).

Drug intoxication may cause the patient to appear acutely anxious or agitated. Some drugs also produce restlessness and akathisia, particularly the phenothiazines. Lithium can produce a tremor similar to that of anxiety. Although the pheno-thiazines and haloperidol are used to calm patients, they may in fact *increase* restlessness and unease. Barbiturates may also cause agitation in children and the elderly.

Serious depression can be masked by anxiety. Here, treating the anxiety alone may deepen the depression. Some psychoses may mimic anxiety states, particularly the "pseudoneurotic" and paranoid schizophrenias.

Treatment

When confronted with a patient presenting with anxiety symptoms, it is not enough to merely declare the diagnosis, as the patient is just as miserable with the label as without it. These patients require a full explanation, support, and reassurance.

Such patients may require many physician contacts and much follow-up. If they do not respond to this type of support combined with antianxiety medication (diazepam, haloperidol, chlordiazepoxide), then the assistance of a psychiatrist should be sought, but it is gratifying how successful a family practitioner can be in managing acutely and chronically anxious patients if he or she takes a positive approach to their management and does not regard them merely as annoying complainers who waste office time.

Acute hyperventilation attacks are best treated by clear explanation of the causative psychological reactions that occur and by explanatory (and ventilatory) psychotherapy. The patient can be taught to recognize the onset of the syndrome and attempt to control the development of symptoms, particularly by learning to control deep breathing. An attack can be precipitated by the physician, getting the patient to hyperventilate for 2 to 3 min, using strong encouragement, to help them understand the syndrome.

Phobic reactions are sometimes controlled by explanation, support, and the use of mild tranquilizers, but behavioral therapy and operant conditioning have been used in recent years with good results and referral to a psychiatrist is usually wise. The best results obtained are in recently developed phobic reactions; the prognosis is poor if they are not treated early. Untreated, patients develop a life pattern altered to fit their phobias, occasionally becoming prisoners in their own home. The prognosis here is poor.

BIBLIOGRAPHY

Hamilton, M. A rating scale for depression. *J. Neurol. Neurosurg. Psychiatry* 23:56, 1960.

Kline, N.S. Depression: Its diagnosis and treatment. In *Treatment in Problems of Pharmacopsychiatry*. 3:67, 1969.

von Brauchitsch, H. Treatment of the hyperventilation syndrome. *Henry Ford Hosp. Med. J.* 22:203, 1974.

Index

A

Abducens n. lesions, 298
Abiotrophies, 677
Abscess, cerebral, 97, 188, 248,
   490-492
  epidural, 97, 489
  lung, 539
  spinal, 489, 685
  subdural, 489-490
Accomodation, failure of, 296
Acid-base disturbances, 538
Acromegaly, 90, 517, 656
Action myoclonus, 225
Acute disseminated encephalomy-
   elitis, 281, 468, 469
Acute inflammatory polyneuro-
   pathy. *See* Guillain-Barre
   syndrome
Acyclovir, 314, 488, 493
Adenoma sebaceum. *See* Tuberose
   sclerosis
Adrenal disease, neurological,
   complications of, 189
Adrenoleucodystrophy, 669
Adult celiac disease, 543
Adversive seizures, 226
Afibrinogenemia, 555
Agitation, 697
Agnosias, 138-141
  anosognosia, 138
  artistic, 139
  auditory, 139, 209

autotopagnosia, 139
body image, 139
simulatagnosia, 139
spatial, 139
tactile, 140
testing, 138-139
visuospatial, 138-139, 209
Akathisia, 564, 597
Akinetic mutism, 174, 178-179
Acquired immunodeficiency syndrome, 474, 488-489
Alcohol
  neurological complications, 188,
   577-584
  amblyopia, 583
  cerebral atrophy, 584
  cerebellar degeneration, 583
  coma, 579
  dilirium tremens, 580
  hallucinosis, 580
  impotence, 384
  intoxication, 578
  myopathy, 584
  neuropathy, 583
  nutritional disorders in, 581-584
  pathological intoxication, 579
  pellagra, 583
  seizures, 580
  symptomatic, 642
  trauma and, 448
  tremulousness, 579
  Wernicke-Korsakoff syndrome, 581-583

Alexia without agraphia, 218
Alpha rhythm, 99, 102
Alternating thermoanalgesia, 146
Alzheimer's disease, 199-200, 209
Amaurosis fugas, 418
Amblyopia, 303
Aminoacidopathies, 457, 464
Amnesia
  anterograde, 186
  hysterical, 208
  post-traumatic, 208
  retrograde, 208
  transient global, 207
Amyloid angiopathy, 196
Amyloidosis, 349, 523, 599
Amyotrophic lateral sclerosis. *See*
      Motor neuron disease
Anaphylaxis, 545
Anergia, 697
Anesthesia
  dissociated, 154-155, 691
  saddle, 156
  dolorosa, 312
Aneurysm
  aortic, 295, 344, 365, 420, 687
  cerebral, 282, 297, 298, 412, 415,
      419, 429-430, 556
    Charcot-Bouchard. 415. 425
  mycotic, 420
Angiography, cerebral, 420
Angina, 314
Angiomas, 523
Ankylosing spondylitis, 365, 548
Anosmia, 71, 278, 567
  traumatic, 278, 447
Anoxia, fetal, 468
Anterior horn cell disease, 588
Anterior spinal a. syndrome, 687
Anterior tibial syndrome, 633
Anticholinergic syndrome, 576-577
Anticoagulants, 434
Anticonvulsants, 231-236
Anton's syndrome, 142
Anxiety, 329, 701-702
Aortic arch disease, 548
Apraxia. *See* dysphasia
Aphonia, hysterical, 72
Apraxia
  constructional, 142
  dressing, 142
  gait, 130
  ideational, 142
  ideomotor, 141
Aqueduct stenosis, 242
Arachnoiditis, 285, 344, 483
Arboviruses, 485
Argyll Robertson pupil, 292, 295
Arnold-Chiari malformation, 88,
      242, 243, 316, 672, 683
Arteriography, cerebral, 110-114
Arteriovenous fistula, 444

Arteriovenous malformation, 427
Arteritis
  cranial (giant-cell, temporal),
      420
  systemic, 295, 420
Arthrogryphosis, 623
Arthus phenomenon, 545
Articulation, 212
Astereognosis, 136
Asterixis, 176, 360, 529, 531
Asthma, 276
Astrocytoma, 510, 675
Ataxia. 41-42, 151. *See also*
      Spinocerebellar degenerations
Ataxia-telangiectasia, 465, 673
Ataxic diplegia, 454
Atheroma, cerebral, 414, 420
Athetosis, 355, 644-645
Atlantoaxial dislocation, 547
Atrial myxoma, 414
Atrophy
  cerebellar, 674
  muscle, 160-161
  neurogenic, 591
  progressive muscular. *See* Motor
      neuron disease
Atypical facial pain, 314-315
Auditory evoked potentials, 103-104
Autism, childhood, 469
Automatism, in epilepsy, 226, 358
Autonomic nervous system
  in depression, 698
  examination, 49-50
  in Parkinsons disease, 639
  toxins and, 571
Autonomic neuropathy, 607, 639
Autoregulation, cerebral, 408

                           B
Back pain, 361-371
  approach to, 362-363
  causes, 363-366
Ballismus, 355
Basal ganglion disorders, 635-650
Basilar a. occlusion, 423
Basilar impression, 87, 536, 677,
      683
Basilar migraine, 182
Basophilic adenoma, 517-519
Battered children, 448, 462
Becker muscle dystrophy, 614
Behcets syndrome, 488
Bells palsy. *See* Nerves. cranial
Bell's phenomenon, 27
Bends, 687
Benign intracranial hypertension,
      242, 248-249, 567
Beriberi, 539, 593
Beta rhythm, 99
Biopsy
  muscle, 107-108

Biopsy (cont.)
  nerve, 107–109
Bladder, 308–381
  automatic, 380
  deafferented, 381
  hypertonic (spastic), 380
  incontinence, 382, 667
  innervation, 378
  in multiple sclerosis, 667
  in spinal shock, 380
  motor paralytic, 381
  retention, management, 381–382
Blepharospasm, 299
Blindness
  causes, 280–285
  hysterical, 71, 283
  See also Visual loss
Body image, 138, 699
Bornholm disease, 624
Botulism, 292, 298, 336, 339, 495,
  631
Brachial plexopathy, 34
Bradykinesia, 355, 637, 699
Brain scans, radionucleide, 109–110
Brain death, 103, 177–178
Brainstem, 143–150
  evoked potentials, 103–104
  reflexes, 80–81
Breath-holding attacks, 181
Broca's area, 130, 212
Broca's dysphasia, 218–219
Bronchiectasis, 539
Brown-Sequard syndrome, 154–155,
  387, 391
Brucellosis, 349, 365
Brudzinski's sign, 14, 56
Brun's gait apraxia, 130, 421
Bruxism, 314
Bulbar palsy, 213, 335–337, 342
Burning feet syndrome, 532, 539

C
Cafe-au-lait spots, 465
Calcification, intracranial, 80,
  95, 465
Caloric tests, 27, 82
Cardiac arrhythmias, 181, 183
Cardiac signs, 161
  valvular disease, 414
  surgery, 414, 541
Cardiomyopathy, 161, 540, 681
Cardiovascular disease, 540–541
Caroticocavernous fistula, 444–445
Carotid a.
  stenosis, 410
  ulcer, 410–411
Carotid sinus hypersensitivity,
  30, 181
Carotid stroke syndromes, 419–421
Carotidynia, 309
Carpal tunnel syndrome, 602–604

in pregnancy, 557
Cataplexy, 182, 275, 419
Cataracts, 280, 303, 457, 536
Catheterization, intermittent
  381–382
Cauda equina lesions, 341
Cavernous sinus
  anatomy, 298
  aneurysms, 295
  thrombosis, 300
Central pontine myelinolysis, 532,
  584
Central retinal a. occlusion, 253
Central serous retinopathy, 283,
  284
Central syndrome, 173–174
Cephalohematoma, 90
Cerebellum, 150–152
Cerebellar disorders, 303, 672–681
  agenesis, 673
  alcoholic, 583
  hemorrhage, 677
  hereditary, 672, 677–681
  in hepatic disease, 529
  infarcts, 677
  inflammatory, 673
  in meningitis, 482
  metabolic, 676
  neoplastic, 675–676
  toxic, 565, 676
Cerebellar examination, 40–42
Cerebellopontine angle tumor,
  316, 325, 326, 333, 516
Cerebral blood flow, 408–409
Cerebral death. See Brain death
Cerebral dominance, 130
Cerebral edema, 243–244, 246,
  281, 438
Cerebral hemispheres, 129–143
Cerebral hypoperfusion, 424
Cerebral hypoxia, 188
Cerebral palsy, 453–459, 484
  associations, 457
  ataxia, 457
  causes, 453–454
  extrapyramidal, 456
  management, 457–459
  spastic, 455
  types, 455–457
Cerebral signs, non-specific, 143
Cerebral venous infarction, 504–506
Cerebro-retinal degenerations,
  464
Cerebrospinal fluid, 94–98
  leaks, 445–446
  lymphocytosis, 97
  in meningitis, 474–475, 477
  in multiple sclerosis, 97
  obstruction, 242–244
  xanthochromia, 97
Cerebrovascular disease. See Strokes

Cerebrovascular dynamics
  anatomy, 405
  collaterals, 400
Cerevical rib, 295, 601, 655
Cervical radiculopathy, 367, 370
Cervical spondylosis, 341, 367-368
Charcot joints, 158, 498
Charcot-Marie-Tooth disease, 592,
    594-596
Cheyne-Stokes respiration, 77
Chiasmal compression, 285
Children
  cranial nerves in, 57, 60
  developmental assessment, 57-58,
    61-63
  head circumference, 56-57
  milestones, 62-63
  motor system, 60-61
  neurological examination in, 54-63
  sensory system, 60-61
Cholesteatoma, 326
Cholinergic crisis, 630
Chorda tympani, 279
Chorea, 355
  dysthyroid, 532
  gravidarum, 554
  Huntington's, 641-644
  in infections, 644
  in pregnancy, 644
  in systemic lupus, 547
  Sydenham's, 644
  toxic, 563-564
Chorioncarcinoma, 554
Choroid plexus papilloma, 510
Choroiditis, 457
Chromophobe adenoma, 519
Chromosome disorders, 464
Chronic obstructive lung disease,
    539
Chvostek's sign, 27, 537, 557, 699
Clonic facial spasm, 322
Clumsiness, 351-353
Cold pressor response, 50
Collagen vascular diseases, 279,
    317, 357, 420, 627, 687
Colloid cyst, 523
Color vision, 20, 286
Coma, 169-177
  alcoholic, 579
  causes, 174
  examination of, 75-83
  grading, 77-78
  in hypothyroidism, 534
  hysterical, 70
  management, 76
  metabolic causes, 172-178
  pathogenesis, 169-171
  toxic causes, 563
  vascular causes, 172
  vigil, 178
Computerized axial tomography, 116-121

Concussion, 174, 188, 438
Conduction dysphasia, 218-219
Confabulation, 582
Congenital myopathies, 617
Coning, 420
Conscious level, 169-183
Contractures, 347, 358
Contralaterality, 129
Contrecoup injury, 439
Contusion, cerebral, 438
Conversion symptoms, 68, 182
Coordination, 4-42
  See also Cerebellar disease
Cortical blindness, 142, 282, 422
Corticospinal tracts, 145
Costen's syndrome, 309, 312
Coxsackie virus, 349, 494
Cracked-pot note, 245
Cramps
  muscle, 340, 358, 532, 573
  occupational, 358
Cranial arteritis, 286, 549
Cranial nerves. See Nerves, cranial
Craniopharyngioma, 90, 285
Craniosynostosis, 86, 244-245,
    249, 462, 463
Crocodile tears, 322
CT scanning. See Computerized
    axial tomography
Cubital tunnel syndrome, 601-602
Cultural deprivation, 462, 468
Cushing's syndrome, 535
Cytomegalovirus, 90, 493

D

Dandy-Walker syndrome, 673
Deafness, 323-327, 534
  acute, 324-326
  causes, 324-327
  hysterical, 72
  sensorineural, 457
  subacute, 326-327
  toxic, 484
Death, cerebral, 103, 177-178
Decerebrate rigidity, 81, 83, 173, 358
Decorticate rigidity, 81, 83, 358
Deep vein thrombosis, 349
Degenerative joint disease, spinal, 91
Dehydration, 357, 468
Deja vu, 228
Delirium, 185-192, 547
  toxic, 560-562
Delirium tremens, 188, 359
Delta rhythm, 99
Delusions, 11
Dementia, 193-201, 542, 547
  causes, 195-201
  in hypothyroidism, 534
  multi-infarct, 196
  toxic causes, 562-563
Depersonalisation, 699

Depression, 194, 278, 437, 534, 642
Dermatomyositis, 626
Dermatomes, 48
Detrusor-sphincter dyssynergia,
    380
Developmental assessment, 61-63
Diabetes mellitus, 176, 551-553,
    687
  neuropathy in, 295, 298, 597
Diabetes insipidus, 446
Dialysis encephalopathy, 188, 532
Diastematomyelia, 684
Diet, in migraine, 262-263
  in multiple sclerosis, 668
Digit span, 9
Digital subtraction angiography,
    114
Diphtheria, 297, 298, 336, 339,
    343, 597
Diplegia
  complex, 456
  spastic, 456
Diplopia, 294, 296-298
  in hysteria, 71
Disc disease, 366-371, 400
Disseminated intravascular coagulation,
    189, 476, 528
Dissociation cytoalbuminologique,
    68
Distal myopathy, 615
Distal weakness, 343-345
Dizziness, 327-331
  causes, 331
  in depression, 698
  with hyperventilation, 331
  See also Vertigo
Dominance, cerebral, 130
Dorsal column stimulation, 399
Dorsal root ganglion disease, 592-593
Dostoyevsky, 228
Down's syndrome, 464
Dressing apraxia, 142
Duchenne dystrophy, 610-614
Dysarthria, 212-213, 424, 529
Dysautonomia, 592
Dysdiadocokinesis, 151
Dysequilibrium syndrome, 532,
    561
Dyskinesia, 337, 564, 650
Dysphasia, 190, 212, 214-220, 529
Dysphonia, 212-213
Dysraphism, 373, 463, 465, 672-673,
    684
Dystonias, 347, 355, 564, 645
Dystonia musculorum deformans,
    645
Dystrophy, genetic muscular, 297,
    341, 610-616
  Beckers, 614
  classification, 611
  distal, 615

Duchenne, 610-614
  facioscapulohumeral, 614-615
  gait in, 375
  limb-girdle, 614
  management, 616
  myotonic, 296, 300, 618
  ocular, 300, 611
  oculopharyngeal, 300, 611
  scapulohumeral, 615

E
Eaton-Lambert syndrome, 630
Eclampsia, 553-554
Elderly, examination in, 65-67
Electroconvulsive therapy, 208
Electroencephalography (EEG),
    98-103
  in cerebral death, 178
  in delirium, 191
  indications, 99, 102-103
  periodic complexes, 501
  stimulation techniques, 98
  waveforms, 99
Electromyography (EMG), 103-106
Embolism
  air, 414, 555
  amniotic fluid, 555
  cerebral, 414
  cholesterol, 286
  fat, 414, 555
  paradoxical, 414
  retinal, 285
  tumor, 414
Emotion
  disorders of, 11
  pathological, 11, 337
Encephalitis, 295, 303, 317, 339,
    485-488
  brainstem, 673
  causes, 486
  clinical features, 487-488
  CSF in, 97
  herpes simplex, 102, 208, 246,
    487-488
  treatment, 487, 488
  von Economo's, 485
Encephalomyelitis
  allergic, 502
  epidemic myalgic, 503
Encephalopathy
  acute toxic, 502
  dialysis, 532
  hypertensive, 424, 540
  metabolic, 526
  portosystemic, 529
  rejection, 244
  toxin-induced, 560-562
  uremic, 531
  Wernicke's, 208-209, 295, 297,
    300, 532
Endarterectomy, 434

Endocarditis
  bacterial, 188, 414, 503-504
  non-bacterial, 528
Endometriosis, 366
Endorphins, 394, 395
Enuresis, 272, 273
Enzyme induction, 574
Eosinophilic adenoma, 519
Ependymoma, 510
Epidemic myalgia, 503
Epilepsy
  adversive, 226
  akinetic, 224
  causes, 229
  in cerebral palsy, 457
  classification, 221-222
  clinical features, 223-228, 352,
    419
  delirium and, 189
  in depression, 700
  febrile, 240
  focal, 225-228, 277
  generalized, 221
  grand mal, 221, 222-223
  hypocalcemic, 526
  hysterical, 70
  Jacksonian, 226
  management, 229-240
  in meningitis, 484
  motor, 226
  myoclonic, 224, 225
  partial, 182, 186, 221, 225-228
  petit mal, 182, 186, 224
  post-traumatic, 447-448
  psychological features, 228
  in pregnancy, 557
  reflex, 227
  sensory, 227
  in systemic lupus, 545
  social management, 231
  status epilepticus, 236-238, 469
  temporal lobe, 207, 384
  toxins and, 529, 562
  in uremia, 531
  visceromotor, 226
Erb's palsy, 600
Erythroblastosis, 462, 468
Essential tremor, 640, 649, 676
Evoked potential studies, 103-104
Examination, neurological, 13-50
  in children, 59-61
  in coma, 75-83
  in elderly, 65-67
  for functional disorders, 68-74
  in infants, 54-59
Exteroceptive sensations, 46
Extinction
  sensory, 49
  visual, 19
Extradural hemorrhage, 246, 441-442
Extrapyramidal syndromes, toxic, 563-564

Eye movement
  abnormality, 294-298
  control, 130
Eye pain, 306

F
Facial nerve. *See* Nerves, cranial
Facial numbness, 315-317
  in hysteria, 72
Facial pain
  atypical, 309, 312, 314-315
  causes, 309
  clinical approach, 308
  local syndromes, 309, 311
  referred, 309, 314
  See also Neuralgias
Facial palsy, 318-322
Facioscapulohumeral dystrophy,
    614-615
Fainting, 179-183, 540
False localizing signs, 298
Fasciculations, 105, 158, 161, 342,
    356, 357
  benign, 633
Fatigability, 105, 159, 342
Febrile convulsions, 225, 238, 240
Fetal irradiation, 468
Fibrillations, 105, 356
Fibrous dysplasia, 90
Foramen magnum lesions, 87-88,
    155-156, 341, 683
Foster Kennedy syndrome, 513,
    514
Freezing, in Parkinson's disease,
    639
Friedreich's ataxia, 678-680
Frontal lobe lesions, 130-135
Functional disorders, 68
  examination of, 68-74
Fundi, ocular, 19

G
Gait
  abnormalities of, 374-377
  apraxia, 130, 421
  ataxic, 375, 376
  in cerebral atrophy, 376
  dyskinetic, 377
  in elderly, 67
  examination, in children, 61
  hysterical, 73, 377
  magnetic, 376
  in muscular dystrophy, 375
  parkinsonian, 376
  spastic, 375
  steppage, 375
  testing, 42, 50
Galactosemia, 462
Gastrointestinal disease, 541-543
Gaze palsy, 301
Gegenhalten. *See* Paratonia

Genetic counseling, 614, 644, 681
Gerstmann's syndrome, 138
Giant cell arteritis. *See* Cranial arteritis
Giantism, 517
Gilles de la Tourette syndrome, 649
Glabellar tap, 27, 137, 637
Glasgow coma scale, 78
Glaucoma, 260, 280-281, 288, 306, 314
Glioblastoma multiform, 509, 511
Gliomas, 509-510
Glomus tumor, 326
Glycogen storage diseases, 347,
    622-623
Gower's sign, 611, 612
Graphesthesia, 136
Guillain-Barre syndrome, 297, 298,
    321, 336, 337, 339, 340, 341,
    343, 597-599
Gum hypertrophy, 233
Gummas, 498

H

Hallucinations
  alcoholic, 580
  analysis of, 11
  auditory, 580
  hypnagogic, 275
  in epilepsy, 228
  olfactory, 279, 700
  visual, 228, 580
Headache
  carotidynia, 257-258
  combined, 258, 265
  classification, 254
  in cranial inflammation, 254,
      260, 267
  exertional, 267
  mechanisms, 253
  migraine, 254-258, 262-265, 277,
      285, 316, 419, 420
    carotidynia, 257-258, 309
    classical, 255-257, 311
    cluster, 255, 306, 310, 311
    common, 256
    complicated, 255
    ophthalmoplegic, 257, 297, 300
    precipitants, 254, 263, 567
    variants, 257-258
    vertebrobasilar, 282
  muscle contraction, 258, 265-266
  from nearby structures, 254,
      260-261, 267
  non-migrainous vascular, 259,
      266
  orgasmic, 258
  sentinel, 431
  tension, 258, 265
  therapy, 262-268
  traction, 259-260, 266
Head circumference, 56-57
Head injuries, 438-448

complications, 208, 297, 320,
    420, 441-448
  management, 439-441
  prognosis, 448
Hemangiomas
  in pregnancy, 556
  of spinal cord, 688
Hemangioblastoma, 523
Hematomyelia, 449, 690
Hemianopsia, 280, 284
Hemiballismus, 355, 649
Hemifacial spasm, 358
Hemiplegia, 340
  pure motor, 424
Hemisensory syndrome, pure, 424
Hemivertebra, 364
Hemochromatosis, 530
Hemolytic disease of newborn. *See*
    Erythroblastosis
Hemophilia, 349
Hemorrhage
  Duret, 415
  intracranial, 413-417
  intracerebral, 425-428, 468
  subarachnoid, 429-433
  See also Strokes
Hepatic failure, 176, 243, 529-530
Herpes zoster, 97, 312, 314, 320,
    325, 402-403, 593
  ophthalmicus, 493
Hiccoughs, 336, 337
Hippus, 290
History, neurological, 5-8
Hodgkin's disease, 523
Holmes-Adie syndrome, 293
Horner's syndrome, 24, 79-80, 145,
    295, 300
  causes, 295, 301
Huntington's disease, 641-644
Hurler's syndrome, 464
Hydranencephaly, 55, 469
Hydrocephalus, 55, 241, 462, 484,
    684
  normal pressure, 242
Hydromyelia, 690
Hyperaldosteronism, 535
Hyperalgesia, 395
Hypercalcemia, 188, 536
Hypercapnia, 188, 242, 244
Hypercoagulability, 574
Hyperemesis gravidarum, 555
Hyperkalemia, 536
  periodic paralysis in, 619, 621
Hyperkinetic syndrome, 459-460
Hyperlipidemia, 414
Hypermagnesemia, 538
Hypernatremia, 188, 535
Hyperostosis, skull, 90
Hyperparathyroidism, 349, 357,
    532, 632
Hyperpathia, 396

Hypersensitivity, delayed, 545
Hypersexuality, 273
Hypersomnia, 273
Hypertension, 244, 281, 298
  encephalopathy in, 188, 243, 246,
    424, 540
Hyperthermia, malignant, 623-624
Hyperthyroidism, 532-533
  neurological complications, 296,
    297, 300, 357, 656
Hyperventilation, 329
  neurogenic, 77
  syndrome, 182, 419, 702-703
Hypoadrenalism, 279, 535
Hypocalcemia, 188, 347, 536
Hypogonadism, 279, 384
Hypoglycemia, 163, 174, 186, 188,
    419, 462, 468, 538-539, 573,
    656
Hypokalemia, 535
  periodic paralysis, 621
Hypomagnesemia, 538
Hyponatremia, 347, 535
Hypoparathyroidism, 90, 349
Hypopituitarism, 246
Hypotension, 281, 420, 687
  idiopathic orthostatic, 181
Hypothalamic lesions, 295, 484,
    522, 547
Hypothermia, 188
Hypothyroidism, 246, 279, 348,
    462, 468, 534-535, 632
Hypotonia, 34, 151
Hypovolemia, 182
Hypoxia, cerebral, 174, 208, 244,
    420, 673
Hypsarrythmia, 227
Hysteria, 68-74
Hysterical personality, 68

I

Illusions, 11, 228
Immunosuppressants, in MS, 666-667
Impotence, 383-385, 571, 665
Inappropriate ADH syndrome, 188
Inattention, sensory, 137
Incontinence, urinary, 134, 382,
    667
Incontinentia pigmenti, 468
Infantile spasms, 102, 224, 226,
    468
Increased intracranial pressure,
    85, 241-252
Infarction, cerebral. See Strokes
Infections of CNS, 472-506
  complications, 502-506
  classification, 473
  post-natal, intracranial, 468
  traumatic intracranial, 445
Infectious mononucleosis. See Mono-
    nucleosis

Influenza, 349, 494
Infratentorial lesions, in coma,
    173-175
Insomnia, 697
Intelligence, 9
Intellect, 193-194
Intracerebral hemorrhage, 425-428,
    444
Internuclear ophthalmoplegia, 147,
    663, 664
Iritis, 260, 283, 306
Isotope cisternography, 110
Isotope brain scans, 109-110

J

Jakob-Creutzfeldt disease, 357,
    500, 671
Jamais vu, 228
Jaw winking, 299, 358
Jendrassik's maneuver, 42
Joint position sense, 46

K

Kayser-Fleischer rings, 646
Kernicterus, 454, 644-645
Kernig's sign, 14, 17
Kerhohan's notch syndrome, 245,
    442
Ketogenic diet, 236
Kline-Levin syndrome, 273
Klumpke's palsy, 295, 600
Korsakoff's syndrome. See
    Wernicke-Korsakoff syndrome
Krabbe's leukodystrophy, 670
Kwashiorkor, 468

L

La belle indifference, 70
Labyrinthitis, 325
Lactic acidosis, 176
Lacunes, 415
Lacunar syndromes, 341, 424-425
Landry-Guillain-Barre syndrome. See
    Guillain-Barre syndrome
Lateral femoral cutaneous n., 605
Lateral medullary syndrome, 147,
    422
Lead poisoning, 462
Learning, 209-210
  disorders of, 460-461
Legionairres' disease, 188
Limbic system, 205-206
Leprosy, 599
Leptospirosis, 349
Leukemia, 349, 483, 523
Leukodystrophies, 464, 597, 670-671
Lewy bodies, 635
Lhermitte's sign, 16, 156-157, 663, 664, 682
Lid lag, 24
Limb girdle dystrophy, 614
Lipid storage myopathy, 623

Lobectomy, frontal, 132-133
Localisation of neurologic disease, 129-164
Locked-in syndrome, 179
Lorazepam, in epilepsy, 237
Louis-Bar syndrome, 465
Lower motor neuron lesion, 152
Lucid interval, 442
Lumbar puncture, 94-98
  contraindications, 94
Lumbosacral plexus lesions, 344-345,
    555, 597, 605
Lymphatic disease, 295
Lymphocytosis in CSF, 97
Lymphomas, 523, 527

M

Macroglobulinemia, 326, 420
Macular damage, 281
  degeneration, 280, 303
Magnetic gait, 376
Malabsorption syndromes, 543
Malignancy
  myopathy in, 632
  non-metastatic syndromes, 526-528
Malignant hyperthermia, 623-624
Malingering, 69
Marche a petits pas, 376
Marchiafava-Bignami disease,
    583
Marcus Gunn pupil, 293
Marfan's syndrome, 617
Mass lesions, intracranial, 507-526
Mastoiditis, 320
McArdle's disease, 62
Medial lemniscus, 145
Medial longitudinal fasciculus,
    145
Median nerve lesions, 602-604
Medulloblastoma, 510
Memory, 204-210
  tests, 9, 205
Meniere's disease, 325, 326, 332,
    333, 419
Meningioma, 513-515
Meningeal carcinomatosis, 483
Meningism, 14, 81, 289, 566
Meningismus, 477
Meningitis, 472-485
  acute, 474-481
  antibiotics in, 478-479, 481
  aseptic, 476-478, 481
  basal, 242, 295, 316, 337, 523
  CFS in, 97, 474, 477
  chemical, 566
  chronic, 483
  complications of, 174, 188, 298,
    454, 484-485
  cryptoccocal, 482
  differential diagnosis, 484
  e. coli, 476
  fungi, 566

gram negative, 476, 481
h. influenza, 476, 479
listeria, 476
meningococcus, 472, 476, 479,
    480
organisms in, 472-476
pneumococcus, 472, 476, 479,
    480
predisposing factors, 474
recurrent, 483
signs in infants, 475
staphylococcus, 476
subacute, 481-483
treatment of, 478-481
tuberculosis, 208, 481-483
uncertain etiology, 481
Meningocele, 242, 684
Mental changes, post-traumatic,
    446-447, 448
Mental retardation, 461
  causes, 462-464
  differential diagnosis, 469
  management, 470
  preventable causes, 462
Mental status examination, 8-12
Meralgia paresthetica, 556
Metabolic causes of coma, 173-177
Metabolism, inborn errors of, 463
Metachromatic leukodystrophy,
    670
Metamorphopsia, 138
Metastatic tumors, 519-520
Metazoal infections, 486
Microgliomatosis, 525, 532
Micturition
  abnormalities of, 378-382
  syncope, 181
  See also Bladder abnormalities
Migraine. See Headache
Miller-Fisher syndrome, 598
Minimal brain dysfunction, 351,
    453, 459-461
Miosis, 292, 568
Mixed connective tissue disease,
    551
Moebius' syndrome, 319
Mononucleosis, infectious, 333,
    349, 494
Moro reflex, 57-58
Morton's metatarsalgia, 606
Motor neuron disease, 319, 336
    341, 343, 357, 628, 651-658
  management, 656-658
Movement disorders, 354-360
Mucopolysaccharidoses, 464
Multi-infarct dementia, 196
Multiple mononeuropathy, 157, 599
Multiple sclerosis, 295, 298, 303,
    317, 319, 325, 341, 419,
    659-670
  CSF in, 97

Multiple sclerosis (cont.)
  and pregnancy, 558
Multiple system atrophy, 678
Multisensory syndrome, 67, 327
Mumps, 349
Muscle
  atrophy, 33
  cramps, 346-348, 573
  diseases, 610-627
      See also Dystrophies, myopathies
  grading of power, 34
  hypertrophy, 342
  innervation, 35-36, 39
  necrosis, toxic, 573
  pain, 349
  tenderness, 349
  tone, 33-34
  wasting, 160-161
Muscle contraction headaches,
      258
Mutism, 214
Myasthenia gravis, 296, 297, 298,
      302, 336, 339, 627-630
  congenital, 627
  with hyperthyroidism, 532
  with malignancy, 528
  in pregnancy, 558
  in systemic lupus, 545
Myasthenic crisis, 343, 630
Myasthenic syndrome, 160, 528,
      630-631
Mydriasis, 292, 568
Myelin diseases, classification,
      659-671
Myelitis, 339, 341, 344, 685-686
Myelodysplasia, 344
Myelography, 114-116, 689
Myeloma, multiple, 349, 525, 599
Myelopathy
  causes, 683-690
  in liver disease, 530
  non-metastatic syndrome, 526-527
  radiation, 688
  in reheumatoid arthritis, 547
  toxic, 565-566
  transverse, 489, 682-683
  traumatic, 687
Myocardial infarction, 181, 276
Myocarditis, 540
Myoclonus, 100, 176, 182, 186,
      336, 529, 531
  palatal, 336
Myofascial pain syndromes, 365
Myoglobinuria, 349, 623, 632-633
Myokymia, 27, 356, 633, 663, 664,
      699
  causes, 357
Myoneural junction, 159-160
Myopathies
  acquired, 624-634
  alcoholic, 349, 584

clinical features, 342-343
in collagen-vascular disease,
    627
congenital, 617
dysthyroid, 339, 533
endocrine, 536, 631-632
inflammatory, 349. See also
    Polymyositis
with malignancy, 528, 632
metabolic, 349, 631-632
ocular, 300, 302, 342
storage type, 622-623
toxic, 349, 572, 632
Myopia, 280
Myositis, 300, 349, 624-627
  classification of, 625
  EMG in, 105
  ossificans, 633
  See Polymyositis
Myotonic pupil, 283
Myotonia, 161, 348, 356
  congenita, 617
  neuromyotonia, 348, 356
  paramyotonia, 619
Myotonic disorders, 617-620
Myotonic dystrophy, 337, 618-619
  EMG in, 105

                N
Naffziger's sign, 368
Narcolepsy, 172, 274-276, 296,
    446
Nasal vasomotor reaction, 261
Nasopharyngeal tumors, 310, 316,
    326
Neoplasms. See Tumors
Nerves, cranial
  abducens, 20-24, 296-298, 319,
      446
  accessory, 31-32
  auditory, 27-30, 323-327, 333,
      569
  clinical examination, 17-33
  facial, 27, 29, 279, 318-322,
      446, 569
  glossopharyngeal, 30-31
  hypoglossal, 31-33
  oculomotor, 20-24, 291-292, 296-297,
      300, 446
  olfactory, 17-18, 278
  optic, 19-20, 280-289, 446, 568
  in systemic lupus, 545
  toxic lesions, 567-569
  traumatic lesions, 447
  trigeminal, 24-26, 308-317, 569
  trochlear, 20-24, 296-298, 446
  vagus, 30-31, 569
  vestibular, 27-29, 327-333, 569
Nerves, peripheral
  axillary, 601
  common peroneal, 345, 605

Nerves, peripheral (cont.)
  lateral femoral cutaneous, 605
  median, 345, 602-604
  obturator, 605
  posterior interosseous, 605
  posterior tibial, 606
  radial, 604
  sciatic, 605
  suprascapular, 601
  ulnar, 345, 601-602
Nerve biopsy, 107
Nerve compression, 339
Nerve conduction studies, 106-107
Neuralgia, 310
  facial, 308, 395
  geniculate, 313
  glossopharyngeal, 312, 313
  post-herpetic, 312-314, 395, 493
  occipital, 309, 313
  trigeminal, 310-313, 664
  vagal, 313
Neuralgic amyotrophy, 340, 343,
      396, 601
Neurasthenia, 339
Neurocutaneous syndromes, 464-467
Neurofibromatosis, 465
Neurogenic claudication, 368
Neurological examination, 13-50
  in children, 54-63
  in coma, 75-83
  in elderly, 65-67
  in functional disorders, 68-74
  scanning, 52-53
Neurological investigations, 85-123
Neurological symptoms, 1-8
Neuroma
  acoustic, 316, 515-517
  trigeminal, 316, 317
Neuromuscular blockade, toxic,
      572-573
Neuromyelitis optica, 281, 670
Neuromyotonia, 348, 356
Neuropathy, autonomic, 607
Neuropathy, cranial. See Nerves,
      cranial
Neuropathy, peripheral, 586-609
  alcoholic, 349
  autonomic, 384, 571, 597, 607
  axonal, 588-594
  causes, 589-591
  Charcot-Marie-Tooth, 594-597
  clinical features, 349
  compression, 584, 600-607
  demyelinating, 530, 594-599
  diabetic, 343, 597
  in diphtheria, 597
  Guillain-Barre syndrome, 297,
      298, 321, 336, 337, 339, 597-599
  hereditary motor, 344, 357, 588, 592
  hereditary motor and sensory,
      287, 594-597
  hereditary sensory, 592-593
  in hypothyroidism, 534
  inflammatory, acute, 597-599
  inflammatory, chronic, 599
  in lead poisoning, 597
  in malignancy, 599
  investigation of, 608
  ischemic, 597, 599-600
  leprosy, 599
  metabolic, 593
  motor, 587
  multiple mononeuropathy, 548
  neuronal, 588-594
  non-metastatic, 527-528, 599
  in polyarteritis nodosa, 548
  in porphyria, 597
  Refsum's syndrome, 596-597
  in reheumatoid arthritis, 547, 596
  sensory, 587
  in systemic lupus, 546
  thin-fiber, 279
  toxic, 570-571, 593
  traumatic, 593
  treatment of, 608-609
  uremic, 531
  varieties, 58
  in vitamin deficiency, 539-540,
      542
Neurotic fatigue, 186
Nieman-Pick disease, 464
Nightmares, 273
Night terrors, 273
Non-metastatic syndromes, 174,
      189, 526-528
Normal pressure hydrocephalus,
      197-199, 637
Nuclear magnetic resonance scans,
      122-123
Nystagmus, 24
  ataxic, 305
  causes, 303
  central, 304, 330
  classification, 303
  direction-changing, 305
  direction-fixed, 304
  jerk, 24, 304
  latent, 305
  optokinetic, 305
  pendular, 24, 304
  peripheral, 330
  positional, 305
  retraction, 150, 305
  see-saw, 305
  toxic causes, 565
  vertical, 305

                        O
Obtundation, 77, $\overline{1}86$
Obturator n. lesions, 605
Occipital lobe, 142-143
Occipital neuralgia, 309, 313

Occupational cramps, 347, 348
Ocular bobbing, 147, 336, 358
Ocular disorders, 290-306
Ocular movements, 20
Ocular muscle weakness, 342
Ocular myopathy, 616
Oculogyric crises, 637
Oculomotor muscles, 22
Oculomotor nerve lesions, 297-298
Oculopharynegeal dystrophy, 300,
        611
Olfactory hallucinations, 279, 700
Oligoclonal banding, 665
On-off effect, 641
Ophthalmoplegia, 533, 569
    plus, 616
    progressive external, 201, 301
Opisthotonos, 474
Opsoclonus, 358
Optic atrophy, 20, 280, 281, 287-289,
        303, 457
    compressive, 288
    ischemic, 286, 288
    Leber's 287
    toxic, 288-289, 568
Optic nerve, 280-289
Optic neuritis, 283, 284-287, 306
Optic neuropathy, ischemic, 286
Orbital neoplasm, 288
Orbital pseudotumor, 296, 306,
        550
Orientation, 9, 194
Oscillopsia, 392
Osteomalacia, 88
Osteomyelitis, 446
Osteoporosis, 366
Osteophytes, 91

P

Paget's disease, 8, 90, 288, 366,
        537-538
Pain, 393-400
    anatomy, 6
    atypical facial, 312
    autonomic, 398
    back. See Back pain
    bone, 362, 364
    clinical approach, 6
    in cord lesions, 396
    cortical, 397
    cramps, 347-348
    deep, 47
    in depression, 698
    in eyes, 306
    facial, 308-315
    gate control theory, 394
    management, 398-399
    muscle, 347-350, 361
    peripheral nerve, 395
    phantom limb, 396
    physiology, 393-394

with plexopathy, 396
    psychogenic, 366
    referred, 362, 365, 397
    root, 361, 395-397
    syndromes, 395-398
    testing of, 46-47
    thalamic, 397
    See also Neuralgia
Painful legs and moving toes, 349
Palatal myoclonus, 336
Palsy
    axillary n., 601
    Bell's, 321-322
    bulbar, 335-337
    common peroneal n., 605-606
    Erb's, 600
    extraocular, 297, 482
    facial n., 318-322
    Klumpke's, 600
    median n., 602-604
    obturator n., 605
    plantar n., 606
    posterior tibial n., 606
    pressure, 600-607
    progressive bulbar, 336, 651-654
    pseudobulbar, 145, 651-653
    radial n., 604-605
    Saturday night, 604
    sciatic n., 605
    serratus anterior, 601
    suprascapular n., 601
    ulnar n., 601-602
Palatal myoclonus, 336
Pancoast tumor, 301, 344
Pancreatitis, 188, 365
Panophthalmitis, 505
Pansinusitis, 317
Papilledema, 20, 289
Papillitis, 285
Papillomacular bundle, 281
Parainfectious syndromes. See
        Acute disseminated enceph-
        alomyelitis
Parameningeal infections, 97, 477
Paraparesis, 340, 341, 546
Paraphasia, 218
Paraproteinemia, 525, 527
Parasellar lesions, 297, 298
Paratonia, 83, 135
Paratrigeminal syndrome, 295,
        316
Parietal lobe, 136-137
Parkinson's disease, 635-641
    etiology, 635-636
    gait in, 639
    post-encephalitic, 637
    Parkinson's plus, 641
    symptom complex, 347
    toxic causes, 529, 564, 637
    traumatic, 446
    tremor in, 638

Parosmia, 278, 446
Partial complex seizures, 186
Pathological emotionality, 337
Pavor nocturnus, 273
Pellagra, 539, 676
Peripheral neuropathy, 586-609
  toxic causes, 570-571
Peripheral nerves, examination,
  16-17
Percussion myotonia, 620
Periodic paralysis, 339, 532, 621-622
  hyperkalemic, 621-622
  hypokalemic, 621
  normokalemic, 62
Periventricular leukomalacia, 456
Pernicious anemia, 287, 541
Peroneal muscular atrophy, 594-597
Peroneal n. lesions, 605-606
Perseveration, 138, 143, 194
Persistent vegetative state, 179
Pes cavus, 595, 680
PET scan, 121
Petit mal epilepsy, 186
Phakomatoses, 464
Phantom limb pain, 396
Phenylketonuria, 457, 462
Pheochromocytoma, 465, 467, 535
Phonation, 212
Photophobia, 212
Photosensitivity, 100
Pick's disease, 200
Pickwickian syndrome, 273
Pinealoma, 242, 305
Pinhole test, 281, 287
Pituitary lesions, 87, 517-519
Platybasia, 537, 683
Pneumocele, 447
Pneumonia, 188
Pneumoencephalography, 114
Poisoning, emergency treatment,
  575-577
Polioencephalopathy, 526
Poliomyelitis, 97, 339, 340, 341,
  343, 349, 493-494
Polyarteritis nodosa, 548
Polyarthritis, 339, 340
Polycythemia, 414, 420, 541
Polymyalgia rheumatica, 260, 340,
  349, 550
Polymyositis, 296, 336, 339, 528,
  624-627
Porphyria, 174, 188, 282, 343,
  543-544, 597
Porter's tip, 600
Portocaval shunts, 530
Portosystemic encephalopathy,
  529
Positional testing, vestibular, 27-28
Positron emission tomography (PET),
  121

Posterior interossesous n., 605
Post-herpetic neuralgia, 312-314
Post-infective encephalopathy,
  188
Post-infective polyneuropathy.
  See Guillain-Barre syndrome
Post-traumatic syndrome, 446-447
Postural hypotension, 180-181,
  183
Pre-eclampsia, 554
Pregnancy, neurological compli-
  cations, 276, 347, 553-558
Pressure palsy, 600-607
Proctalgia, 395
Progressive external ophthalmoplegia,
  301-302, 678
Progressive muscular atrophy. See
  Motor neuron disease
Progressive multifocal leukoenceph-
  alopathy, 501-502, 532
Progressive supranuclear palsy,
  201, 301
Projection, tactile, 138
Pronator sign, 355
Proprioception, 46
Proptosis, 296
Propulsion, 376
Protozoal infection, 486
Prosopagnosia, 139
Pseudobulbar palsy, 145, 337, 546
Pseudohypertrophy, 612
Pseudomyasthenic syndrome, 628
Pseudomyotonia, 161, 534
Psoriasis, 365
Pseudoptosis, 299
Pseudotumor cerebri, 248-249
Pseudotumor orbiti. See Orbital
  pseudotumor
Psychogenic hypersomnia, 699
Psychomotor retardation, 697
Psychoses, 186
Psychosexual disorders, 384
Ptosis, 24, 300
Pulmonary versus thrombosis, 414
Punch-drunk syndrome, 448
Pupils, 290-293
  Argyll Robertson, 292
  examination, 24, 292
  in coma, 78-79
  Marcus Gunn, 293
  myotonic (Adie's), 293
  reflex pathway, 290
Pure sensory stroke, 424
Pure motor hemiparesis, 424
Pure word blindness, 214
Pure word deafness, 214
Pyridoxine deficiency, 462

Q

Quadriparesis, 340

R

Rabies, 488
Radial n. lesions, 694–695
Raeder's syndrome, 295, 316
Raised intracranial pressure, 241–252,
    298, 531, 536
Ramsay-Hunt syndrome, 309, 313–314
Raynaud's phenomenon, 158, 547,
    626
Rebound, 152
Rectal control, 382
Red glass test, 296
Reflexes
    arc, 587
    axon, 50
    Babinski, 44–45
    caloric, 80
    Chaddock, 44
    ciliospinal, 50, 80, 82
    corneal, 24, 80
    deep tendon, 42–45
    doll's head, 80
    in elderly, 67
    flexor withdrawal, 58
    grasp, 135
    glabellar tap, 135
    grading of, 42
    jaw, 24
    light, 79
    menace, 78
    Moro, 57–58
    nuchocephalic, 134
    oculocephalic, 80
    oculovestibular, 80, 82
    palmomental, 135
    parachute, 58
    plantar, 44, 135
    pupillary, 79
    red, 20
    snouting, 81, 135
    suck, 81
    superficial, 43
    tonic neck, 58
Refsum's syndrome, 356, 596, 680
Reinnervation, 356
Renal disease, neurological complications,
    530–532
Respiratory alkalosis, 186
Respiratory failure, 342, 343
Respiratory patterns, 55, 77, 79
Restless legs syndrome, 532, 558
Reticular activating system, 145
Reticulum cell sarcoma, 525
Retinal burns, 281
Retinal detachment, 280, 284
Retinal hemorrhage, 448
Retinopathy
    diabetic, 280, 553
    pigmentary, 283
Retrobulbar neuritis, 285, 542,
    663

Retropulsion, 376
Reversible ischemic neurological
    deficit, 163, 409
Reye's syndrome, 176
Rheumatic fever, 551
Rhinorrhoea, CSF, 110, 445–446
Rheumatoid arthritis, 348, 365,
    366, 547, 655
Rhythias, 360
Rickets, 539
Rigidity, 34, 354, 638
Rigor mortis, 347
Rinne test, 29, 31
RISA scans, 110, 202, 445
Romberg test, 152, 353
Root lesions, 39, 343, 388
Roussy-Levy syndrome, 680

S

Sacral sparing, 156, 390
Saddle anesthesia, 390
Salaam attacks, 468
Salmonellar infections, 365
Sarcoidosis, 97, 483, 551, 599
Saturday night palsy, 604
Scanning neurological examination,
    52–53
Scanning speech, 151
Scheurmann's disease, 364
Schilder's disease, 669
Schizophrenia, 279, 351
Sciatic nerve lesions, 605
Scoliosis, 372–373
Scotomas, 281, 285
Seizures. See Epilepsy
Sensation, cortical, 46, 48–49
Sensory competition (extinction),
    49, 137
Sensory dermatomes, 48
Sensory loss
    alternating, 391
    brachial plexus, 388
    cortical lesions, 136–138, 391–392
    distal, 386–387
    hysterical, 71, 73, 392
    with mononeuropathy, 388
    with root lesions, 388
    with spinal cord lesions, 153,
        390–391
    suspended, 390
    thalamus, 391
Sensory system, 45–49
    in children, 60–61
    testing, 45–47
Septicemia, 18
Serratus anterior palsy, 601
Sheehan's syndrome, 555
Shoulder-hand syndrome, 541
Shy-Drager syndrome, 607
Sickle cell disease, 420
Sinus thrombosis, 247

Sjogren's syndrome, 279, 547, 548
Skew diviation, 301
Skull defects, 89
Skull fracture, 438
Sleep disorders, 270-277
  apnea syndrome, 274
  attacks, 276
  drunkenness, 273, 275
  enuresis, 272
  hypersomnia, 273
  insomnia, 273
  narcolepsy, 274
  nightmares, 273
  NREM sleep, 270
  paralysis, 275
  REM sleep, 270
  sleepwalking, 271-272
  stages, 270-271
Slow virus infections, 499-502
Smell, 278-279
  hallucinations of, 279, 700
  in hysteria, 71
Sodium amytal test, 211
Somatosensory evoked potentials,
    103
Spasmodic torticollis, 648
Spastic diplegia, 456
Spasticity, 34, 667
Speech, 211-220
  areas, 211-212
  tests, 215-217
  therapy, in strokes, 436
Sphenoidal electrodes, 98
Spina bifida. See Dysraphism
Spinal block, 690
Spinal cord, 152-156
  infarction, 423
  lesions, 153-156, 341, 344, 384,
      449-451, 682-694
  trauma, management, 90, 451-452
Spinal disease, 90, 364-365
  compressive, 357
  congenital, 90, 364
  inflammatory, 364
  metabolic, 364
  neoplastic, 364
Spinal muscular atrophy. See Neuropathy,
    Hereditary, Motor
Spinal shock, 449
Spinal stenosis, 94, 341, 368
Spinal trauma, 90, 341, 364, 449-452
Spinal tumors, 341, 344, 688-690
Spinal x-rays, 90-94
  vascular disease, 423-424, 686-688
Spinocerebellar degenerations,
    287, 303, 341, 677-681
Splenectomy, 474
Spondylosis
  cervical, 367-368, 370, 688
  lumbar, 344, 368, 370-371
Spondylolisthesis, 91, 364

Squint, 22
Stance and gait, 42
Startle reflex, 324
Status epilepticus, 236-238
Stereognosis, 49
Stiff man syndrome, 347
Strabismus, 56
Straight leg raising, 16, 363
Striatonigral degeneration, 640
Strokes, 405-437
  arteriocerebral a, 421
  causes, 410-417
  classification of, 409
  hemorrhagic, 246, 413-417, 425-428,
      436
  ischemic, 419-424, 434-435
  lacunar, 341
  management, 433-437
  middle cerebral a, 419-421
  in pregnancy, 555-556
  risk factors, 412-413, 535
  posterior cerebral a, 421
  vertebrobasilar, 418, 421-423
Stupor, 77, 699
Sturge-Weber syndrome, 90, 465
Subacute combined degeneration
    of cord, 341, 542
Subacute myelopticoneuropathy,
    568
Subacute sclerosing panencephalitis,
    102, 500-501
Subarachnoid hemorrhage, 188,
    247, 429-433
  management of, 436
Subclavian-steal syndrome, 180,
    413
Subdural effusion, 484
Subdural hematoma, 188, 195, 248,
    442-443, 457, 462, 532, 584
Subdural hygroma, 444
Subtentorial lesions, 175
Sunset sign, 56
Superior orbital fissure syndrome,
    300
Supratentorial lesions in coma,
    173-174
Swinging flashlight test, 293
Sydenham's chorea, 644
Sympathetic pathway to eye, 294,
    300-301
Symptoms, neurological, 1-8
Syncope, 179-183
  cough, 181
  micturition, 181
Syndromes. See specific names
Syphilis, 90, 420, 496-499
  congenital, 462, 498
  general paresis of insane, 188,
      498
  gummas in, 498
  meningovascular, 498, 687

Syphilis (cont.)
  primary, 496
  secondary, 188, 496, 498
  tabes dorsalis, 498
  tertiary, 325, 485, 675
  tests, 496, 497
Syringobulbia, 301, 310, 316
Syringomyelia, 90, 295, 303, 336,
    344, 655, 690-694
Systemic disease
  complications of, 529-559
Systemic lupus erythematosus,
    545-546
Systemic sclerosis, 550

T
Tabes dorsalis, 287
Tactile discrimination, 136
Takayasu's disease, 548-549
Tardive dyskinesia, 650
Taste disorders, 279
Tay-Sachs disease, 464
Temperature sensation, 46
Temporal arteritis. See cranial
    arteritis
Temporal lobes, 135-136
Temporomandibular joint disease,
    201, 268, 310, 312, 314
Tensilon test, 628-629
Tension headache, 265
Tetanus, 343, 347, 495
Tetany, 348, 358, 537, 557, 702
Thalamic pain, 391
Theta rhythm, 99
Thoracic outlet syndrome, 600
  in pregnancy, 557
Thrombocytopenia, 420, 551
Thrombophlebitis, cerebral, 97,
    504-505
Thrombosis
  cavernous sinus, 504
  cerebral, 410-413
  venous, 349
  venous sinus, 504-505
Thymomas, 627
Thyroid disease, neurological compli-
    cations of, 189
Tick paralysis, 339, 341, 494, 631
Tic douloureux. See Neuralgia,
    Trigeminal
Tics, 360, 564, 697
Time perception, 138
Tinel's sign, 17, 158
Tinnitus, 333
Titubation, 360
Tobacco amblyopia, 289
Todd's paralysis, 228, 410
Tolosa-Hunt syndrome, 306
Tone, 33-34
Torch infections, 454
Touch sensation, 46

Touch testing, 46
Tourette syndrome, 649
Toxic disorders of CNS, 560-575
Toxic encephalopathy, 502, 560-561
Toxoplasmosis, 474, 495-496
Transcortical dysphasias, 218, 219
Transient EEG discharges, 99
Transient global amnesia, 207
Transient ischemic attacks, 163,
    409, 417-419
  causes, 418-419
  management of, 433-434
Transient neurological dysfunction,
    162-164, 419
Transillumination test, 55, 245
Trauma, craniocerebral. See Head
    injury
Trauma spinal. See Spinal trauma
Tremor, 358-360
  action, 360
  anxiety, 358, 359
  causes, 359
  cerebellar, 360
  in depression, 699
  dysthyroid, 359, 533
  essential, 359
  flapping, 529
  hysterical, 359
  intention, 41, 360
  parkinsonian, 360, 638
  pill-rolling, 360
  red nucleus, 360
  toxic, 359, 565
Trichinosis, 624-625
Trigeminal neuralgia, 310-313
Trigeminal sensory neuropathy,
    315-317
  benign, 316
  causes, 316
  toxic, 316
Trigger zone, 363
Triphasic waves on EEG, 530
Trismus, 495
Trochlear n. lesions, 298
Trousseau's sign, 537, 557, 699
Tuberculomas, 673
Tuberculosis, 481-483
  spinal, 90
Tuberous sclerosis, 464-465
Tumors, 248, 507-528
  adenomas, pituitary, 517-518
  angioma, 523
  astrocytoma, 510, 675
  cerebellar, 675-676
  cholesteatoma, 516
  choroid plexus papilloma, 510
  clinical features of, 298, 357,
    508-509
  colloid cyst, 523
  craniopharyngioma, 517
  CSF changes in, 97

delirium in, 189
ependymoma, 510, 675
frontal lobe, 195
glioblastoma, 509
glioma, 509-510, 675
hemangioblastoma, 523, 676
Hodgkin's disease, 523
incidence of, 507
leukemia, 523
lymphoma, 523
management, 525-526
medulloblastoma, 510, 675
melanoma, 519
meningioma, 90, 285, 300, 341,
    465, 513-515, 516, 676
metastatic, 519-520
microgliomatosis, 525
myeloma, 525
nasopharyngeal, 523
non-metastatic syndromes, 526-528
orbital, 295-299
pancoast, 295
pinealoma, 295, 520-522
pituitary, 295
pontine, 319
in pregnancy, 557
reticular cell sarcoma, 525
schwannoma, 515-516, 676
spinal, 688-690
ventricular, 295

U
Ulcer, duodenal, 276, 365
Unar n. palsy, 601-602
Uncal syndrome, 173, 245, 297,
    300
Uncus, 173
Uremia, 176, 349, 357
Urinary tract infections, 188

V
Vagal neuralgia, 313
Vasculitis, 189, 574
Vasovagal syncope, 179-180
Vena cava compression
  in pregnancy, 555
Venous infarction, cerebral, 504-505
Venous lakes, 86
Venous sinus thrombosis, 446, 556
Ventriculography, 114
Vertebrobasilar syndromes, 182-183
    281, 326, 423
Vertigo, 327, 333, 419
  benign positional, 330, 331-332
  central, 332
  central vs peripheral, 329
  clinical approach to, 327-331
  common causes, 331-333
  peripheral, 332
Vestibulitis, 332
Vibration sensation, 47

Virus infections, 485-488
Visual acuity, 19
Visual disorders, 280-289
Visual evoked potentials, 103-104
Visual fields, 19
Visual field loss, 281-285
Visual loss
  field, 352
  in MS, 663-664
Visual symptoms, 280-289
  in hysteria, 283
Visual testing
  in children, 56, 60
Vitamin B12, 841-843
Vitamin deficiency, 188, 582-583,
    539-540
Vitreous hemorrhage, 283
von Economo's encephalitis, 635
von Hippel-Lindau disease, 467,
    523

W
Wada test, 211
Wallerian degeneration, 593
Wasting, muscular, 342
Waterhouse-Friderichsen syndrome,
    474
Watershed infarcts, 424
Weakness, 338-345
  acute onset, 339
  causes, 338
  diagnosis, 160
  distal, 160 343-345
  hysterical, 72
  localized, 340
  myopathic, 159-160
  neurogenic, 159
  painful, 340
  proximal, 160
  respiratory muscle, 342
Weber's test, 29
Wegener's graulomatosis, 550
Wernicke's area, 212
Wernicke's dysphasia, 218
Wernicke-Korsakoff syndrome,
    186, 208-209, 295, 297, 300,
    532, 581-583, 676
West's Syndrome, 224
Whipple's disease, 543
Wilson's disease, 402, 530, 637,
    646-647, 676
Witzelsucht, 133
Writing tests, 217

X
Xanthomas, 599
Xanthochromia, of CSF, 96-97
X-rays
  skull, 85-89
  spinal, 89-90